The
Psychoanalytic
Study
of the Child

VOLUME FORTY-ONE

The
Psychoanalytic
Study
of the Child

VOLUME FORTY-ONE

New Haven
Yale University Press
1986

Designed by Sally Harris
and set in Baskerville type.
Printed in the United States of America by
Vail-Ballou Press, Inc., Binghamton, N.Y.

Library of Congress catalogue card number: 45–11304
International standard book number: 0–300–03767–8
10 9 8 7 6 5 4 3 2 1

Contents

DEVELOPMENT

Contents

The Executive Functions of the Ego

An Extension of the Concept of Ego Autonomy

LEO RANGELL, M.D.

ADAPTATION AND EGO AUTONOMY

IT HAS BEEN COMMON, ALMOST ROUTINE IN PSYCHOANALYTIC writing, for an author to start with a passage of Freud's in which a subject has been laid down but incompletely developed which can then be further explored in depth. Hartmann (1956b) pointed out that Freud made "radical new departures" and reformulations up to his last papers, that he freely admitted to the quality of not being finished, and that there were a number of important chapters "he had not yet come round to" (p. 268). Freud himself continued to expand old ideas as he added new ones. But whatever Freud laid down during his lifetime, a seemingly endless mine was left for others to discover or appear to discover.

The same can be done, although it is far less routine, with the work of Heinz Hartmann. At the Memorial Service for Hartmann, I pointed out that in 1939, the year Freud died, Hartmann published his famous monograph which defined the

Clinical professor of psychiatry, University of California at Los Angeles; clinical professor of psychiatry (psychoanalysis), University of California, San Francisco. Past president, International Psychoanalytic Association.
An expanded version of the Heinz Hartmann Award Lecture of the New York Psychoanalytic Institute for 1985.

direction of psychoanalysis for the next three decades. "The baton had been passed between the two men. Heinz Hartmann stood on a mountain, built just before his time, preserved its space, cleared its top, and built it almost twice as high." While the language was fitting for a eulogy, the thoughts were meant as a scientific assessment. "Each piece of comprehensive writing about some aspect of human behavior was itself an abstract, hard put to contain the ideas which were bursting from its capsule in all directions."

I would like in this presentation to lift out one of the veins exposed by Hartmann but insufficiently pursued since then. Just as Anna Freud (1936) did not discover defenses, but elaborated and systematized what her father had named, and as Hartmann (1939, 1950) expanded ego psychology which had also been set into place by Freud, so would I like us now to work toward a deeper understanding and appreciation of the role of autonomy in human behavior.

While writing centrally of the problems of adaptation, Hartmann included the concepts of autonomy and conflict-free. In the decades since then, however, the mechanisms of adaptation became the primarily discussed theme. While Hartmann's contributions could have been utilized toward elucidating the human aim to shape as well as adapt, historically adaptation— "fitting in" rather than sticking out—clearly became the central thrust. Both Anna Freud's work on the defenses and Hartmann's on the adaptive functions converged on the reactive, leaving an interest in the shaping activities of man for future scientific concern. The ego psychologists from the 1940s to the 1980s concentrated on the ego's reacting to stimuli, stopping short of the immediately subsequent activities of the ego to initiate and direct.

The problems of adaptation need to be followed by an equal interest in initiation. It is into this area that I propose to move. While this shift in direction might seem slight and the movements small, there is a theoretical advance which in my opinion will carry us into a new dimension of relevance and understanding. It is most impressive that this area of human activity has been so slow in being exposed and developed. There has actually been a small but steady edge of crucial research at this border, but at a creeping rate of acknowledgment and acceptance compared to its significance.

Conflict-free and ego autonomy, named by Hartmann, were accepted if not pursued. While the psychoanalytic method is a treatment of conflict (Anna Freud, 1936; E. Kris, 1947; Brenner, 1979), psychoanalytic theory as a general theory, in keeping with Hartmann's view, includes behavior surrounding conflict and independent of it as well. Hartmann (1950) pointed out how primary autonomy can become embedded in conflict formation, and secondary autonomy can arise out of conflict and become reinvolved in it. While the first to formulate and elaborate autonomy, perhaps Hartmann himself also emphasized its limitations, leaving the issue of its executive functions still to be pursued.

Rapaport was one of the few who subsequently wrote of ego autonomy, solidifying its theoretical place in metapsychologic theory. In two papers (1950, 1958) devoted specifically to this subject, Rapaport qualified the term autonomy as "relative," in the first as relative to the force and influences of the drives, and in the second by pointing to the equal restriction on ego autonomy by the pressures of external reality. Taking his cue from Hartmann, Rapaport's aim, while setting into place the role of autonomy, was to preserve the role of drives and of external factors pressing upon the ego from within and without.

The emphasis was to retain the basic discoveries of psychoanalysis and to underscore the limited role to be assigned to autonomous ego capabilities. Each side connected to the ego gave it a degree of independence from the other, but at the same time each impinged on the ego's freedom by its own demands. While the ego's roots in the drives diminished its dependence on the environment, and its connections with reality its dependence on the drives, it could also be said that the drives and the external world each reduced the autonomy of the ego from opposite directions.

With autonomy and conflict-free named but not pursued, the also-new adaptive functions became the key concept occupying the next decades. While the main viewpoint absorbed and stressed by this new emphasis had to do with the ego's interests and methods of adapting to the surrounding world, i.e., the processes of socialization, which had heretofore taken second place in psychoanalytic theoretical concern, adaptation, in its strict sense, as meant by Hartmann, included the ego's dealing with inner conditions as well, with conflicts, restrictions, deficits, and limitations by a variety of adaptive rather than defensive methods.

The psychology of initiation, from simple to the most complex human activities, executed spontaneously or even subsequent to receiving stimuli from any or all directions, was left for the future, or to await another phase, perhaps when its time will have come after the previous new insights had been sufficiently consolidated. This has remained so since the 1950s, with a secondary role granted to autonomous factors. The concept of a conflict-free thrust of motivational behavior, set in place by Hartmann, requires further extension and elaboration to paint that element into the mental canvas in its full colors and to the full extent of its intrapsychic operations. This needs to be accomplished by a removal of the barriers to its more complete acknowledgment and study.

What I am speaking of is "will." This is a word not prominent in psychoanalytic terminology and which I feel is met by a quality of inhibition, as though it places in jeopardy the central contributions of psychoanalytic discoveries and understanding. A few isolated papers have appeared on the subject, especially long ago, such as by Knight (1946) and by Lewy (1961), and a few in modern times, but its role has always been seen as an island and it has never received vigorous or persistent attention. One problem has been the automatic association of the word "will" with the word "free." I will discuss the subject of "free will" to which this subject leads, but will also propose that the automatic linkage between the two words be discontinued, and that each word and concept be separately considered in the service of clarity.

In 1946, Robert Knight saw fit to address the delicate subject of "free will." Keeping in mind what he felt was a strict determinism, which could not be denied or mitigated in the realm of psychology, Knight made room for a freedom of choice, which he saw as occurring in an ego not hampered by neurotic restrictions. While this was a subjective feeling, it was not a spurious one, based as it was on ego-syntonic, "free" choices made by well-integrated persons.

The same vexing subject was approached by Lewy (1961), centering primarily on responsibility, and secondarily but necessarily on the closely contiguous subject of "free will." Confronted by the apparent contradiction of psychic determinism of psychoanalytic theory and the aims of psychoanalysis to develop and strengthen the patient's responsibility, Lewy felt he found the way out of the dilemma by the concept of relative ego autonomy which had emerged from Hartmann's ego psychology. Leaning on both Hartmann's concepts of adaptability and autonomy, and Rapaport's reasoning of the relative independence of the ego, Lewy felt he could support Knight's stipulation that "free choice exists to some extent, provided a person is healthy and integrated" (p. 266f.). This formulation of a limited free will did not interfere with but preserved the requirements of a strict determinism in psychoanalysis. Neither Lewy nor Knight pursued the problem in depth of how determinism was compatible with a relative freedom of choice, or with the free choice which they felt was possible only by the nonneurotic ego.

In a study of the metapsychology of activity and passivity, Rapaport (1953b) mentioned "will" a number of times, but, in a manner atypical for him, never pursued the subject with the depth and penetration characteristic of him. In fact, he tended each time to equate the concept with "voluntary," and by implication with "conscious," and failed to follow up the complexities involved. In the same study, Rapaport mentions that Brenman had suggested to him that he might be speaking of the "metapsychological considerations of the freedom of the will" (p. 535). Freud (1901) wrote of a "special feeling of conviction that there is a free will" (p. 253) in a manner akin to Knight's description and formulation. In one of the few recent papers on this subject, Schwartz (1984) concludes with a formulation that, while intention exists in the unconscious as well as conscious, deliberate choice takes place only in the conscious and preconscious. While this also makes room for the concept of some degree of free choice, a topographic explanation is introduced with which I do not agree. The entire sequence, I will hold, up to and including the final execution of choice, runs its course in the unconscious. Subsequent conscious behavior can then either be consonant with or opposed to the unconscious decision and action.

CONVERGING DIRECTIONS

I will bring to our minds the formulation that "thought is experimental action," a detour on the road to gratification. This is an insight arrived at by Freud (1900, pp. 508ff., 533, 535; 1911, p. 14; 1933, p. 89f.), repeated centrally by Rapaport (1950, 1951b) in his monumental study of the psychology of thought processes, and noted prominently by Fenichel (1945) in his summary of the theoretical background behind psychoanalytic clinical work. This succinct formulation is now regarded as a truism in explanatory theory. Its avowedly teleological nature is accepted without concern. Philosophic and other psychoanalytic considerations may provide caution, but such an explanation fits in well with today's hermeneutic emphasis on meanings and purpose. As a forerunner, however, of my thoughts at this point, which I will develop further, questions are left open, such as who or what conducts the experiment? To what end? What follows and under what circumstances?

The same form of dynamic sequence, to be followed by the same type of questions, is seen in another, even more central formulation of psychoanalytic theory, Freud's (1926) second, signal theory of anxiety. Here again an experimental intrapsychic operation is alluded to. Anxiety now is no longer a result of a build-up of tension resulting from repression. Instead the ego anticipates action to be taken by permitting a small, tentative, instinctual discharge. Anxiety is then a signal the ego produces—Schur (1953) and I (1955) amended this to "experiences"—which indicates danger from the direction of the superego or external world.

A third avenue of approach to the theory I am developing is what I described in a series of papers as the intrapsychic process (1955, 1963a, 1963b, 1968, 1969a, 1969b, 1971a). This was a more microscopic examination of Freud's anxiety theory. In briefest summary, the ego permits a small amount of instinctual discharge and samples the reactions of the superego and external world. If no significant anxiety ensues, the discharge can proceed to full and normal expression. If anxiety or other unpleasurable affect results, producing what I call the first phase, the tentative experimental phase, of intrapsychic conflict, the ego institutes defenses of some type to control the tentative and desired instinctual discharge. If this proves to be successful, stability results and the conflict is at an end. If the defense is insufficient to the pressing instinctual drive, the ego is confronted with a greater disharmony. This brings on the second or major phase of intrapsychic conflict, which challenges the ego for a more viable solution.

A fourth line of psychoanalytic thought I wish to cite is that when we examine ego functions to assess ego strength, we are apt to think of such ego functions as judgment, discrimination, differentiation, etc., but stop short of what happens after the ego judges. Synthesis and integration are usually included in the inventory of ego functions, but these come closest to being thought of as ego goals as well. As goals, however, they are incomplete and do not, in my opinion, accurately reflect the total sweep of ego aims and activities.

Upon what dynamic moment do these various paths converge? In each of the four sequences I have described, the line of reasoning leads in the same direction. What is the result of the experiment which thought represents? What does the ego do after the signal of anxiety has been received? What is the next move of the ego when its initial attempt at defenses proves insufficient? What follows the ego's judgment?

In each case something more is needed. A next step is necessary. An active, decisive move needs next to be made. This is the ubiquitous course of ordinary human life. Lest one feel at this point that I am drifting into a conscious psychology, I wish to state firmly that I am speaking of unconscious mentation, and of processes within the structural view, both hallmarks of central psychoanalytic theory and concern.

Gray (1982) has written of the lag between new theoretical formulations and their applications to technique. Besides historical and cultural inertia, Gray ascribed this to resistance to applying the new knowledge of ego psychology, in particular the necessity to analyze the defenses. I (1982b) have pointed to a wider set of resistances toward the progression of psychoanalytic theory, based on a variety of "transferences to theory," causing recurrent regressions in the steady advance of theory formation. This can take the form of resistances to specific aspects of existing theory, failure to develop or apply necessary advances, or the formation of new systems which abrogate much of what went before.

Such, I believe, has been the case in the failure of fruition of the concept of psychic autonomy. While the conceptual advances enumerated above all culminate naturally in the next necessary step, for the ego to proceed to execute what it is there for, to direct the course and activities of the total organism in its navigation through the surround of its life, furtherance of this understanding has for the most part faltered, or turned back, or has at least been delayed at the threshold of the ego's unconscious decision-making functions. This is exemplified by Hartmann (1947) stating that we do not yet have a psychoanalytic theory of action, as he himself was at the brink of taking that important and necessary step. Such a direction, however, was obviously recognized in its import for the future. He writes, "it seems probable that a theory of action based upon the knowledge of the structural aspects of personality . . . is the most important contribution psychoanalysis will one day be able to make in this field" (p. 38). Preceding action must be the decision to act. Hartmann (1950) stopped short of describing the final mode of action of the ego's executive functions. Although he referred to ego apparatuses, following the ego's original differentiation from the id, as executive apparatuses, Hartmann (1939) never went on to describe their definitive executive functions.

The unconscious decision-making function of the ego is a neglected although not completely overlooked point in the microdynamic series of events which takes place in the interplay of the psychic systems. The problem cannot be averted or better solved by reverting to the organism as a whole as the agent of decision, as is commonly held at this point. It is still the ego, not the self, or the self schema, or the whole person, or consciousness, or the existential "I," which stands at the threshold of executing an act at this decisive moment of the intrapsychic process. Perhaps the occasion of this Hartmann lecture is a fitting time to attempt to extend the articulation and integration of this next crucial step into the psychodynamic series of events, in what I believe can become an advance in theoretical understanding.

Freud, focusing on introducing and defending the crucial, innovative insight of psychic determinism, did not deny the existence of another type of mental activity during the intrapsychic sequence of events, but never gave this aspect his central attention. These organizing and executive functions of the ego were alluded to wherever they became descriptively necessary, although always briefly, glancingly, almost secondarily, and never coordinated into a cohesive and substantive section of theory. In his final *Outline*, describing the two fields of action with which the ego is concerned, Freud (1940) states that "the ego has voluntary movement at its command. It has the task of self-preservation. As regards *external* events, it performs that task by . . . learning to bring about expedient changes in the external world to its own advantage (through activity). As regards *internal* events, in relation to the id, it performs that task by gaining control over the demands of the instincts, by *deciding* [my italics] whether they are to be allowed satisfaction, by postponing that satisfaction to times and circumstances favourable in the external world or by suppressing their excitations entirely" (p. 145f.).

Freud (1940) describes the ego in childhood as "governed in all its *decisions* by the injunctions of a modified pleasure principle" (p. 205; my italics), and later governed toward the same decisions by the reality principle through the now internalized superego as well as the external world. Freud's (1927) emphasis on "the voice of the intellect" as soft but persistent can be taken to express his hope and expectation of ego control. And in 1923, while stating that "Often a rider, if he is not to be parted from his horse, is obliged to guide it where it wants to go" (p. 25), Freud also points out that psychoanalysis aims "to give the patient's ego *freedom* to decide one way or the other" (p. 50n.). In 1926 Freud cautions against making the strength of the id into a Weltanschauung, which would be "an extreme and one-sided view," and speaks for leaving room for independent functioning of the ego (p. 95).

Anna Freud's references to this point also are not copious, or consolidated, yet she takes the same view as Freud of the ego as an organizing and problem-solving agency. In a passage which is also made in passing, after stating that instinctual drives cannot be in conflict with each other but require a formed ego to institute conflict, she states, "the ego develops from a receiving station for dimly received stimuli, to an organized center where impressions are received, sorted out, recorded and interpreted, and action undertaken." Other opinions on the subject vacillate and vary. Rapaport grants freedom of choice to the degree that the ego is within the limits imposed by pressing internal and external events which play a causal role in behavior. Waelder (1960), who feels that Freud saw the ego as a problem-solving agency, also sees the ego as directing purposeful activity, and its processes as "task-solving," attempting solutions (p. 177). To others, e.g., Karl Menninger (1942), free will and responsibility apply only in a legal sense, or as a problem belonging to philosophy to which science can have no answer. Alexander and Staub (1956) consider free will an illusion, and Schafer (1976) as having no place in psychoanalytic discourse.

Aside from such scattered and inconclusive references, the subject has either been unattended or opposed, but it did not remain completely undealt with. I will now return to the intrapsychic sequence in the series I was describing above, which I interrupted at the point at which the defenses were failing to accomplish their intended function. Instead, mounting instinctual pressure leads to the next stage, the major phase, after the tentative, experimental one, of unstable, pressing, intersystemic conflict, as a result of which the ego is confronted with the necessity to choose. This introduces a second type of intrapsychic conflict, which I have called a dilemma or conflict of choice, in contrast to the usual conventional oppositional type of conflict.

Intersystemic conflict becomes superseded at this stage by an intrasystemic conflict of the ego, the necessity to choose between id and superego and/or id and external world. Intention, choice, decision, action enter the unconscious intrapsychic picture. The ego is forced to execute a plan of activity. Normal or pathological outcomes ensue, whether into the external world or the psychic interior, motor act or psychosomatic outcome, symptom, fantasy, or even affect. Or there is the decision not to act, to hold conflicting forces together as long as possible in a state of increasing unstable tension.

UNCONSCIOUS DECISION-MAKING

My own series of papers referred to on intrapsychic conflict and process culminated in a work explicitly on "The Unconscious Decision-making Function of the Ego" (1971a), a function not hitherto included in the official inventory of ego functions by Hartmann, before him by Freud, nor by anyone following. Clinical data came from analysis and everyday life. The vicissitudes of this factor were traced in a particular patient in analysis where it was not an occasional issue but coursed its way through the entire treatment process. However, while the problem was followed in depth during the course of analysis, the phenomenon was to be seen not only in certain patients but in all patients and as part of normal psychic functioning as well.

Autonomy and choice are not, as felt by Knight and Lewy, limited to individuals without psychopathology. Choice of outcome needs to be made during the sequence of intrapsychic events, whether the final external behavior is normal or pathological. Symptoms are as much an unconscious choice as normal behavioral outcomes. While we speak freely of choice of symptoms, we do not as readily acknowledge the unconscious choice to have symptoms at all. I also do not agree with Winnicott's (1958) differentiation between a "false self" subject to psychic determinism and a "true self" able to exercise free will. Every "self"—or ego, to be more precise—functions with a combination of the two, is confronted with deterministic necessities, which are in conflict, following which it has no choice but to choose.

In 1976, I focused on the role of the superego in intrapsychic conflict, especially as operative in group life, which is the "average expectable environment" of everyday life. Before this, the "syndrome of the compromise of integrity" was described (Rangell, 1974), in a scientific not moralistic sense, as another resultant of unconscious ego decision-making, on a par with neurosis in human affairs. Ego-superego tensions and conflicts are as much to be solved, and compromises to be chosen, as between ego and id, or more accurately, between id and super-ego as mediated by the ego.

Unconscious decision-making was introduced in these contributions as squarely anchored within the structural view, not different from the "executive intention" formulated by G. Klein (1970, p. 92) in his "clinical theory," or from the observations or experiments of academic psychology. However, the opposition, or, as I will suggest, the resistance to this concept which I described in the past, continued as before. In 1977, Kohut, as one justification for his superseding the structural view by his new self psychology, stated, "I could find no place [within Freud's model of the mind] for the psychological activities that go by the name of choice, decision, and free will—even though I knew that these were empirically observable phenomena. . . . I had to acknowledge that the theoretical framework at my disposal—classical, mental-apparatus psychology, which conceived of the mind as a reacting machine—could not accommodate them within its realm" (p. 244). This view was of course incomplete.

Other theoreticians concluded similarly that for the inclusion of intention it was necessary to dispose of Freud's meta-psychological model, which included the structural view. G. Klein (1973, 1976), for example, and his followers, felt that Freud's model consisted of two theories, not one; that choice, intention, purpose, meaning belonged in one psychology and that Freud's metapsychological theory, which was an attempt to join psychology to the natural sciences, no longer obtained and needed to be abandoned. Schafer (1976) joined this group in discarding Freud's metapsychological views and developed an "action theory of psychoanalysis" to incorporate the need for intention and action, which he preferred, as did Klein, to attribute to the whole person rather than to a psychic system or part.

Other objections coming from analysts to the concept of unconscious decision-making take several forms. One source of concern is on a philosophical as well as theoretical basis, derived from Ryle's (1949) metaphor of "the ghost in the machine," against the concept of a "homunculus" as the agent of human decision. The latest to express this opinion, widely held by others, is Brenner (1982), who, discussing Waelder's (1930) principle of multiple function, criticizes "Waelder's assumption that the ego is a steering agency—that it is like a little man, a homunculus in a sort of a driver's seat of the psychic apparatus" (p. 117). The same objection caused Klein, Gill (1973), Schafer, Kohut, Gedo (1979), in different ways, to turn away from Freud's metapsychological, especially structural theory, to explanations of psychic decision and action by the person as a whole.

This objection is, in my opinion, a misunderstanding of the meaning of structural theory and a misleading application of Ryle's metaphor to psychoanalytic theory. Actually the opposite is the case. The ego is not the total organism, shrunken down, but an inner structure—a conceptual one, to be sure, but what the development of psychoanalytic theory has come to, for good reasons, over the years—to which this final directing function can be ascribed. The whole person, normal size or diminutive, whether in the new systems designed to replace the structural view, or as erroneously conceived in seeing the ego in this central function as a diminished replica of the total organism, reverses the explanatory power to understand clinical phenomena built up since the advent of psychoanalysis. A diminutive, whole person would still be in need of an explanation as to the specific agency within this new miniature whole which performs this active function. It is not the inert parts of the total organism, or organs or systems serving other functions, which are psychological agents of direction and will, but the psychic system which by agreement over the years has served to clear the way for this final function.

Another source of widespread opposition to this view of ego functioning can be seen in Brenner's (1982) objection that "Waelder's picture of mental functioning impresses the reader as passionless, intellectual, almost mechanical. The ego he depicted could easily be replaced by a computer" (p. 117). This concern of overintellectuality has been used from the inception of psychoanalysis about other psychoanalytic formulations as well, to object to theory in general—see Fenichel's (1941) discussion of the views of Reik—or to Freud's total metapsychological theory which culminated in the structural point of view. The fact is that there is no incompatibility between the most abstract psychoanalytic theory and the understanding of affects or a proper affective approach to clinical psychoanalysis. The opposite is true, as the work of Brenner himself attests. Psychoanalytic theory and the psychoanalytic method each combines the theoretical and clinical. Psychoanalysis consists of a blend between scientific explanation and humanism, just as empathy resides operationally within the analytic attitude. While Brenner feels that Waelder, in presenting his formulation "made no special reference either to anxiety or to psychic conflict," the formulations I have described demonstrate the fusion between affective clinical material and the explanations tracing their course and fate within the operations of the psychic systems. Anxiety and psychic conflict are the material and fuel with which and for which the intrapsychic process continues its dynamic movement. Nor can anyone think that Waelder saw it differently.

What I have been concentrating on in this presentation is the extension of the ego's activities to its next level of functioning and the inevitable outcome and final result. Others react negatively to pursuing ego functions to this extent because of the feeling that extra baggage is being added to a structure already overburdened in a theoretical sense. For a system already credited with being the organ of thought, the seat of affects, the locus of memories, also to be considered the executive agent for the behavior of the individual has elicited a critical reception. Leites (1971), for example, points with strong disapproval to the almost limitless inventory of behavioral functions attributed to the ego, as if the ego becomes synonymous with the person. This shift is made explicitly when the self replaces the ego in a psychology of the self, which takes over for a psychology of intrapsychic structural systems.

The same objections to this persevering and inclusive pursuit of ego functions could be made in the somatic sphere to the organizing and integrative functions of the brain and central nervous system, with their labyrinth of neuronal trunks, pathways, tributaries, and connecting links. In spite of this theoretical asymmetry, however, and a failure to achieve an aesthetic architecture of theory, psychoanalytic theory, with its central executive role of the ego, fulfills its purpose, and has proven useful as a coherent, explanatory system to encompass observational data, which is always the basic foundation upon which theory receives its definitive test.

Still others fail to respond to this aspect of ego functioning out of the feeling that it comes too close to a description of the problem-solving methods of conscious mental life. To this I would point out that the opinions by Freud, the views of Anna Freud, the explicit description of "a steering agency" by Waelder, the data and reasoning I have presented—all point to the existence of a problem-solving function in the unconscious ego that applies to the repressed mental content. Problem-solving is too often met by analysts in a pejorative sense. Such activity takes place in the unconscious routinely, is affected adversely by neurosis, and is to be encouraged and freed from its encumberments rather than regarded with a negative view. The exposure and the stimulation of motivation to seek solutions to unconscious problems do not stand in contradiction to other affective achievements and hermeneutic pursuits.

Freud (1923) initiated this level of insight when he pointed out that not only the id but the ego is unconscious. From there we have come to know, empirically, unconscious defenses, unconscious anxiety and other affects, unconscious fantasies, completely formed and viable, operating outside of consciousness. Then symptoms, character traits, and the most complex psychic formations can be held in repression, even if it is basically the drive components at the heart of each which may provide the central impetus for such global defense.

The topographic divisions into conscious and unconscious do not precisely overlap with Freud's (1911) two principles of mental functioning or primary and secondary process mentation. I have been describing secondary process functioning in the unconscious ego. In a discussion of the ego with Anna Freud, Sandler (1983) notes, and Anna Freud agrees, "The more we know about how the mind works, the more we see the extent to which there is unconscious functioning which involves secondary process" (p. 136). Other writers who have contributed ideas and opinions contiguous to these views include Hendrick (1942) on ego mastery, the Bühlers (1951, 1954) on ego effectance and ego pleasure, Harrison (1984) on the ego as "prime mover," and others who have pointed out the intricate operations of the unconscious ego.

The opposite also is the case—at times and under certain conditions, there are residuals and derivatives of primary process activity operative during conscious life. Contradictions exist and live together in conscious as well as unconscious life. There is no fine line separating the two systems in this regard, even though the preconscious connects them in a neat theoretical sense. People drift, daydream, fantasy when awake, as they can create, be on guard, and solve problems while asleep. The unconscious fantasy, so thoroughly anchored into mental life by Arlow (1969), Rosen (1960), Beres (1962), and others, is more than a cognitive construct. Operative unconsciously during sleep and the waking state, it is an organized cognitive-affective mental complex composed of elements of all three psychic structures and inputs from external perceptions as well.

There is a spectrum from the dream, and even here between deep dream states and REM dreams, hypnopompic hallucinations between sleep and waking, primary and secondary process operations during the day, waking fantasies, alert states, daydreams, and hypnagogic phenomena as one is falling asleep again (Isakower, 1938). All of these mental products, at all stages, during the night and day, are treated by secondary revision as they approach the preconscious and then conscious and alert state. And all are composites of cognitive and affective contents, derivatives of drives and defenses, miniature or intermediate compromise formations, all brought together into one running thought or image as a final, more macroscopic, compromise formation.

Can there be special receptivities and separate creative capacities at the various stages of consciousness from unconscious to conscious? Creativity may be optimum when the two are mixed, perhaps with different types of outcomes with different proportions of each, such as during free imaging, i.e., the admission of primary process thought and affect in the waking state, and secondary process functioning operative during sleep. Einstein, assessing his own creativity, ventured an opinion that his ability and insights came not so much from his capacity to think or remember as to fantasy, i.e., to permit unconscious drive discharge within his waking fantasy life.

The autonomous ego, especially in its unconscious aspects, plays as necessary a role in the creative process as in planned activity. The creativity of which man is capable cannot spring from the conscious alone. Whether the painting of a gifted artist, or a dream created by any individual, or a chemical or mathematical formula arrived at by a creative scientist, the contribution of the unconscious is indispensable, and within this the secondary process revision and integration also are necessary and available at the unconscious level. Creativity is in fact associated with the greatest amount of autonomy, to the point where it can be antiadaptive—an empirical finding which lends evidence to the fact that autonomy and adaptation, both ego functions, do not necessarily overlap.

Individuality, as expressed both in a creative and more planned sense, springs from and rests upon autonomy. In the total fabric of a human life the degree of autonomy, unconscious as well as conscious, is what determines an individual's motivation to develop his own ego style, and directs and propels him along his unique path. From the time of self-object differentiation, this is in fact the pathognomonic determinant toward the development and preservation of the self. Self-differentiation and integration are achieved and maintained by this function of the ego within the self. This can be less understood in the psychology of the self, which obscures this factor by substituting the self for the independent ego.

While all mental functions interrelate, there are specific developmental determinants which may influence the fate of this central measure of ego strength—the ability, when all the data are in, not only to integrate or necessarily to adapt, but to elect to foray, or to strike out anew. This capacity for self expression—to judge, discriminate, differentiate, and then choose—may spell the difference intrapsychically between what in oversimplified terms are called winners and losers. This ability, nurtured or injured from early life on, begins at the earliest stages, is tested constantly, is confronted strongly at certain critical times and ages, and undergoes as many vicissitudes as any other aspect of mental functioning. Its developmental history consists of pro-

gressions and regressions accompanying separations and rap-
prochements (Mahler et al., 1968, 1972, 1975, 1982), and
emerges in a form characteristic for the individual. Hanly (1979)
stresses the developmental aspects of the acquisition of relative
ego freedom. While the developmental or vertical history of this
function is of considerable analytic importance, the function also
exists and is under test during each horizontal moment of
human existence.

Many or perhaps most people remain attached to their surround, as figure to ground, self to object, or individual to the
inevitable group, sacrificing or minimizing this trait in favor of
security. Reality, inner and outer, defines the area within which
choices can be made. Within this area, the ratio between choice
by compulsion and choice with a variable latitude of freedom
separates one individual from another. Weakness or strength in
the capacity to choose or create, whether in a practical or aesthetic sense, stamps the individual character. While the necessity and
therefore the ability to choose are part of all human life and
mentality, the capacity of the ego to roam freely and allow a
creative process to come to pass is achieved by a small minority of
individuals. In the larger perspective, given the restrictions of
everyday life at all levels of society and cultural development, the
capacity to choose with a significant degree of security and freedom is limited and not given to many.

Decisions can take place in the unconscious and remain unconscious. Rationalization is then an unconscious defense made
after the decision which obscures the motivations upon which it
was made. Hartmann (1950) points out that both insight and
rationalization take place in the ego. I would add that both can
take place at the unconscious level. Just as man "knows" more
than he knows he knows, i.e., from memories and thoughts not
permitted into consciousness, so does he decide more than he
allows himself to know he decided. A patient, or people outside
of analysis, may decide and not know it, say they have decided
when they have not, and say they have not decided when they
already have. The analyst, attuned to the unconscious of the
patient, often knows that the patient has decided when the latter
does not yet know it, or that he has not yet decided when he
thinks he has. Contradictions are observed routinely in patients

between conscious decisions and behavior which belies them, and the reverse, actions and behavior which indicate decisions have been made before or without their being consciously acknowledged.

These clinical-theoretical observations have important consequences, including shedding clues as to the explanation of the negative reactions they elicit. It is in this connection that I wish to point out that the ambivalent and contradictory reception accorded this subject since the onset of psychoanalysis can best be understood by psychoanalytic insights themselves. The original opposition to Freud's discoveries and to early evolving psychoanalytic theory was based on the injury to man's narcissism, that he was no longer master of or in control of his behavior. The present theme adds simultaneously an opposite mechanism, affecting not control but responsibility for one's actions. Lewy's (1961) point of departure for his study of autonomy and will was the question of how responsibility was affected. A new resistance to psychoanalytic understanding stems from the fact that man now becomes responsible not for less but for more than he knows. With respect to narcissism, man is traumatized; with respect to an unconscious decision opposing his superego and the external world, he is made anxious and guilty. Both mechanisms of course can and do coexist.

The introduction of the question of responsibility, which flows as a natural extension of the theme we are discussing, moves on to an issue of the widest ramifications in human behavior. A number of applied aspects come into consideration, such as, from the standpoint of the psychoanalyst, the role of responsibility in the therapeutic process, and from the broader perspective, its place in a spectrum from the social relationships of ordinary life to the crucial and ambiguous position of responsibility in the psychosociolegal area. These important applied aspects, in the interest of space, will be pursued in a separate paper, and only the more theoretical stream will be developed further here.

WILL, FREEDOM, AND PSYCHIC DETERMINISM

If the fear of increased responsibility and accountability is the dynamic behind the resistance to autonomy seen in patients and large segments of the public, the lag among analysts in accepting and using this aspect of theory stems from another source as well. Here the conflict involves the need to preserve the concept of psychic determinism, so central a tenet of psychoanalytic theory. Autonomy and determinism have been seen from the start as mutually contradictory, each canceling the other out. Yet just as determinism stands upon an unassailable theoretical and clinical base, the same holds, from both clinical observations and theoretical persuasiveness, with regard to the need for formulations about autonomous functioning. The two appearing to be immiscible, the result has been a theoretical lag. Empirically, from the order of the chronological development, determinism had priority, and autonomy has therefore remained relatively undeveloped.

But continuing phenomenology presses for expansions of theory to accommodate the findings. Observational data leading to a conviction of the presence of both determinism and autonomy are of such ubiquitous and compelling nature as to make any theoretical reasoning which would eliminate either one of them untenable if not absurd.

Theory usually catches up, even if after long periods of time. Of many studies along the lines I have been describing which have not yet coalesced or been brought together, I would mention in particular two centers of such research, one on each coast. Weiss and Sampson (1982) in San Francisco, have come to similar theoretical conclusions, of the routine operation of high-level secondary process functioning in the unconscious ego, from a long-term, experimental approach involving detailed clinical analysis of process notes. On the opposite coast, A. Kris (1977, 1982, 1984, 1985) has postulated the routine presence, stemming from similar observational phenomena, of what he calls divergent conflicts, either-or conflicts, or conflicts of ambivalence, akin to what I have called choice or dilemma types of conflicts. In his case, the same conclusions which from my line of approach stemmed from a microdynamic analysis of "the intrapsychic process" derived from a study of the process of free association.

It would not be amiss, and confirms an aspect of my thesis, to point out that the authors of these studies have felt, not without reason, that their findings have not only been disagreed with, but have been considered controversial. Both have aroused an affective opposition. The reactions to the subject, however, are not negative but ambivalent. There is, in my opinion, a widespread feeling of something having been omitted or at least underplayed. Esman (1985), in a recent brief paper, has elevated Rapaport's 1953 paper on active and passive to the status of a "neglected classic." Noting its immense contribution as well as its fate of having remained unheralded, Esman points out how Klein, Schafer, and others have utilized Rapaport's insights in their own subsequent formulations—in Klein's case, specifically toward a psychology of "will"—without sufficient reference to Rapaport's contribution. Transported back by Rapaport's paper to "the heroic age of ego psychology," Esman found this work helpful not only in his general clinical experience, but specifically in conceptualizing the nature of healthy adolescent development. He also singles out the light it sheds on understanding artistic creativity, "to emphasize the active role of autonomous problem-solving ego functions as opposed to the more conventional notions of passive 'inspiration' based on regression, even if 'in the service of the ego'" (p. 69).

The same combination of special importance coupled with a strange and inexplicable inhibition in furthering the concept is seen at the source in Rapaport himself. In an introduction to the posthumous publication of Rapaport's paper in 1967, Gill notes the surprising fact that Rapaport never published this paper, although it was in careful, finished form since 1953. This was attributed by Gill to "the extraordinary scope of the concept of activity and passivity in Rapaport's mind, [which] he regarded . . . as at the very heart of an adequate conceptualization of the human psyche" (p. 531). It is interesting that Gill himself, a few years later (1973), to achieve the same inclusion of active intention into psychology, joined Klein in abandoning Rapaport's, and Freud's, abstract metapsychological views.

From the arguments and line of reasoning I have adduced, I share Rapaport's opinion of the centrality of the active and directing function of the ego in mental functioning. I also agree with Esman about "the rich, complex, and many-veined lode that Rapaport began to explore" (p. 69) in this paper, which was left aborted. The thrust of this theoretical advance was toward what Brenman recognized as the metapsychology of will. The importance as well as the ambivalent reactions demonstrated to this subject are part of the observable data, and stem, in my opinion, from a push toward and a pull away from deep contradictory unconscious motives which this issue evokes.

I believe that the relationship between autonomy and psychic determinism needs to be clarified and revised. Observational data, the final arbiter, dictate that both need to be fitted together in a harmonious, coherent, and unified theory. Previous studies which have made room for both have not settled on a satisfactory or coherent relationship between the two. Knight, Lewy, and others, for example, include the existence of free will side by side with what they continue to feel is a strict or rigorous determinism in its original sense, without regard for the mutual relations between the two or eliminating the apparent incompatibility between them. I would like, particularly in line with what I believe are subtle new developments since then, to offer a way of thinking about this dilemma which I believe achieves theoretical and scientific consistency.

First, will does not automatically mean free will, as conventional phraseology routinely and literally links the two. Just as I have previously separated conversion from hysteria (1959) and suggested (1982a) that we dissociate self from the concept of borderline or narcissistic, so does the automatic linkage between the pair of words "free" and "will" also need to be discontinued, if clarity of thought in this difficult field is to be attained. As autonomy is relative, so is "freedom" of will. As "free" associations are only relatively free, the same applies to "free" will. Will, as autonomy, is always relatively free and relatively restricted. Hanly (1979) speaks similarly of "grades of freedom."

The concept of autonomy, which is accepted, brings with it the concept of will, which is resisted. Perhaps the recognition and automatic limitation of the human will to the degree of freedom it actually has, while contiguously linked and intimately responsive to its surrounding psychic elements, would reduce or eliminate the immediate rejection it otherwise arouses. I have described with great care the inputs from drives and superego impinging routinely upon the ego before its autonomy can come into its area of functioning. Will has the characteristics of any ego activity, exerts itself after the ego has been subjected to and taken into account motivations from all other sources from within and without.

Will is to be differentiated from the instinctual wish, the wish of early psychoanalytic theory. It is also to be distinguished and separated from a superego demand or requirement. The human will is an ego faculty, a directing capacity following and combining motivations from the three psychic systems, external reality, and the goals and intentions of the ego itself, of which will is its culmination.

The relationship between autonomy and psychic determinism is a complex one, and must take into account the stages by which insights into this area were established. As Freud first discovered the determinism exerted by drives and the unconscious (Breuer and Freud, 1895; Freud, 1900), the role of the latter over what was then known about the ego was the dominant and overriding insight, to be protected and preserved against any minimalization. As the counterforces of the ego in relation to the id were elaborated, the deterministic influence of the id, and later of the superego, on the ego were maintained, while the wider scope of ego functioning was increasingly mapped out (Freud, 1923).

While the developments from then on led Freud to a fuller appreciation of the active in addition to reactive activities of the ego, these were never consolidated into an equally cohesive summary form as had been his earlier discoveries. The way was clearly open, however, for the subsequent work of Hartmann to add the adaptive and, more importantly for our theme, the autonomous functions, without violating, but complementing, what Freud had laid down. From the content and spirit of Freud's writings in this connection, I would say the following. If Freud had done with this subject what he did with anxiety (Freud, 1926), i.e., attempted to coordinate and unify his views of psychic determinism and his cumulative new understanding of the active, directing role of the ego as quoted above in a number of instances, he might well have come to the same conclusion as he did with the two successive anxiety theories. He could have felt, that is, that both views applied, that they seemed at that time to be mutually inconsistent, yet that he did not feel either should be discarded, and that, for the time being, *non liquet.*

And just as I (1955, 1968) concluded with regard to Freud's two anxiety theories that both the first physiological theory and the second psychological signal theory needed to coexist in a unified theory (distinctly a minority view, I might say), I would conclude the same about determinism and autonomy—evidence exists that both concepts apply, and both need to coexist in one harmonious theoretical whole (which also might or might not turn out to be a minority view). Jones (1924), while adducing arguments from philosophy to atomic physics to cast doubt on the scientific credibility of free will, quotes Kant's two forms of truth, his "critical reason" and "practical reason." From psychoanalysis, there are similarly two unconscious truths on the matter of free will and inevitability, from which Jones sees one day "a chance of reconciliation between the two in place of regarding them as an insoluble antimony" (p. 187).

But each concept needs to be clarified on its own, as well as the mutual relationships between them. As autonomy came to be seen as relative, the same can be said to apply to determinism, at least in the original sense of automaticity and compulsion in which Freud introduced the term and concept. Each, in fact, limits, modifies, and influences the other, again thinking of determinism in its original sense. The failure to see this relativity and reciprocity in perspective has led to the usual sequelae of one-sidedness and *pars pro toto* in this area which has been characteristic of the history of psychoanalytic theory during its entire course. Thus Kohut (1977) came to see classic theory as "the domain where the authority of absolute determinism holds sway [as] unlimited" (p. 244), an observation he used in support of his replacement of ego by a new, more flexible self psychology. I do not think that Freud viewed any phase of his discoveries of mental functioning as absolute, as his many changes and modifications attest, but all as a series of checks and balances and interconnecting links. That is why dualism and conflict remained his center. Kohut is correct, however, to the extent that the admission of ego autonomy into psychoanalytic theory and its clinical applications have remained limited and restricted. It was not necessary, however, in order to introduce and integrate choice and intention, to replace ego by self psychology, nor to abandon metapsychology and the structural view in favor of any of the psychologies of the whole as agent, as Klein, Schafer, and others have done.

The subjects of free will and determinism have been among the most debated issues in the intellectual concerns of man from earliest times, occupying the minds of philosophers, religious theorists, ethicists, logicians, and the great psychologists before Freud. The related group of issues woven together in a melange of sophistic and elliptic arguments have included causation, freedom, responsibility, necessity, and that most elusive subject of chance. The opinions offered are all definite, eloquent, well-fortified, and equally convincing on opposite sides of each question. They range from William James's (1897) conclusion for the necessity of free will, espousing pluralism, chance, and indeterminacy in the service of making possible optimism and a moral sense, through Hospers's (1950) arguments against the logical existence of free will, to Wood's (1941) strongly presented conclusion that "a capricious free will—capable of acting independently of antecedent conditions—is a philosophical absurdity" (p. 46). I would like to reflect briefly on how the opinions I have offered from the psychoanalytic viewpoint, most specifically on the function of ego autonomy, relate to these various questions and concerns, and what light they may throw on this perennial area of intellectual controversy and debate.

Autonomy and will are not without motivation, and neither is contrary to the concept of causation, but are included within it. Both take their place as sequences within the causative chain, maintaining the continuity with nature stressed by Hanly (1979), and consonant with Hume's characterization of causation as "the cement of the universe" (in Wallace, 1985a). Thus neither runs counter to the tenets of science as demanded by biologists and psychoanalysts alike. Nor are autonomy and will contradictory to the concept of psychic determinism. In keeping with Knight's requirement that an absolute determinism is intrinsic to science and nature, autonomy, as I have described it in the intrapsychic sequence, also is a psychic determinant of action and thus resides within the domain of psychic determinism. Behavioral outcomes are as much determined by the role of the final autonomous inputs of the ego as by the underlying formative pressures of the drives and superego.

The concept of determinism, however, is seen to have been widened. This is not determinism in the original "id" sense of compulsion with no room for choice and decision, but determinism which includes the ego as well and its final autonomous will and act. Just as external constraints are always present, but are also always circumscribed to a greater or lesser degree, so are internal restrictions always present, but only to a finite degree. "Freedom" of the will lives and exerts itself between these limiting borders. Anchored to its own past history, it is caused and is itself a cause. It is no more capricious, magical, free-floating, or unanchored in history and a surrounding milieu than other psychic elements or agencies, but has its function and power to choose, even if at times it elects to limit, postpone, or abrogate that power.

Will does not make behavior indeterminate, but adds to determinism by compulsion the determinism of choice. Neither does the substitution of probability for absolute predictability impair the concepts of determinism or cause. Probability does not negate causation, but also takes its place among the links of the causative chain. Predictability, another prerequisite demanded by philosophers of science, is present, but in a relative, not absolute sense. Doers fall into groups, which lends some predictability, and within the individual, actions are not independent of antecedent factors, which again provides a means of prediction. But following these preparatory determinants, the autonomy as to final choice, not only within the control of, but required of each separate human individual, prevents predictions from being absolute.

Autonomy, however objective a position one wishes to take toward it, makes for a softer determinism, introducing the factor of human individuality, of choice and direction instituted by an agent of decision. The most elegant expression is contained in Waelder's (1934) concept of ego "transcendence." Referring to man's capacity to rise temporarily above his instinctual and environmental demands, Waelder notes the ability for "objectification of one's self, the attainment of a position above one's own ego" (p. 104). Elsewhere, in a psychoanalytic survey of the entire sweep of human history, Waelder (1967) notes the claims by some of the universality of dominance and aggression in the animal kingdom, from which they would conclude that despotism is a universal law of nature. He states, "Even if this condition were universal, however, it would not prove that man cannot alter it; for man, though rooted in nature, can transcend it to a large degree. As Denis de Rougemont put it: 'Man's nature is to pass beyond nature'" (p. 47).

With the evolutionary development from animal instinct, through intermediate forms to human will, with its intention and direction, a factor is added to biological determinism, coming now from the psychic determinism of the human will, which retains the scientific status of determinism while making it more complex and complete. Human nature, by the combined attributes of intelligence and will, can slow, hasten, prevent, or abort processes in the physical world around it. Waelder (1967) states, "man has since time immemorial changed his environment and disturbed the balance of nature" (p. 285). These capacities have been incrementally accelerated in modern times. Softer deterministic characteristics introduced into physical nature by human nature alter the absolute predictability of the present and future of the physical universe as well as of the human condition contained within it. Wallace (1985b), speaking in favor of a strict determinism, distinguishes determinism from predetermination. The nature of the universe may therefore be not only not predetermined, in the sense pointed out by Wallace; but, now that a relative uncertainty has been introduced by the acts and influence of human nature, it is not subject to determinism or predictability in an absolute sense.

Whatever causative events and determining influences have preceded ego choice in the intrapsychic sequence, it is precisely man's ego autonomy, and the degree of freedom this bespeaks, which defines and makes room for his subsequent assumption of responsibility. Without the possibility of autonomous choice, responsibility for one's actions or behavior is theoretically nonexistent, or in an untenable or ambiguous role, no matter how ardently but inconsistently the opponents of independent will try to include it within their formulations of causation. The factor of responsibility is included by the proponents of all shades of opinion in this area because, by observation and logic, it cannot be left out. Yet its inclusion within the system of reasoning is without a logical and consistent base.

Responsibility, however, is also a gray area, and relative, not absolute, not all or none. Responsibility is directly related to the ratio between psychic compulsion and autonomy, between automaticity and control, however difficult a problem this is to measure clinically or in life. The degree of autonomy and the resultant responsibility are not to be contrasted with the presence of conflict, nor sharply equated with the conflict-free. Will based on autonomy is exercised for cause, expresses motivation, and is instituted equally after the ego is confronted with conflicts as in the absence of these. Nor are this function and capacity related specifically to the degree of psychopathology or its absence, as both Knight and Lewy have suggested. The problem of assessment, of the degree of autonomy with its attendant responsibility, exists in all behavioral functioning. Accountability may not overlap or coincide with responsibility, but may be wider or narrower than the latter. Society and legality add their own criteria. A person may be held accountable even if not responsible, and in some instances the reverse.

"Will power," a colloquial expression which resonates with meaning to the average person, connotes an intuitive recognition of this decisive ego force. It is man's will which gives him the power to direct the path to be taken by the self, to decide, to execute, to do, to act. The role played by "the will to recover" in the psychoanalytic process has been traced by Nunberg (1926). The "will to win" is well known as it influences outcomes, from competitive sports to the games of business and living. It is recognized how, in times of severe crisis, the "will to survive" can determine life or death. "Brainwashing," a term used to connote the elimination of this force under conditions of oppression, is not a solution of cortical cells of the brain, but a dissolution of the will while the brain remains intact. The decision of the victim to allow this to happen is a psychological defense, typically preconscious, or unconscious, or even conscious, in the service, in fact, of preserving the existence of body and brain somatically. The uncritically accepted and commonly agreed-upon misnomer for the syndrome of submission, making it instead a physical process, defends and excuses the ego decision, with which all can identify, made by the captive against odds.

Freedom and necessity, both of which occupy a central place in the reflections of philosophers, are reciprocally restricting, and both are relative, not absolute, even in more fortunate societies. Necessity is relative, not absolute even in an oppressive environment. Heroic acts, choosing for or against self-preservation, point out that from the mundane to the extreme, even after necessity comes the necessity to exercise choice. To execute this, the will of the ego takes its place in the sequence of the instinctual wish and superego demand as an element in the causative psychological chain.

Democracy is also "free" only to a certain degree, within the boundaries of rules and restrictions necessary to preserve an orderly and sufficiently predictable life. Predictability is subjected to a softer view from this line of observation and reflection. As Rapaport and Gill (1959) point out, although autonomy has an antecedent history of its own, its actions cannot be predicted as the sum total of its history. No matter how much is known of an individual's previous patterns of behavior, the outcome to a current, particular combination of stimuli is always uncertain, even more so in an environment which prides itself on the attainment of a "free society." Given the fresh confrontation and exposure to the ego's will, the result can never be predicted in an absolute and infallible sense. This is characteristically human.

Limitations of predictability have recently been indicated by scientific reflection even in the physical and biological worlds, where causation and predictability had previously held absolute sway. Much has been made in recent years by social scientists, philosophers, theologians, and ethicists who wish to preserve man's freedom of choice, of the introduction of unpredictability into the world of physical matter by Heisenberg's (1958) principle of uncertainty in the movement from Newtonian physics to quantum mechanics. Random occurrences among subatomic particles have been assumed to be paralleled by random, or at least independent, choice by whatever each psychological system considers the human agent to be. While I agree with Hartmann (1959) that psychoanalysis, or psychology for that matter, need not be bound by the laws or requirements of the physical, including the somatic, world, similar end points, arrived at independently by research in each field, each by their own paths and criteria, would seem to convey a special impact.

Waelder (1967) includes the role of chance in his thorough list of the determinants of history. Chance is part of nature and of science, Max Born is said to have said to Einstein. Social scientists, with the concurrence of nuclear physicists interested in applying their new knowledge, have stressed the role of accident and chance, some to the point of developing the chaos theory of social progress and regress. And Darwin has demonstrated the role played by chance in the random mutations along the course of the evolutionary scale. Chance is minimized but not eliminated by active choice, and continues to play a causative role outside of ego control. This applies to an equal degree to the physical, biological, and psychological chains of events impinging on the course of human history. Not all illnesses, for example, are psychosomatic, nor all accidents brought about by an accident-prone victim. Reality, as Hartmann (1956a) points out, is more than man's unconscious.

The history of an individual life is not determined entirely by causative events within the psychic self, without influence by physical occurrences external to it and outside of its control. Conversely, with man now having within his power the capacity to unleash energy of a magnitude to significantly alter the physical arrangements in the external world, the history of the physical world is to a certain extent dependent on the vicissitudes and choices of the human will. The latter, I have been saying, cannot be predicted with certainty. As a culmination of these views about the sequence of thinking and affect within the intrapsychic process of man, the influences which play upon it and those which derive from it, I would say that human history, individual and collective, results from a combination of determinism, random occurrences, and the guided event.

Freud discovered that unconscious forces determined psychological history more than was known. This never proceeded to an opinion by Freud that determinism, in the sense of compulsion in which it was first considered, was thereby absolute. Nor did it follow that all aspects of behavior are determined outside of the control of the subject doer, a fallacy fallen into by many who erroneously attributed this view to Freud. There is no evidence that Freud ever set himself against what strict determinists call "nonnecessitated choosing." Autonomy and will are part of the chain of psychic determinism, as I have described. Both are included in unconscious mentation, as well as the conventional association of these with conscious functioning. Just as defenses are unconscious, so can decisions be equally kept from consciousness. The motive, as always, is to ward off anxiety, in this case from the unconscious ego decision and action having been made counter to the interests of the superego, with the usual fear of punishment resulting. Consciously, in such instances, either the person denies that a decision has been made, or its external presence is attributed to other motives. Such a sequence of decision-making and rationalization is commonplace in life.

While improved choices on a conscious basis are expectable and acknowledged as an outcome of analysis, a more subtle achievement is an effortless solution of intrapsychic conflicts by autonomous activity of the unconscious ego. The psychoanalytic process makes the intrapsychic process less disturbed and disruptive, and more efficient during its entire course. Changes after insight do not take place automatically. With the increased freedom available to the ego, the patient needs next to act. Waelder (1960) is one of the few authors on technique whose formulation leaves room for the factor of choice, although this is not elaborated upon in an explicit way. After insight, the patient has "a *possibility* of working out a viable, nonneurotic, solution" (p. 46; my italics), Waelder states. Glover (1949) writes of "freed will." The decision, however, then remains with the patient to proceed with the possibility. While some patients do, others introduce further difficulties at this point, which may either be dissolved or, with further analysis, open new possibilities, which may then be chosen to effect a change.

Without the inclusion of unconscious forces, cognitive psychologies limited to conscious intention are incomplete. Without the inclusion of the role of ego autonomy in the unconscious, psychoanalytic theory also remains incomplete. Such an omission adversely affects the analytic situation and the theory of therapy which guides it. A psychic determinism which does not include the roles of unconscious decision and choice makes psychoanalytic treatment untenable and incomplete, and defeats its goals from the start. I cannot visualize practicing psychoanalysis without having within my therapeutic armamentarium the interpretation that "you have a choice," or "you had a choice, and chose this or that," or at least that "you set up the conditions which made such-and-such a decision necessary or inevitable." Without the inclusion of such concepts and tools, understanding the past and influencing and guiding the future life of the patient must remain incomplete.

Clinical psychoanalysis decreases the determinism emanating from id and superego and increases the scope within psychic determinism of unconscious ego autonomy and choice. This expanded view of Hartmann's ego autonomy, which, in my opinion, has been aborted in psychoanalytic theoretical development, is necessary to achieve the full meaning and applicability of the concept in psychoanalytic theory and practice. With its successful inclusion into the total psychoanalytic goal, psychoanalysis joins other conscious psychologies in including deliberation and direction in the chain of causative events. It would then, however, be the only psychology which also includes its unconscious scope of operation. Without an unequivocal role given to autonomy and choice, with their attendant assumption of responsibility for behavior, the Sartrean existential criticism of "bad faith" leveled at the psychoanalytic view of psychic causation acquires credibility. The widespread acceptance of this critique of psychoanalysis is at least partly due to the awareness of this common omission in psychoanalytic theoretical and practical discourse.

A patient expressing repetitive, uncontrolled anger against indiscriminate targets, displaced from repressed rage against his father, comes to see the irrationality of his behavior, not only of the present inappropriate objects of his aggression but even in the part he played in the original development, what he contributed to bring about his father's aggressive acts. During the progressions and regressions of this insight, the patient himself introduces a metaphor to reinforce his accumulating insight, "You can't blame the caddy for giving you the wrong club. In the end, it was I who swung the club." As he returns to this repeatedly

with each new incident, we are awaiting the time when he solid-
ifies this insight and learning, that he should and can swing the
club differently, and finally that he does so. His affects as actions
will also then be under greater control.

To return to a colloquial phrase I referred to above, one might
say that psychoanalysis increases "will power," an equivalent of
Freud's, and Fenichel's, pointing to the increased operation of
the rational ego. Hartmann (1956a), pointing out the "bewilder-
ing . . . complexities [behind each] basically simple question" (p.
267), hoped for such a time when "we may reach a decidedly
more beautiful and satisfactory stage, when simple formulations
will become of equal or superior value" (1958, p. 313). That time
has not yet come and, in view of the history and course of the
applications of psychoanalytic insight, may be far off. For the
time being, limiting ourselves, as an example, to the subject under discussion, recognition of the autonomous functions of the
ego has had a greater effect on the conduct of an analysis than
their discovery has had on psychoanalytic theory.

We will end with a passage of Freud's quoted by Hartmann
(1950, p. 141), in connection with Hartmann's "synchroniza-
tions and reformulations" of Freud's psychoanalytic theory of
the ego. "There is no need," writes Freud (1926, p. 160), com-
menting on his own changes in the theory of anxiety, "to be
discouraged by these emendations. They are to be welcomed if
they add something to our knowledge, and they are no disgrace
to us so long as they enrich rather than invalidate our earlier
views—by limiting some statement, perhaps, that was too general or by enlarging some idea that was too narrowly formulated."

BIBLIOGRAPHY

ALEXANDER, F. & STAUB, H. (1956). *The Criminal, the Judge and the Public*, rev.
ed. Glencoe: Free Press.
ARLOW, J. A. (1969). Unconscious fantasy and disturbances of conscious experience. *Psychoanal. Q.*, 38:1–27.
BERES, D. (1962). The unconscious fantasy. *Psychoanal. Q.*, 31:309–328.
BRENNER, C. (1979). The components of psychic conflict and its consequences
in mental life. *Psychoanal. Q.*, 48:547–567.
——— (1982). *The Mind in Conflict*. New York: Int. Univ. Press.

34 *Leo Rangell*

BREUER, J. & FREUD, S. (1893-95). *Studies on Hysteria. S.E.*, 2.

BÜHLER, C. (1954). The reality principle. *Amer. J. Psychother.*, 8:626–647.

BÜHLER, K. (1951). On thought connections. In *Organization and Pathology of Thought*, D. Rapaport, pp. 39–57. New York: Columbia Univ. Press.

ESMAN, A. H. (1985). Neglected classics. *Psychoanal. Q.*, 54:66–69.

FENICHEL, O. (1941). *Problems of Psychoanalytic Technique*. New York: Psychoanalytic Quarterly.

_____ (1945). *The Psychoanalytic Theory of Neurosis*. New York: Norton.

FREUD, A. (1936). The ego and the mechanisms of defense. *W.*, 2.

FREUD, S. (1900). The interpretation of dreams. *S.E.*, 4 & 5.

_____ (1901). The psychopathology of everyday life. *S.E.*, 6.

_____ (1905). Three essays on the theory of sexuality. *S.E.*, 7:125–243.

_____ (1911). Formulations on the two principles of mental functioning. *S.E.*, 12:213–226.

_____ (1916–17). Introductory lectures on psycho-analysis. *S.E.*, 15 & 16.

_____ (1923). The ego and the id. *S.E.*, 19:3–66.

_____ (1926). Inhibitions, symptoms, and anxiety. *S.E.*, 20:77–175.

_____ (1927). The future of an illusion. *S.E.*, 21:3–56.

_____ (1933). New introductory lectures on psycho-analysis. *S.E.*, 22:3–182.

_____ (1940). An outline of psycho-analysis. *S.E.*, 23:141–207.

GEDO, J. E. (1979). *Beyond Interpretation.* New York: Int. Univ. Press.

GILL, M. M. (1963). *Topography and Systems in Psychoanalytic Theory*. Psychol. Issues, Monogr. 10. New York: Int. Univ. Press.

_____ (1973). Introduction to George Klein's "Two theories or one?" *Bull. Menninger Clin.*, 37:99–101.

GLOVER, E. (1949). *Psychoanalysis*, 2nd ed. London: Staples Press.

GRAY, P. (1982). "Developmental lag" in the evolution of technique for psychoanalysis of neurotic conflict. *J. Amer. Psychoanal. Assn.*, 30:621–655.

HANLY, C. (1979). *Existentialism and Psychoanalysis*. New York: Int. Univ. Press.

HARRISON, I. B. (1984). Function pleasure and Freudian theory. Unpublished manuscript.

HARTMANN, H. (1939). *Ego Psychology and the Problem of Adaptation*. New York: Int. Univ. Press, 1958.

_____ (1947). On rational and irrational action. In *Essays on Ego Psychology*, pp. 37–68. New York: Int. Univ. Press, 1964.

_____ (1950). Comments on the psychoanalytic theory of the ego. Ibid., pp. 113–141.

_____ (1956a). Notes on the reality principle. Ibid., pp. 241–267.

_____ (1956b). The development of the ego concept in Freud's work. Ibid., pp. 268–296.

_____ (1958). Comments on the scientific aspects of psychoanalysis. Ibid., pp. 297–317.

_____ (1959). Psychoanalysis as a scientific theory. Ibid., pp. 318–350.

HEISENBERG, W. (1958). *Physics and Philosophy*. New York: Harper.

HENDRICK, I. (1942). Instinct and the ego during infancy. *Psychoanal. Q.*, 11:33–58.

Hospers, J. (1950). Free will and psychoanalysis. In *The Problem of Free Will*, ed. W. F. Enteman, pp. 195–215. New York: Scribner's, 1967.

Isakower, O. (1938). A contribution to the pathopsychology of phenomena associated with falling asleep. *Int. J. Psychoanal.*, 19:331–345.

James, W. (1897). The dilemma of determinism. In *The Will to Believe*, pp. 145–183. New York: Longmans, Green.

Jones, E. (1924). Free will and determinism. In *Essays in Applied Psychoanalysis*, 2:178–189. London: Hogarth Press, 1951.

Klein, G. S. (1970). *Perception, Motives, and Personality*. New York: Knopf.

—— (1973). Two theories or one? *Bull. Menninger Clin.*, 37:102–132.

—— (1976). *Psychoanalytic Theory*. New York: Int. Univ. Press.

Knight, R. P. (1946). Determinism, "freedom," and psychotherapy. *Psychiatry*, 9:251–262.

Kohut, H. (1971). *The Analysis of the Self*. New York: Int. Univ. Press.

—— (1977). *The Restoration of the Self*. New York: Int. Univ. Press.

Kris, A. O. (1977). Either-or dilemmas. *Psychoanal. Study Child*, 32:91–117.

—— (1982). *Free Association*. New Haven: Yale Univ. Press.

—— (1984). The conflicts of ambivalence. *Psychoanal. Study Child*, 39:213–234.

—— (1985). Resistance in convergent and in divergent conflicts. *Psychoanal. Q.*, 54:537–568.

Kris, E. (1947). The nature of psychoanalytic propositions and their validation. In *Selected Papers of Ernst Kris*, pp. 3–23. New Haven: Yale Univ. Press, 1975.

Leites, N. (1971). *The New Ego*. New York: Science House.

Lewy, E. (1961). Responsibility, free will, and ego psychology. *Int. J. Psychoanal.*, 42:260–270.

Mahler, M. S. (1972). Rapprochement subphase of the separation-individuation process. *Psychoanal. Q.*, 41:487–506.

—— & Furer, M. (1968). *On Human Symbiosis and the Vicissitudes of Individuation*. New York: Int. Univ. Press.

—— & McDevitt, J. B. (1982). Thoughts on emergence of the sense of self, with particular emphasis on the body self. *J. Amer. Psychoanal. Assn.*, 30:827–849.

—— Pine, F., & Bergman, A. (1975). *The Psychological Birth of the Human Infant*. New York: Basic Books.

Menninger, K. (1942). *The Human Mind*. New York: Knopf.

Nunberg, H. (1926). The will to recovery. In *Practice and Theory of Psychoanalysis*, 1:75–88. New York: Int. Univ. Press, 1948.

Rangell, L. (1955). On the psychoanalytic theory of anxiety. *J. Amer. Psychoanal. Assn.*, 3:389–414.

—— (1959). The nature of conversion. *J. Amer. Psychoanal. Assn.*, 7:632–662.

—— (1963a). The scope of intrapsychic conflict. *Psychoanal. Study Child*, 18:75–102.

—— (1963b). Structural problems in intrapsychic conflict. *Psychoanal. Study Child*, 18:103–138.

———— (1965). The scope of Heinz Hartmann. *Int. J. Psychoanal.*, 46:5–30.

———— (1968). A further attempt to resolve the "problem of anxiety." *J. Amer. Psychoanal. Assn.*, 16:371–404.

———— (1969a). The intrapsychic process and its analysis. *Int. J. Psychoanal.*, 50:65–77.

———— (1969b). Choice-conflict and the decision-making function of the ego. *Int. J. Psychoanal.*, 50:599–602.

———— (1971a). The decision-making process. *Psychoanal. Study Child*, 26:425–452.

———— (1971b). Obituary, Dr. Heinz Hartmann. *Int. J. Psychoanal.*, 51:567.

———— (1974). A psychoanalytic perspective leading currently to the syndrome of the compromise of integrity. *Int. J. Psychoanal.*, 55:3–12.

———— (1976). Lessons from Watergate. *Psychoanal. Q.*, 45:37–61.

———— (1980). *The Mind of Watergate*. New York: Norton.

———— (1982a). The self in psychoanalytic theory. *J. Amer. Psychoanal. Assn.*, 30:863–891.

———— (1982b). Transference to theory. *Annu. Psychoanal.*, 10:29–56.

RAPAPORT, D. (1950). On the psychoanalytic theory of thinking. *Int. J. Psychoanal.*, 31:161–170.

———— (1951a). The autonomy of the ego. *Bull. Menninger Clin.*, 15:113–123.

———— (1951b). *Organization and Pathology of Thought*. New York: Columbia Univ. Press.

———— (1953a). On the psychoanalytic theory of affects. *Int. J. Psychoanal.*, 34:177–198.

———— (1953b). Some metapsychological considerations concerning activity and passivity. In *The Collected Papers of David Rapaport*, ed. M. M. Gill, pp. 530–568. New York: Basic Books, 1967.

———— (1958). The theory of ego autonomy. *Bull. Menninger Clin.*, 22:13–35.

———— (1959). *The Structure of Psychoanalytic Theory*. Psychol. Issues, monogr. 6. New York: Int. Univ. Press, 1960.

———— & GILL, M. M. (1959). The points of view and assumptions of metapsychology. *Int. J. Psychoanal.*, 40:153–162.

ROSEN, V. H. (1960). Some aspects of the role of imagination in the analytic process. *J. Amer. Psychoanal. Assn.*, 8:229–251.

RYLE, G. (1949). *The Concept of Mind*. New York: Barnes & Noble.

SANDLER, J. & FREUD, A. (1983). Discussion in the Hampstead Index of *The Ego and the Mechanisms of Defense. J. Amer. Psychoanal. Assn. Suppl.*, 31:19–146.

SCHAFER, R. (1976). *A New Language for Psychoanalysis*. New Haven: Yale Univ. Press.

———— (1978). *Language and Insight*. New Haven: Yale Univ. Press.

SCHUR, M. (1953). The ego in anxiety. In *Drives, Affects, Behavior*, ed. R. M. Loewenstein, pp. 67–103. New York: Int. Univ. Press.

SCHWARTZ, W. (1984). The two concepts of action and responsibility in psychoanalysis. *J. Amer. Psychoanal. Assn.*, 32:557–572.

WAELDER, R. (1930). The principle of multiple function. In *Psychoanalysis*, ed. S. A. Guttman, pp. 68–83. New York: Int. Univ. Press, 1976.

——— (1934). The problem of freedom in psychoanalysis and the problem of reality testing. Ibid., pp. 101–120.

——— (1960). *Basic Theory of Psychoanalysis.* New York: Int. Univ. Press.

——— (1967). *Progress and Revolution.* New York: Int. Univ. Press.

WALLACE, E. R. (1985a). *Historiography and Causation in Psychoanalysis.* Hillsdale, N.J.: Analytic Press.

——— (1985b). Determinism, possibility, and ethics. *Psychoanal. Q.,* in press.

WEISS, J. & SAMPSON, H. (1982). Miniseries, Postgraduate Education Committee, San Francisco Psychoanalytic Institute. Unpublished manuscript.

WINNICOTT, D. W. (1958). *Collected Papers.* London: Tavistock.

WOOD, L. (1941). The free-will controversy. In *The Problem of Free Will,* ed. W. F. Enteman, pp. 32–46. New York: Scribner's, 1967.

PSYCHOANALYTIC THEORY

Disposition and the Environment

SAMUEL ABRAMS, M.D.

IN THE 1960S, AN ADOPTION AGENCY FOUND ITSELF INVOLVED WITH the placement of several sets of identical twins and, guided by a variety of influences, chose to separate the members of each set. Of the guiding influences, clinical considerations were central. The prevailing scientific literature of the time had been discovering features about twins that were bound to attract the attention of any serious practitioner in the mental health field. Those features included the following: (1) the parenting of twins was burdensome, so that care giving was often compromised; (2) the children invariably faced specific developmental hazards that appeared directly attributable to the twinship; and (3) they also appeared more vulnerable to a wide variety of pathological disturbances (see, e.g., Karpman, 1951; Burlingham, 1952; Gardner and Rexford, 1952; Demarest and Winestein, 1955; and Panel, 1961). Once the placements were made, for ethical reasons, the agency could tell neither the adoptive parents nor the children of the existence of a twin, lest that knowledge impair the family-child bonding that was expected to evolve and is recognized as so necessary for growth and development.

It soon became clear that an extraordinary research opportunity had presented itself, the study of identical twins reared apart in *prospect*. For the first time—and as far as anyone knew this really was the *first* time—it would be possible to follow sys-

Clinical professor, The Psychoanalytic Institute, New York University Medical Center.

Presented in a somewhat modified form as "The Victor Calef M.D. Memorial Lecture," San Francisco, Sept. 29, 1985.

Derived from a study (Christa Balzert, Ph.D., project director) supported by the Philip and Lynn Straus Philanthropic Fund and the Tappanz Foundation, Inc.

tematically children with shared biological heritages as they
grew up in different households. Among other things, the study
promised to cast a brighter light upon the nature-nurture issue:
how much is owed to disposition and how much to the
environment?

To be sure, that issue had been joined in prior studies of
separated twins. But such studies had been *retrospective* ones; the
twins who were investigated were not examined until their adult
years. The examination generally included several interviews, a
few standardized tests, and the recording of physiological data.
The findings were often used to appraise the weight of nature
and nurture by comparing outcomes in terms of health and
disease. As for developmental features, the records of the child
rearing each had received were accessible only through recall;
consequently, they were clouded by the usual limitations of retrospective falsification and reorganization. Because of this,
questions remained about the reliability of the resultant hypotheses, especially as they concerned *developmental* questions. Furthermore, in many instances, the separation of the twins had
occurred late in childhood after they had been involved with one
another for some time and had shared a common milieu. This
blurred the boundaries of nature and nurture even further. (For
an extensive review see Farber, 1981). A *prospective* study of twins
separated early in infancy and carefully followed with a multi-
disciplined approach as they grew up in different households
was seen as overcoming many of the methodological limitations
of the earlier investigations.

A research team headed by Peter B. Neubauer was put together. It brought to the uniqueness of the circumstances a systematic attention to detail within a clinical, psychoanalytic, and
developmental framework. An extraordinary quantity of data
soon followed: direct observations, films, psychological tests,
parent interviews, sibling interviews, school reports, child interviews, integrated discussions, impressions, hypotheses, findings—all captured in the minutes of almost a thousand weekly
conferences.

It would be difficult to convey adequately the feelings generated in those conferences. Frequently dominated by excitement,
they were often invaded by disbelief, occasionally by wonder.

There were even moments of distress when some long-cherished views about human development suddenly seemed quite vulnerable. The findings yielded fresh ideas. I will describe the first 10 years of the lives of one of the sets, Amy and Beth,[1] to demonstrate the excitement and to illustrate at least one new discovery. I will outline the detailed appraisals of their disposition, the parenting each received, what their siblings were like, the different family values they were offered, and the special circumstances they encountered. I then will delineate how each child turned out at age 10 and how we attempted to solve the puzzle of the unexpected outcome.

AMY

Amy was the first of this pair of twins born after a 39-week gestation. The labor and delivery were unremarkable. She weighed 6 pounds, 12 ounces and was 19½ inches long.

Initially, she was viewed as a well-formed, fair-skinned, somewhat small and slender infant, with dark blond hair and blue-grey eyes, a small oval face, and a slight snub nose. At 6 weeks, she was sent to a "good" foster home with her twin. Her head was still a bit "floppy" when she arrived and it was felt she needed careful handling. The foster mother, a former nurse, was known to be warm, engaging, sensitive, and intelligent, and unusually capable of tendering physical care to infants. She was often observed talking to Amy and she kissed her frequently. She reported these impressions: Amy "did not relate as closely as some babies"; she had difficulty getting herself comfortable when handled; she required several formula changes before she began eating heartily; she was prone to vigorous mouth movements; she readily averted her eyes from light and, by 3 months, she still was not focusing them quite appropriately. Three features, expressions of dispositional leanings, were catalogued by the research team: a tendency toward inner-directedness, a shortcoming in engaging persons and things, and some limitation in her integrative capacities.

1. Barbara Abrams was primarily responsible for the organization of the data on this set of twins.

When she was 3 months, 26 days, Amy was adopted by a family of modest means; her twin had been adopted 5 weeks earlier. The family consisted of a mother, a father, and a biological son, who was 6½ years old when Amy was brought home. All three were described as warm, engaging, and eager to receive the child. By the end of the first year it appeared as if she was fully accepted and a source of pleasure especially to her mother and older brother. She was motorically active, not particularly responsive to outside stimuli, a placid child who imposed herself minimally upon the environment. Her affective tone tended to be negative, and from time to time she was described as tense or anxious.

In her second year, more clearly defined problems surfaced and one difficulty or another was to be reported regularly thereafter. The mother-daughter relationship became increasingly problematic in spite of what could only be described as a sincere attempt on the mother's part to be responsive. Amy was clingy and demanding. She always needed someone around. Eating problems, nail biting, thumb sucking, and the use of a blanket for tension relief all began in earnest during the second year and stayed with her throughout the period of formal study. She was bowel-trained easily at the age of 24 months. Nighttime bed-wetting continued until her fourth year. There were occasional daytime urinary accidents from her fourth to sixth year. Everyone noticed that she required lots of sleep. Amy's mother began to look upon her as "different" from the other members in the family, citing poor eating habits and lack of diligence. Amy's father thought she was stubborn; and he reacted with distress to her being such a puzzle to her mother. Between the ages of 3 and 6 things improved between the father and daughter, but by the seventh year it worsened again and he occasionally referred to her, somewhat playfully, as his "little witch."

In her fourth or fifth year, it was reported that she was definitely right-handed.

Nightmares appeared in Amy's fourth year and continued through the eighth. She also expressed discrete fears, e.g., the dark, loose dogs, bumblebees. When she was 8 she refused to go to the back of the house by herself and by the time she was 10 she had hypochondriacal tendencies. She was prone to imitating and role play; this gave her a kind of artificial quality. These features, along with a strangely discoordinate quality to her figure drawings and moments of real gender confusion, led to the impression of poor self-integration.

Outside the family, Amy's relationships did not fare much better. She was shy and uninitiating with children. She was an indifferent student during her school years. She was inclined toward "figurative" learning, manifesting itself as literalness, minimal interest in the novel, and limited creativity. She had a disturbance of thinking noted clinically and in tests. She developed a fairly serious learning disorder. By her tenth year, toward the end of the period of formal study, it was recognized that she was a child who was not appropriately involved with the tasks of latency. Judged by the usual criteria, i.e., peer relationships, reduced symptoms and conflicts, the capacity to give up earlier positions, self-integration, the availability for expansion, and more complex adaptive proclivities, she was found seriously wanting.

AMY'S FAMILY

Amy's family, the nurture side of the equation, was studied with equivalent attention to detail.

Amy's mother was amiable and gracious but somewhat socially awkward, matronly, and in a continuing struggle with her weight. She was affectively low-keyed, even a bit phlegmatic, and not sharply defined. She regarded herself as poorly educated and she felt unattractive. She seemed fair-minded, loyal, compassionate, and, despite occasional periods of tension in her marriage, respectful and warm toward her husband. However, she frequently expressed concern about her own ability to mother, especially where Amy was concerned. She was viewed as a bit "clingy" herself so that she was not disposed to encourage separateness easily. In addition, she was intolerant of expressions of hostility or negativism and often called Amy "stubborn" when she simply disagreed with her. She was an ineffectual disciplinarian. Sexuality may have been troublesome for her. For example, she withheld Barbie dolls from Amy because she felt such dolls encouraged sexual feelings. She found Amy's attrac-

tiveness appealing but she openly expressed disappointment
about her poor schoolwork. At least in her words and phrases,
she frequently set Amy apart from the other members of the
family. Judging her competence during different phases of development, the research team felt this about Amy's mother: she
had adequately accepted the caretaking role in the first year or
so, had been unable to reinforce Amy's emerging sense of herself because she exaggerated the differences between them so
much, was intimidated by Amy's aggressive and budding sexual
feelings at ages 4 through 7, and did well in actively urging peer
involvement in the later years, although the urging proved relatively ineffective. There was little doubt about her desire to be
helpful and the sincerity of her feelings.

Amy's father invariably gave the picture of competence—in
his work, in social contacts, and within the family setting. Although he earned only a modest income, he thrived in his role as
the provider in the family and was the most compelling figure in
the household. Relaxed and comfortable most of the time, he
was somewhat committed to the view that serenity could best be
achieved by avoiding confrontations with feelings. As a result he
often appeared ingenuous or even secretive. His own past had
been dominated by a troublesome relationship with his mother
and a period in his childhood when he was viewed as a ne'er-do-
well. As a husband he was supportive of his wife. Some discord
between them surfaced in the last years of the study. His relationship to Amy varied. He was remote in the early period,
became warmer and more attentive when she was between the
ages of 3 and 6, often encouraging her to cuddle in bed with him
as the two watched TV together, and resentful and teasingly
disparaging thereafter. Judging his competence at fathering
over different developmental periods, the study group felt that
he was adequately available to mitigate some of the early mother-
daughter discord, was sufficiently warm and affectionate albeit
at times perhaps a bit overly stimulating, but eventually unable
to resist accepting the view of Amy as a disappointment, "different," and an important source of family discord.

Amy's brother was tall, thin, handsome, of pleasant mood,
academically successful, and openly affectionate. When comparisons were made between Amy and her brother, she failed in

every area with the possible exception of looks. Despite the openness of such comparisons, Amy seemed unresentful. Her brother was warmly responsive to her from the time she arrived and expressed almost a paternalistic pride during her growth. He would often playfully "roughhouse" with her, although mother disapproved because she saw overtones of sexuality in the behavior. When her brother entered his teen-age years and became less involved with her, Amy was noticeably chagrined.

In short, the family as a unit was intact, in stable equilibrium with the societal surround. It featured a surface tranquillity eroded by mother-daughter discord, latent marital problems, and reluctant—albeit emphatic—reports of distress. It was once characterized by some members of the research team as a well-knit threesome—mother, father, and son—and a less involved, alienated Amy. Values included academic success, low-keyedness, the containment of feelings, tradition, and simplicity.

In spite of the observations of problems, discord, and distress, some members of the research team felt that the family had provided more or less "average expectable" conditions for growth. They held that it should have been possible for an adequately equipped child to develop properly within such a setting. Others were more impressed with what they viewed as potential pathogenic features in the surround, at least when viewed from the psychological perspective of the developing child. They offered a different set of hypotheses for Amy's disorder. One proposal: an unfortunate mother-daughter match had left Amy's affective contact blunted. Another: the separation-individuation phases had been poorly negotiated partly because of mother's difficulty with hostility and negativistic behavior, partly because she seemed unempathic to Amy's need for closeness. A third: unconscious jealousy may have impacted upon the oedipal period. It seemed to them a misfortune of fate that Amy's brother was so able and she so intellectually limited. It was also seen as regrettable that educational achievement happened to be such a high family value. The members of the research team who structured the data in this fashion surmised that it was possible to look upon Amy's disordered latency as caused predominantly by deficiencies in nurture. The poor environmental setting had made separation-individuation unnegotiable and the oedipus complex unsolvable. They hypothesized that if Amy had only had a mother who was more tolerant of her limitations, less overcome with her difficulties, and more openly forthcoming, how much better life would have been for her. If her father had only been more consistently available and affectionate and her mother less rivalrous, then perhaps the oedipus complex might have had a chance. If her brother had set lower standards of achievement, she would have been spared the mortification implicit in the inevitable comparisons—or, at least, if the family had only valued academic achievement less.

BETH

Beth was the second of this pair of twins born after a 39-week gestation. Again, the labor and delivery were unremarkable. She weighed 6 pounds, 9 ounces and was 19 inches long. (Amy's weight and height advantage over Beth never changed throughout the first 10 years of the study.)

Initially, Beth was described in terms identical to those used for Amy: well formed, fair skinned, somewhat small and slender, with dark blond hair and blue-grey eyes, a small oval face, and a slight snub nose. At the age of 6 weeks, she was sent to the same "good" foster home as her twin, but stayed a much shorter time. The sensitive foster mother noted that Beth, like Amy, had some "floppiness" to her head when she first came, had trouble focusing, "did not relate as closely as some babies," had digestive difficulties in general and with solid foods in particular, needed "careful handling," averted her eyes from the light excessively, and regularly engaged in vigorous mouth movements. The same three features observed in Amy were catalogued as dispositional leanings in Beth: inner-directedness, problems in effectively engaging persons and things—although she was somewhat more involved with persons than was Amy, and a limitation in integrative capacities.

When she was 2 months, 18 days, Beth was adopted by an upper middle-class family. The parents had adopted two other children before, a boy who was 7 years older and a girl who was 3 years older. The mother was eagerly looking forward to the new baby, hoping that Beth would provide some respite from the many problems she was having with her son; in fact, Beth was promptly christened "the fun child." From the start and right on through the 10 years her mother viewed her in these ways: she was wonderfully easy to care for; she was interested in all people, not just those she was familiar with; she cried rarely; she did not impose herself upon others; she made few demands; she was relatively unassertive; and she maintained a positive mood most of the time.

Toward the end of her first year—just about the same time similar observations were being made with Amy—eating problems surfaced along with nail biting, thumb sucking, and the use of a blanket for tension relief. The eating problems faded in her fourth year, but the remaining symptoms persisted thereafter. Like her twin, she was bowel-trained easily and at the same age, 24 months; nocturnal bed-wetting persisted for some years more than for Amy, until age 9. Beth, too, required long periods of sleep, especially in the earlier years. She soon developed an important relationship with her mother, which the latter described as close rather than clingy. She could also be alone for what her mother assumed to be fantastic periods of time. Such reports of her ability to play by herself and greater peer relationships contrasted somewhat with Amy's behavior. Despite mother's frequent comments about Beth's independence, the closeness between the two of them did not wane until Beth's tenth year. Beth also developed what was called a "special tie" to her brother during her second year and became "daddy's girl" at about the same time; her relationship to the two of them was maintained evenly thereafter. Her behavior with her sister was also described as positive, at least by her mother.

She became left-handed.

By the time she was 4, Beth was suffering from diffuse hypochondriacal concerns and a fear of the dark. When she was 7 several specific anxieties such as fear of death or of being left alone crystallized. Difficulties in integration abounded. Beth was also prone to imitating and role playing a good deal; this left her with a certain artificial quality somewhat more marked than Amy's. She was seen as a "performer" who tried on feelings rather than being able to experience them directly. She was surprisingly uninvolved with the high levels of tension that erupted about the house at times, especially those evoked by her brother's wayward behavior. She did poorly in school, being viewed as unmotivated and somewhat of a daydreamer. She, like Amy, was inclined toward figurative learning. She was assessed as having a thinking disturbance noted clinically and confirmed in psychological tests. She also had specific difficulties in reading and math. By her ninth year, it was evident that she, too, was a child who was insufficiently involved with the tasks of latency. While her peer relationships were broad, they were also quite shallow, and an excessive closeness to mother periodically reappeared. Was it, like Amy's, clinginess after all? A host of symptoms and a predilection for immaturity persisted; furthermore, she too was found seriously wanting in the areas of self-integration, readiness for expansion, and adaptive proclivities. Her overall mood seemed somewhat more positive than Amy's; however, on psychological tests she voiced an abiding feeling of sadness and a longing for maternal care in terms almost identical to those expressed by her twin.

BETH'S FAMILY

Beth's mother was described as pleasant, youthful, chic, slim, poised, and self-confident, occasionally forcefully cheerful and dynamic. She defined herself primarily in terms of traditional female roles but participated in a variety of activities outside of the home and enjoyed a broad social life. She was clearly the dominant parent in the home. She ignored unpleasantries. When her son's problems were at their worst, she would speak of his good nature and fine intellect. She blurred the differences between herself and Beth. For example, she dyed her own hair the same color as Beth's to accentuate the similarity between them. She consistently exaggerated Beth's positive features and ignored her shortcomings. Viewing her competence as a mother in different phases of her daughter's development, the research team saw her as adequately accepting the early caretaking role, insufficiently able to reinforce Beth's emerging sense of herself because of her tendency to blunt differences between them, and helpfully leading her to peer relationships by acting as an effective role model for social interaction.

Beth's father, like Amy's, saw himself as the family provider.

He was a competent worker and enjoyed financial success. Like Amy's father, he was not the preferred parent for the child, but he was more emotionally available for Beth, more involved with her, and more even in his temperament. Like his wife, he was prone to deny problems; for example, he was an apologist for Beth's difficulties at school, accounting for her learning disorder as an indication of her independence. He seemed to be a private person, although he never quite gave the impression of secretiveness like Amy's father. The marital relationship was secure. Judging Beth's father over different developmental periods, the study team concluded that it was regrettable that he had been unable to add a necessary note of reality to his wife's tendency to ignore distressing features and that the indiscriminate evenness of his response to Beth over time was not useful.

Beth's older brother was a source of family grief. At first he simply had memory and learning problems, but as the years went on he became more psychologically troubled, was expelled from several schools, and eventually came into direct conflict with the law. His relationship to Beth was characterized by a certain paternal pride and in a pleasure in physical play with her, especially when she was younger. His attentiveness to her was in sharp contrast to his behavior with his other sister, with whom he was in constant rivalry. That sister was a rather inhibited but capable girl who was prematurely thrust into an adult role by her mother. Oddly enough, there were few observations or reports of her relationship to Beth.

The family as a unit was characterized as having a high activity level; at times the word "frenetic" would not have been inappropriate. They harmonized well with the surrounding societal requirements. The parents were compatible in their views and complemented each other's judgments. The home was *au courant* and attractive; materialism was clearly a value, and education was not especially promoted. Disagreeable feelings were put aside and pleasantries, even artificial ones, were emphasized.

Some members of the research team were also prepared to view this family as "average expectable"; they noted that there had been no major mishandling, no truly traumatizing disruptions in the form of catastrophic illness or circumstances. It should have been possible, these observers maintained, for Beth to find sufficient nutrients for normal growth in this household, providing her inherent equipment was adequate. Others saw the family as something less than average expectable. For them, hypotheses about Beth's difficulties were readily couched in terms of object relationships, separation-individuation, and unconscious conflicts. One theory: her mother's inability to engage differences and recognize limitations interfered with differentiation and burdened the separation-individuation process; self-definition and affective mobilization were blunted as a consequence. Another: the oedipus complex could find no kernel of genuine rivalry or opposition about which to crystallize; being "daddy's girl" at 2 never evolved into an organized triad of affective intensity. Another: father's inability to intervene psychologically between the poorly differentiated mother-daughter interaction was unfortunate as far as Beth's development was concerned. His view that his daughter's poor schoolwork merely showed her independence probably interfered with her ambition and only further solidified her poor performance. As for Beth's siblings, there were speculations about unconscious resentments arising from each one, for different reasons. Furthermore, it could hardly have been beneficial for Beth to have had such a disturbed boy as an admired older brother. These theories all implied something of the following: if mother had only been more confrontative, more aware of Beth's difficulties, had made more demands upon her; if only she had concentrated on some of the differences between them instead of exaggerating the similarities—how different her development would have been. If father had only been a bit more reactive in his feelings, even a bit stimulating with Beth, and not so undifferentiatedly tuned into the alleged tranquillity of the household, how helpful that would have been for separation-individuation and the oedipal period. If Beth's brother had only set higher standards for her to emulate, how much more studious she might have become.

AMY AND BETH: A COMPARISON

Amy and Beth are children with serious disorders. Furthermore, the two are *equivalently* pathological: they share a limited development; they share a timetable of emergence, an excess of expression, and a channelization of symptoms; they share character disturbances; they share a quality of shallowness and a limited self-definition; they are poorly integrated; they share comparable cognitive deficiencies. To be sure there are differences: Beth is somewhat more involved with persons, happier, and a bit less confused. However, she is also more artificial and less connected to her feelings.

If Amy and Beth had been just any two children and not identical twins, many clinicians and researchers would have readily linked their disorders to deficiencies in the environment. They might even have speculated along these lines: if Beth had only had the dominant features of Amy's family—the confrontative mother, the strong father, the successful brother, the value of academic achievement—or if Amy had only had the dominant features of Beth's family—the overly accepting mother, the evenly attentive father, the less successful brother, the lack of concern about education—how much better each would have fared! Speculative theories linking environmental stimuli with pathological outcomes have been cultivated in decades of research efforts and validated in countless therapeutic settings over time. Such proposals underscore the contribution of object relationships, the family, and the social milieu to outcome. And for good reason. The environment is a critical factor in growth and development. It impacts in a variety of ways on virtually all areas. Clinicians and researchers are understandably prone to focus upon the influence of nurture in prospect and in retrospect. The surround has powerful influences. Before turning from the environment, it seemed wise to review those influences.

The Environment: A Metapsychological Survey

The environment is comprised of the stimuli in the surround; this is an *economic* view of the environment. Some of the stimuli originate from random sources and only secondarily are placed into structures and meanings; this is particularly true of stimuli that arise from inanimate objects—so important for the development of imagination and cognition, but it also holds for much of the stimuli from animate, human, or societal sources. Other stimuli originate within more structured offerings and are designed to convey specific meanings. This is a *structural* view of the environment.

The interaction between stimuli derived from the environment and the perceiving and organizing components of the mind of the growing child creates products, necessary nutrients for development. (Essential products for development also result from the interaction between the mind and stimuli arising from somatic sources on the one hand and from within the mind itself on the other.) For development to proceed, the environmental stimuli and the perceptual and organizational capacities of the mind must fall within certain limits. This is a *developmental, genetic* (i.e., *historical*), and *economic* view of the environment.

The environment is also the organized setting within which the tools of adaptation are deployed in the service of survival. This view entails certain assumptions about the optimal nature of a social organization at different stages of development and in adulthood; and of features that facilitate and features that inhibit the emergence of an expectable repertoire for existence. This is the *adaptive* view of the environment.

The environment also contains the people and events that are acted upon in a *dynamic* sense. The resultant representations are characteristically drawn into the inevitable conflicts that arise in the course of growth. The conflicts and the strategies designed to deal with the conflicts leave their residue in the tendency to organize the residual random and proposed environmental stimuli into a recurrently perceived selective "reality."[2] For many persons, the environment becomes restricted to just such a construction of the outside world, i.e., a continuous expression of unconscious conflict. And, regrettably, what is misrepresented often proves more calamitous than what is unknown.

The environment, in sum, is a codeterminant of nutrients that yield products for development. It is a setting for adaptation, imparting a facilitating or encumbering influence. It is a codeterminant of conflict formation and resolution. And it is an

2. For a comprehensive review of the history of "reality" in psychoanalysis, see Wallerstein (1983).

existence that goes beyond all of these components, both a random and organized wonder of stimuli.

With the environment impacting so broadly and in so many ways, it is no wonder that disposition is frequently neglected when explanations to account for clinical disorders are proposed. There is either the feeling that endowment, in comparison to the readily observable outside circumstances, is probably a negligible factor or that very little can be done about it anyway. For those members of the research team who were prepared to assign the source of Amy's and Beth's difficulties to nurture, the view of the families as so very different precipitated a dilemma. If children share a common biological heritage and the surround is so important for development, one would imagine that substantive differences in the environment would inevitably yield substantive differences in outcome. But Amy and Beth turned out to be remarkably similar at every step in the study and at the end of the formal period of study as well. Their differences were merely stylistic, not substantive, or they were accountable on the basis of other factors such as congenital influences. The hypothesis was proposed that an inherent component was at work, one that arose early and exerted a continuing effect upon development as growth went on. For those who had insisted that the families had provided very different stimuli, the hypothesis was particularly felicitous because it could account for the similiarities in the face of such different nutrients. For those who had seen the families as average expectable all along, the hypothesis offered the promise of defining the faulty equipment with greater specificity. But what could it be in disposition that so readily overrides environmental offerings at virtually every step in the developmental sequence, that produces such a thoroughgoing abnegation of either an average-expectable milieu or one filled with opportunities or impediments? And how does our theory of normal development permit us to understand such a pathological formation?

NORMAL DEVELOPMENT

Normal development proceeds in an expectable sequence of progressive hierarchical organizations in accord with a biological blueprint and driven by an inherent impetus. The sequence of organizations provides progressive complexity, differentiation, and integration, assuring that there will be the necessary transition from more concrete responses to the environmental stimuli to responses that increasingly take on more abstract meanings. Anna Freud's (1965) developmental lines rest upon this conceptual framework. For example, it is the underlying, evolving, developmental organizations that permit children progressively to redefine what is good and what is bad as they grow older. Initially, for infants, "good" is the concrete experience of pleasure or relief from pain; it becomes the feeling of power, then the idea of "maleness," and finally the moral precept, what is "right." "Bad" is pain, then it is helplessness, then "female" when a child attributes a distorted meaning to the perceived anatomical differences between boys and girls, and finally the "bad" becomes the concept of what is "wrong" in its budding ethical sense. These steps, expressions of emerging developmental organizations, may also be looked upon as an illustration of the gradual shift in the determinants of behavior, a shift from more concrete physical causes to more abstract psychological meanings.

This description of discrete steps implies sharp demarcations in the underlying, evolving, developmental organizations. However, in nature, the impetus and blueprint rarely yield such sharply defined products. Several variations within the range of normal are known: in addition to relatively sharp demarcations, the organizations may interweave, overlap, or coexist; they may show greater or lesser fluidity in the progressive-regressive balance, or they may be more fixed; there may be a precocity or a retardation in the pace (Flapan and Neubauer, 1975; Neubauer, 1980). Whatever the variations, however, with further growth a normal child continues to attribute more sophisticated meanings to the stimuli in the surround. These meanings are both useful for adaptation and necessary for further progressive differentiation. Similarly, as new developmental organizations emerge, the persons in the environment are apt to clothe the proposed stimuli in specific meanings, partially as a reflection of who they are, partly in response to the child's newly advancing positions and individual characteristics. The readiness of the child to make use of such dressed-up meanings in a facilitating or injurious way rests to a considerable degree on the inherent competence of the underlying process that guides the emerging phases. That process, fashioned by its inherent impetus and blueprint, is central to the inevitable progressive recycling of meanings.

We know of a few pathological outcomes attributable to a breach in this process. There is one developmental deviation that is caused by a disharmony between one aspect of mental development and another, the ego and the instincts, for example. A more moderate degree of such a disharmony in which ego outstrips id is known to be one predisposing factor for obsessional neuroses. The so-called neuroses, however, are not disorders of the developmental process, although disorders dominated by neurotic mechanisms can cause varying degrees of inhibited development. Neuroses arise when certain constellations of drive and ego become entrapped in earlier developmental organizations because of conflict and therefore cannot participate in the transformations of structures and functions as new hierarchies emerge.

A NEW DISORDER

Amy's and Beth's disorders are not caused by a disharmony and they certainly were not a neurosis. They appear to share *an impairment in the inherent impetus*,[3] the pull forward that ordinarily permits the blueprint of development to become actualized by the stimuli afforded in the environmental context. As a consequence of the impairment, the entire developmental sequence of emerging phases and recycled meanings is disrupted. The resultant organizations lack structural integrity. The children are left with diffuse impediments to integration, they remain tilted toward the concrete, they fail adequately to transform stimuli into expectable meanings, they struggle to adapt with earlier modes of relating, their symptoms are more expressions of a mind struggling to sustain some stability rather

3. Peter B. Neubauer was the first to call attention to the disorder and to recognize it as a circumscribed entity.

than one engaged in unconscious conflicts. It is a serious disorder, a kind that seems unlikely to be undone even by the "second chance" of adolescence. While, in this case, the evidence points to the disturbance as arising from defects in the native equipment, it is possible that the disorder may also be promoted by extreme situational factors. We recognized that it was possible to propose other hypotheses to account for our observations, but none of them were as parsimonious or as consistent with the bulk of our findings and with other generally recognized principles of development.

DISPOSITION: THE DEVELOPMENTAL PROCESS

As often occurs in research, a disabling disorder can clarify normal variations and less disruptive pathological entities. Amy's and Beth's disturbance underscores the concept of the developmental process, the progressive sequence of hierarchical organizations with its inherent impetus and blueprint. Clinicians are schooled to attend to the drives, the ego, the object relationships, the self, familial and social settings, and potential traumas. Such attention is entirely appropriate; it permits an understanding of conflicts within and between systems and of the ways in which relationships and circumstances facilitate and inhibit growth. These are valuable categories to engage a wide variety of clinical disorders. However, this aspect of the twin study demonstrates that it is also valuable to add the dispositional perspective of the maturational basis for *developmental organizations* to the list. Such a perspective is useful for appraising the shapes that behavior takes, degrees of structural coherence, the stability of sequence, and other clinically relevant features. The belief that little can be done for a dispositional component is insufficient reason to ignore the possibility that it exists; furthermore, the belief may be an unwarranted one anyway. The perspective of the shape of pull of developmental organizations may also be of use in designing therapeutic strategies, for example, for distinguishing an intervention that explains a cause from one that interprets a meaning. Freud (1940) outlined such points of reference for the libidinal phases of development. Few analysts, however, have tried to exploit the clinical applicability of such perspectives or to extend them beyond the libidinal. (For an exception, see Neubauer, 1980.) The effective use of the category of developmental organizations in clinical work may have been further compromised in recent years because the term *developmental* is ambiguously defined and because the concept of the developmental *process,* as well as the word *process* itself, is frequently misunderstood. The disorder of impaired impetus may turn out to be an infrequent one; however, it will be of value to clinicians despite its rarity if it serves as a reminder that there is a viable concept of developmental process beyond the highly controversial and ambiguous term *developmental.*

SUMMARY

I have tried to describe the growth of two girls, Amy and Beth, identical twins reared apart, to highlight some of the methodological and conceptual problems encountered in the course of studying them. I have proposed a metapsychological outline of the environment, extended the view of disposition as it is ordinarily understood, described a new disease entity, and suggested that there may be some clinical applications of the maturational aspect of the developmental process.

Nature can be differentiated into many discrete components, partly an expression of inherent blueprint, partly determined by congenital factors. Some of the components of nature are evident almost at once; others do not assert themselves until later, perhaps much later. Nurture includes the animate and inanimate, the structured and the random, stimuli that are mere excitations and those that are ripe with meaning. Nature and nurture, disposition and the environment, are potentials waiting to be realized. Each exacts a continuing influence upon the other, transforming potential into shape and substance. And, while the concept of a complementary series is a most useful one, there is still much that can be learned when attention is drawn to the polar extremes.

BIBLIOGRAPHY

BURLINGHAM, D. (1952). *Twins.* New York: Int. Univ. Press.
DEMAREST, E. W. & WINESTEIN, M. (1955). The initial phase of concomitant treatment of twins. *Psychoanal. Study Child,* 10:336–350.

FARBER, S. (1981). *Identical Twins Reared Apart.* New York: Basic Books.

FLAPAN, D. & NEUBAUER, P. B. (1975). *The Assessment of Early Child Development.* New York: Aronson.

FREUD, A. (1965). Normality and pathology in childhood. *W.*, 6.

FREUD, S. (1940). An outline of psycho-analysis. *S.E.*, 23:141–207.

GARDNER, G. E. & REXFORD, E. N. (1952). Retardation of ego development in a pair of identical twins. *Q. J. Child Behav.*, 4:367–381.

KARPMAN, B. (1951). A psychoanalytic study of a fraternal twin. *Amer. J. Orthopsychiat.*, 21:735–755.

NEUBAUER, P. B. (1980). The life cycle as indicated by the nature of the transference in the psychoanalysis of children. *Int. J. Psychoanal.*, 61:137–144.

PANEL (1961). The psychology of twins. E. Joseph, reporter. *J. Amer. Psychoanal. Assn.*, 9:158–166.

WALLERSTEIN, R. S. (1983). Reality and its attributes as psychoanalytic concepts. *Int. Rev. Psychoanal.*, 10:125–144.

The Contributions of Child Psychoanalysis to Psychoanalysis

E. JAMES ANTHONY, M.D.

THE GRADIENT FOR LEARNING, IN THE NORMAL COURSE OF EVENTS, extends from the experienced adult to the inexperienced child, and this proclivity then becomes a built-in model for the transmission of knowledge. Extrapolated to the professional sphere, the same inclination is assumed to hold: that professionals who work with children derive their knowledge base from those who work with adults, whether they be child psychiatrists, child analysts, or pediatricians. In psychoanalysis, however, where the nuclear tenet is that the child is father to the man, one would take it for granted that the analysis of children, together with the analytic observation of children, would have something basic to offer that might not otherwise be available. For the field to advance as a whole, there needs to be an essential understanding between the two component parts and for this to happen, competition must be eschewed, efforts must be cooperative. Adult and child analysts must work together in professional synergy.

THE CONJOINT CONTINUOUS CASE CONFERENCE: REPORT FROM THE CANDIDATES

In some institutes, unfortunately not all, continuous case seminars are conducted jointly by an adult and child analyst, and this is what takes place in my institute. Candidates soon learn that the retrospective and prospective analytic vision brings different

---

Training and supervising analyst; director of the Division of Child and Adolescent Psychoanalysis, St. Louis Psychoanalytic Institute.

types of material into focus which often offer a more complete picture of the patient and his conflicts. At times, the two viewpoints work together to enrich the understanding, but at other times, some unusual divergences may appear. According to the candidates, the child analyst presents the following differences: (1) his analytic interest veers almost imperceptively but predictably toward the preoedipal period where he seems to be "at home" with the pregenital content; (2) his analytic eye is very easily caught by the mother transference, and he will seem to give it an undue amount of attention, particularly its negative aspects and the ambivalent dependency; (3) although alive to the psychosexual vicissitudes of libido, there is greater emphasis on aggressivity and its endless displacements and reversals; (4) the analysis of defenses is often more systematically undertaken and more meticulously explored than in the case handled by the adult analyst; (5) the transference neurosis is not so easily recognized and the early symptoms of this are often missed; (6) there is more recognition of the "real" analyst and the "real" environment containing parents, siblings, spouses, and families; (7) trauma is looked at with a fairly wide-angled lens so that what looks at first like a single disturbing event is expanded into an entire stage of development, implying that one enema does not create a fixation or regression; (8) because of the nature of childhood and the temporospatial limitations set to the horizon, the here and now is brought very much to the forefront of technique, there is altogether less reliance on memory work and reconstruction, and the child analyst is more content to work with nonverbal cues and communications; (9) insight is not pursued as relentlessly and understanding is left in a more nebulous and feeling state with very little of the "ah-ha" drama about it; (10) the child analyst always appears peculiarly sensitive to the most miniscule countertransferences and prepared to detect their operations at all levels of the analysis; (11) there is much less hurry, on the part of the child analyst, to translate the dynamic process continuously in flux in the analytic situation into the language of structure.[1]

1. It should be emphasized that this was an informal, nonobtrusive study in which 30 candidates were invited to discuss their reactions to the joint seminar

WHAT IS AND MIGHT HAVE BEEN: THE CONTRIBUTIONS OF CHILD ANALYSIS TO PSYCHOANALYSIS ACCORDING TO ANNA FREUD

For Anna Freud, the new perspective offered by child analysis was a most important feature. As she put it, it was hard to convey "how dramatic was this period in the history of psychological treatment." For the first time "what had been merely guessed at and inferred became a living, visible, and demonstrable reality. . . . The oedipus complex was seen displayed toward the living parents in the external world as well as in ongoing fantasies and in the transference." Furthermore, what had appeared in reconstruction with the adult patient as a single traumatic event revealed itself in child analysis "as a sequence of such upsets, telescoped by recollection into cover memories" (1970, p. 210f.) This first-hand view of the nuclear complex allowed the analyst for the first time to take a closer look at all the preoedipal events that led up to the oedipal combination. Yet, Anna Freud was surprised and very disappointed by the reactions of the adult analyst. One might have anticipated, she thought, that they would not only be "highly interested in these findings" but eager to have a grandstand view themselves and thus compare what emerged directly in child analysis and indirectly in reconstructive work. In brief, one might have imagined the plethora of candidates applying for child analytic training, but this was far from being the case. Adult analysts remained "more or less aloof" from child analysis, "almost as if it were an inferior type of professional occupation" (p. 211) (child psychiatrists will recognize a similar reaction in their adult colleagues). It is of course, true that child patients were more difficult to obtain than adult ones; it was harder for them to attend during school hours; the parents had to bring them and found this onerous; and the work with the parents involved a lot of extra effort. The most striking, and perhaps unfair, indictment of child analysis was that it lacked a clear-cut technique that could be systematically put into

---

in open forum focusing on differences between the two teachers. They appointed their own chairperson and reporters who summarized consensus opinions after a 2-hour group discussion.

practice. Anna Freud felt that all the excuses were "shallow"; these adult analysts "vastly preferred the childhood images which emerged from their interpretations to the real children in whom they remained uninterested" (p. 211f.) This is not the whole story. There are many adults who have lost the connection with their childhood or have set it aside as a regressive interlude about which they felt vaguely ashamed and which they preferred to forget. Furthermore, additional training does act as a deterrent. As one candidate remarked to me: "It would be nice to learn directly about sources, but I simply could not afford another three or four years more of time and money." Why, indeed, would they want to learn a technique where free association was nonexistent, where transference was shared with the parents, where there was a minimum of insight, a maximum of resistance, where the therapeutic alliance was unstable and precarious, where parents were needed to keep the child in treatment, where action took the place of words, and where the analyst's attention could not be concentrated on the patient exclusively but needed to be extended to his environment (A. Freud, 1970).

But where else could one learn directly about the psychosexual stages, about the process of separation-individuation, about the changing nature of defenses, about the emergence of ego functions and self-attributes, and about the origins of structure? It is only the beginnings that are susceptible to a preventive approach, and it is in the beginnings that one can observe the gradual making of the personality.

THE CONTRIBUTIONS OF CHILD ANALYSIS TO PSYCHOANALYSIS ACCORDING TO FREUD

Like many offspring, the birth of child psychoanalysis was something of an "accident," somewhat unexpected; and it certainly was not expected to grow to maturity. When Freud undertook the supervision of the first child analytic case of little Hans, he regarded it as a serendipitous event with little therapeutic significance since it was a matter of pure chance that a psychoanalytically oriented physician was father to a phobic child and enthusiastically interested in treating him under Freud's guidance. How did this first child analysis make a contribution to psychoanalysis? Freud's response (1909) was clear: "Strictly speaking," he said, "I learnt nothing new from this analysis, nothing that I had not already been able to discover (though often less distinctly and more indirectly) from other patients analysed at a more advanced age" (p. 147). However, this first analysis of a child offered confirmatory evidence and this was a contribution. It was the confirmatory value that he stressed and reiterated most frequently. "It was *a very great triumph* when it became possible years later to confirm almost all my inferences about the analysis of very young children—a triumph that lost some of its magnitude as one gradually realized that the nature of the discovery was such that one should really be ashamed of having had to make it" (1916-17). This brings up an interesting if speculative question: if childhood is the prerogative of the child analyst, and if Freud had started as a child analyst, would he have discovered the oedipus complex more quickly and with less effort? He remarked on another valuable contribution, that of consolidating psychoanalytic tenets: "Every analysis of a child strengthens the convictions upon which the theory of psycho-analysis is founded, and rebuts the re-interpretations made by both Jung's and Adler's systems." Here child analysis was being used not only to confirm Freudian theory, but also to disconfirm rival systems.

When Freud worked on the case of the Wolf-Man (1918), his enthusiasm for new therapeutic departure became even more pronounced. He began to compare and to contrast the retro-spective and prospective modes of analysis, pointing to the ad-vantages and disadvantages of both approaches. For example, it seemed to him that the analysis of the child appeared to be more trustworthy, although the material often lacked in richness. Fur-thermore, not only were there linguistic and cognitive limita-tions, but the child's inability to introspect rendered the deepest strata of the mind impenetrable to consciousness. It was true that adult analysis was relatively free from these impediments, but, on the other side, the method of recollection involved distortion and confabulation. It may be, he concluded, that child analysis furnished more convincing results, but adult analysis was far more instructive. Here he makes a subtle distinction that is not easy to grasp, but one takes it to mean that conviction can be based on bare facts, provided they stand out clearly, directly, and uncontaminated by the elaborate superstructure that the mind builds up defensively over time and that renders the adult analysis such a maze of complexity. One learns much more than the bare bones of the nuclear complex: the entire apparatus of the mind and all its endless ramifications are brought into play; accordingly, one stands to learn a great deal more: hence, the accent on "more instructive."

At this point, he recognized that the difficulty of feeling one's way into the mental life of the child set the analyst "a particularly difficult task"; but even allowing for such built-in obstacles, he maintained that the analysis of a child's neurosis would "claim to possess a specially high theoretical interest" since they provided a better understanding of adult neuroses in the same way as children's dreams complete our understanding of adult dreams. But then Freud touched on a point that continues to buoy child analysis. Admittedly, he said, the task may be difficult, but "so many of the later deposits are wanting in them that the essence of the neurosis springs to the eyes with unmistakable distinctiness" (1918). It is this distinct, close-up view of the relatively undefended neurosis that will allow the child analyst to delineate the disorder more distinctly and thus make an invaluable contribution to the nosology of the neuroses.

By 1919, Freud was becoming more aware of the significance of child analysis as a *therapeutic contribution* and even made a suggestion on analyzability. "Children for whom there is no choice between running wild or neurosis may be made capable by analysis" (of gaining greater control and working more effectively). Children who run wild, but are not hyperkinetic are more amenable to analytic treatment than adults who "run wild." But clearly the treatment was eminently worthwhile because he predicted that at some future date, the state would recognize its efficacy and ensure that children would be treated analytically without cost.

In 1933, he pointed out that child analysis had made a *contribution to psychoanalysis* by confirming "on the living subject what we had inferred (from historical documents, as it were) in the case of adults. But the gain for the children was also very satisfactory.

It turned out that a child is a very favourable subject for analytic therapy; the results are thorough and lasting" (p. 148). He did acknowledge (presumably after much discussion with his daughter) that adult technique must be modified for children since the latter were psychologically different. Their consciences, their associative capacities, their transferences (since the real parents were still around) were still in the process of development; in addition to the internal resistances encountered in adult analysis, in children the child analyst was also faced by external difficulties constituted by the parents.

He seemed to be much better acquainted with the potentials of child analysis now that he shared offices with his daughter and observed the growth of her work. He was thus able to say that even small children could be analyzed without risk, and he pointed to the pleasure of analyzing a preschool child and the decreasing pleasure of dealing with the child during latency. ("I have an impression," Freud remarked with delightful candor, "that with the onset of the latency period they [children] become mentally inhibited as well, stupider. . . . many children lose their physical charm" [1926, p. 215]. My own impression is that many children who suffer from latency disorders do seem to regain their charm with analysis.)

By 1925, looking back on the patchwork of his life's labors, Freud added a postscript about child analysis that had gained "a powerful momentum owing to the work of Mrs. Melanie Klein and of my daughter, Anna Freud" (p. 70).

By this time, child analysis was on a voyage of discovery and he downplayed its confirmatory and secondary role to psychoanalysis. The educator could call the psychoanalyst in for help when dealing with a particular child, but child analysis was not a substitute for education, he said. The analytic situation, unlike the didactic situation, required the presence of certain psychical structures and a particular attitude on the part of the analyst. He was quite intrigued by some of the insights covered by child analysts. "Among the observations made by child psychoanalysis, there is scarcely one that sounds so repugnant and unbelievable as that of the boy's feminine attitude to his father and the fantasy of pregnancy that arises from it." He seemed a little surprised by this contribution and one wonders why since it represents a piece of psychopathology that could very well be recovered from an adult analysis.

He had been much impressed by this burgeoning new discipline and predicted that it would become still more important. *"From the point of view of theory, its value was beyond question. It gave unequivocal information on problems that remained unsolved in the analyses of adults; and it thus protects the analyst from errors that might have momentous consequences for him."* So here we have the founder of psychoanalysis emphasizing the following points regarding the contribution of child psychoanalysis to psychoanalysis:

1. He foresaw that it would become even more important as time went on.

2. Theoretically, it had become invaluable in giving unequivocal information on problems that remained unresolved in the analyses of adults and alerted the adult analyst to possible errors in his work.

3. It permitted us to observe neurosis in the making when the picture was still relatively uncontaminated by subsequent psychological developments.

4. It could be applied to children who had no clear-cut neurotic symptoms but were moody, refractory, inattentive, nervous, anorexic, or sleepless—indications which went well beyond the simple phobia that had initiated the whole child analytic movement.

5. Of even greater importance was the fact that if children with incipient neuroses were treated analytically, adult analysis might become unnecessary. A child analysis could then become "an excellent method of prophylaxis."

Freud did not think that every analyst could or should become a child analyst, but that the treatment was best carried out by those who were not embarrassed to find themselves in the child's world and not at a loss to find their way into the child's mind. This latter comment was a far cry from a recommendation he had made about 20 years earlier when he referred a child to Binswanger and suggested that he should be treated, analytically, as in the manner of little Hans, by a nurse who had sustained a serious neurosis and had recovered with the help of analysis. In 1933, he had made the point that children had turned out to be very favorable subjects for analytic therapy and that the results were comparable to those of adults and lasting. The external difficulties were certainly present, but psychoanalysis might still be able to count the analysis of children among its greatest successes.

In his last great work, *Moses and Monotheism* (1939), which he carried with him to London, he stated that "the analytic study of the mental life of children has provided an *unexpected wealth of material for filling the gaps in our knowledge of the earliest times*" (p. 84; my italics). What greater tribute could there be to the contributions of child analysis to psychoanalysis? Moreover, consider that Freud started with a view that did nothing more than confirm what was already known to the point when he believed that it made an invaluable contribution to psychoanalysis both theoretically and technically, and that potentially it might make adult analysis unnecessary. Ernest Jones (1955) noted the leap in Freud's assessment, beginning with his cautious statement about the case of Little Hans. "The brilliant successes of child analysis . . . prove that here Freud's customary insight had deserted him. It seems a curious thing to say of the very man who explored that child's mind to an extent that had never before been possible that he should nevertheless have retained some inhibitions about coming to too close quarters with it. It is as if some inner voice had said thus far and no farther. We remarked earlier on the slowless with which Freud was willing to admit the existence of infantile sexuality, particularly in its allo-erotic aspects, and to the end of his life he displayed certain reservations about the limits of what it was possible to accomplish in child analysis and the exploration of the more remote and hidden regions of the earliest mental processes" (p. 261).

I do not agree with this comment at all. As I see it, Freud responded positively to each step in the development of child analysis, and if Jones could say that he had inhibitions about coming close to infantile sexuality, one needs only to remember that mankind before him (and many after him) suffered from the most repressive inhibitions; and if he displayed some reservations about the limits of child analysis, one needs to remember that there are many adult analysts today who are much more dubious about its value and who question its authenticity as an analytic method. There are many today who find it difficult to listen to child analytic material, read it, or even begin to understand it; and there are many institutes in which child analysis continues to receive short shrift and where child analysts are treated with quite a degree of condescension. As always, so it seems to me, Freud was amazingly ahead of his time. Even back in 1909, while he thought that "the investigation of childhood life will for some time yet be dominated by the knowledge we gain from adults," he added: "but that is not the ideal state of affairs." Distance may bring enchantment to the view, according to the poet, but it also brings obscurity and obfuscation. Yet the view from childhood itself was not entirely flawless and he wondered to what degree the parent's neurosis built a wall around the child's neurosis.

BEYOND THE ANALYTIC COUCH, OR THE ADAPTATION OF PSYCHOANALYSIS TO CHILDHOOD

In the last years of her life, Anna Freud was stressing the importance of collaboration between child and adult analysts and instituted a series of annual meetings whereby major psychoanalytic concepts could undergo mutual examination, with one side stimulating the other to further contributions. The discourse was not only of a high order but it was novel in combining both retrospective and prospective viewpoints and attempting to synthesize them. There seemed to be an inherent belief that the two viewpoints were essential for the healthy and productive growth of psychoanalysis. The forum was conducted without rivalry and acrimony and each party appeared to profit from the experience. I would hope that every psychoanalytic society would create a similar type of forum to tackle some of the present unknowns in psychopathology.

There is no doubt that technical difficulties, as Freud pointed out, often help to open up new theoretical considerations regarding the essential nature of the psychoanalytic process and the structure of the psychic apparatus. At first reading of the classical child analytic literature, one must logically conclude that the child is unanalyzable. He is not aware of suffering, not motivated to getting better, not prepared to postpone gratification, not inclined to seek help, not equipped to develop insights, not yet independent of his parents, not able to form a sustaining therapeutic alliance, nonintrospective, incapable of free association, inept at working through or working with dreams, and scarcely (or only rarely) able to experience a transference neurosis that can be systematically interpreted—in fact all the reasons, quoted earlier, why adult analysts refrain from becoming child analysts. There are further anaclitically off-putting tendencies on the child's part, such as eschewing the couch, remaining face-to-face, keeping on the go, and making predominant use of nonverbal communications.

All these have raised questions even in the minds of adult analysts benignly oriented toward child analysis as to whether the child is truly analyzable and whether child analysis is at best applied analysis or at worst "wild" analysis. How then can one do psychoanalysis without using prescribed psychoanalytic methods? How can good practice with children be bad practice with adults and vice versa? And how can one carry out psychoanalysis with children when the parents are constantly hovering intrusively over one's efforts? As mentioned earlier, Freud eventually became convinced that not only was child analysis genuine psychoanalysis as he had more or less shaped it, but that children were often more successful analysands than adults and that the unconscious urge to complete development on the part of the child represented a stronger therapeutic factor than the conscious motivation of the adult patient to get well.

The history of child analysis can be understood as an extraordinary attempt to render the apparently nonanalyzable analyzable, and the success of this venture had its repercussions on other seemingly nonanalyzable groups of patients such as delinquents, psychotics, borderline patients, and severe character disorders with a large narcissistic component. All of these are currently being subjected to psychoanalysis through the use of so-called "parameters" in the child analytic situation since its technique must, of necessity, undergo changes from stage to stage and yet remain psychoanalytic in essence and correctly regarded as psychoanalysis and not psychoanalytically oriented psychotherapy. Although the "parameters" used by adult analysts for poorly analyzable patients have received a certain amount of discussion, there have been heated arguments about whether the diagnosis was correct and whether the technique was genuinely psycho-analytic. Child analysis could perform a basic service to psycho-analysis by defining and clarifying the dimensions and bound-aries of what constituted a psychoanalytic approach. Child analysis has become something of a paradigm for cases that do not respond to the "classical" adult mode of treatment.

In the early years of child analysis, Anna Freud (1927) intro-duced the ideas of a "preparatory phase" that could help to make a child analyzable, but today this is no longer deemed necessary except in rare instances. Aichhorn (1925) had already pointed out that delinquents were not susceptible to the usual technique and needed "preparation" during which the analyst attempted to make himself indispensable to the patient and to cultivate a gratifying relationship through the portals of pa-thology. At a certain point, the approach was reversed, with the analyst assuming the posture of relative neutrality, precipitating a neurotic crisis in the delinquent subject which then became amenable to psychoanalysis. Eissler (1958) applied a similar method and rationale to another hard-to-reach group with some success.

The Contributions of Child Psychoanalysis to the Analytic Situation

Let me try to itemize the areas in which child analysis has made a contribution to a better understanding of the analytic situation:

1. There is the area of the "real" relationship in the analytic situation which is an acceptable and workable phenomenon in child analysis when, from time to time, the analyst, as the child perceives him, seems to step out of his transference role to be-come a real person, belonging to a real world, and obviously functioning in a real manner. This occasional shift from the deeper image that is becoming part and parcel of the internal conflict carries with it a certain degree of reassurance. I believe that child analysis, through Winnicott, has demonstrated that there is not only an internal analyst and an external analyst, but, in some intermediate area, a transitional analyst who can medi-ate between inside and outside, between fantasy and reality, and, in the situation of mutual play, can help the child patient to deal

with his conflictual situation more creatively. In the same context, Greenson (1972) asked whether adult patients suffering not from structural conflicts but structural deficiencies in the formation of the ego and essentially "preneurotic" should be afforded stable or real objects to build up a stable ego as a prerequisite before a conflict-uncovering analysis could be undertaken. Winnicott (1954b), speaking as a child analyst, advocated some degree of "management" in such cases interspersed with psychoanalysis, and Anna Freud (1965), also with the perspective of a child analyst, had this to say: "With due respect for the necessary strictest handling and interpretation of the transference, I still feel that somewhere we should leave room for the realization that analyst and patient are also two real people, of equal adult status, in a real personal relationship to each other," but she recognized that such a comment might be regarded as "technically subversive" and to be "handled with care!"

2. Next we come to the "real" environment as it encroaches on the encapsulation of the analytic situation, thereby, according to purists, contaminating it. In my own analytic work with children, I practice encapsulation and teach it as a necessary but not essential condition for a fuller unfolding of the transference, but even then I keep a wary eye on the environment, especially in its familial part (Anthony, 1980, 1981). Anna Freud (1965) knew that child analysts could be plotted along a spectrum at the one end of which the environment was almost totally disregarded from the intimacy of treatment along with all its distracting appurtenances such as parents, while at the other end the parents and the environment were included in the treatment, even permitted to participate in some sessions, and utilized as a "news service" from the outside. The analyst located at this latter pole was able to learn something of the subtle and complex interplay between the home situation and the analytic situation, and the fact that the child habitually externalized his intrapsychic conflicts made his behavior in analysis easier to understand. Children, in fact, have a limited capacity for internalization and an inordinate capacity for externalization, but there are many adult patients who present in a similar fashion. Anna Freud (1965) pointed out that adult analysts have been trained to exclude the environment and focus their attention on the psyche. She

viewed them as "too eager" to see all current happenings in terms of resistance and transference and to discount their value in reality. For her, there was more balance in the analysis of children and such adult patients who are in a pressing relationship with the object world and the associated environmental influences, such as borderline cases where it may be important to take into account not only the internal fantasies but also current events, family quarrels and upsets, frustrating and anxiety-arousing actions, and ongoing sexual problems. As she put it, "The child analyst who interprets exclusively in terms of the inner world is in danger of missing out on his patient's reporting activity concerning his—at the time equally important—environmental circumstances" (p. 51). And this would be true of some disordered adult patients. How to do this with due psychoanalytic procedure is something that the analyst can hope to learn from the child analyst.

3. The process of free association has aroused much analytic attention since Freud first introduced it as an integral part of the psychoanalytic method. The degrees of "freedom" show a wide variability among adult patients: some seem to fall into it very readily as if saying what came into their minds as part of their general spontaneity in life; some acquire it during the course of analysis when their defenses and resistance to the process have been adequately dealt with; some manifest it during termination leading analysts to regard it as a criterion for stopping treatment; and some obsessional types seem never to acquire it at all. Its relation to the primary process has never been clarified; did it indicate that the patient was in touch with his unconscious life or was it simply a "cognitive style" typifying "liberated" personalities? Could child psychoanalysis throw any light on its origins and connections? Schiller regarded it as a tool of creativity and Freud's first reading of it in the literature suggested that "anyone" might become creative if they allowed their free-floating minds to hover over a blank sheet of paper! Sir Francis Galton (1882), the prominent Victorian scientist, experimented with free association and concluded that it was analogous to exploring a house: there was life upstairs but quite another kind of life downstairs, the "antechamber of consciousness," and if you pursued the process further, it *invariably* carried you not only into

the area of plumbing and sewage, but also into the childhood past—not quite the place for a Fellow of the Royal Society! It seemed to represent a kind of adult play in an easy relationship with fantasy and symbolic functioning, and it was therefore not a big step for child analysts to take to regard it as not alien to childhood but as the very quintessence of the early years. The component parts were all familiar to this age: play, daydreaming, symbolism, spontaneity, creativity. Was the child not nearer to unconscious processes than the adult? Did not Piaget (1922) demonstrate (and present to Freud) the fact that the child's thinking was intermediate between primary and secondary process and was characteristically syncretic, juxtapositional, transductive, and egocentric, all of which, it might be argued, were ingredients of free association.

Klein (1927), pointing to the accessibility of unconscious fantasies and symbols, felt that play was equivalent to free association and therefore treated it similarly as an analytic communication. One could agree that young patients talk more freely, spontaneously, and less defensively in the language of play since they seem to regard this special realm, preconsciously, as once removed from the pressures and demands of everyday life. When the connection is pointed out to them, a "disruption" in their communication may occur and they may switch to a less playful and more banal approach in a manner not dissimilar to the adult's retreat into reality when his free associations are understood at a more latent level by the analyst. The child analytic world is much more than a world of words. The patient makes use of both words and activities as in play and will move from the "microsphere" of little family and household figures to activities with water, play, drawing, and acting. What one finds is that the associations to a dream, for example, may make their appearance successively in all these different media so that the discerning therapist can follow the chain of ideas throughout a session. For analytic purposes, this represents an invaluable mode of "free" communication. Having observed this, one can begin to see that the nonverbal activities of the adult patient on the couch may continue a train of associations that have apparently dried up in the verbal sphere. The child analyst may be able to help in elucidating some of the vagaries and connections that are covertly contained in the free associations. The child analyst, specializing as he does in the area of nonverbal communication, can help to sensitize adult analysts to the nuances of this rich, parallel communication system that is so often overlooked in the predominantly verbal analyses of adults (Anthony, 1977).

4. There is another phenomenon of the analytic situation that has become a cornerstone of psychoanalytic treatment, namely, the transference, with its almost inevitable and ubiquitous counterpart, the countertransference. In the beginning, transference was somewhat left out of child psychoanalysis. Although it was clear that Little Hans projected a strong transference onto Freud as the invisible and omniscient interpreter and explicator, nothing was made of this in the treatment since the concept was still generating in Freud's head. When formal work with children began in the 1930s, the emphasis was more on the immaturity of the child and the consequent deficiencies in his analytic functioning. There was thus a tendency to assume what he was unable to do rather than to take note of what he was able to do in the analytic situation. Since the therapeutic alliance was considered to be the prominent factor in the child's treatment, the negative transference was "tucked away under the carpet" to prevent it from interfering with the formation of the alliance, which gave the reports of child analysis an unreal quality. The child patients appeared to do better than they should. The crucial development of the transference neurosis was theoretically excluded from the analytic situation with the child because his real parents were waiting outside to take him home. As transference became a major issue in child psychoanalysis, it was looked at in novel ways. During development, the child's parental needs, particularly with respect to the mother, showed a gradient with the greatest need for the actual parent located in the earliest years and with a gradual tapering off during the school years into adolescence. The gradient for transference would seem to be the opposite of this: as the actual parents become less essential to the daily life of the child, the psychic recreation of the parent in the transference increased. This suggested that transference was not entirely a function of the repressed unconscious operating at the culmination of the nuclear complex: the availability of the actual parents and their necessity to the child also

played important roles. Child analysts also investigated the transferences from the current parents which might possibly operate in two steps: the transference from the deeply buried oedipal parents to the contemporary parents, and a displacement from the latter to the analyst. The mechanisms are probably easier to explore in child analysis, and the findings may be applicable to the adult case.

It is sometimes said that the countertransference generated in analytic work with children is more intense and pervasive than any encountered in adult work. The analyst may take the child as a transference object, or react to the child's transference to him as manifested erotically or aggressively; or he may identify with the child's parents and become overcontrolling or oversolicitous, or he may find incestuous fears and fantasies stirring as a result of direct body contact with the child. Such countertransferences are the daily bread-and-butter of the child analyst, and if he is as insightful about himself as he is about his patient, he will be alert to such reactions constantly, and at times even able to utilize them for a better understanding of the analytic process. One would like to say that this area of analysis has been illuminated by contributions from child analysis, but unfortunately the reverse is true. Child analytic publications rarely mention the phenomenon, clearly regarding it, at all times, as a contaminant. This is especially surprising in view of the mutuality of the therapeutic relationship in child analysis. It has been left to those working with psychotic patients, like Searles (1965), to scrutinize this element objectively as a complex ingredient of the analytic situation and peculiarly tied to the vicissitudes of transference. As Glover (1955) once remarked, in all case reports, we are only being presented with one-half of the analytic story. The "toileting" of countertransference stimulates insights in the analyst in parallel with his patient. There is no doubt that child psychoanalysis could make a significant contribution to this mutually evolving interplay in insights.

5. The insights that one encounters in child analysis are of a different order to those found in adult work. If insights are a product of affect and cognition working in unison, one would expect developmental trends, and one finds them. For true insight, there needs to be some understanding of causality, some

degree of operational thinking, in Piaget's terms, and some sense of responsibility. At the intuitive level of development, true insight is not expectable, and in its place one often encounters what Neubauer (1979) calls "uncanny feelings"—a diffuse mixture of knowing and not knowing it affectively but not cognitively. If the child is challenged about a supposedly insightful pronouncement, he will invariably deny it because he is unable to recognize it. If his analyst reformulates his "belly feelings" in the full array of secondary process thinking, it will be forthrightly rejected. During latency, especially early latency, insights may have a transient quality, even when couched in very concrete and verbally simple terms. For example, the statement "You're mad with me because you saw my patient outside in the waiting room, just as you were mad with your mom when she brought your baby brother home from the hospital; you're very jealous now, you must have been very jealous then" may be accepted at first hearing and then totally rejected subsequently, or vice versa, and the acceptance-rejection does seem to reflect the state of the transference. Since child analysts are working with the rudiments of insight, they could help to clarify the various categories of insight (since the childhood varieties are also met within the nascent insights of adults), the vagaries of insight, and the relationship between the insights generated by the patient within himself and the insights that are conveyed by the analyst's interpretation. In both child and adult analysis, the analyst's insights into himself and into his patient are helpful to the ongoing analytic process even when the patient has failed to acquire any insights for himself. There is still a feeling of reassurance that "at least someone knows what is happening in this murky situation!"

THE CONTRIBUTIONS OF CHILD PSYCHOANALYSIS TO PSYCHOANALYTIC PSYCHOLOGY

There are two areas of psychoanalysis that have profited especially from child psychoanalysis—the ego and its mechanisms of defense. In both, the efforts of Anna Freud have been in the forefront. Since many of the patients in the early phase of child analysis were latency children, the developing and consolidating defense structure was very apparent and yielded maximum information about the variety of strategies that the embattled ego erects against the onslaughts of conflict. Whether the child analyst will eventually be able through his observations in treatment to outline a chronology of the defenses that cover the personality like a series of onion skins remains to be seen, but it would represent a contribution that would be of help to the adult analysts in their use of defense analysis.

Since analysis of children provides a grandstand view of the development and resolution of the oedipus complex, it also supplies a vantage point for observing the construction of the mental apparatus, particularly with regard to the emergence of the moral (superego and ego ideal) system, and along with this the beginnings of shame, disgust, and guilt. In dealing with the problem of disgust, Freud (1950) pointed out that direct observation in nurseries could tell us something of the coprophilic phase that preceded the development of disgust; in his work on shame (1950), he retrospectively discovered the existence of a shameless period; presumably there also is a guiltless period antecedent to later guilt. All these transformations, so crucial for our understanding of psychosexual development, might be observed in the nursery by highly sophisticated observers, but there could be no better laboratory for investigating this than in child analysis. As Freud would have undoubtedly agreed, this would be an important offering to the field.

The analysis of very young children, taken on in increasing numbers, promised to bring new analytic knowledge of the obscure preoedipal stage that appeared to be so cut off from the reaches of adult analysis. Not all child analysts, however, have an interest in exploring this phase of development. Anna Freud (1965) had this to say: "So far as I am concerned, the study of this darkest of all ages has never been my predilection. I have always preferred as my subject those phases of development where assumptions can be checked against verbalized material recaptured from the unconscious by the analytic method, or against the facts which are open to view in the direct observation of infants." Other child analysts felt differently, having less compunction at making analytic inferences some of which have startled adult analysts into feeling that there was a lack of psychoanalytic discipline and rigor about the techniques used by child analysts. Klein (1930) took note of the earliest reality when "the world is a breast and belly which is filled with dangerous objects, dangerous because of the child's own impulse to attack them." She elaborated a view of this world that had a huge impact on adult analysts drawn to this quasi-psychotic external reality which is largely a mirror of the child's own instinctual life as it appears in the analysis of children between 2½ and 5 years. Whether one agrees with the approach or not, it is a powerful presentation that appears to make sense to the adult analyst confronted with a psychotic or borderline patient. Also brought into psychoanalysis were new conceptualizations regarding object relations: for these very small children, side by side with their relations to real objects are parallel relations to unreal images that are viewed as excessively good or bad, and these two kinds of object relations intermingle and color each other to an ever-increasing degree in the course of development (Klein, 1934). Adult analysts who espouse these Kleinian ideas—and those who do, do so passionately—would be the first to declare that these contributions from child analysis completely dominate their theory and practice of psychoanalysis.

Mahler's (1966) contributions to our understanding of the preoedipal phase has certainly had an impact on the dynamic approach to child development in the United States, although we are still too close to the situation to decide whether the effect has been equally profound on psychoanalysis in providing it with a developmental substratum and so helping to fulfill Hartmann's dream of a general psychoanalytic psychology. Based on direct observation of toddlers but *not* on their analysis, the primary focus as with Klein was on the mother-child relationship and the intrapsychic struggles of the child within this dyad. It is of special interest that the two child analysts, Klein and Mahler, both emphasized the significance of depression (a normative depressive "position" and a "basic depressive mood" during the critical rapprochement crisis) that needed to be resolved before an orderly classical psychosexual development could ensue. As a result, the general psychoanalyst has become more accepting of the concept of depression as a primary affect that makes its presence felt from the earliest years and contributes to later psychopathology. Winnicott, another child analyst, had two other offerings for the general field. The wide-ranging concepts of transitional phenomena and playful creativeness have both been assimilated into psychoanalysis operationally. For him, the distinction between child and adult psychoanalysis is reduced to a simple but compelling formula: both types of work are done in the overlap of two play areas, that of the patient and that of the analyst. Play is the major criterion for treatability and analyzability. "If the therapist cannot play, then he is not suitable for the work. If the patient cannot play, then something needs to be done to enable the patient to become able to play" (Winnicott, 1974). What Winnicott has to offer the general psychoanalyst is not systematic theory or details of technique but exciting ideas that are steeped in rich clinical experience. His influence lies in his free-floating and spontaneous approach to psychoanalysis and to patients. What he has to say invariably has meaning for both children and adults, as if he was constantly dealing with the child in the adult and therefore not prepared to differentiate too sharply between them.

Erik Erikson (1950) is a child analyst who has wandered freely through the adult domain and made himself at home in every one of the seven ages of man. This represented a much wider span than workaday analysts were prone to include in their usual frame of reference but within the context of the "wider scope," this psychoanalytically oriented psychosocial theory could quite possibly find a niche in a general psychoanalytic psychology that is still struggling to be born. With its historical, anthropological, literary, and artistic facets, the Eriksonian system has helped to make psychoanalysis more acceptable to a more general public.

All these child analysts have attempted to rewrite small or large portions of psychoanalytic theory and many have introduced startling new insights that have been at variance with classical theory yet, at the same time, keeping faith with the general body of psychoanalytic knowledge. They continue to regard themselves as doing no more than extending traditional conceptualizations.

Generally speaking, child analysts have not done too much with oedipal psychopathology and have not discovered anything new or different regarding the hysterias. Understandably, because of their predominant focus on mother and child, they have added considerably to the preoedipal psychopathologies, just as they have contributed to a wider and deeper understanding of preoedipal development.

The origins of depression viewed prospectively have added to the insights stemming from the work of Freud, Abraham, Bibring, and others. Making use of the Hampstead Index (another significant contribution from child psychoanalysis to psychoanalytic research), Joffe and Sandler (1965) found nine pathognomonic items characterizing depression in children and tried to distinguish this clinical reaction from the more basic depressive response and "unhappiness." Unhappy children protest against pain-producing situations, whereas depressed children capitulate and retreat from it. What they discovered in cases of depression was a discrepancy between the actual state of the self and an ideal state of well-being or primary narcissism. The latter is connected with feelings of security, satiation, and contentment, whereas the former has links to chronic discomfort, unrelieved hunger, and frustration. According to them, certain predisposed individuals under certain conditions respond to the latter situation by the development of a primary psychobiological state that represents the ultimate reaction to the experience of helplessness in the face of unremitting pain. Like Bibring (1953), approaching the issue from the later part of the life cycle, their focus was on the element of helplessness, seen by Bibring as a "narcissistic shock" and by the child analyst as a painful capitulation and retreat. For Mahler (1966) the depressive mood originates during the separation-individuation process and is an exaggeration of the basic depressive response, similar to anxiety, that evolves at this time. During the "practicing" phase, toddlers show a phase-specific elation, but with the next development, depression appears when the toddler becomes more aware of himself and of his parents as separate people, and of his mother no longer administering immediately and magically to all his needs. She is still the omnipotent one, but deliberately withholding her power from him. Based, therefore, on careful, systematic observation and not child analysis, Mahler noted the occurrence of depressive-like reactions, with mental content, in the latter part of the second year of life and considered these to be the first reactions that could be related to later depression. Klein (1935) carried the notion of a normally occurring depression into the earlier part of the first year of life with the formation of a "depressive position," and this again was not unlike the "depressive constellation" postulated by Benedek (1956) reaching back inferentially to the infant in the first 6 months from the viewpoint of adult retrospection. Both point to the same frustrating alimentary experience, the use of introjection-projection mechanisms, to conflicts based on ambivalence, and, when there is a failure at working through, a persistence of a proclivity toward adult psychopathology. Anna Freud, although unwilling, as mentioned earlier, to elaborate on detailed mechanisms at this early stage of life, did point to the way in which the little child tried to establish rapport with a depressed mother by reflecting her mood (1965), and this found support from Winnicott (1954a) whose clinical focus was always on the mother-infant relationship and the feeding experience. The infant, according to Winnicott, is concerned about two things: what happens to the mother before and after feeding, and what happens inside him as a personal inner experience. He talks of the "complex ideas" at work in the infant's mind. When Freud (1909), an adult analyst, said, "I am aware that I am attributing a great deal to the mental capacity of a child between four and five years of age," there were many skeptics to doubt him, and today, when the child psychoanalyst is making the statements about the "thinking" of infants in the first year of life, there are disbelievers among both adult and child anaysts. However, there would be general agreement that child analysts, working through analysis and observation, have opened up a far more complex picture of the preoedipal phase and its disorders than could conceivably be uncovered by the adult analyst. One should add that even in the field of general psychology, infants are now being regarded as far more "competent" than was thought a few decades ago.

But there was more to come, as child analysts delved deeper and earlier, and explored the question of where the relatively common adult sense of persecution originated. It certainly seemed to have no place in the oedipus complex, as classically constituted. Its primitive characteristics suggested a much ear-

lier birth. The child analyst, with his hyperempathic resonances
to the infant and small child, is inclined to view the torrential
weeping of the helpless baby as a daily but distressing disaster.
As Winnicott (1952) put it, "We allow the infant this madness,"
particularly because he is unable to distinguish between inside
and outside; but if he were an adult, we might not hesitate to
label him truly mad (p. 224). At the moment of this tempestuous
disorganization, Winnicott becomes concerned with the baby's
precarious position and the danger of "irreversible disintegration." He is considered to be in the Humpty Dumpty situation
and not too well put together, and at any moment could come
apart. This represents a "paranoid potential" which is a little
different from the more complex, not to say convoluted "schiz-
oid-paranoid position" described by Klein to which the classical
analyst has taken great exception. The child analyst who treats
psychotic and borderline children is constantly aware of how
close he is to feelings of persecution and the accompanying anxieties. Winnicott (1952) stated this more strongly: "It is a world
of magic, and one feels mad to be in it. All of us who have treated
psychotic children of this kind know how mad we have to be to
inhabit this world, and yet we must be there, and must be able to
stay there for long periods in order to do any therapeusis" (p.
227). I would guess that this would immediately tax the free-
floating serenity and neutrality of the general psychoanalyst
who would regard this attitude as overinvolved, countertrans-
ferential, and nonproductive in the service of resolving high
degrees of anxiety.

As mentioned earlier, child analysts have their fair share of
countertransference, but, oddly enough, this seems to allow
them not to become unduly disconcerted by the "monsters" encountered in the small child's murky psyche where the comforts
of structure are absent. What child analysis is doing here, as a
contribution to analysis in general, is to call attention to the
origins of the haunting sense of persecution that stays with some
individuals all their lives as well as the black depressions that
appear and disappear to old age. With the help of the child
analyst, the general analyst can trace the red thread that runs
sometimes on the surface and more often subterraneanly from
infancy onward. It is my strong belief that psychoanalytic psy-

chopathology can be most rewardingly studied by a combination of direct and reconstructive strategies, which implies, of course, a fruitful collaboration between child and adult analysts. How can psychoanalysis learn more fully about the acquired capacities for working through mourning, about the earliest vicissitudes of narcissism, about the growth of the sense of reality, about the development of the self, about the earliest manifestations of transference, about the prestructural activities of the moral system with the interactions of shame and guilt, about depression and paranoia and a host of other human phenomena at manifest and latent levels, except through this collaborative process. For psychoanalysis, the child analyst is "Our Man in Havana" who can spy on the hidden systems and provide detailed information on the entangled network of forces that work in the shadow of the preoedipal period. So much of this appears to be taken for granted by the adult analyst as the given data of analysis, but these "givens" are already complex developments and need to be disentangled further.

Finally, it may be presumptuous on my part to say that one of the most important contributions of child analysis to psychoanalysis is to keep it in continuous and close touch with the dynamic unconscious since, with our current preoccupations with the ego and the self, we may be in danger of losing contact with it, and, in a sense, forgetting from whence we came when Freud made his first seminal discoveries. It is through the world of play, make-believe, symbolic functioning, and fantasy that the child analyst lives next door and keeps constantly in touch with the bottomless reservoirs of life's energy and drive.

BIBLIOGRAPHY

Aichhorn, A. (1925). *Wayward Youth*. New York: Viking Press, 1935.
Anthony, E. J. (1977). Nonverbal and verbal systems of communication. *Psychoanal. Study Child*, 32:307–325.
—— (1980). The family and the psychoanalytic process. *Psychoanal. Study Child*, 35:3–34.
—— (1981). Psychoanalysis and environment. In *The Course of Life*, 3, ed. S. I. Greenspan & G. H. Pollock. Washington, D.C.: DHHS.

BENEDEK, T. (1956). Toward the biology of the depressive constellation. *J. Amer. Psychoanal. Assn.*, 4:389–427.

BIBRING, E. (1953). The mechanism of depression. In *Affective Disorders*, ed. P. Greenacre, pp. 13–48. New York: Int. Univ. Press.

EISSLER, K. R. (1958). Notes on problems of technique in the psychoanalytic treatment of adolescents. *Psychoanal. Study Child*, 13:223–254.

ERIKSON, E. H. (1950). *Childhood and Society.* New York: Norton, rev. ed., 1957.

FERENCZI, S. (1931). Child analysis in the analysis of adults. *Int. J. Psychoanal.*, 12:468–482.

FREUD, A. (1927). Four lectures on child analysis. *W.*, 1:3–69.

—— (1965). Normality and pathology in childhood. *W.*, 6.

—— (1970). Child analysis as a subspecialty of psychoanalysis. *W.*, 7:204–219.

FREUD, S. (1909). Analysis of a phobia in a five-year-old boy. *S.E.*, 10:3–149.

—— (1916–17). Introductory lectures on psycho-analysis. *S.E.*, 16 & 17.

—— (1918). From the history of an infantile neurosis. *S.E.*, 17:3–123.

—— (1919). Lines of advance in psycho-analytic therapy. *S.E.*, 17:157–168.

—— (1925). An autobiographical study. *S.E.*, 20:3–74.

—— (1926). The question of lay analysis. *S.E.*, 20:179–258.

—— (1933). New introductory lectures on psycho-analysis. *S.E.*, 22:3–182.

—— (1939). Moses and monotheism. *S.E.*, 23:3–137.

—— (1950). Extracts from the Fliess papers. *S.E.*, 1:175–280.

GALTON, F. (1882). *Inquiries into Human Faculty and Its Development.* London: Eugenesis Society, 1951.

GLOVER, E. (1955). *The Technique of Psychoanalysis.* New York: Int. Univ. Press.

GREENSON, R. R. (1972). Beyond transference and interpretation. *Int. J. Psychoanal.*, 53:213–218.

JOFFE, W. & SANDLER, J. (1965). Notes on pain, depression, and individuation. *Psychoanal. Study Child*, 20:394–424.

JONES, E. (1955). *Sigmund Freud.* London: Hogarth Press.

KLEIN, M. (1927). Symposium on child analysis. In *Contributions to Psycho-Analysis 1921–1945*, pp. 152–184. London: Hogarth Press, 1948.

—— (1930). The psychotherapy of the psychosis. Ibid., pp. 251–253.

—— (1935). A contribution to the psychogenesis of manic-depressive states. Ibid., pp. 282–310.

MAHLER, M. S. (1966). Notes on the development of basic moods. In *Psychoanalysis—A General Psychology*, ed. R. M. Loewenstein, L. M. Newman, M. Schur, and A. J. Solnit, pp. 152–168. New York: Int. Univ. Press.

NEUBAUER, P. B. (1979). The role of insight in psychoanalysis. *J. Amer. Psychoanal. Assn. Suppl.*, 27:29–40.

PIAGET, J. (1922). Symbolic thought and the thought of the child. *Arch. Psychol.*, 18:273.

SANDLER, J. & JOFFE, W. G. (1965). Notes on childhood depression. *Int. J. Psychoanal.*, 46:88–96.

SEARLES, H. F. (1965). *Collected Papers on Schizophrenia and Related Subjects.* New York: Int. Univ. Press.

WINNICOTT, D. W. (1952). Psychoses and child care. In *Collected Papers*, pp. 219–228. New York: Basic Books, 1958.

———— (1954a). The depressive position in normal emotional development. Ibid., pp. 262–277.

———— (1954b). Metapsychological and clinical aspects of regression within the psycho-analytical set-up. Ibid., pp. 278–294.

———— (1974). *Playing and Reality*. London: Tavistock Publications.

Causal Explanation in Science and in Psychoanalysis

Implications for Writing a Case Study
MARSHALL EDELSON, M.D., Ph.D.

IN RESPONSE TO THOSE WHO DEMAND EPIDEMIOLOGIC AND EXPERI-
mental tests of psychoanalytic theory (e.g., Grunbaum, 1984), I
have argued that the case study, now held in disrepute, is nevertheless necessary to test psychoanalytic hypotheses and, if
properly formulated, can indeed test, not merely generate, hypotheses (Edelson, 1984). I have in addition described various
kinds of scientific arguments relating hypothesis and data that
can be used in case studies to provide support for the credibility
of psychoanalytic propositions (Edelson, 1985).

In this paper I do not take for granted, as I have previously,
the current standard paradigm of explanation and hypothesis
testing. Instead I take as a starting point Freud's own view of
what science is all about and the strategy of explanation he used
in his case study of the Wolf-Man (1918). There he tells a causal
story. He makes use of a causal pattern rather than a covering
law model of explanation. He makes use of both etiological explanations, in which a cause is external to its effect, and constitutive explanations, in which a cause is a relation among inter-

Professor of psychiatry, Yale University; director of research in the Outpatient Division of Yale's Community Mental Health Center; and member of the
Western New England Institute for Psychoanalysis.

This paper owes something to the oral discussions and written presentations
of Eric Bilsky, Stuart Dunbar, David Edelson, Kurt Feigl, Erika Geetter, Daniel
Kosoy, and Scott Masters, members of a college seminar on Freud's case studies
I taught in the fall of 1984 at Yale University.

nal constituents of an effect. Any evaluation of the validity of one of Freud's explanations should take into account the kind of explanation it is.

I write this paper to confound psychoanalysts (especially of a hermeneutic bent), philosophers of science, methodologists, and other members of the academic community who doubt that the psychoanalytic case study can provide support for the scientific credibility of psychoanalytic theory. (It is also true that I write in part because I believe that, regrettably, most case studies in the psychoanalytic literature are not written in such a way that they meet criteria for such support.)

I argue three points: (1) Freud's intent in his case studies was to provide empirical evidence for causal claims. Although he was not always successful in achieving this objective, there is something to learn from his example even when he ran into difficulty. (2) Freud's strategy of explanation, although it involves reference to psychological entities, is based on the same conception of the causal structure of the world that informs causal explanation in the natural sciences—notwithstanding that his work does not conform to the paradigm of explanation (and ideas about hypothesis testing that go with this paradigm) dominating contemporary philosophy of science. (3) The psychoanalytic case study, when it successfully meets—as often it does not—*criteria of adequacy* implied by my analysis of Freud's explanatory intent and strategy, can indeed provide evidence capable of supporting not only the scientific credibility of empirical generalizations in psychoanalysis but the credibility of causal explanations involving theoretical entities as well.

FREUD'S STRATEGY OF EXPLANATION

THE PROBLEM OF THE RETROSPECTIVE STUDY

Freud begins by issuing some disclaimers. He acknowledges that a study of a childhood illness based on a later account of it by an adult patient, although instructive, is not as likely to be as convincing as a study of the child's illness at the time he suffered it. He points out, however, that the study of the child has disadvantages; the material is less rich, especially because words and thoughts have to be supplied to the child.

The issue here has to do with the many problems which have to be addressed in establishing both facts and causal connections retrospectively. It is difficult to argue convincingly from the retrospective reports of an analysand alone that particular childhood events (actual or imagined) such as "the primal scene" really did occur and occurred at particular times. Even if one accepts that an event did occur, it is even more difficult to argue from such reports alone that the event was in fact the cause of the analysand's much later behavior or symptoms.[1] Freud struggled with these difficulties throughout the Wolf-Man's psychoanalysis, and the strain is evident in the case study. The extent to which these problems are at least partially solved in a retrospective case study determines how credible its conclusions are.

THE PROBLEM OF PRESUPPOSITIONS

Freud makes a somewhat more sweeping disclaimer—one which might be taken as made to evade the consequences of failing to construct a convincing argument. He has not published the case study, he writes, to convince those who are skeptical and refuse to accept the word of the scientific investigator, but has published it only to provide new facts for those already convinced by their own clinical experiences.

About what is this conviction Freud mentions? He is not explicit. Surely, not his conclusions, which he will argue follow from the data he presents in his case study. Does he mean that the reader for whom he writes is one able to accept that the facts are as the investigator reports them to be? If the facts are the patient's reports, as they are in this case, and not empirical generalizations, then Freud's expectation of his reader does not seem unreasonable. However, questions might arise if a reader were to distrust the investigator's memory or written reconstructions of what the patient has reported.

More probably, Freud expects that his reader will be able to accept, at least provisionally, inferences made in the course of

1. Just how difficult this is in a psychoanalysis, Kris (1956a, 1956b) shows. But Gould's (1986) Darwin-as-a-historical-methodologist showed what scientific arguments can make hypotheses about time-remote events scientifically credible.

the argument about the patient, when these inferences are based on what the patient reports in conjunction with parts of psychoanalytic theory that are presumed to have previously been shown to be scientifically credible. For example, Freud makes inferences in interpreting the wolf dream that presuppose his theory of dreams.

This expectation remains troublesome, because, even if a certain knowledge of psychoanalysis (whether based on clinical experience or not) is necessary, the convictions of a knowledgeable reader too may be groundless. That is, by objective scientific standards the presupposed propositions may not previously have been adequately established as scientifically credible. Furthermore, even a knowledgeable reader can be skeptical about the status of such propositions. If questions about presupposed propositions are likely to arise in a reader's mind, the author should refer him to some other study or studies in which there is at least some valid argument for the scientific credibility of these propositions—not, as is so often the case, merely an enumeration of anecdotes or vignettes that are consistent with them.

A CAUSAL STORY

Freud tells a *causal* story. He links particular causes to particular effects. A particular cause may not generally (in all other cases) produce this particular effect, although psychoanalytic theory may postulate that a particular cause *of this type* may in general produce a particular effect *of this type*.

Those regarding psychoanalysis as a hermeneutic discipline regularly overlook that the story told is a *causal* story, which makes causal claims. These claims require substantiation.

1. *The existence of causes.* The causes must be shown to exist. The noun "cause" refers to an actual event, state of affairs, or entity that possesses the power to produce an effect. The verb "cause" refers not to a conceptual or logical relation between facts but rather to a brute existential connection between facts. A causal connection is not part of a thought about what is out there in reality; it is a part of what is out there in reality.

Freud, believing that unconscious psychological entities are causes, exerts himself to demonstrate that these entities actually exist in the patient's mind; they are not just conceptual fictions or mere figures of speech. The ability of an investigator to intervene and manipulate causes, especially when these causes are hypothetical, and even to use hypothetical entities to produce effects in domains other than those in which they serve an explanatory role, argues for their existence (Hacking, 1983). For this reason, the importance of the role of hypnosis in the origins of psychoanalysis cannot be underestimated, for here the investigator is able to implant an idea which clearly has causal efficacy with respect to the subject's subsequent actions, although throughout the course of these actions the subject remains unconscious of it.

Freud is constructing a causal account, not simply arguing for the therapeutic efficacy of a procedure. Therefore, he is rightfully concerned in this case study with his patient's immediate and long-term responses to his interpretations. His interventions are meant to influence the properties and powers of unconscious entities, which actually exist in the patient's mind.[2] The efficacy of interpretative interventions is a major argument in psychoanalysis for the existence of the unconscious ideas it postulates as causal. Establishing that efficacy in studies of the analysand's responses to interpretation throughout the psychoanalytic process should, therefore, have a high priority in psychoanalytic research.[3]

Freud's treatment of causes in this case study is of major importance to psychoanalytic theory, because here the question of the relative roles of external traumas and fantasies looms large. One of Freud's few discussions of the kinds of criteria that might be used to distinguish memories of actual events from memories based on fantasies occurs in this case study. Following Freud's

2. So Freud (1918) mobilized his patient's incredulity, and "then had the satisfaction of seeing his doubt dwindle away, as in the course of the work his bowel began, like a hysterically affected organ, to 'join in the conversation,' and in a few weeks' time recovered its normal functions after their long impairment" (p. 76).

3. "The patient accepted this [construction]. . . , and appeared to confirm it by producing 'transitory symptoms'. A further additional piece which I had proposed . . . had to be dropped. The material of the analysis did not react to it" (Freud, 1918, p. 80).

conjecture that the sudden change in the patient's character
after the summer of his third year was in part at least the result of
a supposed castration threat by the patient's governess during
that summer, the patient reported some dreams, which involved
material concerned with aggressive actions against his sister or
governess and punishments he received because of these. But
the content was vague, and the dreams gave the impression of
making use of the material in different ways. Freud concludes:
"the correct reading of these ostensible reminiscences became
assured: it could only be a question of phantasies, which the
dreamer had made on the subject of his childhood at some time
or other, probably at the age of puberty, and which had now
come to the surface again in this unrecognizable form" (p. 19).
On the other hand:

> . . . his seduction by his sister was certainly not a phantasy. Its
> credibility was increased by some information which had never
> been forgotten and which dated from a later part of his life,
> when he was grown up. A cousin who was more than ten years
> his elder told him in a conversation about his sister that he very
> well remembered what a forward and sensual little thing she
> had been: once, when she was a child of four or five, she had sat
> on his lap and opened his trousers to take hold of his penis
> [p. 21].

2. *The time relation between cause and effect.* Causes must be
shown to exist prior to or simultaneously with their putative
effects. The relation between cause and effect is not symmetrical
as is, in contrast, the relation between variables in generalizations about co-occurrence or correlation. Establishing the facts
of chronology is especially important when cause is held to be
prior to effect. Just one way to demonstrate chronology is, as in
an experiment, to intervene and manipulate the cause, and observe what follows this intervention. This way is, however, not
available in the psychoanalytic situation, where a retrospective
reconstruction of chronology is at issue.

There can be no question that Freud was well aware of the
importance of chronology to a causal account. For example, he
questions whether one attitude in his patient existed simultaneously with, or replaced, another.

Whether these contradictory sorts of attitudes towards animals were really in operation simultaneously, or whether they did not more probably replace one another, but if so in what order and when—to all these questions his memory could offer no decisive reply. He was also unable to say whether his naughty period was *replaced* by a phase of illness or whether it persisted right through the latter [p. 16].

The incessant attention to chronology that Freud pays throughout the Wolf-Man case is not motivated simply by his wish to show that the facts of the case favor his own explanation of phenomena, as caused by sexual experiences and motives stemming from *very early* periods of childhood, over Jung's explanation of the same phenomena, as caused by difficulties in coping with current tasks in *adult* life and especially failures in fulfilling high cultural aspirations. Much more, Freud's attention to chronology is motivated by the necessity to substantiate causal claims.

In his attempt to derive the chronology of remote events from a much later account of them, Freud was not, as one should expect, completely successful. His struggles with the problem are manifested in inconsistencies and contradictions in the way he dealt with it. In the text he writes "*certainly* before his fourth year," whereas the editor notes that "In the editions before 1924 this read '*perhaps* in his sixth year'" (p. 13; my italics). The comment "He *must* have been very small at that time" is followed by this note: "Two and a half years old. It was possible later on to determine almost all the dates with *certainty*" (p. 14; my italics). Freud does not reveal his method for determining any of the dates with such certainty. This omission is serious with respect to his argument that the data of the case study support his causal account, because even the plausibility of much of his causal account—to say nothing of its credibility—so much depends on chronology.

Indeed, any psychoanalyst can confirm how difficult it is in fact to establish chronology with any certainty in the psychoanalytic situation. The difficulty is exemplified by many passages from Freud's account (see pp. 15, 37, 76). However, his frequent claims of certainty about chronology cannot help but

shake the reader's confidence in the accuracy, perhaps even the
honesty, of Freud's account of the facts, leaving aside the question of his explanation of them.[4]

I do not myself believe that the problem here lies in Freud's
character but rather with a limitation in his conceptual preferences and knowledge. He is concerned to maintain a strict determinism, and statistical reasoning and probability, so much a part
of contemporary science, and so necessary in dealing with uncertainty, do not seem available to him. He rarely relativizes his
conclusions to current knowledge: this is what I can assert now,
but I do not know what other factors may eventually turn out to
make a difference or how much of a difference they might make.
That there are irreducibly random processes in the world is, of
course, a notion he rejected.

Now we can say that it would have been better if Freud had
indicated even roughly the probability that supposed states of
affairs had occurred in the way he supposed, and in each case
exactly what evidence led him to even an estimation of that
probability. The moral for the writer of a case study, if he wishes
to retain the reader's confidence, is to avoid Freud's example
here, acknowledging uncertainty where it exists and qualifying
his conclusions accordingly. (Such a stance is, of course, just what
one would expect a psychoanalyst to have as he offers explanations to an analysand in the psychoanalytic situation.)

It is also possible that Freud at times is so positive about a
chronological inference on theoretical grounds. He has inferred
a chronology from parts of psychoanalytic theory that he regards as not in question in this case study. For example, we have
the following passage. "I naturally assumed that these obvious
symptoms of an obsessional neurosis belonged to a somewhat
later time and stage of development than the signs of anxiety
and the cruel treatment of animals" (p. 17). Freud does not refer
the reader to the grounds for his assumption. Even though the

---

4. "*No doubt* was left in the analysis that these passive trends had made their
appearance at the same time as the active-sadistic ones, or very soon after
them" (p. 26; my italics). "Since Christmas Day was also his birthday, it now
became possible to establish with *certainty* the date of the dream and of the
change in him which proceeded from it. It was immediately before his fourth
birthday" (p. 35; my italics).

reader with some knowledge of the psychoanalytic theory of development may guess what these grounds were, I do not recommend that a writer follow Freud's example here either. Psychoanalysis is a body of knowledge that is important to a wider intellectual and scientific community than that comprised by psychoanalytic practitioners. In its documentation, it should follow the scholarly practices, and accept the standards, of that community.

3. *Causal powers.* The writer of a case study must show that a cause has the power to produce its effects by virtue of its structure or properties, and also just how—by virtue of what processes or mechanisms—its causal influence is propagated from one space-time locale to another.

Freud attributes properties and causal powers to unconscious mental contents and processes different from those possessed by conscious mental contents and processes.[5]

He describes *mental operations* (mechanisms), which his causes set into motion. These mental operations transform psychological entities. Such operations are not exhausted by a list of defense mechanisms. Examples are:

a. Substitution of one object for another as the object of a mental state or event. Examples: the patient replacing his sister with his governess as the object of his anger; replacing his sister with his nurse, and then his nurse with his father, as the object of his sexual wishes; replacing others with himself as the object of his sadistic wishes; replacing himself in his fantasies with unidentified boys or an heir to the throne as the object of his sadistic wishes.

b. Substitution of one kind of mental state or event for another. Examples: replacing one kind of wish (to play with his penis) with another (to torment others); replacing *memories* of himself as a passive victim with *fantasies* of himself as an active aggressor.

---

5. "Our bewilderment arises only because we are always inclined to treat unconscious mental processes like conscious ones and to forget the profound differences between the two psychical systems . . . the whole process is characteristic of the way in which the unconscious works. A repression is something very different from a condemning judgement" (p. 78ff.).

c. Altering the intensity or importance of a mental state or event. Example: exaggerating his love for his nurse.

Use of mental operations may be motivated (caused) by a wish to avoid a painful state of affairs—e.g., states of affairs in which loss, shame, or guilt are experienced.

4. *Rival explanations.* The investigator must argue that it is more likely, given his data and the way they were obtained, that what he claims produced the effect in which he is interested did in fact cause it, rather than some other factor which might have done so.

Freud argues that the data of his case study favor his explanatory account of all the phenomena over Jung's and others' (1918, pp. 7, 48–60, 103). His account gives causal priority to childhood traumas or fantasies occurring well before culture impinges in any direct way on a child and well before the child aspires to realize "higher" cultural values and aims. The rival account, which gives causal priority to cultural influences, postulates that the fantasies a patient reports are formed later in life and merely carried backward to childhood.

Freud also argues that data favor his explanatory account of such specific phenomena as the patient's inveterate heterosexual object choice and the patient's sudden change of behavior in his third year of life. Adler would have given another explanation of the former (p. 22f.), and the boy's relatives do give another explanation of the latter (p. 15).

Freud's determination to refute rival views is not, from the point of view of science, a fault. Case studies that have a strong impact, changing the beliefs held about a particular domain, almost always achieve this effect because of a convincing argument that the data reported favor the investigator's conjectures over rival conjectures. An investigator should make explicit what rival conjecture he is attempting to eliminate and what data provide a warrant for dismissing it.

COVERING LAW MODEL VS. CAUSAL MODEL

The telling of a causal story as an explanation bears little resemblance to the received view of scientific explanation, the so-called covering law model. "According to the 'received view,' particular facts are explained by subsuming them under general laws, while general regularities are explained by subsumption under still broader laws" (Salmon, 1984, p. 21). Grunbaum (1954) contrasts the covering law model of explanation with causal explanation in the following passage:

> It is crucial to realize that while (a more comprehensive law) G entails (a less comprehensive law) L logically, thereby providing an explanation of L, G is *not* the 'cause' of L. More specifically, laws are explained *not* by showing the regularities they affirm to be products of the operation of *causes* but rather by recognizing their truth to be special cases of more comprehensive truths [p. 14].[6]

In the Wolf-Man case, Freud certainly does not seem to be subsuming the particulars of his case under some general law, from which—given particular circumstances ("initial conditions")—they might be deduced, and which might be said then to explain them. He is describing a pattern of cause-effect connections; phenomena are explained by the way they are fitted into this pattern.[7]

In explaining phenomena in the Wolf-Man case, Freud moves freely among interrelated but essentially independent theories. These theories are not deducible from each other or from one small set of axioms, postulates, or basic laws. He makes use of the psychoanalytic theory of dreams (e.g., in interpreting the wolf dream as evidence for a primal scene experience or fantasy early in childhood); the psychoanalytic theory of psychosexual development (e.g., in dating the chronology of symptoms); and the psychoanalytic theory of neurosis (e.g., in explaining disturbed behavior as the result of a regression from later to earlier kinds of sexual wishes). Psychoanalytic theory is clearly demonstrated in this case study to be a *concatenated* theory, whose components "enter into a network of relations" and, "typically, converge upon some central point, each specifying one of the factors which plays a part in the phenomenon which the theory is to explain," rather than a *hierarchical* theory, which "is a deductive

---

6. The covering law model of explanation is trenchantly criticized by Cartwright (1983) and Salmon (1984).

7. Kaplan (1964, pp. 327–336) gives a general account of the pattern model of explanation.

pyramid, in which we rise to fewer and more general laws as we move from conclusions to the premises which entail them" (Kaplan, 1964, p. 298f.).

The fruits of Freud's strategy of explanation should be evaluated with this distinction in mind. In the received view (covering law model of explanation, hierarchical theory), deducing particular facts from empirical generalizations, and empirical generalizations or less general laws from more general laws, is a major method for testing conjectures. If a more general law is true, what is predicted—because it follows—from it, is expectable (certain or at least highly probable). If the prediction fails, the more general law is falsified. However, deducing predictions is not necessarily the way to test theory if it is concatenated, as psychoanalytic theory is, and if one uses, as Freud does, a causal pattern model of explanation.

ETIOLOGICAL VS. CONSTITUTIVE EXPLANATION

Freud uses different kinds of causal explanation in his case study. In some instances (e.g., in detailing the responses of the patient to an external trauma—his sister's seduction of him), Freud makes use of *etiological* causal explanations. In other instances (e.g., in explaining a phobic or obsessive symptom as an expression of an internal constellation of conflicting motives), he makes use of *constitutive* explanations.[8] Salmon (1984, pp. 269–270, 275) gives a general account of this distinction.

Etiological explanations postulate causal connections in which cause and effect are at the same level, and causes are external to and impinge upon the system whose properties are to be explained. A given fact is explained "by showing how it came to be the result of antecedent events, processes, and conditions" (Salmon, 1984, p. 269). Example: the effect of one moving medium-sized body upon the motion of another with which it collides.

Constitutive explanations postulate causal connections in which cause and effect are at different levels, and causes are internal to, or constituents of, the system whose properties are to

8. Grunbaum (1984) evaluates psychoanalysis as if its main causal claims were etiological.

be explained. Such explanations exhibit the internal causal structure of what is to be explained. Examples: pressure inside a container is caused by the impact of moving molecules on the sides of a vessel (pressure *is*, or is an expression of, such impacts); temperature is a function of, and is caused by, the velocities of molecules (temperature *is*, or is an expression of, such molecular velocities).

One of Freud's explanations—of the patient's marked change in character during his third year—seems to be a mixture of etiological and constitutive explanation. The patient had repeatedly heard during his adult illness that he had exhibited a marked change of character. Before the summer of his third year, he had been good-natured, tractable, quiet, but after that summer during which he was in the care of an English governess he became discontented and irritable; easily offended, he often screamed in rage. The patient remembered becoming upset when he was not given double presents one Christmas, which was also his birthday. He also remembered tormenting his nurse, whom he loved.

Members of the family offered two explanations of this change in him: the governess irritated him; dissension between the governess and his nurse upset him. Freud implies that these explanations are discredited by the fact that there was no change in the boy's unbearable behavior after the governess was sent away. (This is an example of Freud's use of a datum to exclude alternative explanations of a phenomenon.)

Freud explains the boy's change of character as follows. An external trauma (seduction by his sister, who was also his rival) was a state of affairs some of the aspects of which caused pleasure (penis being touched) and some of the aspects of which caused pain (loss of masculine self-esteem resulting from his passivity). The external trauma caused a wish for a state of affairs that would cause the same kind of pleasure without causing the same kind of pain. That wish motivated (caused) a mental operation (substitution of nurse for sister in the state of affairs desired). An attempt to satisfy the transformed wish caused a new external trauma (nurse's rebuff and castration threat). The new external trauma caused a wish to avoid a repetition of this painful state of affairs. This wish in turn motivated (caused) various mental operations: substitution of father for nurse in the state of affairs desired; substitution of one kind of wish for another (wish to torment others for wish to masturbate); substitution of one object for another in the new desired state of affairs (himself for another as the one to be hurt). His naughty behavior had multiple internal causes—principally, his wish to torment his nurse and others; and his wish to provoke his father into beating him. By a chain of such external and internal causal connections, Freud explains the change in the boy's character.

In another explanation—of the patient's phobic symptoms—Freud gives an essentially constitutive explanation. (He tends to use "express" rather than "cause" when a constitutive explanation is given: "the symptoms express an unconscious conflict.") The phobic symptoms were caused, Freud explains, by the patient's retrospective interpretation of a memory or fantasy of seeing, at a very early age, his mother and father having intercourse, in the light of later sexual researches (and his preoccupation with castration); his simultaneous realization that gratification of his wishes for passive pleasure from his father seemed then to entail his being castrated; the fear of his father aroused by this realization; and displacement of this fear to animals.

PSYCHOANALYTIC EXPLANATION

It is a common mistake to suppose that because psychoanalysis is concerned with meanings or purposes it is not concerned with causal explanation (Edelson, 1985, esp. p. 87). Some writers automatically assume that an explanation in terms of wishes and beliefs cannot be a causal explanation; they mistakenly contrast motivational and causal explanation. But, of course, motives are among the causes of psychological phenomena, as this paper has endeavored to demonstrate.

Often the mistake seems to rest on equating "causal" and "mechanistic" and then "mechanistic" and "machinery." The notion of man as a machine is derided as nineteenth-century science and contrasted with a humanistic view of man. But a mechanistic explanation, no matter what the content, is essentially any explanation that attempts to answer the question "How?"—by what steps, involving what causal processes? An explanation that employs such concepts as "mental operations," "shifts in emphasis," and "alterations in representations" to account for how a cause produces an effect is a mechanistic explanation.

A similar mistake, as Freud emphasized over and over, rests on equating "what is mental" with "what is conscious." This equation is usually made because the possibility that there really are unconscious mental entities is rejected. It is assumed instead that talk of unconscious mental entities must really be talk about neural events. The conviction here is that true causes cannot be mental but must be physical. It is the burden of this paper that this is not so.

To have explanatory knowledge is to have more than descriptive or predictive knowledge. It is to have a knowledge of underlying mechanisms. To understand a cause-effect relation is to know what the causal connection between them is.[9]

A *causal process* is a process that transmits its own structure, its own features, and changes in its own structure from one space-time locale to another, and is therefore capable "of propagating a causal influence from one space-time locale to another" (Salmon, 1984, p. 155). One event *produces* or causally influences another event by means of the causal process connecting them. A causal process *propagates* causal influence from one space-time locale to another. There may be successive intermediate events between cause and effect; these are connected by spatiotemporally continuous causal processes. Both an arrow flying from bowman to target and a memory are examples of causal processes.

I maintain that Freud regards psychological entities as causal processes. These transmit their own structure or features, and changes in their own structures or features, through time. The

9. The account of causality and causal explanation in this paper is from Salmon (1984). Salmon refers primarily to the natural sciences in his discussion of scientific explanation. However, his view of science and scientific explanation is in many ways close to the view one may infer from the Wolf-Man case that Freud himself held. Both adhere to a causal rather than a covering law model of explanation. Both believe in the reality and the causal efficacy of theoretical (nonobservable) entities. ("Atoms" and "unconscious wishes" are nonobservable entities.) Both are "mechanistic."

significance of his abandoned Project was that it served him, even after he abandoned it, as a *model*, exemplifying cause-effect relations. His metapsychology was an expression of his commitment to causal explanation. A case study, such as the Wolf-Man case, tells a causal story; it is a causal explanation of the Wolf-Man's symptoms and their interrelations.

It is especially important to note that causes and effects in a causal story are particulars: "A causal process is an individual entity, and such entities transmit causal influence. An individual process can sustain a causal connection between an individual cause and an individual effect. Statements about such relations need not be construed as disguised generalizations" (Salmon, 1984, p. 182).

A *causal interaction* occurs when two causal processes intersect in space-time and modify each other's structures. The modifications in structure are produced by the interaction and propagated by the causal processes after the interaction. Cause and effect here are *simultaneous*. Both two colliding balls which modify each other's motion and the seduction of the Wolf-Man by his sister (each one a causal process) are examples of causal interactions. (Freud, interestingly enough, goes to some length to describe what happened subsequently to the sister as well as to the Wolf-Man—how each of them might have been modified by this interaction.)

Simpler interactions include the coming together and *fusion* of two causal processes, resulting in one ongoing causal process; and the *bifurcation* of a single causal process, resulting in two ongoing causal processes. Salmon (1984) gives as an example of fusion a snake swallowing a mouse, and as an example of bifurcation an amoeba dividing to form two amoebas. Just so, *condensation*, a mental process, may be considered an example of causal fusion of mental contents, each one of which before fusion was a separate causal process. And Freud certainly seemed to have some kind of causal bifurcation in mind when he spoke of *displacement* as involving the splitting of a mental content and its associated affect, with the content and the affect then as separate causal processes undergoing different vicissitudes. Similarly, differentiations in psychological development may result from causal bifurcations, and the blurring of boundaries between self representations and object representations in introjections and identifications may involve causal fusions.

Two or more causal processes that are physically independent of one another and do not interact with one another but that arise from the same set of conditions are said to have been produced by a *common cause*. Cause here is *prior* to effect. A causal story or pattern may include such constituents as the following: two independent causes produce a common effect; a common cause produces two causal processes that have a common effect.

Although causal processes and interactions may be governed by laws of nature, the same cannot be said about the origination of two or more independent causal processes by a common cause, which involves de facto conditions and nonlawful facts.

Salmon (1984) gives as examples the coincidence that two students' papers are identical, because as it turns out they both independently copied from the same paper, and the coincidence that a number of people became ill at the same time, because as it turns out they all independently ate from the same pot. A similar kind of coincidence, often observed in a psychoanalysis, occurs when an analysand utters exactly the same rather unusual phrase in a number of very different and apparently completely unrelated contexts in the same session, inviting inference to a common cause—e.g., a hypothetical unconscious state of the analysand.

What is needed here now is an account of psychoanalytic explanation—however tentative, crude, or inadequate at this time—that will fit Freud's strategy of explanation in his case study, and that at a minimum will at least approximate the kind of explanations given by a psychoanalyst to an analysand.

The domain of psychoanalysis is comprised by psychological entities, and some of their properties and relations.[10] Psychological entities are intentional—i.e., they include as constituents mental states or events that are *directed to, about,* or *of* some object or state of affairs.[11] Some examples of psychological entities are:

10. My position is that psychoanalysis, like other sciences, explains a limited domain. It is a theory of motivation and therefore cannot explain "everything." It is not a "general psychology" (Edelson, 1986).

11. In this account of intentional entities, I more or less follow Searle (1983).

thinking or believing something; having a feeling about a thing, someone, or some state of affairs; wishing for or wanting something; perceiving something; remembering something; imagining something; planning to do (including to say) something; and intending to do (including to say) something.

The *structure* of a psychological entity consists of three components: an *agent;* a *mental state* or *event* that is directed to, about, or of some object or state of affairs; a *representation* of that object or state of affairs. (The structure of a state of affairs consists of an object and a property, or of a number of objects and the relation between or among them.) A representation may be linguistic, a linguistically interpreted image, or—questionably—nonlinguistic. The object or state of affairs to which a mental state or event is directed may itself be a psychological entity. Examples: I feel guilty about this wish. I want to do it.

Psychological entities have *conditions of satisfaction.* For example, they are satisfied if a certain object exists or state of affairs obtains. A perception is satisfied by the existence in the here and now of what is perceived. A belief is satisfied by adequate evidence for the existence of a state of affairs that corresponds to what is believed. A memory is satisfied by the past existence of the state of affairs remembered. A wish is satisfied by the existence of a state of affairs that corresponds to what is wished. It is sometimes part of an etiological explanation in psychoanalysis to attribute the origin or exacerbation of pathology to the fact that conditions of satisfaction do not exist.

A psychological entity is *comprehensible* (either to an agent or to another) if it is in accord or consistent with a set of beliefs and wishes that are easily accessible to the agent's consciousness.

Psychoanalysis seeks to explain *inhibitions, compulsions, representational or other anomalies,* and *mistakes or failures.* Examples of these are: neurotic symptoms, dreams, and parapraxes (e.g., slips of the tongue or pen, forgetting something or forgetting to do something one planned to do, doing just the opposite of what one planned to do). What this turns out to mean is that psychoanalysis seeks to explain particular kinds of properties that psychological entities may have.

Inhibitions, compulsions, representational or other anomalies, and mistakes or failures are appropriate subjects of psychoanalytic explanation insofar as they are not explicable, given present knowledge, as the effect of a defect in the design of the physical organism (genetic endowment); a lesion of the physical organism; or environmental conditions (e.g., inaccessibility of opportunities, facilities, or resources). A stronger requirement would be that the explicability of a phenomenon is inconceivable in terms of such causal factors. The paradigm is a conversion symptom that makes no sense in terms of well-established knowledge about anatomy.

Another way to express this idea is that when there is "something wrong" at the psychological level, and there is no condition, event, or process fitting the description "something is wrong" at the neurophysiological level or in the social situation that is sufficient to produce the "something wrong" at the psychological level, we have a psychological phenomenon that is an appropriate subject of psychoanalytic explanation.

This is not to say that no physical or situational factor is *causally relevant* in an explanation of such phenomena. Endowment may determine an agent's capacities and, therefore, what defensive strategies he is likely to use. The example of, or identifications with, others may also influence what defensive strategies he is likely to use. Causal relevance means that the presence or absence of a factor (like the presence or absence of oxygen in getting a fire started) makes a difference, but that factor does not in itself necessarily have the power to cause a phenomenon. It may be correlated with the occurrence of the phenomenon, but there is no mechanism by virtue of which it in itself can produce the phenomenon.

The identification of a phenomenon as an appropriate subject for psychoanalytic explanation then presupposes knowledge about the causal powers of neurophysiological and environmental factors. (This does not imply, however, that psychoanalysis as a scientific discipline is responsible for or capable of generating such knowledge.) The set of what is to be explained by psychoanalysis is a fuzzy set with fluid boundaries, for its members may change as knowledge of physical organisms and the causal efficacy of situational factors changes. There will always be borderline cases. It is assumed, however, that it is also true that there always will be unequivocal cases whose features are such as to defy explanation in terms of neurophysiological or situational factors, given what is already securely known about such factors.

In explaining inhibitions, compulsions, representational anomalies, or mistakes or failures—regarded as properties of psychological entities—psychoanalysis tries to answer two kinds of questions. *Why* does a psychological entity have such a property? This is a question about what motives (what other psychological entities) cause psychological entities to have such properties. *How* do these motives cause psychological entities to have such properties? This is a question about causal powers—about mental mechanisms or operations.

In general, psychoanalysis explains a psychological entity (easily accessible to consciousness) as a substitution for a set of unconscious psychological entities. Mental operations have effected transformations upon a set of unconscious psychological entities, and this process has produced the psychological entity to be explained.

1. The psychoanalyst infers the existence of unconscious psychological entities. The mental states or events that are constituents of these unconscious psychological entities are directed to imagined states of affairs (fantasies).

2. There are two kinds of imagined states of affairs, those the analysand wishes to actualize and those the analysand wishes to avoid. The imagined states of affairs the analysand wishes to actualize are states of affairs in which the analysand is experiencing sexual or sensual pleasure.[12] The imagined states of affairs the analysand wishes to avoid are states of affairs in which the analysand is experiencing pain: helplessness; loss of love, of a needed other, of a body part, of whatever might be needed to achieve pleasure; shame (he is being exposed, ridiculed, or belittled); guilt (he is being scolded or criticized).

3. The psychoanalyst infers the existence of unconscious beliefs that states of affairs the analysand wishes to actualize will inevitably be followed by states of affairs he wishes to avoid, or will make impossible other states of affairs the analysand wishes to actualize. In other words, the psychoanalyst infers the existence of unconscious conflicts and dilemmas.

12. To avoid difficulties discussed elsewhere (Edelson, 1986), I omit here mention of aggressive wishes.

4. The psychoanalyst infers that the analysand is tempted to actualize a state of affairs that he believes will have one or more of these dread consequences, and that his unconscious realization that he is so tempted generates anxiety. The psychoanalyst infers that the anxiety motivates the analysand to develop and carry out strategies for resolving the conflict or dilemma in such a way that anxiety may be avoided.

5. The psychoanalyst infers the nature of these strategies—what mental operations the analysand has used upon what psychological entities to achieve this resolution. The psychological entities to be explained realize a state of affairs which to some extent and in some way yields pleasure, and yields it in such a way that the analysand is able to some extent and in some way to escape the consequences he wishes to avoid. The state of affairs resulting from the use of these mental operations is to some extent and in some way a realization of the conditions of satisfaction for unconscious wishes.

The usual list of defense mechanisms does not exhaust the possible strategies. In addition, defense mechanisms are often confused with mental operations which come into play in any unconscious mental processes; the use of such a mental operation does not necessarily serve defense. Possibly, condensation is such a mental operation (Edelson, 1982).

How does psychoanalysis explain that a particular mental operation has been used by an agent? Often, it postulates that a relation among the representations belonging to more than one psychological entity causes a choice of mental operations. Paradigmatic example: This representation reminds the analysand of that representation, because of certain similarities between them, similarities that are relevant to his wishes and fears. Therefore, the mental operation of displacement is used. Furthermore, mental operations are used which fulfill at one and the same time a number of wishes or resolve a number of conflicts or dilemmas. Constraints on the choice of strategies or mental operations include the analysand's psychological capacities (e.g., cognition, language, memory, perception), knowledge of which is presupposed, not generated, by psychoanalysis (Edelson, 1986).

An analysand may maintain eternal vigilance—always prepared to avoid what is feared and to grasp what is desired—in order to avoid anxiety. The analysand can perceive any situation as one involving or at least promising pleasure or pain by focusing on characteristics (imagined or real) of others in his situation that are relevant to his wishes and fears, and by attributing to others in his situation motives, intentions, or attitudes toward himself. Interpreting then every situation in such a way that it yields some pleasure and enables him at the same time to evade an imagined danger becomes a strategy for effecting a resolution of an unconscious conflict or dilemma. So the patient appears compelled to experience the same state of affairs over and over.

Here, of course, is the basis for the importance of transference phenomena in both psychoanalytic therapy and research. Grunbaum (1984) argues that the psychoanalyst is begging the question when he uses here-and-now transference phenomena as evidence for etiological causal explanations. The psychoanalyst claims that current mental representations of particular past events or fantasies are constitutive causes of current behavior, and then goes on to claim that therefore past actual events or fantasies are etiological causes of the analysand's symptoms. However, the characterization of transference phenomena as involving a transfer from the past to the present assumes that the past occurrences existed, and furthermore that their causal influence has been propagated through time by accurate mental representations of them. But the truth of these assumptions is the very question at issue.

Transference phenomena are nevertheless nonquestion-begging evidence for constitutive explanations. Such explanations involve inferences about causally efficacious psychological entities existing or occurring in the here and now (including, e.g., memories or fantasies of the past, in which early important objects play a part in the states of affairs represented). Explaining the origin of such causally efficacious psychological entities is logically independent of the constitutive explanation.

6. The psychoanalyst may offer a genetic explanation. He may locate the origin of present unconscious wishes and beliefs in the analysand's infantile experiences with his body and with parents and siblings, and attempt to show how the influence of these was transmitted and altered through time by developmental and

environmental factors. However, genetic explanations are at a different level from constitutive explanations, in which cause lies in the presence of an unconscious conflict or dilemma in the here and now, even if current unconscious wishes for pleasure are postulated to be infantile (the kind of wishes a child might have).

It is true that Freud and others do try to explain the existence of unconscious conflicts and dilemmas in terms of origin in early childhood; as a statement of remote etiology, such formulations are part of psychoanalytic theory. However, the Wolf-Man case has features (e.g., difficulties in establishing chronology of remote events) which suggest that the psychoanalytic case study might in general offer stronger evidence for the scientific credibility of constitutive explanations (a current symptom is caused by or expresses a currently existing and active unconscious conflict)—or for etiological explanations which involve very recent, putatively causal events (a recent event, perhaps occurring in the psychoanalytic situation itself, causes a phenomenon such as an intensification or transient appearance of a neurotic symptom)—than it can offer for the scientific credibility of etiological explanations which involve remote, putatively causal events.

7. The psychoanalyst also may show an analysand what consequences the resolution he has attempted has for adaptation. This kind of explanation, too, is at a different level from his constitutive explanation of the analysand's resolution as an effect of an internal complex of unconscious psychological entities and mental operations, for here the analysand's resolution itself becomes the cause of other effects—his relations with external reality—and these effects in turn may act as causes of additional difficulties for the analysand.

In summary, the phenomena to be explained—inhibitions, compulsions, representational or other anomalies, and mistakes or failures of the kind described—are psychogenic or, to use Wollheim's felicitous term (1981), ideogenic. Their causes are unconscious psychological entities and the transformations effected upon these by unconscious mental operations. In every case, the existence of a phenomenon is explained as to some extent and in some way an actualization of the conditions of satisfaction of unconscious psychological entities.

IMPLICATIONS FOR PSYCHOANALYTIC RESEARCH: WRITING A PSYCHOANALYTIC CASE STUDY

A psychoanalytic case study may be written to support an empirical generalization, or to tell a causal story.

EMPIRICAL GENERALIZATIONS

A psychoanalyst might want to establish that certain kinds of observable phenomena co-occur or are correlated, and what the strength of their relationship is.[13] (Freud's Wolf-Man case has no such objective.) The requirements for such a case study are:

1. An empirical generalization, which goes beyond the particular observations made, is clearly and prominently stated.

2. The phenomena are, in principle at least, intersubjectively observable, and documented in such a way that different judges can agree independently of each other about what they are. Durable records of a psychoanalyst's and an analysand's utterances meet this requirement.

3. The author specifies what observations would count against the generalization, and recounts the attempts he has made to discover if these exist. If he discovers any such facts, and does not reject the generalization, he uses them to limit its scope—he specifies under just what conditions, in which observations might be made of this case, he would expect the generalization to hold.

4. Hypotheses are underdetermined by data. That is, no set of data can decide that one and only one hypothesis is true. (Many different lines can be drawn through the same sample of points.) Since there are many empirical generalizations that will account for the same observations, the author gives some argument why his observations are better evidence for his empirical generalization than for at least one comparable competing or rival one. For example, he may claim that he makes a higher proportion of correct guesses to incorrect guesses with this generalization than with some other about as yet unobserved phenomena (in later

---

13. Luborsky's studies (1967, 1973, 1974) are valuable exemplars of this kind of study in psychoanalysis and they are discussed as such by Edelson (1984).

sessions, if the generalization has been made on the basis of data from earlier sessions). To make this argument, he must keep count of his incorrect guesses as well as his correct guesses. Other arguments, many of which are nonquantitative, are also available to an author (Edelson, 1984, 1985).

5. His observations and the way they have been obtained may favor his over a rival generalization. However, he still must consider what factors in the situation of observation could have resulted in his obtaining just these observations even if his generalization were false. He presents some argument—it may be a nondesign argument—for dismissing at least one such factor as a plausible alternative explanation of his having obtained the data he claims favor his empirical generalization over a rival.

6. He makes clear in what other cases or kinds of cases he claims the same generalization will hold, and offers some grounds for this claim.[14]

If the relationship thus established has not in addition been demonstrated to be a causal relationship, it is not an explanation of anything. If it were true that most of the time if an analysand talks about fire and water early in a session, he talks about ambitions later in that session (Meehl, 1983), such an empirical generalization (even if it held universally rather than assigned some probability to the later event) would not be an explanation of the fact that an analysand in a particular session talked about ambition later in a session in which he had earlier talked about fire and water. The generalization (together with the occurrence of the antecedent event) entails that the later event will occur (with some degree of probability), but it does not *explain* its occurrence. Nor does the occurrence of the prior event itself explain the occurrence of the later event.

Such an empirical generalization—even if one were able to represent it, which seems unlikely, by a sophisticated mathematical equation, describing a functional relationship among quantities—is, at most, a regularity or a pattern in nature to be explained, not by subsuming it under some more comprehen-

14. That these six requirements can be met in a case study is argued in Edelson (1984, 1985). But for reasons to have some reservations about this use of the case study in psychoanalysis, see Danziger (1985).

sive generalization in a deductive argument, but by discovering the causal nexus in which it is embedded. What the writer of this kind of case study has achieved—it is not a small achievement— is to establish that such a regularity does in fact exist, and that it calls for explanation.

One could well argue that it is the facts of psychoanalysis that are most in question in the scientific community, and that such studies as these are badly needed to establish the scientific credibility of psychoanalytic theory. I have already reviewed recent developments in the methodology of the single case study (1984), which make it feasible to use single case studies to demonstrate empirical generalizations. However, contrary to what some might think, establishing empirical generalizations is not the sine qua non of science. For those who think so, a case study such as Freud's must be baffling indeed.

WRITING A CAUSAL STORY

1. The writer organizes a set of facts about a case so that they tell a story about causes and effects. A fact in such a story is neither just something to be explained nor something that explains, but is usually cause in relation to some effect(s) and effect in relation to some cause(s)—a constituent in a pattern of cause and effect relations. Such a pattern may be, but need not be, a time-ordered sequence of events; feedback loops, for example, may also belong to such a pattern.

The writer may begin by specifying the phenomena that he intends to explain, essentially by showing how they are causally interconnected.

> What was the origin of the sudden change in the boy's character? What was the significance of his phobia and of his perversities? How did he arrive at his obsessive piety? And how are all these phenomena interrelated [Freud, 1918, p. 17]?
> But if we put together as the result of the provisional analysis [of the dream] what can be derived from the material produced by the dreamer, we then find before us for reconstruction some such fragments as these:
> *A real occurrence—dating from a very early period—looking—immobility—sexual problems—castration—his father—something terrible* [p. 34].

The difference between facts and inferences is sometimes glossed over in a psychoanalytic case study (Edelson, 1985, esp. p. 83f.). As Freud has intimated in his beginning disclaimers, it is in connection with what is presented as fact and what is presented as inference (rather than in connection with the causal story itself) that the reader is most likely to boggle. Freud goes to some length to show why propositions from his theory of dreams conjoined with statements of the analysand's seem to him to entail the inferences underlined in the passage above, which he then treats as facts whose interrelations will be explicated by his causal story. The writer should follow his example, carefully differentiating facts and inferences, and giving some justification for treating what is inferred as fact.

After presenting a set of facts, the writer then tells a causal story that explains these facts—that is, that places them in a pattern of cause and effect relations. "Story" is an apt term. Cause and effect are events. Each of these occurs in a space-time locale. The process that connects them—producing an effect by propagating causal influence from one space-time locale to another—does so by transmitting its own structure from one space-time locale to another.

2. Locating or specifying a common cause may be an element in a strategy of causal explanation.

a. If improbable events occur—even more improbably—together, the writer infers to a common cause. He notices a coincidence—the occurrence of two improbable events, which supposedly arise from physically independent causal processes, and whose joint occurrence, given the probability of the occurrence of each one, is therefore highly improbable. He infers—since the probability of their joint occurrence, which has in fact occurred, is evidently not so low—that they must have an antecedent common cause.

In other words, if they have a common cause, then the probability of their joint occurrence is greater than would be the case if they were truly independent. The probability of the joint occurrence of independent events is the probability of the occurrence of one multiplied by the probability of the occurrence of the other. If one is able to count the number of occurrences of each kind of event participating in a series of such coincidences and the number of such coincidences, one can calculate the relevant relative frequencies and show that the probability of joint occurrence is greater than would be expected if the events were truly independent. Statistics in a causal framework are evidence (but surely not the only kind of evidence) for causal relations (Salmon, 1984, p. 261).

b. The writer then locates and specifies the common cause, and demonstrates that its structure or features are such as to give rise to causal processes producing the events in question.

c. If the common cause is nonobservable, he justifies the assertion that it is in fact the explanation of the coincidence by describing with as much precision as possible its structure and features, and then using this description to describe how it produces still other causal processes, which lead to still other events—of very different kinds—that can be and are observed.[15]

In general, then, the author should make use of heterogeneous data in writing a causal story—data that are different in kind and that, given background knowledge, there is no reason to assume have any connection with each other. In the Wolf-Man case, Freud explains a behavior change; different symptoms, beginning at different ages; a type of heterosexual object choice—and their interconnections.

A strong argument is made when the same inference (that particular unconscious psychological entities currently exist) can be made from the very different kinds of information available to the psychoanalyst. Examples of such kinds of information include: responses to interpretations, including exacerbation of symptoms or the temporary appearance or reappearance of symptoms; memories, including the analysand's memories of what he has been told about his past by others (what Freud calls

15. The principle of the common cause can be used to justify claims that nonobservable entities, such as unconscious psychological entities, exist. If such a claim is true, different independent methods should lead to the same state of affairs or value. When this in fact happens, that it should be a coincidence is so highly improbable that science proposes instead to accept as credible the existence of the postulated nonobservable entity as the common cause of reaching in each case the same state of affairs or value (Salmon, pp. 211–238).

"direct tradition"); dreams; parapraxes; what the analysand reports of his responses to extra-analytic intercurrent events; daydreams; and the analysand's responses to aspects of and events occurring in the psychoanalytic situation, including his speculations and fantasies about the psychoanalyst.

Similarly, the author of a case study uses the very different parts of a concatenated theory such as psychoanalytic theory to make inferences about nonobservable entities and to forge causal links. Different (interrelated but independent) parts of the theory sometimes suggest different causal factors and different causal connections as the author attempts to tell a causal story. Different parts of the theory may also converge on the same nonobservable psychological entities or mental operations (causal processes or modes of propagation of causal influence).

3. Another element in a case study writer's strategy of explanation, similar to that involving inference to a common cause, involves inferring a causal interaction when modifications in causal processes are observed to be correlated—for example, changes in the Wolf-Man and his sister following their interaction (the seduction).

4. Gaps in a causal story, like coincidences or correlations, call for explanation. The writer notes where there are gaps in his causal story, and infers to causal processes that propagate causal influence in order to close such gaps. Freud, of course, inferred to unconscious psychological entities and processes to account for gaps in the continuity of conscious mental life—gaps, where he looked for causal relatedness between mental contents in consciousness.

5. Another explanatory strategy a writer may use is analogy. He shows, or tells how it has been shown, that an event of a particular kind causes another event of a particular kind. Then he argues by analogy that, since the event he is explaining is similar to that effect, it is caused by a similar cause.[16]

A special case of an argument by analogy is the use of a *model*

16. Salmon (1984, p. 233f.) shows how causal arguments and argument by analogy are used to argue from observables to nonobservables, arguments similar to those used by Freud in arguing for the existence of unconscious entities.

(Cartwright, 1983). A model is a concrete or abstract exemplification of a set of causal relations. Events in the model are interpreted by or coordinated with events in the case study. Causal processes are interpreted by or coordinated with causal processes in the case study. Outcomes of interventions are predicted from the model. Since the model does not include any de facto conditions or nonlawful facts, the predictions usually turn out to be only approximately correct. However, the model, which is a kind of metaphor, is fertile; it suggests what kind of changes in it will result in more accurate predictions. An imaginative application of a sophisticated model (catastrophe theory) to psychoanalytic clinical case material can be found in Sashin (1985).

A model is an idealization. Statements describing entities and their relations in a model are not strictly true of anything but the model itself. However, a model is useful in organizing facts in a system under observation. It raises new questions. It suggests what kinds of things and what properties of these things are causes, and how causal influence is propagated. Mainly, the ability to predict facts, events, or values with ever increasing accuracy, as the model is modified in various attempts to apply it in specific cases, determines just how useful a model is. The use of a model calls for a series of case studies.

ARGUING FOR THE VALIDITY OF A CASE STUDY

1. The writer is careful to distinguish between etiological explanation and constitutive explanation. In general, the case study can give more powerful arguments for accepting a constitutive explanation than for accepting an etiological explanation, especially if the etiological causal factor is remote from the effect of interest. Such an etiological explanation will be strengthened if evidence for intermediate causal connections can be found, but Freud's strenuous and perhaps unique effort in this direction possibly demonstrates the difficulty in supporting such an etiological explanation with data from a case study alone. There is no reason not to write such a case study if it is clear that acceptance of its conclusions must wait for the convergence by other methods of investigation upon the same conclusion.

At the moment, it is not clear what these methods might be, although direct observation of children, despite the drawbacks Freud points out, can surely make a contribution. Epidemiological and experimental evidence is, of course, welcome on specific points; such evidence will have bearing not on the particulars of the causal story but on the theory that has been used for the purposes already described in constructing it. Glymour's bootstrap method (1980), applied by him in explicating one of Freud's arguments in the Rat-Man case, has implications for both etiological and constitutive explanation.

Similarly, the author of a case study will find it difficult to justify explanations of phenomena, where cause or effect is adaptation or maladaptation to extra-analytic reality, using data obtained in the psychoanalytic situation alone. Here, the effect of the analysand's symptoms and character traits upon his relation to external reality is at issue, as well as the extent to which his character traits are the result of responses or adaptation to reality (external etiological causes). It is easy to confuse cause and effect in dealing with such problems. Are impaired object relations, for example, cause or effect?

2. What exactly is the role of rival explanations in justifying a causal story? I do not think that causal stories are underdetermined by data in the same sense that empirical generalizations are. If I tell a causal story in which a bowman shoots an arrow from a taut bow, the arrow flies from one space-time locale to another, and pierces its target, what is the alternative explanation of the effect on the target? It is just the particularities of a causal story, in contrast to mere instances of an empirical generalization, that raise questions in my mind about the underdetermination thesis.

Nevertheless, it is important to ask the following question, at least when there is another *comparable* explanatory account of the same data. What leads to the judgment that an explanation of a phenomenon is a better explanation than a rival explanation of that phenomenon? The writer may make one or more of the following arguments.

a. No rival explanation exists, or a rival explanation exists but is not truly comparable. It may, for example, offer a rival explanation of one or another phenomenon, but it does not offer an explanation for the set of phenomena—one that shows the interrelations of all the facts.

It is, of course, always possible to think up different explanations for each part of a causal story. However, to prefer a congeries of rival explanations for different data, all of which are explained by a causal story, violates the principle of parsimony. It also violates the principle of the common cause; that all these different explanations should be correct seems much more improbable than that one causal story is correct.

Freud emphasizes that his objective is not simply to explain the Wolf-Man's behavior change, phobia, and obsessive piety. Using a covering law model of explanation, one might explain all three of these by one law, e.g., a law involving the causal impact of constitutional defects—or each one of them may be explained as a positive instance of three different laws. But Freud seeks to do something other than that. He seeks to explain the interrelations among the three. He does not explain them as the manifestations of one diagnostic entity or even as three different effects of one cause. He wants to explain how one event, the effect of one set of causes, leads together with additional causes to another event, and this event together with still other causes to another.[17] Here we have the hallmark of dynamic as opposed to nosological explanation.[18] An explanation that purports to ac-

---

17. For an example of this kind of explanation, see the summary of Freud's explanation of the Wolf-Man's symptoms (pp. 63–70, 106–19). As part of his explanatory strategy, Freud distinguishes between the cause of a neurosis and the cause of an attack of a neurosis or of an intensification of a neurotic symptom. "The obsessional neurosis ran its course discontinuously; the first attack was the longest and most intense, and others came on when he was eight and ten, following each time upon exciting causes which stood in a clear relationship to the content of the neurosis" (p. 61). "We already know that, apart from its permanent strength, it [the obsessional neurosis] underwent occasional intensifications" (p. 68).

18. "The genetic approach in psychoanalysis does not deal only with anamnestic data, nor does it intend to show only 'how the past is contained in the present'. Genetic propositions describe why, in past situations of conflict, a specific solution was adopted; why the one was retained and the other dropped, and what causal relation exists between these solutions and later developments" (Hartmann and Kris, 1945, p. 17).

count for phenomena but not for their interrelations is not a comparable rival to an explanation that accounts for both.[19]

b. A more fertile explanation is preferred to a less fertile one. The author's explanation leads to important and interesting questions—in fact, generates an entire research program.[20] Freud's explanation in the Wolf-Man case, for example, leads to such questions—still largely unanswered—as: What determines an agent's choice of mental operations, in general, and with respect to a particular psychological entity at a particular time? Not only why, but how, does a psychological entity become unconscious?

c. The author's inferences, unlike those in a rival account, result in increasingly detailed, precise descriptions of the structure and properties of nonobservable entities; such knowledge leads to new findings and/or an improved fit between case and model. Similarly, an author's constitutive explanation may be more complete than a rival account. It makes use of all the properties of psychological entities that theory suggests are important. It addresses the difference that topographic, economic, dynamic, and structural properties of psychological entities make to a causal story—that such entities are unconscious, that they are ordered on dimensions of priority and intensity, that they are of different kinds and have different and often competing or conflicting conditions of satisfaction.

d. The author's explanation results in the interpolation of causal connections where other accounts leave gaps. Here, Freud's injunction in the Wolf-Man case that an interpretation of a dream must account for all details of the dream comes to mind.

e. The author is able to render implausible claims that his data

19. "I am of course aware that it is possible to explain the symptoms of this period (the wolf anxiety and the disturbance of appetite) in another and simpler manner, without any reference to sexuality or to a pregenital stage of its organization. Those who like to neglect the indications of neurosis and the *interconnections* between events will prefer this other explanation, and I shall not be able to prevent their doing so" (Freud, 1918, p. 107; my italics).

20. "On these issues I can venture upon no decision. I must confess, however, that I regard it as greatly to the credit of psycho-analysis that it should even have reached the stage of *raising* such questions as these" (Freud, 1918, p. 96).

are favorable to his over a rival explanation simply because of factors in the situation or in the way he obtains his data. Although suggestion is one possible such factor often mentioned (for example, by Freud himself throughout his writings; and by Grunbaum, 1984), it does not seem to me that it is reasonable to offer it as an alternative way to account for the data obtained in a case study without taking note of a careful documentation—if one exists (as, of course, ideally, it should)—of factors that count against the plausibility of such an alternative account. These include: the content and sequence of the psychoanalyst's interventions; the extent of the analysand's knowledge of psychoanalytic theory; the degree to which the psychoanalyst is unprepared for, surprised by, and even unbelieving about what the analysand reports (as Freud shows he is in the Wolf-Man case), even when it is consistent with the theory; the degree to which the psychoanalyst not only pays attention to the analysand's disagreements with him but ends up accepting the analysand's views (as Freud reports he does in the Wolf-Man case);[21] and the very long periods during which the analysand stubbornly and persistently rejects, ignores, forgets, and fights about not simply an explanation but the very reports he himself has given which the psychoanalyst offers in support of it.

It is noteworthy in this connection that Freud makes clear that he has confidence in an interpretation just to the extent that the interpretation makes use of, or that the response to the interpretation includes, particular idiosyncratic details *which the psychoanalyst could not have predicted from the theory (i.e., from general formulations)*. Nothing could make clearer how far Freud is from a covering law model of explanation.[22]

21. "I could not succeed, as in so many other differences of opinion between us, in convincing him; and in the end the correspondence between the thoughts which he had recollected and the symptoms of which he gave particulars, as well as the way in which the thoughts fitted into his sexual development, compelled me on the contrary to come to believe him" (Freud, 1918, p. 62).

22. In attempting to explain his patient's recurrent memory of being seized with fear of a butterfly, Freud puts forward "the possibility that the yellow stripes on the butterfly had reminded him [the patient] of similar stripes on a piece of clothing worn by some woman." The patient's associations, however, indicate that the stripes on the butterfly in fact reminded him of a pear, the

f. An important point with respect to the validity of explanations is that explanations of phenomena, based on limited data—a limited subset of the total set of relevant data—are less likely to be valid than explanations based on a larger subset of these data. An advantage of the psychoanalytic study is that it makes use of data obtained in the psychoanalytic situation, which are otherwise unavailable. Such data, for example, cannot be obtained in experimental and field-questionnaire studies. Imagine testing hypotheses such as Freud's thesis that "a man's attitude in sexual things has the force of a model to which the rest of his reactions tend to conform" (1909, p. 241) by methods which do not afford access to intimate facts a person is reluctant to communicate even when he is conscious of them. Examples are: the content of masturbation fantasies; and under what circumstances such fantasies are excited. Given a stream of "purposeless" communications, the relation of such intimate information to facts about "nonsexual" areas of life can be inferred from sequences, contexts, or metaphoric and other linguistic linkages.

The argument that the investigator has selected his facts to suit his explanation is feckless. It is just these facts that he intends to show can be fitted into a causal pattern. His challenger must show that these facts—along with others—may better be fitted into some other causal pattern; he gives other factors, kinds of events, or entities, for example, a causal status, or causally relates the same facts in a different way. The investigator, writing with his rival in mind, must accept the obligation to include in his account any facts which are relevant to his rival's purposes—

name of which was the same as the name of a nurserymaid who, it turned out, was important in his life. Freud mentions this "as an illustration to show how inadequate the physician's constructive efforts usually are for clearing up questions that arise, and how unjust it is to attribute the results of analysis to the physician's imagination and suggestion." That "the opening and shutting of the butterfly's wings" had looked to the patient "like a woman opening her legs, and the legs then made the shape of a Roman V, which . . . was the hour at which, in his boyhood, and even up to the time of the treatment, he used to fall into a depressed state of mind" were associations which, Freud declares, he could never have arrived at himself. Freud also mentions deprecatingly his own "facile suspicion that the points or stick-like projections of the butterfly's wings might have had the meaning of genital symbols" (p. 89ff.).

especially events that are not encompassed by his causal pattern but which might well be encompassed by his rival's. He argues strongly, of course, if he is able to show that he is able to encompass the facts that are most relevant to his rival's purposes but that his rival is not able to encompass those most relevant to his own. An examination of Freud's *Interpretation of Dreams* (1900) will show that Freud so argued against the view that the choice of content and other properties of dreams are determined solely by somatic or external stimuli.

One who thinks in terms of a covering law model of explanation and who intends to use it to explain one phenomenon may argue that all the rich data collected by the psychoanalyst might well be irrelevant for the explanation of a neurotic symptom, for example, and that the psychoanalyst's use of them simply results in a "fairy tale" (an epithet one of the critics of Freud's case studies is especially fond of using). However, these data are not irrelevant if they are produced unexpectedly by the analysand with a kind of particularity and detail that along with other characteristics of the situation tend to render implausible the supposition that they are suggested by the psychoanalyst; if they are relevant to a consideration of the kind of thesis of Freud's exemplified by the one (a central one) quoted above; and if the investigator's theory—or set of concatenated theories—enables him to fit them into a causal pattern which has no comparable rival.

CONCLUSION

A psychoanalyst will distinguish between using a case study to establish facts (empirical generalizations) and using a case study to tell a causal story (i.e., to give a causal explanation of phenomena and their interrelations). No matter which is his objective, he will pay attention to the necessity of arguing for the scientific credibility of his conclusions. In particular, if he attempts the kind of causal explanation Freud offers in the Wolf-Man case, he will not only pay attention to the power of his explanation (how many facts it encompasses and how elegantly it does so), but will include in his case study some appropriate argument, based on theoretically relevant evidence, for the scientific credibility of that explanation.

Some psychoanalysts are fond of claiming that psychoanalysis is different from other sciences and has its own rules of evidence, but they are often at a loss to explicate in just what sense it is different and just what these rules of evidence are. A strong argument can, in fact, be made that scientific methodology (e.g., hypothesis-testing) is not independent of theory (Danziger, 1985). Theoretical presuppositions about the structure of the world underlie methodological rules (e.g., the rules of statistical inference). Such presuppositions include that a system of phenomena has the same *structure* as the numerical system, or that relations among phenomena are of the same type as relations among numbers. These presuppositions, therefore, determine what constitutes evidence and which limited class of theories will be considered suitable for testing at all.

It may be true, as Danziger claims, that the rules about what constitutes evidence are neither independent of theory nor fixed forever, and that different methods are required to establish the scientific credibility of different kinds of theories. But that does not necessarily imply that there is no general characterization of science in terms of methodology, which holds across different disciplines or domains. For example, I know of no theory, no matter how complex, that does not at least involve *classification* of entities, states of affairs, or events, and at a minimum the kind of *measurement* that makes use of dichotomous yes-no, on-off variables. At a minimum, a scientific theory will attempt to explain why an entity has one of at least two values, "has the property" or "does not have the property"; why a state of affairs has one of at least two values, "exists" or "does not exist"; or why an event has one of at least two values, "occurs" or "does not occur."

If we offer a causal explanation such as Freud offers in the Wolf-Man case, it is still so that some carefully reasoned (and, with respect to the kind of theory at issue, appropriate) argument must be provided as to just why, given a body of empirical evidence (also, with respect to the kind of theory at issue, appropriate), we should believe this causal explanation has indeed captured at least some of the features of, or in some way reflects, the causal structure of the psychological no less than of the physical world. Such an argument is the irreducible methodological imperative of any scientific enterprise—and psychoanalysis, as Freud well knew, perforce must yield to it.

BIBLIOGRAPHY

CARTWRIGHT, N. (1983). *How the Laws of Physics Lie.* New York: Oxford Univ. Press.

DANZIGER, K. (1985). The methodological imperative in psychology. *Phil. Soc. Sci.,* 15:1–13.

EDELSON, M. (1982). Language and dreams. *Psychoanal. Study Child,* 27:203–282.

———— (1984). *Hypothesis and Evidence in Psychoanalysis.* Chicago: Univ. Chicago Press.

———— (1985). The hermeneutic turn and the single case study in psychoanalysis. In *Exploring Clinical Methods for Social Research,* ed. D. N. Berg & K. K. Smith, pp. 71–104. Beverly Hills, Calif.: Sage Publications.

———— (1986). Heinz Hartmann's influence on psychoanalysis as a science (in press).

FREUD, S. (1900). The interpretation of dreams. *S.E.,* 4 & 5.

———— (1909). Notes upon a case of obsessional neurosis. *S.E.,* 10:155–318.

———— (1918). From the history of an infantile neurosis. *S.E.,* 17:3–122.

GLYMOUR, C. (1980). *Theory and Evidence.* Princeton: Princeton Univ. Press.

GOULD, S. J. (1986). Evolution and the triumph of homology, or why history matters. *Amer. Scientist,* 74:60–69.

GRUNBAUM, A. (1954). Science and ideology. *Sci. Monthly,* 79:13–19.

———— (1984). *The Foundations of Psychoanalysis.* Berkeley: Univ. California Press.

HACKING, I. (1983). *Representing and Intervening.* Cambridge: Cambridge Univ. Press.

HARTMANN, H. & KRIS, E. (1945). The genetic approach in psychoanalysis. *Psychoanal. Study Child,* 1:11–30.

KAPLAN, A. (1964). *The Conduct of Inquiry.* New York: Harper & Row.

KRIS, E. (1956a). The personal myth. *J. Amer. Psychoanal. Assn.,* 4:653–681.

———— (1956b). The recovery of childhood memories in psychoanalysis. *Psychoanal. Study Child,* 11:54–88.

LUBORSKY, L. (1967). Momentary forgetting during psychotherapy and psychoanalysis. In *Motives and Thought,* ed. R. R. Holt. Psychol. Issues, 18/19:177–217. New York: Int. Univ. Press.

———— (1973). Forgetting and remembering (momentary forgetting) during psychotherapy. In *Psychoanalytic Research,* ed. M. Mayman. Psychol. Issues, 30:29–55. New York: Int. Univ. Press.

———— & MINTZ, J. (1974). What sets off momentary forgetting during a psychoanalysis? *Psychoanal. & Contemp. Sci.*, 3:233–268.

MEEHL, P. E. (1983). Subjectivity in psychoanalytic inference. In *Testing Scientific Theories*, ed. J. Earman, pp. 349–411. Minneapolis: Univ. Minnesota Press.

SALMON, W. C. (1984). *Scientific Explanation and the Causal Structure of the World.* Princeton: Princeton Univ. Press.

SASHIN, J. (1985). Affect tolerance. *J. Social Biol. Struct.*, 8:175–202.

SEARLE, J. R. (1983). *Intentionality.* Cambridge: Cambridge Univ. Press.

WOLLHEIM, R. (1981). *Sigmund Freud.* Cambridge: Cambridge Univ. Press.

Child Analysis, 1947–1984

A Retrospective
MARJORIE HARLEY, Ph.D.

I APPRECIATE THIS OPPORTUNITY TO WRITE A PAPER HONORING
Marianne Kris. She was a valued teacher, a uniquely loyal friend,
and one to whom I owe much in many ways. With the passage of
time, I have been able to perceive with increasing clarity how
much the theory and technique of child analysis to which I, and I
am sure others also, adhere are basically consonant with the
principles which Dr. Kris instilled in us novices at the Child
Development Center in 1947 and in her continuing supervision
of our work with older children outside the center. Further, she
was among the first to assimilate new findings as they came into
being, and, with those of us who moved forward with her into
the 1950s, she shared the enrichment of her knowledge gained
through her sustained contact with Anna Freud and the Hampstead Clinic and through her continuing grasp of the contributions of Hartmann, Ernst Kris, and Loewenstein to the expand-
ing ego psychology of that period. I well recall, for instance, a
supervisory hour when, as I was describing a child's play, Dr.
Kris helped me to perceive firsthand, as it were, the act of neu-
tralization.

   For the moment, however, I shall turn back to the period from
1947 to 1950 and summarize how in those days, and with Marianne Kris as our chief illuminant, we defined and practiced

The Fourth Marianne Kris Lecture read at the Twentieth Meeting of the
Association for Child Psychoanalysis, Chapel Hill, March 31, 1985.

   Faculty member and supervisor of child and adolescent analysis, Baltimore–
D.C. Institute for Psychoanalysis; faculty member, Division of Child and Adolescent Analysis, Columbia Center for Psychoanalytic Training and Research.

child analysis. In short, we were taught that there was but one analytic method which, to state the obvious, was based on an overall emphasis on the patient's inner psychic life and which entailed interpretation of resistance and defense, reconstruction, working through, and so on. At this point my omission of transference is deliberate.

Of particular importance was the distinction Dr. Kris made between the analytic method and the techniques employed to implement this method; and it was here that she introduced the concept of *adaptation* of technique to child analysis. In this concept lay her emphasis on the differences between child and adult analysis, and, in the tradition established by Anna Freud, she stressed the necessity for the analyst to be ever mindful of the level of ego development attained by a given child at a given time. This involved not only cognitive development and modes of communication—knowing the "language of the child," as she put it—but respect for the vulnerabilities attendant on the child's relatively immature ego: the extra caution and patience required in dealing with the child's defenses and in assessing the degree of frustration he might tolerate; the importance of underscoring the ego aspect when addressing areas of conflict as an aid in conveying the analyst's role as an ally in combating id forces, in facilitating the reinternalization of externalized conflicts, and in avoiding the promotion of externalization; the necessity for attunement to, and verbalization of, the child's feeling states, whether these were expressed directly or through play characters and stories, whichever the case may have been.

Finally, Dr. Kris drew a sharp distinction, on the one hand, between those adaptations of technique which were designed to attain compatibility with the analytic method and, on the other hand, modifications of technique which, subject to their nature and degree, might impinge upon and, in some instances, even disrupt the analytic process. Numbered among such modifications were, for example, interventions by the analyst aimed at changing the patient's environment, including advice to parents, educational measures intended to correct the child's sexual confusions, or other misconceptions before the underlying fantasies could be sufficiently analyzed; and undue gratifications, including the wholesale answering of questions, especially when the analyst was at a loss to find the appropriate interpretation. I would underscore, however, that Dr. Kris's admonitions were tempered by the demand for constant flexibility and discrimination so as not to provoke a power struggle or stalemate which, in and of itself, would obstruct the analytic process.

At first glance, the foregoing would seem not unlike our contemporary views on the theory of child analytic technique, albeit the exclusion of transference is of no mean significance. But in point of fact there were contained in these adaptations of 1947 practices which most of us today would regard as modifications or parameters, and other practices which some of us today, myself included, would challenge, even though there are those who would accept them as standard procedure. In the first group I have in mind, for example, the fact that in those days we not infrequently took a child even as old as 4 or 5 to the store to choose a Christmas or birthday gift, or to buy ice cream. On one occasion, I took a 5-year-old, who was eminently analyzable without need of recourse to any special technical measures, to the St. Patrick's day parade during her analytic hour, this constituting a compromise between her not missing her appointment and not being deprived of the parade. As I recall, it was a cold day and we stopped for hot chocolate! In the second group, that of potential disagreement, we relied excessively, I believe, on extra-analytic information from parents and other sources. This was doubtless often justifiable with the younger children we were treating but not in its extension to latency and even prepubertal children. What might be regarded, but perhaps not by everyone, as an overemphasis on this extra-analytic information may in part, and I underscore in part, have reflected a reaction to Melanie Klein's equation of child and adult without regard for the greater potential for the child's daily events to insert themselves into any given analytic hour.

It was at the end of the 1940s that transference came to play a role in Marianne Kris's thinking and teaching. Until then it had been generally accepted as a rather hard and fast fact among non-Kleinians that, owing primarily to the continuing presence of the original love objects, children simply did not form transferences. Here also it is possible that Melanie Klein's wholesale application of so-called transferences to child analysis may have

contributed to the delay in acknowledging or recognizing transference phenomena in children. We did sometimes speak of
transference reactions, but by this we meant not transference in
the traditional sense of a repetition of past relationships and
their attendant revisions and distortions, but rather a simple
displacement of current attitudes directed toward the parents.
When, toward the close of the 1940s, the analytic observations of
the then newly found Hampstead Clinic revealed that transference did, indeed, play a role in child analysis, Dr. Kris was
among the first of the senior analysts and, I am reasonably certain, the first in the New York area, to explore and then embrace
this finding. She now added the contamination of the transference to those factors inherent in the technical modifications
which she saw as posing a danger to the development and/or
preservation of the analytic process. Regrettably, this distinction
between the two terms, *adaptation* and *modification* of technique,
has not been universally adopted; rather, the two are not infrequently used interchangeably. To my mind, this may mar the
perception of child analysis in the eyes of the uninitiated.

So much for this introduction. I trust it is evident that I cannot
compress a review of child analysis encompassing almost four
decades in a way as comprehensive as the perhaps ill-chosen title
of this paper may imply. Rather, my aim is to highlight, mainly
from the vantage of the theory of technique, only some of the
added dimensions and amplifications of our basic data which
have resulted from the accumulation of knowledge over the
years.

In pondering how to proceed, I concluded that transference,
the associated therapeutic alliance, and reconstruction might
prove useful. All three at one point or another meet and interact; all three have connotations for the theory of technique;
all three have been subjected repeatedly to scrutiny from different perspectives; and, in certain respects, all three still involve
unsettled issues. But we scarcely need a second glance to acknowledge the enormous expansion of the developmental viewpoint. This has not only given us a far broader understanding of
the child within our psychoanalytic developmental framework,
but also has had far-reaching significance for many facets of the
whole of analysis. Therefore, even though I have placed this

developmental viewpoint at the end rather than the beginning of this admittedly arbitrary order, it is clear that developmental factors are part and parcel of those topics placed first. I would add that the writing of this paper has inevitably turned my attention to children I analyzed in the far as well as near past, and thus has made me keenly aware of my own changing angles of vision, something I assume is the usual accompaniment of continuing experience. For that reason, it has seemed to me unavoidable that some of my own thoughts will intrude themselves into what follows.

I turn now to transference. Our awareness of the child's potential for transference and, somewhat later, of his capacity to form a therapeutic alliance, was fairly widespread among the majority of child analysts in the 1950s, and certainly by the 1960s, and led to revisions of no small import in our theory of technique. There were (and perhaps still are), however, at least a few colleagues who tended to force almost the whole of the analytic material within a transference framework, the rationale being that intrapsychic conflicts could only be sufficiently analyzed through the transference. In reflecting on this aftereffect of the discovery of transference developments in children, I was struck by the fact that child analysis at that time had not yet attained the respect it now has. It may be, then, that those who overplayed, as I would put it, the role of transference were, consciously or unconsciously, attempting to place child analysis on a par with adult analysis, although I feel impelled to add that I number myself among those who believe that extratransference interpretations also play a significant role in the analysis of adults. In any event, the acceptance of transference as an intrinsic ingredient of the analytic process in children soon became fairly universal. In addition, Frankl and Hellman's (1962) important paper, which demonstrated the child's capacity to form a therapeutic alliance, influenced our technique in the handling of the transference significantly. We now recognized that in most cases this alliance allowed the child to withstand phases of negative transference which we could interpret as such, and afforded us a greater freedom to interpret the positive transference resistance when indicated. To many of our younger child analysts it may seem strange that for some time we had felt it indispensable to maintain only a positive transference, yet that was the state of affairs in those earlier days of child analysis.

Throughout the 1960s and extending even into the 1970s, transference remained a lively issue in respect to the nature and degree of the child's potential for transference developments. These differing opinions were more or less reconciled by fairly general accord on well-known developmental considerations, so well-known they scarcely bear repetition: that is, the parents, the original objects with whom his infantile relationships were formed, and around whom his infantile fantasies were woven, were still very much a part of the child's life. Coupled with this was the fact that the child's ego structure lacked the cohesiveness of that of the adult and, as a corollary, that the processes of internalization were not so stable. For these reasons, transference in child analysis was considered not to be the equivalent of that in adult analysis, and this distinction is still widely held.

There is, nonetheless, a more recent unsettled issue in respect to transference which may deserve special comment, and that is the tendency among some child analysts to extend the term *transference* to encompass habitual modes of relating, that is, aspects of what we would commonly call character traits, and to the extension into the analytic situation of current relationships to the primary objects (Sandler et al., 1980). As for the first of these, that is, habitual modes of relating or character traits (Harley, 1971a), I am unable to look upon them as transference unless or until that point is reached where the repressed component elements which resulted in their formation have been revived and are experienced in relation to the analyst.

In trying to understand the rationale for subsuming under transference the displacement onto the analyst of current relationships, I must own that I continue to be confounded. I should like, however, to thank the Tysons (1984) who attempted to clarify the problem for me. They stated that "influences from the past are important in the selection of which apparently current conflicts appear in the transference" (1984). For my part, I would regard the extension into the analysis of apparently current conflicts in the relationship with the parents, but which contain elements of the past, as reflecting a transference to the original objects rather than to the analyst. I would inject here that although the concept of the parents as possible transference objects, especially in young children, is now by no means a novel one, already in 1968[1] Blum (1971) suggested that one could theoretically postulate transference to a parent.

The Tysons (1984) also stated that a current conflict can reactivate an old one and that "subtle but important elements from the past are reflected in those situations which are transferred in this way," that is, by the extension into the analysis of current conflicts. I would rather be inclined to see these elements as comprising transference potentials. But however way this question may be put, I am still puzzled and unable to perceive the validity or usefulness in enlarging the term *transference* in such a way as to modify or blur its traditional meaning of a repetition, albeit by no means an exact facsimile, of the past. And I am still more comfortable in viewing analysis of current conflicts, which have been shaped by past conflicts, not as a form of transference but, as I have said, as containing the potentials for transference developments which then more often than not do materialize. At least for me, this question of broadening the concept of transference still remains debatable.

To turn back now to a discussion of transference in its more limited but more usual definition, transference in children is often characterized as more diluted than in adults. From one aspect this is quite justifiable; yet from another it may be misleading due to the variations in intensity and in duration of transference manifestations, not only between children, but also within the same child in different phases of his analysis. In this connection, it should be emphasized that internalization tends to become more stable with the child's advancing age. Further, the fact that early libidinal and aggressive strivings and their concomitant fantasies, which have been reanimated by the analytic process and directed toward the analyst, are then, in larger or smaller measure, redirected to the original objects need not, in my experience, preclude their continuing and varying expression in the transference. Or, the different aspects of the transference may be divided between analyst and parents. Also, there

1. At a Panel of the American Psychoanalytic Association on "The Current Status of the Transference Neurosis."

is no little diversification with regard to the frequency of alternating cathectic shifts between analyst and parent, and not
rarely I have encountered instances where a seeming shift from
the analyst to the parent is not, in fact, a shift back to the parent
but rather a defensive displacement of the continuing transference to the analyst. If this is not interpreted as such, the
transference developments may be temporarily aborted.

Another aspect of transference I would touch upon is the
question of whether a given patient, child or adult, may sometimes come to analysis with a preformed transference, or invariably comes only with at most a transference potential. I incline
toward the probably minority view that preformed transferences may occur. From this vantage, we might then ask whether
or not a child's frequent expectations that the analyst will right
all his ills may not contain elements deriving from the time when
the parent was perceived as omniscient and omnipotent, and
whether these then may not evolve into a transference resistance. Even more to the point is what I am certain others
besides myself have encountered in prepubertal children:
namely, an adoption fantasy pertaining to the person of the
analyst and which is already in the making at the very time of the
initial contact. I have experienced three such instances with prepubertal girls. One of these was the oldest of four children,
spaced approximately two years apart, whose mother was well
along with still another pregnancy. On the way to her first hour,
the child wondered aloud to her housekeeper if any of the people on the bus might think she was adopted, although the idea of
myself as the adoptive parent was still unconscious.

Understandably, such fantasies in relation to the analyst stir
loyalty conflicts which may complicate and even threaten the
analysis unless and until they are worked through. In my own
mind, I have included them within the context of transference,
relating them to Freud's (1909) family romance where he points
to prepuberty as the time when this fantasy flourishes. It should
perhaps be noted that the idea of the analyst as the adoptive
parent is a reverse variation of Freud's version in which it is the
real parents who are the adoptive ones. To extend to the girl
child Freud's statement, in which he speaks particularly of the
boy and his relationship to the father, and to paraphrase it, one

might then say that the turning away from the mother of today is actually the girl's wish to rediscover the loved mother of the earlier years, and in one sense is an expression of her regret that those happy days are gone. These illustrations of possibly pre-formed transferences are admittedly controvertible and may even be unsustainable, but they warrant consideration.

The aforementioned adoption fantasies, of course, usually involve a number of dynamics as, for example, a phase-specific defensive displacement onto the analyst so as to avoid the phase-specific regressive pull to the preoedipal mother; or, a defensive splitting of the phase-specific ambivalence toward the mother, and so forth. Nonetheless, I have found it technically useful to first interpret this fantasy along the lines borrowed from Freud (1909) in that this intervention has served to alleviate the loyalty conflict sufficiently to enable the analysis to proceed. I might add parenthetically that I have also found this kind of interven-tion at times helpful in respect to those comparable transference fantasies that not rarely occur when the prepubertal girl's analy-sis is well underway, although I have only known them to be discernible when the analyst is a woman. But their counterpart may occur in boys with male analysts.

These possibly preformed, or ready-made, transferences should not be confused with the fantasies and expectations re-garding treatment before it begins, a topic which Anna Freud addresses in the extremely thought-provoking book on tech-nique as practiced at the Hampstead Clinic (Sandler et al., 1980). Such fantasies and expectations, Anna Freud notes, are not pro-duced by transference, but they may become linked with subse-quent transference developments. This has often been borne out in my own experience. For example, one of a 9-year-old boy's fantasies on entering analysis was that his parents had sent him to me because they had little interest in communicating with him, although they did so profusely with his younger sister. Yet, as he magnanimously put it, they were conscientious enough to acknowledge he was entitled to someone with whom he could talk! This fantasy, in and of itself, could by no means be labeled transference, yet it opened the way to analyzing, in the trans-ference, many of the elements comprising this fantasy: to name but some, the patient's jealousy of his sister; his belief not only that she was preferred by virtue of being a girl but because, unlike himself, she did not masturbate; and his strong masochistic strivings which led him to cherish this belief and by his own behavior to make it well-nigh impossible, indeed, for his parents to communicate with him.

As I have said, the child's capacity for transference developments gained increasing acceptance during the 1950s and 1960s, although for some time it was a subject for continuing clarification and revision, especially in respect to whether or not oedipal material was repeated in the latency child's transference, something we no longer question. Moreover, these discussions on transference were enriched by Anna Freud's enumeration of the ways in which the child makes use of the analyst other than as a transference figure. But any discussion of transference would not be complete without mention of the transference neurosis which evoked even livelier discussions.

At a Panel (1966) on "Problems of Transference in Child Analysis," the participants noted a paucity of reported transference neuroses in children to date, and revealed that our understanding of the concept, and how it should be applied, was still confused and lacked uniformity. By implication one definition was that a transference neurosis was in effect when the child no longer manifested his disturbance outside the analysis, while reliving past conflicts with the analyst. Such a case was presented by Fraiberg, but it is noteworthy that her patient relived only pregenital and preoedipal conflicts, a point to which I shall return.

Today most of us have concluded that transference neurosis does occur in children, although it is more fluid, less cohesive, and of shorter duration than its adult counterpart. It is now most commonly defined in quantitative terms, that is, as put by the Tysons (1984), it is the "extensive concentration of the child's conflicts, repressed infantile wishes and fantasies on the person of the analyst, with a relative lessening of their manifestations elsewhere." The Tysons, however, add a qualitative aspect. The latter refers to the fact that these earlier conflicts, fantasies, and so forth are indubitably expressed in a revised form. This revision predictably results from the accumulation of genetic experiences and developmental transformations that have occurred over the course of time, usually with a correlation between the extent of the time span and complexity of the revisions. This qualitative aspect, as I see it, applies to all transferences and is not limited to transference neurosis.

Insofar as I have been able to ascertain in perusing the literature, more recent explications of transference neurosis in children would seem to de-emphasize, if not omit, the factor of the infantile neurosis, though possibly it has been thought that this factor is so universally known, it no longer needs to be stated. Nonetheless, I shall here restate that despite our emphasis on preoedipal development and its contribution to the texture and fabric of the oedipal constellation itself, a neurosis per se continues to derive its driving force from the oedipal conflicts. Therefore, I do not see how we can speak of a transference neurosis without the inclusion of at least some aspects of the infantile neurosis.

Occasionally, one comes across a transference neurosis more cohesive and occupying a longer time period than one would normally expect in children. I have had only two such cases, both latency girls, one with a dog phobia on whom I reported many years ago (Harley, 1971b) and the other one whom I analyzed more recently. Both these children developed transference neuroses which lasted 15 and 9 months respectively, and which receded when the oedipal distortions arising from preoedipal disturbances had been analyzed. I should add that both these cases have been unique in my experience.

In the past, when alluding to the first case, I suggested that the transference neurosis might have been augmented by a propensity for displacement since displacement itself is so bound up in the structure of a phobia. Now this suggestion seems to me less than adequate. In the course of further reflection, it occurred to me that one clue might lie in the fact that the complex of conflicts which comprised both these children's neuroses was more tightly integrated than is expectable in early latency, and that this might have indicated a precocious development of the integrative function. This is but a tentative thought, nor would it anyway comprise a total explanation.

A few words about the therapeutic alliance and the changed thinking about it over the years are now in order. I earlier referred to Frankl and Hellman's (1962) paper and the technical implications of the child's ability to form a therapeutic alliance, especially for our handling of the transference. Originally, this therapeutic alliance was seen as quite distinct from transference in that it pertained to those aspects of the ego not involved in conflict. This coincided with the concept of the therapeutic alliance as set forth by Zetzel (1956) and which, in turn, was based on the earlier formulations of Sterba (1934) and Bibring (1937). In its purest sense, one might still conceptualize the therapeutic alliance in this way; and the essence of Frankl and Hellman's statement that "one element in the ego keeps touch with the reality of the analyst and his real role" (p. 335) would still be correct. But we have come to see that it is not so easy to draw a neat line between the therapist as new object and in his real analytic role on the one hand, and as an object for transference distortions and habitual, neurotic attitudes on the other, since these different aspects not only intermingle but at times seem almost to commingle.

Sandler et al. (1984) offer two ways in which to view the therapeutic alliance: the narrower is compatible with what I have just outlined and is described as arising from the patient's awareness of his illness and the wish to do something about it, these factors being linked with the ability to tolerate the effort and pain attendant on facing internal conflicts. The other is a broader one, and includes a number of other elements such as love for the analyst, object hunger, and so on (see also Curtis, 1979). The authors' admonitions in respect to the importance of attunement insofar as possible to what they view as the different ingredients of the therapeutic alliance I believe cannot be overstated. In addition, although these other elements may at certain times combine with the therapeutic alliance per se to strengthen it (for example, the positive libidinal transference, the wish to please, or even some belief in the therapist's magic), they must be assessed in terms of degree: that is, a little bit of one or the other of these is doubtless useful, especially when the alliance is strained or temporarily aborted, an occurrence which we know too well is more usual in children than in adults, although this factor, too, must be assessed with regard to the stages of the child's analysis and his ongoing development. But the more space these elements occupy in their relation to the therapeutic alliance in its purer sense, the more they are tantamount to transference resistances.

In his deeply thoughtful paper on the analytic process in children, Ritvo (1978) refers to a basic transference which has bearing on the therapeutic alliance. He says: "Just as the parent invests the toy for the young child in the interest of . . . play, so the adult invests the analyst for the child in the interest of the relief of discomfort or suffering. In this way the basic transference of the analytic situation is initiated" (p. 300). Ritvo goes on to say, "Even if the analyst cannot count on the child's active conscious participation in the analytic process or on his ability for reflection and self-observation, the basic transference provides a directional force for the child to present his conflicts and symptoms" and the child turns to the analyst for help as to a parent (p. 301).

This eventuality appears to be very much an outgrowth of the parents' alliance. The term *basic transference,* however, brings to mind Greenacre's (1954, 1968) concept of the basic transference which she views as a replica of the patient's earliest experiences with the mother and out of which she sees arising that basic trust in the analyst indispensable to the therapeutic alliance. As she puts it, the basic transference may catalyze the therapeutic alliance, while its regressive elements may simultaneously act as contaminants. In my judgment, any discussion of the therapeutic alliance should include this concept of a basic transference.

Ritvo's reference to the parents is a reminder that their alliance is often a necessary adjunct to the child's alliance. In fact, I see this as the chief rationale for any continuing contact with the parents, although admittedly we still need extra-analytic information in respect to the very young child, that is, up to the age of 3 or 4. Additionally, to exclude the parents from the treatment situation of the preschool or younger latency child, who needs to feel that at least one parent is in accord with the analysis, is akin to a neglect of the child's developmental needs. But with advances in ego development, and the concomitantly increasing stability of the therapeutic alliance, many of us have observed over the years that we can count on the child himself to maintain the analysis and, I would add, to provide the material for the analysis of his intrapsychic conflicts.

Moreover, we must be mindful that parents are liable to the same memory distortions, repressions, and screening devices as are our patients and that these may act as impediments to our understanding of the child's past and to our reconstructive efforts. To cite but one example, an apparently single trauma may be used by the parents to screen another trauma to which they have attached more guilt; or it may be used to obscure stress traumas to which their attitudes may have subjected the child. Not infrequently, such isolated screening traumas are of a dramatic nature, allegedly unknown to the child, but their derivatives appear early in the analysis and with increasing frequency so as to threaten to preoccupy the analyst. When the reconstruction has been made, the child now also uses this trauma in the same way as the parents (or parent), that is, as a screen, and the reconstruction of what lies behind is by no means easily achieved. This phenomenon doubtless contributes to the adult's personal myth as elaborated by Ernst Kris (1956a).

This leads directly to the topic of reconstruction in child analysis. In 1971, Kennedy introduced an issue around reonstruction which still remains an unsettled one: she questioned, in the light of developmental factors, the value of reconstruction in child analysis. Kennedy underscored in particular the child's greater concern with solving his problems in the here and now rather than in looking back. (I would add that this extraction from her paper is extremely condensed and does not do justice to the argument she presented in support of her thesis.) More recently, Rees (1978) has written, from the standpoint of cognitive development, about the child's difficulties in forming connections between past and present prior to adolescence. Also in 1971, however, Furman gave convincing examples of reconstructions in child analysis which augmented the progress of the analysis. More specifically, she described how, in the analysis of a boy between the ages of 5 and 9, already in the first year of his analysis, and then again when he was 6½, she was able to make meaningful reconstructions dating back to his toddlerhood and including the meaning of an event which had occurred in his third year.

In my discussion of Kennedy's paper at the time she presented it, I affirmed, and here reaffirm, my belief not only in the technical value and validity in general of the genetic viewpoint, but in particular of the value and validity of reconstruction in selected instances. As Kennedy said, the major aim of child analysis is to enable the child to resolve those conflicts which are impeding his further development. But from my vantage, if we are to accomplish this, the child's optimal understanding of his conflicts, and his working them through, often rests on his awareness of how the past is operating in the present. Indispensable to the value of the reconstruction is the recovery of the affective components of what is reconstructed. As an 8-year-old once said: "The feeling helps me to believe and not just understand."

For a number of years I have been privileged to be part of a Study Group on Reconstruction[2] in both child and adult analysis. From the very rich contributions of the members of this group, three concepts emerged which had particular meaning for me. The first one was the fact that not only is the integrative function essential to the patient's understanding of reconstruction, but reconstruction itself contributes to the development of the integrative function through the linkages thus made, something of special consideration in terms of fostering the child's development. The second concept was that while it is the analytic process that makes possible the reconstruction, the latter, in turn, promotes the analytic process, thus often enabling us to amplify the reconstruction. And the third was that reconstruction may entail the near or even immediate past, especially so in children for whom time subjectively proceeds at a much slower pace,[3] and who are more prone to quick denials and repressions.

These last two concepts were illustrated in an 11-year-old girl who complained that an older neighborhood boy had threatened her with a "dangerous" stick. She was adamant in her insistence she had done nothing to provoke this, and I believed her. By way of her dream and fantasy material, I dared to suggest she might have encountered an exhibitionist, a suggestion she eventually confirmed but with a notable absence of affect,

2. Under the auspices of the Psychoanalytic Research and Development Fund, Inc.

3. It is a matter of common knowledge that the faster the pace of development, the slower the subjective sense of the pace of time.

although neither isolation nor denial of affect were habitual defenses. This event apparently had happened over the weekend preceding the Monday on which she brought up the matter of the stick and was something she said she had forgotten. Whether the child had withheld this information consciously or had denied and/or repressed it I cannot say with certainty, but I am very much inclined to think her anxiety, fear, and guilt had actually eventuated in her having forgotten it.

When I was able to interpret the child's defense against the terribly frightening and uncomfortable feelings this incident must have evoked in her, she was gradually able to reexperience these and, in the hours following my suggestion that it was as though a great big, dangerous, angry penis had been coming at her, primal scene innuendoes began to emerge in the analysis. This ultimately led to a reconstruction of an event which had lent an added force to this more recent one: that is, in early latency, also on a weekend, she had opened her parents' door as they were about to have intercourse, whereupon her father, out of his own surprise and anxiety, had walked toward her with his penis erect, and in a way which she perceived as having been altogether menacing. I cannot here go into the various oedipal strivings and accompanying anxieties which then constituted even further elaboration of the reconstruction, but it was apparent that they had become amalgamated with the phase-specific enhancement of her penis envy and sadomasochistic fantasies so characteristic of prepuberty.

I believe we have ample evidence of the ability of children 5 years and older to make use of reconstruction, though the younger the child, the simpler must be the manner in which the reconstruction is phrased, the more limited are the linkages which the child can comprehend, and the smaller must be the dosages of our reconstructive elaborations. What I have just said is very much in line with Abrams's (1980) contribution to the child's different ways of knowing as he makes his way up the developmental scale. But a question we might ask, and one raised by Abrams,[4] is: how old must a child be to utilize recon-

4. At the Study Group on Reconstruction, under the auspices of the Psychoanalytic Research and Development Fund, Inc.

struction? Inasmuch as I have not treated any children under 5 for very many years, I shall turn back to a child who was at the Child Development Center during our days there with Dr. Kris. Incidentally, this was the child who in the late 1940s drew our attention to the capacity for transference developments in children.

This boy was not quite 2 when his brother was born, at which time he became sad and withdrawn, a mood which had lifted by the time he had entered the center where if anything he was seen as exuberant. When he was approaching 3½ and had been in analysis for over a year, I became ill and was absent for almost a month. During this period, he once more became withdrawn and depressed, reflecting the same mood he had shown around his brother's birth. In response to his inquiry, the nursery teacher told him I was being cared for by a nurse. Upon my return, he associated my having had a nurse to the fact that his mother had had one when his brother was born. He told how his dog had to be sent away because she was going to have a baby. He added angrily that all ladies seem to have nurses when they have babies. The fantasy that I had gone away to have a baby was interpreted and linked with the birth of his brother, and in the ensuing weeks we worked on restoring his feelings of abandonment and sadness as these related to the original experience. These affects he clearly relived in the analytic situation. But I am quite sure he could not, in any cognitive sense, connect the earlier experience with his reaction to my absence. Moreover, when we uncovered some of his fantasies surrounding the advent of his brother, these were organized around phallic and phallic-oedipal material, thereby not only indicating that his entry into a new developmental phase had altered and colored his original perception, but also depicting a merging of past and present which Kennedy (1979) has referred to as characteristic of very young children. I realize this one illustration does not answer the question of how young a child may be to make use of reconstruction, and, for me at least, it still remains an open one.

Both these vignettes serve as a reminder of the opportunity that reconstruction in children affords us to see aspects of past history undergo alterations eventuating from developmental transformations and new experiences at the time these are occurring. If we resort to the much used metaphor of the telescope, we might say that while in the adult all of its segments are fitted together, in the child we can view some of these segments in the process of being fashioned and assembled. The following example illustrates this with special clarity.

This boy began treatment when he was 9 years old and his analysis extended well into his adolescence (Harley, 1961). In the oedipal phase, and in a sudden burst of exhibitionism aimed at his mother, he had attempted to leap from a dock onto a boat. He slipped, fell into the water, knocked his chin against the side of the boat, and bit his tongue, which bled profusely. His father jumped into the water to rescue him, whereupon the child struggled desperately against him. When he was 6 years old, in a bid for his teacher's recognition, the patient went to fetch her a cup of tea. Cup in hand, he stumbled, fell, and cut his lip, all of which evoked laughter from the other children.

When the memory of the original trauma first emerged in his analysis, its most predominant feature seemed to reflect the shock that the child had sustained as exemplified by his description of the glaring sunlight which had blinded his eyes as he fell into the water. There then followed, in subsequent sessions, the castration implications of the trauma from the sides of both positive and negative oedipal positions, that is, his having construed his father's rescue to be a homosexual attack. Although the factor of humiliation was an ingredient in the meaning of his fall with the teacup, the injury to his lip seemed more in the foreground and provided a link to the castration connotation of his accident on the dock.

In adolescence, when this boy was especially sensitive to any real or imagined ridicule by girls, he began to accuse me repeatedly of ridiculing him. Through a dream, his mishap on the dock again emerged in the analysis, but now its most striking meaning for him was that of humiliation. Whether this aspect was a part of the original experience, or whether it had become associatively linked with it through the teacup episode, I cannot say. In either event, one could clearly perceive the changed emphasis of meaning which corresponded with his particular adolescent sensitivity.

Last, I come to the developmental viewpoint. In contemplating the totality of the vast amount of developmental data which has been accumulated since the early 1950s, both from analytic practice and observational research, one finds oneself well-nigh overwhelmed.[5] Yet, as Abrams (1978) noted, the genetic viewpoint, as it appeared until very recently in the literature, for the most part stressed historical continuities rather than developmental transformations. In this regard, Abrams offered two useful alternatives: either to add another metapsychological viewpoint, namely, a developmental viewpoint; or to change the genetic viewpoint to a genetic-developmental viewpoint.[6] It is noteworthy that Abrams refers to the idea of a genetic-developmental viewpoint as deriving from Marianne Kris.

In his recent and extremely helpful elucidation of Anna Freud's developmental lines, Neubauer (1984), within the context of an emphasis on progressive sequences, also points to the importance of transformations versus continuity, that is, while new functions and new structures supersede old ones, all past experience is still available.

The developmental approach is useful in keeping us ever mindful of the child's ongoing and evolving developmental processes, not only in helping us assess which changes reflect developmental transformations and which are a result of our analytic work, but also as an aid, though by no means a fool-proof one, in determining both the need for analysis and analyzability. Yet, also inherent in this developmental approach is the danger of shifting the balance of our therapeutic efforts too much to the side of assisting development in ways not central to the analytic method, and thereby sliding over into psychotherapy. For example, the knowledge that the analyst is a new object whom the child may utilize to fulfill certain developmental needs may tempt the analyst to swerve from his analytic stance, and con-

5. These data have led to a broader comprehension of ego development, including the contribution of the aggressive drive and an extension of our knowledge of object relations. I would therefore raise the question of whether the concept of regression and fixation, which is limited to the psychosexual sphere, in itself is sufficient for a full understanding of neurotic development.

6. It should be stated that Kennedy (1971) was the first to make a distinction between the genetic and developmental viewpoints. However, at that time she did not take into account the question of continuity versus discontinuity.

sciously or unconsciously attempt to fulfill such needs. If the analyst maintains an analytic atmosphere, and concentrates on the analytic process and on his transference role rather than on that of real or new object, the child will nonetheless use him in these other ways, but the gains thus derived I would judge to be by-products of, rather than central to, the analytic method.

In the earlier years, I well recall Marianne Kris saying that she feared a particular child's diagnosis might be more than a neurosis, by which she meant a childhood schizophrenia or frank psychosis. In other words, that huge middle ground of deviations in structural development had not entered our thinking. In this respect, one should, nonetheless, recall Annemarie Weil's (1953, 1956) pioneering work which she began in the early 1950s, but which had not yet received widespread recognition.

Today our knowledge of structural deviations arising from skewed development, and/or developmental arrests, has become an integral part of our diagnostic thinking and of our efforts to define the limitations of the analytic method. It has, however, led, in some quarters, to attempts to recast rather than to broaden the principles on which analysis rests; and to treatment methods still labeled analysis, but based on theoretical assumptions incompatible with the mainstream of psychoanalytic developmental theory. If I am correct, these so-called analytic endeavors, which rest on a simplism apparently appealing to some, are to be found more in adult analysis than in child analysis. Therefore, it seemed to me a bit ironical to recall Anna Freud's (1970) comment that child analysis "lacked the decisive technical prescriptions which govern adult analysis and keep its practitioner on a straight and narrow path" (p. 211). Today, I think we might say that the situation has been somewhat altered.

As Blum (1981) has said, "contemporary psychoanalytic interest does not involve reductionist repair of structural 'deficiency,' but does consider dimensions of the psychoanalytic situation and process which, preceding and co-acting with insight, might lead to developmental advance and mastery" (p. 56). I would add that those milder ego deviations which are present in many of our analyzable patients may often be alleviated to greater or less degree by the auxiliary aspects inherent in the analytic situation. Further, I would think this factor would apply especially to children for whom in many ways development is a more open system. But as Blum cautions and as I have already mentioned, it is fraught with danger lest it lead to nonanalytic procedures.

Another problem arising from our increasing awareness of developmental deviations has to do with the danger of mistaking these as the cause for apparent ego deficiencies, which, in fact, are the outcome of neurotic conflict. The opposite is undeniably also often operative, that is, we may view neurotic conflict as a cause for pathology which actually is a reflection of structural deviations. I would add that I have always found it difficult to conceptualize structural conflicts as superimposed on whatever basic developmental deviations may exist. Rather, I tend to see these deviations as entering into and influencing the very nature and patterning of the later conflicts. It is clear that this whole realm of deviational development is still one in which we have much to learn. The answers we shall ultimately come by will derive not only from the therapeutic study of such patients, but also through observational research.

The utilization of data from direct observational studies is still an open question, however, in both child and adult analysis, but perhaps more so in adult analysis. It has to do with the assets as opposed to the hazards involved, and has been addressed incisively by Solnit (1975). Psychoanalytic technique, he says, and direct observational studies are essential and mutually dependent in the study of the child. He adds that the barriers between the two are artificial, and that the psychoanalytic treatment process can correct for tendencies of observational studies to speculate beyond reasonable limitations. Further, the questions which may be raised by direct observational studies can be explored by the psychoanalytic process, and thus augment the theory-building capacity of the psychoanalytic method. It is here pertinent to note that Marianne Kris played a leading role in the Yale Longitudinal Study which was the first to utilize observational data in conjunction with direct analytic data.

In the context of the usefulness of observational studies, I would refer to Mahler's (1979) research on separation-individuation. At least as I see it, her work, valuable as it is, has been overused and abused in a way I am sure she by no means intended it to be. To amplify this, there are those who have tended to give too much space within the whole of things to Mahler's important findings, thus overlooking the multiplicity of developmental and genetic processes; or else, to take too great and artificial a leap back to this early period, to the neglect of the intervening developmental and genetic factors. For that reason, and out of my respect for Mahler's contributions, I offer the following vignette to show how unresolved developmental conflicts of the rapprochement subphase may combine with other antecedents toward influencing the character of the oedipal phase, as preoedipal factors become organized and integrated within the oedipus complex.

This little girl entered analysis at the age of 8. When she was 18 months old and her mother was 7 months pregnant with her brother, she had a tonsillectomy, staying alone in the hospital overnight. Upon her return, she had little emotional contact with her mother, as had been the case previously, inasmuch as the mother had remained irritable and withdrawn through most of her pregnancy. The child was therefore much in the company of a maid, fairly new to the household, with whom she obviously had not formed a strong attachment. She had been, and continued to be, witness to violent altercations between her parents and had been overstimulated in various other ways; the groundwork was fast being laid for sadomasochistic relationships, especially with her father. As we can see, a number of factors by that early age already were contributing to her pathology. But here I wish to emphasize the child's understandable inability to sufficiently weather the rapprochement crisis and how this eventuality then played a part in her phallic-oedipal development and concomitant oedipal distortions.

The interferences with this child's attainment of optimal separation-individuation resulted in a relatively mild self-boundary problem and a concomitant proclivity, though a not all pervasive one, for primitive identification; the prolongation of her omnipotence strivings led to an intensification of her strong penis envy and to her endowing the phallus with the omnipotence she so strenuously sought to attain. Oedipal ambivalence toward her mother was compounded by the persisting image of the bad mother of the rapprochement subphase. Her positive oedipal strivings were not only burdened by an abundance of sadomasochism, but her tendency for primitive identification mechanisms contributed to oedipal distortions as object love for her father merged with identification. Further, her positive oedipal position was also marred by her sadistic, aggressive wish to attain the father's phallus. This wish, at the same time, derived an additional increment through her not infrequent use of an illusory phallus as a defense against the conflict-laden, regressive pull toward reengulfment by the mother. The force of this regressive pull, in turn, was augmented by her fierce fantasies surrounding the oedipal father.

The foregoing vignette is excessively streamlined with a number of genetic-dynamic factors omitted. Yet I trust it demonstrates that untoward happenings in the rapprochement subphase, although by no means causing the whole of the oedipal problems, contributed to a heightening of them.

Despite commonly recognized obstacles, more often than not children do enable the analytic process to evolve. The reasons for this are well known: the child's wish for relief of suffering, his ability to form a therapeutic alliance, and so on. It may be, however, that we should consider another factor. We know that some degree of regression is a natural accompaniment of development. In addition, both Ernst Kris (1956b) and Greenacre (1968) have characterized the analytic process as involving *essentially* a progression of growth, its regressive features notwithstanding. I find it therefore tempting to speculate that in some further sense, and perhaps beyond conscious awareness, the child somehow may know that this process itself will support his innate need to complete development.

In the preceding pages, I have tried, albeit in rough and rapid outline, to convey some of the changes which have taken place in child analysis since 1947, with special attention to the theory of technique. Along the way I have raised some controversial points, but, as Hartmann (1939) stated, the roots of ego growth are to be found not only in internal peace but also in conflict. I am sure that, basically, internal peace prevails among us and also that as older issues are resolved, newer ones will arise in endless fashion, thus enabling child analysis to continue its own growth and development.

Much of what I have said I think Marianne Kris would agree

with. Those statements with which she might not agree she would forthrightly oppose, at the same time respecting my autonomy. And if in this paper I have conveyed what her example and teaching instilled in me—an adherence to and respect for the analytic method—then I shall have achieved my aim.

BIBLIOGRAPHY

ABRAMS, S. (1977). Genetic point of view. *J. Amer. Psychoanal. Assn.*, 25:417–425.

———— (1978). The teaching and learning of psychoanalytic developmental psychology. *J. Amer. Psychoanal. Assn.*, 26:387–406.

———— (1980). Therapeutic action and ways of knowing. *J. Amer. Psychoanal. Assn.*, 28:291–307.

BIBRING, E. (1937). Therapeutic results of psychoanalysis. *Int. J. Psychoanal.*, 18:179–189.

BLUM, H. P. (1971). Transference and structure. In *The Unconscious Today*, ed. M. Kanzer, pp. 177–195. New York: Int. Univ. Press, 1971.

———— (1981). Some current and recurrent problems of psychoanalytic technique. *J. Amer. Psychoanal. Assn.*, 29:47–68.

CURTIS, H. (1979). The concept of therapeutic alliance. *J. Amer. Psychoanal. Assn. Suppl.*, 27:159–192.

FRANKL, L. & HELLMAN, I. (1962). Symposium on child analysis. *Int. J. Psychoanal.*, 43:333–337.

FREUD, A. (1970). Child analysis as a subspeciality of psychoanalysis. *W.*, 7:204–219.

———— (1981). The concept of developmental lines. *Psychoanal. Study Child*, 36:129–136.

FREUD, S. (1909). Family romances. *S.E.*, 9:237–240.

FURMAN, E. (1971). Some thoughts on reconstruction in child analysis. *Psychoanal. Study Child*, 26:372–385.

GREENACRE, P. (1954). The role of transference. In *Emotional Growth*, 2:627–640. New York: Int. Univ. Press, 1971.

———— (1968). The psychoanalytic process, transference and acting out. Ibid., 2:762–775.

HARLEY, M. (1961). Some observations on the relationship between genitality and structural development at adolescence. *J. Amer. Psychoanal. Assn.*, 9:436–460.

———— (1971a). The current status of transference neurosis in children. *J. Amer. Psychoanal. Assn.*, 19:26–40.

———— (1971b). The analysis of a phobia in a latency child. In *The Unconscious Today*, ed. M. Kanzer, pp. 339–362. New York: Int. Univ. Press, 1971.

HARLEY, M. & WEIL, A. (1979). Introduction. In *The Selected Papers of Margaret S. Mahler*, 2. New York: Aronson.

HARTMANN, H. (1939). *Ego Psychology and the Problem of Adaptation*. New York: Int. Univ. Press, 1958.

—— (1950). Psychoanalysis and developmental psychology. In *Essays on Ego Psychology*, pp. 99–112. New York: Int. Univ. Press, 1964.

KENNEDY, H. (1971). Problems in reconstruction in child analysis. *Psychoanal. Study Child*, 26:386–402.

—— (1979). The role of insight in child analysis. *J. Amer. Psychoanal. Assn. Suppl.*, 27:9–28.

KRIS, E. (1956a). The personal myth. In *The Selected Papers of Ernst Kris*, pp. 272–300. New Haven: Yale Univ. Press, 1975.

—— (1956b). On some vicissitudes of insight in psychoanalysis. Ibid., pp. 252–271.

MAHLER, M. S. (1979). *The Selected Papers of Margaret S. Mahler*, 2. New York: Aronson.

NEUBAUER, P. B. (1984). Anna Freud's concept of developmental lines. *Psychoanal. Study Child*, 39:15–27.

PANEL (1966). Problems of transference in child analysis. H. Van Dam, reporter. *J. Amer. Psychoanal. Assn.*, 14:528–537.

REES, K. (1978). The child's understanding of his past. *Psychoanal. Study Child*, 33:237–259.

RITVO, S. (1978). The psychoanalytic process in childhood. *Psychoanal. Study Child*, 33:295–305.

SANDLER, J., KENNEDY, H., & TYSON, R. L. (1980). *The Technique of Child Psychoanalysis*. Cambridge, Mass.: Harvard Univ. Press.

SOLNIT, A. J. (1975). Developments in child psychoanalysis in the last twenty years. In *Studies in Child Psychoanalysis*, 5:1–13. New Haven: Yale Univ. Press.

STERBA, R. (1934). The fate of the ego in analytic therapy. *Int. J. Psychoanal.*, 15:117–125.

TYSON, R. L. (1984). Personal communication.

TYSON, R. L. & TYSON, P. (1984). Transference. *J. Amer. Acad. Child Psychiat.* (in press).

WEIL, A. P. (1953). Certain severe disturbances of ego development in childhood. *Psychoanal. Study Child*, 8:271–287.

—— (1956). Some evidences of deviational development in infancy and childhood. *Psychoanal. Study Child*, 11:292–299.

ZETZEL, E. R. (1956). The concept of transference. In *The Capacity of Emotional Growth*, pp. 168–181. New York: Int. Univ. Press, 1964.

On "Merging" and the Fantasy of Merging

IRVING B. HARRISON, M.D.

THE PARADIGM FOR THE TERM "*MERGING*," AS IT IS USED BY psychoanalysts, is the assumed mental state of the satiated infant as he falls asleep at his mother's breast. The term is also used, somewhat loosely, to describe subjective experiences in childhood and later, characterized by a sense of diffusion or dissolution of the usual ego boundaries with respect to the separateness of oneself from one's surroundings or from the discreteness of one's place in time. Although the term has not long been common in the psychoanalytic literature, it has precedent as a theoretical concept. *Unity* and *fusion* have been used more or less synonymously.

Anna Freud (1960) used the verb *merge* in conceptualizing an event in the psychic life of the infant in which an "object—to use an expression introduced by W. Hoffer—is drawn wholly into the internal narcissistic milieu and treated as part of it to the extent that self and object merge into one" (p. 56). Mahler (1968) cited Anna Freud's comment with the parenthetical observation: "This corresponds to what I name the symbiotic dual-unity stage of primary narcissism" (p. 221n.). In Mahler's early writings on the separation-individuation phase of infant development, she emphasized the infant's intimate relation with its mother. Her book's first sentence, pertaining to symbiosis, described "a close functional association of two organisms to their mutual advantage" (p. 7). Her account further underscored the original separateness, in the description of a transition from physiological

Faculty, The New York Psychoanalytic Institute.

interactions to psychological interactions. From that perspective, use of terms such as *dual unity* and *dyad,* widely incorporated into current theory, acknowledges at least tacitly that the infant's psyche is a discrete and unique entity. In the same volume, however, Mahler alluded to the primal psychic state of the infant, prior to the earliest memory traces, as "the hitherto 'oceanic feeling' of complete fusion and oneness with the mother" (p. 44) and to "primal mother-infant unity" (p. 169). In a recent description Mahler and McDevitt (1982) alluded to an initial mother-infant "dual unit" (p. 828), and also to "the originally fused symbiotic self-object schemata" (p. 830). The extent of the leap from an infant's intrapsychic process to symbiotic mother-infant dual unity seems now to have been largely forgotten. These terms have tended to replace Freud's concept of absolute primary narcissism. The assumption that the psyche of the infant is "fused," "symbiotic," or in "dual unity" at the time of its "origin" is in fact a radical departure from Freudian thought, which I believe reflects the influence of the studies of psychotic children on Mahler's theories.

There is no basis for the assumption that the oceanic feeling exists in normal infants or children, nor in the presumed intrauterine tranquillity of absolute (i.e., never disturbed) primary narcissism.[1] The oceanic feeling as observed in adults is a symptom, incorporating a defensive maneuver, comparable to a delusion denying the fact of intense distress. The hallucinationlike imagery of oneness with the Universe, of being one with the Divine Mother, etc., associated with the oceanic feeling, is unique, in that absolute primary narcissism, to which the subject fantasizes a return, is devoid of content and so cannot provide a memory trace on which to base a hallucination. Nothing is returned to, in the extreme regression of the oceanic feeling, except in fantasy. Inevitably, the early experiences of the infant (some of which must have been positive, for psychic survival) provide the potential for the fantasy of a return to the ideal mother, e.g., the Eternal Feminine, just as the occasional agony

1. Freud described absolute primary narcissism in the *Outline* (1940). It referred to the whole *available* quota of libido. He added, "It lasts till the ego begins to cathect the ideas of objects with libido" (p. 150).

of acute, severe, physical discomfort may be experienced as the threat of annihilation by an evil, devouring, maternal figure. We know nothing about the circumstances, in infancy or in adult life, that determine whether a merging fantasy will take the manifest form of annihilation, Paradise regained, or elements of both, as with Ramakrishna (in the passage from which Rolland is believed to have extracted the term *oceanic feeling* [see Harrison, 1979]). In any event, the fact that some adults experience oceanic feelings does not imply that they represent the original psychic state of the neonate.

The concept of an original dyad was first presented by Jacobson (1964). On one occasion Lewin (1973) seemed to have assumed that a "fusion" of infant with mother exists at the breast, which he likened to the fusion of ego and superego in mania (p. 64). He too, as had Jacobson, drew theory from observations on psychotics. In that context he did not consider whether or not the infants' alleged fusion was primary—i.e., original. Lewin was customarily extremely sensitive, however, to the need to question such manifest experiences as that of "pure" pleasure, and one can see in his account of the dream screen his conviction that a secondary, hallucinatory wish is responsible for such illusions as that of primal fusion.

In many recent theoretical innovations incorporating the idea of an initial mother-infant unit, the perspective is lost which is essential if psychoanalytic theory is to rest on the solid ground of biology. One purpose of the present essay is to emphasize the dangers that arise as a result of conceptualizing the human psyche as originating in a nebulous entity such as the "*psychic field consisting originally of the mother-child (psychic) unit*" (Loewald, 1971, p. 118).[2] The dangers are not confined to theory construction. There is a directly related, although subtle, shift in conceptualizing the psychoanalytic process. The essence of the shift is

---

2. Loewald (1981) brilliantly delineated the regression which is appropriate to psychoanalysis. He wrote: "In analysis, in order to facilitate this instrumental function of regression, we analyze defenses interfering with that resumption, those that impede the regressive movement itself (impede the unfolding of the transference neurosis) and those defenses that stand in the way of renewed progression" (p. 24). Subsequently Loewald recommended the potential benefits of regression far beyond those limits, however (see p. 41f.).

that the human yearning for easing of tension has come to be regarded as requiring the analyst to endeavor to gratify that yearning. An entire volume has recently appeared with the title *The Search for Oneness* (Silverman et al., 1982), in which an analyst-author seems to regard the analyst's task as a successful facilitation of that search and in which, for those admittedly beyond the reach of the suggested psychoanalytic approach, meditation and jogging are noted as therapeutic.

Buie (1981) has presented an example of this danger. He observed that Kohut's view of empathy is mystical, noting views of Olden and of Kohut that imply "a unique and special means of knowing another person's experience which does not depend on usual sensory perception" (p. 284). Amplifying his critique of empathy, he noted that the alleged capability is said to be based upon a presumed primitive resonance, anterior developmentally to a functioning ego and independent of normal perception. He observed that those who maintain that empathy is a special innate capacity for perceiving the inner experiences of others trace this to "the symbiotic stage of infancy, which theoretically is characterized by merging of the infant with its mother. . . . Our problem with this view [of '*primary empathy* with the mother' (Kohut, 1966, p. 262)] is that implicitly it treats the phenomenon of merging, or fusion, literally, as if somehow there were a genuine intermixing, blending of one person's personality with another's" (p. 285). Buie's conclusion is correct and fundamental: "merging in the symbiotic phase is qualitatively similar to merging in healthy later life; at both points it is illusory" (p. 286).

The etymology of the term *merge* is of some interest. Originating in the French *merger,* earlier translated simply as "to drown," as a transitive verb, current usage has evolved from French law, meaning, according to the Oxford English Dictionary, "To sink or extinguish (a lesser estate, title, etc.) in one which is greater or superior. Hence, *gen.* to cause (something) to be absorbed into something else so as to lose its own character or identity; to sink or make disappear." It should be noted that the transitive usage contrasts sharply with psychoanalytic applications.

Merging lends itself, in its ambiguity, to usage which leaves unclear or seems to obviate the distinction that I noted earlier. In general use, *merging* may involve units which retain their individuality, as in "merging traffic," or may indicate the absorption or diffusion of one unit into another, as happens in corporate mergers. Similarly, *emergence*, a term central to Mahler's view of the "psychic birth" of the human infant, may imply the appearance of a new entity—as when a butterfly emerges after metamorphosis from its cocoon—or imply a simple change in locale, from an enclosure to the surrounding world.

Freud's writings offer no grounds for positing an initially fused or merged state. He wrote (1914) that the adult retains some energy resulting from the initial disruption of primary narcissism leading to "a vigorous attempt to recover that state" (p. 100).[3] There is no hint in Freud of dual unity. He used the word *fusion* to describe an intrapsychic process of the ego with the superego in mania, and not an interpsychic one. He attributed the concept of the Nirvana Principle to Barbara Low (1920), who had described it as the wish to return to infantile omnipotence.

Beyond question, however, the imagery inherent in the concept of Nirvana is very close to that of merging. Freud wrote of an overarching tendency toward the extinction of tension—i.e., he advanced a quantitative theoretical hypothesis—but one can readily recognize, in the adoption of the term *Nirvana*, the influence of a strong, subjective wish to merge. This relates to Freud's lifelong dread of abandonment and his fascination with the Eternal Feminine, both documented by Schur (1972). Goethe's romantic imagery had great appeal for Freud; it is awesome that, despite subjective vulnerability to longings for her embrace, Freud kept his theoretical writings, excepting only aspects of death instinct theory, free from the influence of mystical ideas. Freud's views of the infant's psychic origin in the disruption of absolute primary narcissism lend themselves to integration with conclusions drawn from current research on neonates. This con-

3. Freud expressed this insight in many forms, and it has led to two complementary series of studies. Chasseguet-Smirgel (1976) observed about the child: "Separated from his narcissistic omnipotence he senses within himself a gap which he will seek to fill throughout his life" (p. 348). Rangell's attention (1982) was directed to the disruption of original narcissism, in a general critique of self theory, and a particular criticism of Kohut.

trasts with such concepts as original dual unity. Stern (1983) in particular has cast doubt on the latter assumption. (He also expressed reservations about important elements of specifically Freudian theory, but the comments to be cited do not relate to those.) He has challenged the assumption of an autistic phase:

> If *autistic* means uninterested and unregistering of external stimuli, then the infant never was autistic and cannot become less so. Rather, the infant's intrinsically determined social nature simply continues to unfold [p. 10].
>
> [Moreover:] The distinction between cognitive and affective knowledge may have little substance until a language-based semantic system emerges. . . . The central point is that once the assumed "cognitive" incapacity, and the assumed "emotional" need to see self and other as a dual unity have been deeply mitigated, then the central unit of a "normal symbiotic" phase has been removed. The infant need not differentiate from an initial symbiotic position [p. 14].

I find these conclusions, in the context of the data from which they were drawn, very persuasive.

Lester (1983), who has strongly supported Mahler's contributions to psychoanalytic theory, nonetheless observed:

> The two first stages as defined by Mahler do not account for the totality of functions, changes, and phenomena taking place during this age (covering approximately the first five months of life). The terms autism and symbiosis, originally used to describe severe pathological states, exercise a certain constraining influence in our thinking. . . . The term (normal) autism is used to describe a total lack of self-object awareness, i.e., a primary undifferentiated state. Mahler (1967) and other analytic writers (Pine, 1971; Settlage, 1971; Kernberg, 1976) refer to the stage of normal autism in negative terms, by emphasizing what is not there, and by seeing autism solely as a period preparatory to the next stage of symbiosis. Mahler specifically conceives of this stage as a "state of primitive hallucinatory disorientation," associating this to the view of the sensorium as an "autistic shell," a sensory barrier that isolates and protects the immature apparatus of the neonate from a barrage of stimuli [p. 135].
>
> The concept of stimulus barrier has persisted in psychoanalysis despite the fact that evidence challenging the idea of a protective shield in early life has been appearing at an ever-

increasing rate during the last ten to fifteen years . . . the infant, from birth on, far from being within an autistic shell, is able to respond to a great variety of stimuli from the environment [p. 136].

Mahler and McDevitt (1982) recognized only one possible alternative to their view of an original mother-infant unit, namely, that the neonate initially differentiates himself from others, a view which they of course rightly rejected. The almost nonexistent capability of the newborn for orientation with respect to time, place, and person precludes that he conceptualizes the actuality of his being an entity at his mother's breast, i.e., that he differentiates the sources of his feelings and sensations on the basis of whether they arise, objectively speaking, from within or outside. These authors did not endorse a different alternative, however, namely, Freud's hypothesis that the infant's earliest differentiation was, after the first disruption of tranquillity, between his retained pleasure (the core of his being, as the pure pleasure ego) and an experienced discomfort, felt as foreign, hence, "outside" the core of the ego. This hypothesis, enunciated in 1930, continues to be tenable in every respect: "A tendency arises to separate from the ego everything that can become a source of such unpleasure, to throw it outside and to create a pure pleasure-ego which is confronted by a strange and threatening outside" (p. 67).

Weil (1976) provided a luminous account of the infant's experiencing maternal cardiac and respiratory rhythms *in utero*. These are aspects of the initiation of a reciprocity in which the mother is also responding to fetal activities. Subsequent to birth, "the environment shapes the infant—but the infant also shapes the environment" (p. 251). Weil's account of these processes is lucid and precise.[4] Her precision is the exception, however, rather than the rule. Her effort at clarification of Mahler's use of the word *symbiosis* in the context of normal development implied that the word could be a source of confusion, which seems clearly to relate to the idea of merging. Greenacre also questioned the concept. In 1971 she suggested that the infant does not neces-

4. Her adherence to the term *dual unity*, however, is misleading, in my opinion.

sarily experience the apparent contentment, during the normal "symbiotic" phase, which is the basis for assumptions about pleasurable merging. She also said (1979): "the degree of separateness is so uncertain and fluctuant that the infant seems to attribute to another person or thing the hurts which have originated in his own activities" (p. 126). The basic problem inherent in the use of the term symbiosis was highlighted in Buie's observations, as I have indicated.

Mahler's statements about the infant's psychic origins often approach those of Jacobson who explicitly expressed her assumption of original psychic "unity" of infant and mother (1964, p. 38). Moreover, what Jacobson recognized as fantasy, she related to what she believed had originally existed, as evidenced by the phrases "fantasies . . . expressive of wishes to re-establish the lost unit" and "elements of happiness derived from the feeling of return to the lost, original union with the mother" (p. 39).

It is essential to differentiate fantasy from assumed actuality. Merging *fantasies* are common in awe experiences among healthy children and adolescents. This was vividly illustrated in a passage I cited (1975) in which "earth and sky and tree and windblown grass and the child in the midst of them came alive together . . . I in them and they in me, and all of us enclosed in a warm lucent bubble of livingness" (p. 185). Such awe experiences are probably indispensable for full development of the superego. The example just quoted is unusual in its repeated allusion to vitality, but it originates in a volume devoted to experiences facing death (Austin, 1931).

Many merging fantasies of adult life are attended by particularly intense feelings, which may be either of transcendent calm or of dread and horror. Both seem to reflect the response to severe stress among individuals with a particular vulnerability. In some clinical instances it can be conjectured with a fair degree of probability that a genetically or constitutionally determined psychological defect made the early experiencing of trauma inevitable. This was probably true in a case to be described below.

The merging fantasies attended by feelings of dread and horror can often be related readily to early trauma, which inevitably contaminates the infant's view of his mother. This occurs even when the trauma had nothing to do with the mother's actual deficiencies, and may of course remain as only one deeply repressed complex of images, separate from others which may be conscious and positive. In the other case, it may seem paradoxical that children who suffered trauma, perhaps directly resultant from the mother's inability to provide adequate mothering, so consistently long for a "return" to "oneness" with her. The paradox is resolved by the recognition that what is longed for is the tranquillity of the prenatal state, which is presumably devoid of content and certainly of object representations, and that this is regularly extended to the mother. The process is that to which Anna Freud referred, suggested also in Weil's description, of the harmonious integration of the earliest self and object representations into a (secondary, rather than original) merged state. The following examples illustrate the clinical relevance of intense merging fantasies and wishes, and their apparent relation to early trauma which resulted in a distorted memory of the mother.

The first account of a merging fantasy is related to a distorted awe experience. It is taken from the life of Tolstoy as told by his biographer Troyat (1967). Tolstoy's dying mother had asked to see her infant son. "In his nurse's arms little Leo, twenty-three months old, screamed in terror at the sight of the livid mask whose eyes, full of tears, were fixed upon him with unbearable tenderness. He did not recognize his mother. He hated this strange woman" (p. 13).

As is later chronicled, Tolstoy at the age of 17, after having "plunged into the dark, moist forest" one day, had an experience of wondrous awe. That evening as he settled himself for sleep, "every thing took on a different meaning. He dreamed of the ideal woman."

His biographer explains that what then happened is taken from Gusev's *Tolstoi in His Youth:* but "something told me that SHE, with her bare arms and searing embrace, was by no means all the happiness in the world and that even my love for HER was by no means the only good. The longer I stared up at the moon, high in the sky, the more it seemed to me that true beauty and true happiness were still higher, more pure, closer to HIM . . . and tears of joy, an unfulfilled, straining sort of joy, came to my eyes. . . . It seemed to me that nature, the moon and I were one and the same" (p. 50).

Here the residue of a profound infantile trauma complicates

an intense conflict on the oedipal level. Despite Tolstoy's determination to hold onto an awesome deified father figure as a protection from the regressive pull toward the ambivalently experienced mother, he revealed the fantasy of merging with her in his oneness with nature and the moon. The latter element is easily distinguishable from his oedipal-level fantasy, which can be seen to include a feminine identification. Simon and Simon (1972) have described a momentous change in the life of Bertrand Russell when the tragic death of a mother figure gave rise to an intense mystical feeling with similar implications. In the essay which provided the account of wondrous awe described above, Plank (1957) included other examples with more fearsome aspects.

Chasseguet-Smirgel (1971) has delineated the passive anal and aggressive conflicts which influenced the works of Edgar Allan Poe. She also commented on the insufficiency of Marie Bonaparte's concept, in which a "dead-living" woman was said to be the key element influencing Poe's writings. While Chasseguet-Smirgel has enriched our understanding of Poe's pathology and its influence on his creative work, her emphasis on anal and aggressive content deflected attention from the unique quality and characteristics of Poe's creativity, evident especially in his short stories. Symbolic material can be shown to relate to the oral and phallic phases as well as the anal. What is most distinctive about his tales, and some of his poetry, however, is their uncanny and awesome-horrific quality. Often this relates to a gruesome death or a calamity. In these fantasies the consistent concern, made explicit in *The Raven,* is one of hopeless abandonment and the longing for merger. In them, the merging fantasy is even more deeply immersed in dread and horror than was Ramakrishna's, in his experience of oceanic feeling.

An illustrative example of clinical material reflecting the aftermath of early trauma follows. In supervising the analysis of a young woman I learned that when she was 6 she spent about a year in analysis with a noted child analyst. Both the maternal grandmother and the maternal grandmother's father had had shock treatment for depression and two other close relatives on the maternal side had had severe psychiatric problems which had not responded to analytic efforts. She alone of several siblings suffered from severe 3-months colic without any medical (or psychosocial) reason having been discovered. The child's symptom, bed wetting, which had begun after the birth of a sibling, had been cured in the first analysis, and her parents had been told that she was often very sad and was finding treatment too painful; perhaps when she was grown up she would desire further analysis. Early in her adult analysis she described having felt wretched because of harsh treatment by her parents, which seemed inconsistent with available data. Symptoms suggestive of depression included a feeling of helplessness in a variety of situations. She had been an affectionate, lovable, and apparently often happy child who had, moreover, shown many talents. Indeed, no one, including herself, suspected the depth and tenacity of her disorder until she left college, in her second year, because of agitation and depression. Efforts by her parents to get her back into analysis failed, and she found solace in mystical or religious movements. All of these had, in a more or less disguised way, the ideal of merging. They sustained her conviction that her "real" transcendent identity was coextensive with time itself, and that she was usually conscious of only one facet of her being. She related in the ongoing analysis an experience which had astonished her; while someone in a group therapy session was describing seeing people starving in India, she had suddenly become aware that she was crying and experiencing intensely severe abdominal cramps. She had known the history of her infantile colic and assumed that the incident must have been related. I surmise that the colic was a major contributing factor in the psychoetiology of her depression.[5] If, in turn, she was predisposed to a physiological expression of profound malaise on a genetic basis, that might tend to refute the criticism of "genetic fallacy," in that a genetic vulnerability to depression may have been responsible for the early somatic expression of inherent distress. Further data seemed to suggest that this early infantile experience skewed her perception of her mother as well as of herself. It goes without saying that serious and deep-rooted conflicts were delineated in the analysis, and that these

5. See Gaensbauer (1982) for a description of depression at 3 months and speculation about possible consequences.

played a neurosogenic role. My emphasis on the preconflictual, traumatic elements of these conflicts is consistent with Green-acre's view (1979). Referring to nonverbal behavior by analy-sands, she commented: "Frequently these are understood as part of a transference reaction or of some concurrent problem and conflict. This is true, but from experience I have found that patients who have had undue disturbances early show such reactions more plentifully and more sharply than others and often have rather florid physical complaints, formerly often referred to as 'hypochondriac.' The body participates in the analytic situation to an unusual degree, *essentially with a primordial cry to get back to an illusory comforting mother*" (p. 139; my italics). Further, after noting the presence in these patients of symptoms indicative of oedipal conflicts, castration fears, and penis envy, she added: "They are, however, oriented toward narcissistic aims with a weakness in object relatedness" (p. 139f.).

An apparently later source of infantile trauma is suggested in the following instance. A 17-year-old girl came to see me, most reluctantly, at the insistence of her parents. They, in turn, overcame their own aversion only at the urging of the family lawyer, their long-time friend. They found everything about psycho-analysis distasteful. The girl's adolescent years had been stormy, culminating in an accident caused by her drunken driving. Her own car had been taken from her by her parents and she had "borrowed" a car of a friend without his knowledge. After the accident she fled from the scene without discovering whether or not she had injured anyone.

Despite her callous veneer and uncooperative attitude, there was a mute appeal and a profound sadness in her appearance. In what little she volunteered, she had a slight peculiarity of speech remotely suggestive of a German inflection. One of the few details that I obtained from her without difficulty was her un-disguised detestation of her mother, based on flimsy explanations such as the mother's "snobbishness." It was also possible to surmise that her wildly defiant and dramatically amoral behavior had, as a partial explanation, a variant of a wish to merge: when she had enough to drink (which was important not only for its inebriating effect but for the warm internal glow), she sought genital intercourse for the feeling of warmth and closeness the body contact provided. These symptoms and her behavior were the only overt hints at the existence of a merging fantasy. I suspected that she was barely succeeding in deflecting the suicidal wish to realize such a fantasy in death.

She wished to terminate the consultation when it began, and I asked to see her parents. They seemed to be "stonewalling," and I then met with each parent alone. Again the mother provided no significant information. The father kept fingering a disfiguring scar while talking to me, however, and when I asked him what had caused it, he broke down and wept for several minutes and then related that the severe and unusual illness which had caused the scar followed immediately upon the sudden death of their first-born child during the patient's first year. He and his wife agreed to remove every trace of the dead child from their home and never to allow the surviving baby to know that she had existed. Their German domestic servant was subsequently discharged in the patient's second year because her own grief was so painful to the parents. The patient's father had thought that they had been entirely successful in rising above their tragedy. The patient and her subsequent siblings had seemed to be "good" children, compliant and attractive.

I advised her parents to share the details which they had hidden from the patient and she seemed amazed to learn the facts. I myself suggested to her the probable explanation of her speech peculiarity which she had previously thought of as "weird." She seemed to have a change in attitude about therapy for a short time, but was not able to tolerate any further efforts. A few years later, in a chance encounter, the patient's mother volunteered the information that the daughter's wild behavior had ceased and that she was about to marry. Those who have worked with adolescents will undoubtedly wonder how much improvement one can attribute directly to her new knowledge about her infancy. Possibly many chance events could have helped her to stop her misbehavior. But I cannot doubt the relevance of the drama during her first year nor of the speech patterns of the mother figure she lost before the age of 2, to the severe depression which had been concealed from her parents until it gave way to the destructive behavior in adolescence.

Although it is not possible to provide other examples as clear-cut as Buie's demonstration (1981), it seems very likely that many of the current modifications recommended for psychoanalytic technique reflect the influence of the concept of an originally merged state encompassing mother and infant. I will conclude the essay with an example which seems to me to underscore the turning away from a psychoanalytic focus upon reconstruction and interpretation, in a direction which is strongly suggestive of that influence.

The specific example is taken from an essay which, as is true of so many new technical proposals, dealt with the analysis of very ill patients. Limentani (1977) described a case in which there were months of silence. He accepted notes from the patient which he felt helped him "establish transitional space" and were valuable in preventing acting out. Up to that point, the classical Freudian must be inclined to accept the view of an eminent colleague that a parameter may have been necessary in order to create or to maintain an analysis. In what seems, however, to mark a transition from the use of a parameter for that purpose to a radical departure from it, Limentani asked (p. 179): "Are words . . . all that important to the psychoanalytic process?" Without words, how can a specifically analytic cure be possible?

Many other current recommendations, e.g., for "persuasion," consistent with the assumption of a "new era" reflecting a humanist trend (Friedman, 1982, p. 365), also depart from Freud's modest request as to what should be labeled as psychoanalytic. In all of these departures, the potential for gratifications of regressive longings exists for both parties to the transaction. Such regressive gratifications further sleep, to paraphrase Lewin's famous analogy. In that sense, I conclude that technical innovations in the direction of gratifying the analysand's regressive wishes all have in common the implicit assumption that ideal comfort lies at the end of a regressive route. That is the essence of the concept of merging, whether it is presented at the far end of life or at its commencement.

SUMMARY AND CONCLUSIONS

The assumption of an original state of mother-infant unity is now widely accepted as a fact of individual psychic development.

That assumption is shown here to incorporate a concept of merging. Merging was originally advanced and understood as a primitive intrapsychic activity whereby the early ego blended sensations and impressions from diverse and nondiscriminated sources. It has become confused with an alleged capability of two individuals to "merge" to some extent, based on processes which are either more primitive than, and developmentally anterior to, perception via the senses (Kohut, 1966), or (Loewald, 1981) existent in a realm of "psychic fields" beyond the observable events of human physiology. The distinction between merging and the fantasy of merging has been explicated.

Many recent theoretical and technical innovations in psychoanalysis reflect the influence of the assumption of an original mother-infant unity. The goal of efforts to promote empathy and to encourage regression in pursuit of the merged state is here contrasted with the Freudian technique in which regression has the exclusive goal of facilitating the analysand's access to his repressed conflicts so that a connection can be established between these and his conscious (verbal) ego.

BIBLIOGRAPHY

AUSTIN, M. (1931). *Experiences Facing Death.* Indianapolis: Bobbs Merrill.

BUIE, D. H. (1981). Empathy. *J. Amer. Psychoanal. Assn.,* 29:281–308.

CHASSEGUET-SMIRGEL, J. (1971). *Pour une psychanalyse de l'art et de la creativité.* Paris: Payot.

———— (1976). Some thoughts on the ego ideal. *Psychoanal. Q.,* 45:345–373.

FREUD, A. (1960). Discussion of Dr. John Bowlby's paper. *Psychoanal. Study Child,* 15:53–62.

FREUD, S. (1914). On narcissism. *S.E.,* 14:67–104.

———— (1915). Instincts and their vicissitudes. *S.E.,* 14:117–140.

———— (1920). Beyond the pleasure principle. *S.E.,* 18:1–64.

———— (1930). Civilization and its discontents. *S.E.,* 21:57–146.

———— (1940). An outline of psycho-analysis. *S.E.,* 23:139–208.

FRIEDMAN, L. (1982). The humanistic trend in recent psychoanalytic theory. *Psychoanal. Q.,* 51:353–371.

GAENSBAUER, T. (1982). The differentiation of discrete affects. *Psychoanal. Study Child,* 37:29–66.

GREENACRE, P. (1971). Notes on the influence and contribution of ego psychology to the practice of psychoanalysis. In *Separation-Individuation,* ed. J. B. McDevitt & C. F. Settlage, pp. 171–200. New York: Int. Univ. Press.

────── (1979). Reconstruction and the process of individuation. *Psychoanal. Study Child,* 34:121–144.

HARRISON, I. B. (1975). On the maternal origins of awe. *Psychoanal. Study Child,* 30:181–195.

────── (1979). On Freud's view of the infant-mother relationship and of the oceanic feeling. *J. Amer. Psychoanal. Assn.,* 27:399–421.

────── (1985). A fresh look at the regulatory principles. Unpublished essay.

JACOBSON, E. (1964). *The Self and the Object World.* New York: Int. Univ. Press.

KOHUT, H. (1966). Forms and transformations of narcissism. *J. Amer. Psychoanal. Assn.,* 14:243–272.

LESTER, E. (1983). Separation-individuation and cognition. *J. Amer. Psychoanal. Assn.,* 31:127–156.

LEWIN, B. D. (1950). *The Psychoanalysis of Elation.* New York: Norton.

────── (1973). *Selected Writings of Bertram D. Lewin,* ed. J. A. Arlow. New York: Psychoanalytic Quarterly.

LIMENTANI, A. (1977). Affects and the psychoanalytic situation. *Int. J. Psychoanal.,* 58:171–182.

LOEWALD, H. W. (1971). On motivation and instinct theory. *Psychoanal. Study Child,* 26:91–128.

────── (1981). Regression. *Psychoanal. Q.,* 50:22–43.

LOW, B. (1920). *Psycho-Analysis.* New York: Harcourt, Brace & Howe.

MAHLER, M. S. (1968). *On Human Symbiosis and the Vicissitudes of Individuation.* New York: Int. Univ. Press.

MAHLER, M. S. & McDEVITT, J. B. (1982). Thoughts on the emergence of the sense of self, with particular emphasis on the body self. *J. Amer. Psychoanal. Assn.,* 30:827–848.

PLANK, R. (1957). On "seeing the salamander." *Psychoanal. Study Child,* 12:379–398.

RANGELL, L. (1982). The self and psychoanalytic theory. *J. Amer. Psychoanal. Assn.,* 30:863–891.

SCHUR, M. (1972). *Freud.* New York: Int. Univ. Press.

SILVERMAN, L., LACHMAN, F., & MILICH, R. (1982). *The Search for Oneness.* New York: Int. Univ. Press.

SIMON, B. & SIMON, N. (1972). The pacifist turn. *J. Amer. Psychoanal. Assn.,* 20:109–121.

STERN, D. (1983). Implications of infant research for psychoanalytic theory and practice. In *Psychiatric Update,* ed. L. Grinspoon, 2:8–21. Washington: American Psychiatric Press.

TROYAT, H. (1967). *Tolstoy.* Garden City, N.Y.: Doubleday.

WEIL, A. (1976). The first year. In *The Process of Child Development,* ed. P. B. Neubauer, pp. 246–265. New York: Meridian.

The Empathic Wall and the Ecology of Affect

DONALD L. NATHANSON, M.D.

AFFECT THEORY

MODERN AFFECT THEORY BEGINS WITH THE WORK OF SILVAN TOMkins (1962, 1963). Observing the face of his newborn son, Tomkins saw what looked like "emotion" displayed on the face of an organism with none of the history, none of the life experience we have always considered necessary for the development of emotion. "Certainly the infant who emits his birth cry upon exit from the birth canal has not 'appraised' the new environment as a vale of tears before he cries" (Tomkins, 1982, p. 362). Nonetheless, the crying infant looks quite like a crying adult—this cry of distress must have been *available* to the infant courtesy of some preexistent mechanism triggered by some stimulus acceptable to that mechanism.

Tomkins sees nine of these mechanisms, a group of primarily facial responses which he calls "innate affects," as operating from birth. The positive affects are *interest* or *excitement, enjoyment* or *joy,* and *surprise* or *startle.* The negative innate affects, also present from birth and visible on the face of the newborn, are

Attending psychiatrist, the Institute of Pennsylvania Hospital.

Portions of this paper were presented at the International Symposium on Denial, Jerusalem, 30 January 1985.

I am deeply indebted to Dr. Léon Wurmser for his constant support and encouragement and for the many theoretical discussions which allowed clarification of my ideas.

distress or *anguish, fear* or *terror, shame* or *humiliation, dissmell,*[1] *disgust,*[2] and *anger* or *rage.*

Tomkins assumes that the affects are triggered by the way information comes into the brain through neural pathways—it is the number of neural firings per unit time, what he calls the "density" of neural firing, which is responsible for affect activation. Once activated, the subcortical program then begins to produce affect, which itself triggers more affect. It does not matter whether the stimulus comes in on the auditory, visual, or kinesthetic track—in this theory the affects are essentially neutral with respect to their activators. Thus he postulates that a stimulus which begins at a low level and increases gradually produces the affect *interest,* which affect at its higher levels of intensity is experienced as *excitement. Distress* is activated by stimuli which are at a relatively constant but higher than optimal level, and *anger* by stimuli which are constant but at a still higher nonoptimal level. *Enjoyment* accompanies the sudden reduction of any stimulus, and *surprise* will be activated when the stimulus gradient is sudden and upwards, as with a pistol shot. Babies are thus equipped from birth with perceptual and protective systems which allow them to react to stimuli that they will not "understand" for quite some time.

Affective behavior patterns are inherited programs available to the infant. These may be combined with each other and with the experiences which triggered them to form complex patterns, just as the letters of our alphabet may be combined to form words and words combined to form sentences. Memory, for instance, can produce the shock of recognition, which involves

1. The sense of smell allows us to evaluate a distant entity by its emitted odor. What functions initially as a drive auxiliary, protecting us from unchecked and therefore potentially dangerous hunger, becomes an affect later in development. This is seen in such expressions as "turning up one's nose at" and calling the object a "stinker."

2. Taste is the final sentinel of the gastrointestinal tract, allowing us to "spit out" something before it gets into the gut. Tomkins also views disgust as an affect which developed from a drive auxiliary. Nausea, vomiting, and diarrhea are the other mechanisms protecting the gut from noxious substances—although presenting frequently as emotion equivalents, they are not displayed on the face and do not rank as primary affects in Tomkins's system.

an affective response to the suddenness with which various higher cortical systems presented an association. These affect programs involve a host of bodily systems, including of course what we have always called the "muscles of expression" in the face, but also the endocrine and exocrine glands and nearly any group of odors, postures, and colors. Basch (1976, 1983a, 1983b) has suggested that we use the term "affect" to refer to biological events, "feeling" to our awareness of these events, and "emotion" to the complex interrelationships formed by the experience of an affect and our associations to it. "Emotion," he suggests, "when developed, is evidence of neocortical activity of a highly sophisticated sort" (1976, p. 770).

Buck (1984) suggests that the emotions evolved in three phases. Arising first as subcortical mechanisms concerned with bodily adaptation and the maintenance of homeostasis, they operated completely out of awareness (Emotion I). In the second phase, the affects became expressed in externally accessible behaviors as spontaneous expressions of internal states, perhaps useful for the coordination of behavior in a species (Emotion II). The final phase of development (Emotion III) involves the direct subjective experience of the state of certain neurochemical systems. It is this last adaptation which has allowed the linkage of the phylogenetically earlier subcortical affect mechanisms with higher cortical function to form the type of emotion with which we are most familiar in psychoanalytic thinking.

PSYCHOANALYTIC CONCEPTS

The historic focus of psychoanalysis on cognitive, intrapsychic function has tended to underemphasize the importance of affect expression and affective communication. Yet, as Modell (1978) has said, "assuming that psychoanalysis is a study of meaning, meaning itself is determined by the communication of affects" (p. 170).

It is in the nature of evolution that existing systems are recruited for new functions—we should not be surprised that the affects evolved into a quite sophisticated communication system. That the affects are displayed on the signboard of the face is not limited to man, as any dog owner can testify. Our pets convey messages of the most remarkable complexity by a combination of intentional gesture and affect display. Affective communication in the human is of even greater complexity, and nowhere is this more important than in the relationship between mother and infant.

Although it suited the purpose of previous generations of theorists to view the infant as entirely self-involved, it has become clear that the baby spends a considerable portion of his time observing mother with rapt attention. To Winnicott has been attributed the comment that there is no such thing as a baby—there is only the baby and his mother. Mother and infant are linked in a dyadic relationship. Lichtenberg (1981) states, "The overwhelming weight of evidence from infant research indicates that the neonate begins life in an interactive dialogue with his mother. From the beginning, for both partners, this dialogue has models of perceptual organization that activate the responsiveness of the other. Within this dyadic communicative exchange there is no distinction between affect response and perceptual-cognitive ordering" (p. 333). From the moment of birth the infant is delivered into the climate of mother's affect. Any competent theory for the development of the infantile ego must include systems for the processing of affective communication.

Anna Freud (1936) may have alluded to this when she wrote, "The efforts of the infantile ego to avoid 'pain' by directly resisting external impressions belong to the sphere of normal psychology. Their consequences may be momentous for the formation of the ego and of character, but they are not pathogenic. When this particular ego function is referred to in clinical analytic writings, it is never treated as the main object of observation but merely as a by-product of observation" (p. 71). In this communication I wish to refocus our attention on such ego functions, and to demonstrate their relevance to our clinical work.

EMPATHY

The term for an affective linkage forged during psychotherapy is "empathy." As Basch (1983a) has so convincingly demonstrated, while it is affect which is transmitted in empathy, we experience this empathic perception as emotion because of our associations to the particular affect transmitted. We never really share the other person's emotion because each of us has lived too complex a life, has formed associations to these innate affects based on experiences which are different despite their general similarity. Your experience of shame is not mine, your anger is not my anger. Yet through empathy I may clench my jaw when you feel angry, and look away in embarrassment when you are shamed. Many clinicians are loathe to diagnose depression in a patient who does not make them *feel* depressed; similarly we accept without comment that mania is infectious.

The psychoanalyst is a paradigm of the "good" audience. Indeed, for many people, therapy provides the first life experience in which they feel heard, in which they feel real. So highly do both therapists and patients value this feeling of being known on an affective level that a significant underlying truth has been obscured. We consider the absence of empathy normal, and the presence of it special. The most mature among us do not live in a world of shared emotion. Maturity implies a certain degree of isolation from the emotions of others.

THE EMPATHIC WALL

Rather than asking how the message of happiness, grief, resentment, anger, or distress is *transmitted,* we should consider how such transmission is *blocked.* How is it that we are not more often taken over by affect so broadcast? When infectious disease was the frontier of science, such transmission was called contagion of affect (Scheler, 1912; Sullivan, 1954). One has only to watch dispassionately the flow of laughter through an audience, or the flow of anger through a mob, to wonder how the normal human develops immunity to this contagion; how do we learn to remain ourselves in the presence of the affect of the other?

These and many other questions may be answered by the introduction of a new ego mechanism to which I have given the apparently paradoxical name the "empathic wall." The empathic wall allows us to monitor our affective experience and determine whether the affect of the moment is generated from within or without, thus defining the difference between self and other. It may be the root mechanism for a host of normal and pathological defensive operations of the ego.

Rather than considering all experience of affective transmission to be synonymous with empathy, I would agree with Basch (1983a) that *mature* empathy involves the intentional acceptance of such transmission. It is my feeling that mature empathy can occur only in a person with a healthy empathic wall mechanism, who is in addition capable of relaxing this ego function in order to merge briefly with the affective broadcast of the other. In our analytic work this lapse into primary process, which is analogous to other examples of the creative process, is followed by a return to secondary process accompanied by data about the other learned during the empathic link. In the remainder of this paper I will focus on the development of the empathic wall and its relationship to denial, projection, and the phenomenology of certain psychopathological conditions.

INFANT RESEARCH

That infants reward the smile of the mother with a smile of their own is an indication of the relationship between mimesis and affective transmission. Emde et al. (1976) have written extensively about affect mutualization between mother and infant. The infant's smile makes the mother feel good, which sense of pleasure may be communicated to the child; conversely, the infant's cry of distress activates distress in the mother. Demos (1982) describes the infant as scanning his environment with interest, accepting it as a provider of stimulation. When this stimulation begins to produce distress, "he will attempt to decrease the level of stimulation by turning away from the object" (p. 565). One form of stimulation is, of course, the affect available in his environment; I believe that such activity of turning away represents the early beginnings of the empathic wall.

Beebe and Sloate (1982) describe the attempts of an infant to handle the affective onslaught of a psychotic, intrusive mother. By 3 to 4 months the child had lost her fascination with mother's face and demonstrated extensive gaze aversion. "It can be hypothesized that the pattern of extensive looking away was already being used by this infant to help modulate inappropriate stimulation that was experienced as aversive" (p. 606). At 8 months, "She tuned out and withdrew from mother's attempts to engage her in play, turning her back, looking out the window, behaving as if she did not hear her mother" (p. 616). Adequate data are given in this case material to allow the conclusion that the infant was avoiding mother's affect, using what I believe to be the blocking function of the empathic wall mechanism. Beebe and Sloate explain this by reference to Rubinfine's (1962) comments "on the child's use of denial to conserve the object relation in situations where the mother has taken on the properties of an aversive stimulus" (p. 616).

Selma Kramer (1983) has suggested that, in the normal child, the appearance of stranger anxiety marks achievement of an ego mechanism which can allow him to recognize the difference between the affective transmission of mother and of anybody else. Awareness of the difference between such transmission sets may be one way the infant learns to recognize individuals; more important for our purposes here, it certainly may provide the analogue for recognizing the difference between self and other on the affective level. Emde et al. (1976) note that by this time the "transactions between mother and infant have differentiated to the point where both are 'tuned in' to a mutually specific attachment. . . . As a stranger approaches [the infant] looks with an expression of interest which then becomes one of sober perplexity. This is followed by what is rated as a fearful expression, with frowning and then crying . . . accompanied by gaze aversion and a turning away of the head and body" (p. 145).

DENIAL AND PROJECTION

Both denial and projection involve application of skills learned in the formation and operation of the empathic wall mechanism. The child has learned to evaluate intense experiences of affect by checking to see whether a feeling has arisen from within self or other. In the face of intense, perhaps unacceptable affect broadcast by the mother, the empathic wall allows the child to succeed in the struggle to maintain affectional ties while *separating from the feeling*. Proper use of the empathic wall allows the child to remain self while leaving broadcast feelings outside the self. The case of Beebe and Sloate (1982) cited above represents an extreme example of the affect blocking provided by the empathic wall mechanism. Thus, denial and projection are part of the normative functioning and not limited to being in the service of pathological defense mechanisms.

Here, then, is a mechanism which allows the individual to sample his own affective state and determine its source, a mechanism valuable for an organism whose perceptual and communicative apparatus are not developed adequately to allow symbolic communication. If such a mechanism can allow the child to wall off external affect, to feel that this affective state comes from outside the self and rightly should remain outside the self, then that mechanism is capable of being recruited for further use when unpleasant affect derives from *inner* conflict. The child can wall off the feeling, even to the extent that the feeling is viewed as an intrusion from the outside, the result of affective transmission. Denial utilizes the affect-blocking portion of the empathic wall, while projection makes use of its ability to perform a "vector analysis"—to determine from which direction a particular affect originated.

Useful as this mechanism may seem in allowing the individual to disavow some portion of the meaning of an event or a percept in order to reduce the associated painful affect (Weisman and Hackett, 1961), it alters rather than solves the problem. As Waelder (1951) said, even if projection shifts the focus from self to other, "the denied instinct remains in the limelight; he who projected his aggressiveness onto others has his mind occupied with aggressiveness, albeit somebody else's" (p. 174). The noxious affect is still being experienced, but it is attributed to the other.

PROJECTIVE IDENTIFICATION

Kernberg (1967) comes close to my understanding of the empathic wall mechanism in his discussion of projective identification; he states that the patient's aggression, although projected onto the object, remains active. "This leads such patients to feel that they can still identify themselves with the object onto whom aggression has been projected, and their ongoing 'empathy' with the now threatening object maintains and increases the fear of their own projected aggression. . . . In summary, projective identification is characterized by the lack of differentiation between self and object in that particular area, by continuing to experience the *impulse* as well as the fear of that impulse while the projection is active, and by the need to control the external object" (p. 669; my italics).

But it is affects, not impulses which are projected. Further, in the language developed here, it is through a defensive misuse of the empathic wall mechanism that one has attributed an affect to the object and decided that one is experiencing this uncomfortable affect by affective transmission from the object. What Kernberg calls "empathy," I see as affective transmission, which by its nature is a transient or reactive state; identification, which implies a move toward likeness to another person including the adoption of interests, ideals, or mannerisms of the other, is therefore a much more lasting phenomenon. It would appear, in view of our current understanding of affect, that the term "projective identification" is a misnomer at many levels. Perhaps the actual phenomena involved would be described better by the terms "subjective naming" and "objective naming," to take into account the situations where our idea of the other derives from our own, subjective sources, or from the object seen clearly.

INTERPERSONAL ASPECTS OF DENIAL

An often ignored yet supremely important matter is the interpersonal aspect of denial—what denial does in and to a relationship. We take it for granted that in a good, healthy object relationship the participants share reality. But as Dorpat (1983) has said so well, "The dynamic defensive function of denial is carried out by the active exclusion of information from focal attention, i.e., explicit conscious awareness" (p. 48). What if, through denial, one member of a dyad acts as if some piece of information, taken for granted by the other, and the competent subject of focal attention by that other, does not exist?

Our observation is that each belief system produces its own characteristic affective display—i.e., we wear on our faces the feeling state, or mood which derives from the sum of our knowledge, whether conscious, preconscious, or unconscious. When the intimate other senses, by affective transmission, the disparity between the two belief systems, anxiety is produced. This anxiety causes interpersonal tension which must be resolved if the relationship is to endure at the previous level of intimacy. Each relationship has a characteristic mode of tension resolution, ranging from friendly inquiry to open hostility and fighting. Denial seems to work better in the privacy of one's defenses. Thus denial in the subject causes anxiety in the object, verifying again Waelder's (1951) observation that, at least in a relationship, there may be no such thing as "successful" denial unless there is a fit of one person's denial with the needs or tolerances of the other person in the close relationship.

CLINICAL ILLUSTRATIONS

CASE 1

Karen, a 24-year-old graduate student, entered therapy in an attempt to interrupt a recurring cycle of unhappy romantic liasons. Men flocked around her in bars and at parties; she was courted impulsively by suitors who responded to her with a degree of sexual intimacy and openness one might expect in a more developed relationship. She remarked, "They seem to be turned on, ready for sex when I am just getting to know them. The first couple of guys who said 'Come on, I know you want it too' made me furious. But enough men have said something like that, and I thought I should bring it up here."

What excited those men? Karen noted with some interest that although in intercourse she experienced a considerable degree of vaginal anesthesia, and that she did not look forward to intercourse, she was aware of nearly constant vaginal wetness unassociated with conscious sexual ideation. That she had disavowed sexual excitement as a compromise settlement of oedipal conflicts became apparent to her much later; what helped her at this stage in treatment was the recognition that men were sexually aroused by her denied arousal. Knowing that her body was responding to unconscious forces with which she was not yet ready to deal, she was better able to integrate relationships with men now that she understood that portion of their behavior deriving from her denied arousal. Late in her fourth year of therapy, when she was well on her way toward healthy object relatedness, beginning to be involved in genital sexuality with a loved and loving partner, she commented that during sexual excitement she was aware that her facial expression was reminiscent of the facial set which, before therapy, she had displayed nearly constantly.

Sullivan (1954) commented that lust appears as a drive in early adolescence. It is during this period in development that sexual ideation becomes connected to its affective component. Parents of adolescents know this best, for children previously unsuspected of sexual ideation "suddenly" are seen as being "sexy." "Sexiness" is an affective broadcast. I have confirmed this observation in clinical practice on countless occasions—men and women who are read by others as sexually exciting are themselves, at that moment, involved in their own sexual excitement. This is normal affective transmission, handled, as Anna Freud said, by the ego functions which monitor external impressions.

The hysteric is decidedly uncomfortable with the oedipal ideation which has produced her sexual excitement, and has used the affect-blocking portion of the empathic wall mechanism to keep this complex of affects out of awareness. The fact that she is condemned by this defensive decision to be the object of sexual pursuit confirms Waelder's observation that denial is not freedom.

Finally, this case illustrates the relationship between denial, projection, and the empathic wall, for Karen's denial does not eradicate her own sexual excitement, which is still being triggered, but now by forces of which she is not aware. This affect remains in the interpersonal field, where it may be confused with normal affective transmission from the object. Both the hysteric and the paranoid see the disavowed, unacceptable affect as emanating from the object. The difference lies in the competence of the vector-analyzing portion of the empathic wall mechanism. The hysteric has blocked the feeling, and remains relatively free of it—the sexual excitement and ideation are attributed to the object through a defensive misuse of the empathic wall. The paranoid, whose empathic wall is weaker than that of the hysteric, continues to experience the affect, but blames the object for "influencing" him.

Any ego function can be eroded in the schizophrenic process—indeed, study of the schizophrenias has taught us much about the range of normal ego functions. If a breach in the empathic wall has been forced by illness, the patient may complain that the feelings of others are being experienced as an unwelcome intrusion. Wurmser (1981) reports the statement of Blanche, 3 years before an overt schizophrenic psychosis, trying to defend against terrible discomfort in the presence of others, "I try consciously to get to know them, but it's as if I lack empathy" (p. 140). Later, during the worst of her illness she reported, "I'm so dependent on what other people think. I wanted to get away from people—to be myself, to feel my own feelings. Why do other people affect me that much?" (p. 140). This failure to block broadcast affect also may be interpreted by the patient as fantasies of telepathic power, or delusions that one is the subject of messages broadcast from another's space ("outer space").

Failure of the empathic wall ego mechanism is seen in "psychotic insight," which involves involuntary empathic acceptance of affective and gestural communication otherwise denied by the sender. Such insight is considered psychotic because the patient either is unable to use the empathic wall to return to self, or cannot use other ego mechanisms to integrate this new information about the other for the purposes of normal interpersonal relatedness.

Another patient, Jocelyn, complained bitterly that in the company of others she was unable to maintain her own emotions. If a friend seemed upset about something Jocelyn had said, she too would begin to feel upset; if a companion were to be gleeful, she would feel inappropriately gleeful, then confused and angry as she felt a loss of her own identity. The experience of affective resonance was quite unpleasant for her. Concomitantly she was extraordinarily restricted in the display of her own emotions. I will take up two facets of her relationship with her mother in an attempt to explain the development of what she regarded as her most uncomfortable symptoms.

Jocelyn avoided contact with her mother, whom she described as an affective steamroller whose rages and sulks dominated the family. The family dog was severely beaten whenever it soiled a floor or rug, despite the fact that no attempt at housetraining was ever made. The patient was often awakened to hear her mother screaming at her father. In dreams the mother usually was represented as a dark figure, frequently a witch, always an object of terror. Such a parent provided an environment overloaded with unmodulated affect, depriving the growing child of the opportunity to develop an adequate empathic wall, rendering the child susceptible to external impression.

By age 11 Jocelyn had discovered lying, which gave her some sense of distance from her mother. Later she learned to control her own affective output around her mother, developing first a sort of facial flatness and then a number of elaborately conceived and practiced pseudoemotional behavioral entities which we came to call "affective modules." By maintaning (initially consciously, later unconsciously) her facial musculature in a mask-like state, she reduced the affective resonance which so upset her, for the face is the major display board of the affect system. This served another function, for, as she described interactions with her mother, "Unless I am in complete control of my emotions when I am around her, she takes over my emotion. I can't be in a bad mood, or she will not only be in a bad mood, but it will be her bad mood, and she will tell me what I should do. After I am around her for a little while when one of these things is happening, I feel crazy because I can't even remember why I was in a bad mood to begin with, let alone what I was really feeling." I suspect that this mother's problems with affect modulation bear some relationship to a defect in her own empathic wall mechanism.

In treatment Jocelyn gave up the defensive flatness only when she had thoroughly and repeatedly tested my ability to maintain a calm, warm manner despite her attempts within the transference to see me as volatile. A breakthrough of enormous importance came in the third year of therapy when she decided to stand before a mirror experimenting with facial expression. As she mimicked the expressions of anger, distress, shame, joy, surprise, and disgust, she felt herself flooded with feeling which she could now control by turning off the expression. Through a year-long series of exercises she worked through a wide range of affects, building her ability to tolerate emotion. Growth in therapy strengthened her ability to handle her own affect as well as that broadcast by others. Now, in her fifth year of treatment, she has begun to develop a good sense of self and a healthy need for privacy appropriately bounded by shame.

INTEGRATION WITH OTHER THEORIES

In his microanalysis of the mechanism of denial, Dorpat (1983) determined the following "four phases of denial reactions: (1) preconscious appraisal of danger or trauma, (2) painful affect, (3) cognitive arrest, and (4) screen behaviour" (p. 47). He explains that "cognitive arrest is brought about by unconscious fantasies of destroying or rejecting whatever he considers to be the cause of his psychic pain (or what I have termed 'the painful object')" (p. 47). I believe that it is the normal function of the empathic wall to sense that the pain one is experiencing derives from the object by affective transmission. Dorpat has come quite close to my concept in his suggestion that an affective state deriving from inner conflict has, through denial, been attributed to pain caused by another.

Basch (1982) points out that *Verleugnung* is properly translated as disavowal, rather than denial, for disavowal implies the vernacular use more central to Freud's meaning—the unconscious version of the self-serving socially acceptable evasions of everyday life, in which there is no hint of psychotic distortion of thought process. He shows that Freud meant to designate disavowal "as the mechanism which defends against traumatic external reality, whereas repression deals with unacceptable instinctual demands" (p. 135). "Disavowal," he continues, "prevents the union of affect with percept, without, however, blocking the percept from consciousness" (p. 147).

Finally, Basch states that "conceptual clarity would be served if the term 'denial' was used as a collective term for those psychotic or nonpsychotic mechanisms that actually interfere with the perceptual interpretation of sensory signals, while following Freud, using the term 'disavowal' only to describe that situation in which the affectively toned meaning that a percept would be expected to have for the self is unconsciously repudiated" (p. 146). Both senses of *Verleugnung* fit well with the concept that they are preceded by skills learned in the use of the empathic wall mechanism. The empathic wall conforms to Basch's requirement for a mechanism which "interferes with the perceptual interpretation of sensory signals" as long as one understands that affective resonance is a sensory analogue.

The relationship between affective transmission and the repudiation of the "affectively toned meaning of a percept" requires further discussion. Just as affect display can be mimicked—as it is normally in affective resonance and intentionally in the experiment of Ekman et al. (1983)—it can be mimed for the purpose of conveying a false communication. The "confidence man," the salesman, and the seducer pull us into a trusting relationship by their use of the verbal tone and facial affect display of affection and caring. The mature person ignores these messages in order to focus better on the verbal, symbolic content of the communication. It is the ability to resist affective transmission which protects us from such sales techniques. Philosopher Alan Watts (1970) called this "ig nor' ance," the healthy ability to ignore. Disavowal of an affective percept is initially the function of the empathic wall.

As the head turns and the eye blinks to shield the retina from intense light, so the growing ego is protected by a host of mechanisms from overly intense affect, whether generated from within or impinging on the child from the interpersonal environment. The mental mechanisms are not some sort of refuge for the weak. They are a group of protections built into the organism itself, protective systems inherent to the nature of man, defenses accumulated through the ages of evolution, recruited even today in the life of an organism struggling for survival.

SUMMARY

The nature and significance of affect and of affective transmission are examined, and a new ego mechanism, called the empathic wall, is described to explain the organism's adaptation to affective resonance. The earliest form of communication is the sharing of affect; the infant needs some way of differentiating between affect experienced as the result of (maternal) transmission and that resulting from purely inner sources. The empathic wall mechanism provides a primitive form of affect blocking and allows attribution of experienced affect either to subject or object, thus providing the substrate on which both denial and projection are formed. The psychoanalytic understanding of empathy is reviewed in terms of the empathic wall. Clinical material is provided to demonstrate the use of this concept in our understanding of patients and in therapy.

BIBLIOGRAPHY

BASCH, M. F. (1976). The concept of affect. *J. Amer. Psychoanal. Assn.*, 24:759–777.
———— (1982). The perception of reality and the disavowal of meaning. *Annu. Psychoanal.*, 11:125–163.
———— (1983a). Empathic understanding. *J. Amer. Psychoanal. Assn.*, 31:101–126.
———— (1983b). The concept of "self." In *Developmental Approaches to the Self*, ed. B. Lee & G. Noam, pp. 7–58. New York: Plenum.
BEEBE, B. & SLOATE, P. (1982). Assessment and treatment of difficulties in mother-infant attunement in the first 3 years of life. *Psychoanal. Inqu.*, 2:601–623.
BUCK, R. (1984). *The Communication of Emotion.* New York: Guilford Press.
DEMOS, E. V. (1982). Affect in early infancy. *Psychoanal. Inqu.*, 2:533–574.
DORPAT, T. L. (1983). The cognitive arrest hypothesis of denial. *Int. J. Psychoanal.*, 64:47–58.
EKMAN, P., LEVENSON, R. W., & FRIESEN, W. V. (1983). Evidence for autonomic reactions in specific emotions. *Science*, 221:1208–1210.
EMDE, R. N., GAENSBAUER, T. J., & HARMON, R. J. (1976). *Emotional Expression in Infancy.* Psychol. Issues, monogr. 37. New York: Int. Univ. Press.
FREUD, A. (1936). The ego and the mechanisms of defense. *W.*, 2.
FREUD, S. (1921). Group psychology and the analysis of the ego. *S.E.*, 18:67–143.
KERNBERG, O. (1967). Borderline personality organization. *J. Amer. Psychoanal. Assn.*, 15:641–685.
KRAMER, S. (1983). Personal communication.
LICHTENBERG, J. (1981). The empathic mode of perception and alternative vantage points for psychoanalytic work. *Psychoanal. Inqu.*, 1:329–356.
MODELL, A. H. (1978). Affects and the complementarity of biologic and historical meaning. *Annu. Psychoanal.*, 6:167–180.

RUBINFINE, D. L. (1962). Maternal stimulation, psychic structure, and early object relations. *Psychoanal. Study Child,* 17:265–282.

SCHELER, M. (1912). *The Nature of Sympathy.* Hamden, Ct.: Archon Books, 1972.

SULLIVAN, H. S. (1954). *The Psychiatric Interview.* New York: Norton.

TOMKINS, S. S. (1962). *Affect/Imagery/Consciousness,* 1. New York: Springer.

———— (1963). *Affect/Imagery/Consciousness* 2. New York: Springer.

———— (1982). Affect theory. In *Emotion in the Human Face,* 2nd ed. ed. P. Ekman, p. 362. Cambridge: Cambridge Univ. Press.

WAELDER, R. (1951). The structure of paranoid ideas. *Int. J. Psychoanal.,* 32:167–177.

WATTS, A. (1970). Personal communication.

WEISMAN, A. & HACKETT, T. (1961). Predilection to death. *Psychosom. Med.,* 23:232–256.

WURMSER, L. (1981). *The Mask of Shame.* Baltimore: Johns Hopkins Univ. Press.

TRAUMA

On Trauma

When Is the Death of a Parent Traumatic?
ERNA FURMAN

AS MY CONTRIBUTION TO THE PANEL ON TRAUMA REVISITED (E.
Furman, 1984), I was asked to discuss the potentially traumatic
effects of parental bereavement in childhood. This assignment
gave me the opportunity to trace again, for myself, the history of
the term *trauma* as an analytic concept, to review the material
gained from the treatments of traumatized children, both my
own cases and those of my Cleveland colleagues, and to formulate some thoughts as well as questions about the topic. Although
I shall limit the case examples and most of the discussion to
children who had lost a parent through death, my thinking is
also based on data derived from the analytic study of other traumatic experiences, such as sexual and aggressive abuse, life-
threatening accidents, illness, injury, and medical/surgical
procedures.

WHAT IS A TRAUMA?

In analytic papers the term "trauma" is frequently used in the
sense of connoting a severe stress, and a child's parental bereavement is commonly referred to as a traumatic experience. I do not
wish to minimize the crucial importance for a child of his loss of a
parent through death or to underestimate the potentially devastating effects this may have on his personality, but I feel it is
necessary to differentiate instances where a parent's death is

From the Cleveland Center for Research in Child Development, the Hanna
Perkins Therapeutic Nursery School and Kindergarten, and the Department
of Psychiatry, Case Western Reserve School of Medicine.

traumatic from those where it is stressful, because the impact on the psychic system and the means the personality employs in dealing with the tragedy differ, and this in turn affects therapeutic handling as well as preventive measures. This differentiation is in keeping with A. Freud's (1964) view. She urged us to use the term trauma according to its original analytic definition, "to rescue it from the widening and overuse which . . . lead inevitably to a blurring of meaning and . . . abandonment and loss of valuable concepts," and she suggested that we exclude "notions of the accumulative, the strain, the retrospective, the screen trauma . . . [because they make it difficult] to differentiate between adverse, pathogenic influences in general and trauma in particular" (p. 222).

According to Freud (1920) and A. Freud (1964), the essence of trauma is an influx of stimuli from within or without which wholly or partly breaks through the ego's protective shield and floods the system with excitation. Such an occurrence may be caused by the sheer quantity or nature of the stimuli, and/or by the relative lack of preparedness of the system through prior hypercathexis, and/or by the system's inadequacy in coping with stimuli, due to immaturity, anomaly, pathology, or individual variations in the level of tolerance for excitation. In the youngest children the traumatic break through the stimulus barrier may be related to insufficient availability of the protective containing function of the "holding" environment, a point repeatedly stressed by Winnicott (1960a, 1960b, 1962, 1963a, 1963b, 1963c) or, as A. Freud puts it, a failure in the mothering person's function as her infant's auxiliary ego. Since thus a trauma may be caused by factors in the id, ego, and external world, and since these factors are usually closely related and mutually dependent, it is difficult, if not impossible, for the outsider to determine what the cause or causes may have been unless they become revealed in the course of an analysis. We therefore need to heed A. Freud's reminder to herself, "I shall remember not to confuse my own with the victim's appraisal of the happening" (p. 239). This applies to parental bereavement as the potential cause of trauma. We can never say before treatment that the death of the parent as such was traumatic. The later case vignettes will illustrate that, in each instance, different combinations of internal and external factors proved to have been traumatogenic—the circumstances of the death, the incapacitation of the ego through bodily injury at the time of loss, the antecedent experiences, existing ego mechanisms and instinctual impulses, the role of the environment, developmental factors, and many more.

Irrespective of the varied individual causes of trauma, however, its immediate effect on the organism is always the same. The ego and pleasure principle are put out of action when the psychic system is either altogether overwhelmed by the excess of excitation or cannot prevent the pouring in of stimuli through a limited breach in its protective shield. In the case of total flooding, all ego functions are suspended, the entire defense organization which served as the protective shield becomes inoperative, and the mental apparatus is reduced to what A. Freud (p. 238) calls "physical responses via the vegetative nervous system taking the place of psychic reactions," or what Yorke et al. (1980) term "vegetative excitement" which may behaviorally resemble a temper tantrum. In the case of a breach in the protective shield, the reparation process, according to Freud (1920), begins at once by a massive anticathexis which drains off all the available energy and extensively reduces or paralyzes the remaining functions. This manifests itself in states of shock (Freud), in states of paralysis of action and/or numbness of feeling (A. Freud), in battle exhaustion (Yorke, et al.), in some types of apathy (Greenson, 1949; E. Furman, 1974), and in some forms of depersonalization.

These traumatic or immediately posttraumatic states may last for minutes, hours, days, months, or years. They may recur, even recur repeatedly under certain conditions, a point I shall return to. When we can actually observe these states in patients, they can serve as one indication that the patient experienced a trauma. However, since these states sometimes last only for brief periods and since both the patient and others may not notice them or may misinterpret them, such observations are often omitted from the personal history and from reports on current behavior. Moreover, even professionals find it hard to differentiate posttraumatic states from other disturbances, especially in prelatency children. I know of two cases misdiagnosed as "minimal brain damage and retardation" and several others termed "psychotic" (E. Furman, 1956).

The Process of Recovery

After the catastrophic event, the psychic apparatus is faced with the problem of binding, or mastering, the noxious excess of stimuli and of restoring all areas of ego functioning and their phase-appropriate maturational progression.

According to Freud (1920), the gradual process of binding takes the form of repetition compulsion until all stimuli have been mastered and brought under the domain of the pleasure and/or reality principle. Among manifestations of this process Freud includes certain forms of children's demands for repetition and passive into active play, repetitive dreams, fate neuroses, and analytic transference phenomena. Yorke et al. (1980) further include children's pavor nocturnus and stage IV nightmares and their accompanying motoric discharges.

A. Freud (1964) points out that we should differentiate between two types of repetition. One is a pre-ego process, i.e., the repetition compulsion; the other is an ego mechanism "repeating an experience with variations suitable for its assimilation, such as turning a passive experience into an active one" (p. 237) or employing defenses such as denial. Such a transition from pre-ego mechanisms to ego mechanisms indicates a progression in the recuperative process.

Another measure of the nature and rate of recovery mentioned by A. Freud is the reemergence of ego functions—either residual or reinvested—and how fast or slowly they reach their pretraumatic level and pick up their phase-appropriate maturational momentum.

The nature and role of anxiety are other important elements in our understanding of trauma and of posttraumatic developments. Freud relates the failure of signal anxiety, and aspect of the system's preparedness, to the occurrence of trauma and views the need to repeat as an endeavor "to master the stimulus retrospectively, by developing the anxiety whose omission was the cause of the traumatic neurosis" (p. 32). Yorke and Wiseberg (1976) and Yorke et al. (1980) trace the developmental line of

anxiety from vegetative excitation which is bodily, to ter-
ror/panic which is primitive mental, to signal anxiety. Winnicott
emphasizes two further stages in the development of anxiety
which follow the purely vegetative excitement and precede the
essentially mental terror/panic. Both of these anxiety states combine mental and bodily responses. The first (Winnicott, 1960a,
1963c), the developmentally earlier one, happens when the traumatic impingement awakens the ego's awareness to experience
an interruption of its "going-on-being" (1963c, p. 256). The
second, later one is characterized by annihilation anxiety or "unthinkable anxiety." Its contents are "(1) Going to pieces. (2) Falling for ever. (3) Having no relationship to the body. (4) Having
no orientation" (1962, p. 58). I am uncertain as to the developmental point in earliest infancy when vegetative excitement begins to be accompanied by the mental experience of an interruption in "going-on-being." Clinical experiences with babies
suggest that the second stage, annihilation anxiety combined
with bodily responses, is present in the latter half of the first
year.

Some of my analytic patients have clearly described the overwhelming fears Winnicott lists during their recurrent states of
traumatic overwhelming. These take the form of awake episodes
of terror and frantic motor discharge, sometimes accompanied
by bodily distress of nausea, abdominal discomfort and an
urgency to urinate or defecate, and sometimes ending in total
bodily collapse in a fetal position with paralysis of all functions.
In the most severely affected patients any excess of stimuli, e.g.,
a minor change in their environment, can trigger such a recurrence of the traumatic state. They are sensitized to trauma in
general. Their reparative measures include withdrawal, avoidance of all stimulation, and insistence on sameness; preoccupation with things as opposed to people—the latter being less predictable and controllable; a frantic separation anxiety, using the
mother as a protective auxiliary ego. At a later point denial and
passive into active may be used, for example, in the form of
actively bringing on the traumatic state to avoid being surprised
by it and to "traumatize" the helpless onlookers. It also is a sign
of the healing process when these patients' traumatic states begin to occur in response to specific stimuli or situations which in

some ways remind them of the original trauma, and it is further progress when the recurrences take place primarily or exclusively in the analysis and are linked to the transference. Some patients are at the stage of situation-specific traumatic recurrence when they start treatment, and it is not always clear whether they ever were generally sensitized to trauma or perhaps experienced only a brief period of that stage during the immediately posttraumatic time. The next milestone in the recuperative process is reached when, in the course of the analysis, and sometimes prior to it, these states of situation-specific annihilation anxiety become linked with and supplanted by later developmental anxieties and by contents which apply directly to the original trauma.

These clinical experiences have led me to regard the presence of annihilation anxiety in its various forms as another manifest indication that a trauma did occur, and to view the defenses against annihilation anxiety as well as its gradual change to other forms of anxiety, or even an admixture of other anxieties, as a measure of the ongoing reparative process.

Let me now turn to another aspect of trauma damage and the healing process which has seemed particularly important to me. In her study of adult analysands who were raped during childhood, A. Katan (1973) found that these patients were most severely affected in two areas, impairment of integration and drive defusion. These damages permeated their personality structures and functioning and could not be improved much through analytic treatment. My own work with children who could not feel good showed that these patients invariably also suffered from marked difficulties with drive fusion, integration and ability to develop and maintain neutral interests and to be creative in whatever form. All these characteristics proved to be psychically related to one another, and one of the genetic causes was the experience of trauma. In 1985, I attempted to trace the mutual dependence of these characteristics, discussed the factors which facilitate and impede their development, and suggested some clinical approaches to the problems they pose for the afflicted patients and their analytic work. In the context of the present focus on trauma, one finding is especially pertinent: Drive fusion can take place only when there is a sufficient quantity of libido in relation to aggression and when the libido is sufficiently bound to be securely under the sway of the pleasure principle. Binding the libidinal energy and indeed all stimuli is, in part if not wholly, accomplished through the function of integration. At the same time, integration depends on bound, as opposed to free-flowing, libido because it draws on this very source of energy to fuel its own functioning. Freud pointed out that the impact of trauma, the break through the ego's protective shield, and the flooding of the organism with excessive stimuli put the ego and the pleasure principle out of action. This means that drive fusion can no longer be maintained and that the integrative function which helps to bind excitations is totally or largely incapacitated. The damaging effect of trauma on drive fusion and integration is therefore particularly severe. The clinical manifestations of defusion and impaired integration are especially prominent in the personality functioning of traumatized children. This is most marked in those who experienced trauma during their earliest years because in them drive fusion and integration were interfered with during the initial, most vulnerable phases of development. As a result, drive fusion and integration fail to mature normally and cannot appropriately contribute to the progression of other areas of personality growth.

Yet it is just in these two most damaged areas of drive fusion and integration that we also can most readily follow the reparative process. It takes the form of gradually integrating the traumatic noxious excess of stimuli by libidinizing them—bringing them under the domain of the pleasure principle—and, at the same time, accomplishing the first steps in drive fusion. This shows itself in increasing sexualization of the traumatic event, alteration in some of its features, and linking with other more adequately mastered life experiences. In this form the trauma may be incorporated in anxiety dreams and nightmares with an element of wish fulfillment (succeeding the mere repetition compulsion of pavor nocturnus and stage IV nightmares with motor discharges); it often becomes the content of masturbation fantasies; it infiltrates behavior patterns and actively provokes interactions with others which partly serve instinctual gratification; it affects the formation of the superego and instinctualizes its interaction with the ego; it may even libidinize the posttraumatic forms of anxiety. The primitive degree of fusion attained through this aspect of the reparative process is usually of a crudely sadomasochistic nature. This may be clinically distressing for the patient, his loved ones, and the analyst, and may indeed lead to secondary pathology, yet it represents definite strides in assimilating the trauma and in restoring maturational progression of drive fusion and integration.

TRAUMA IN PARENTALLY BEREAVED CHILDREN

Since the publication of *A Child's Parent Dies* (E. Furman, 1974), the original number of 23 parentally bereaved children treated by my Cleveland colleagues and myself has more than doubled. In assessing which of these patients were traumatized by their experience of the parent's death or by factors related to it, I have used the criteria listed above which indicate traumatic or post-traumatic responses. With some patients the data were gained during analyses that took place after the loss; with others, whose parent died during their treatment, the data include the actual time of bereavement. Many patients did not experience the death of the parent as a trauma. A number did. From among these I shall briefly describe four, to illustrate some of the earlier points and to raise further questions.

Miriam was the eagerly welcomed, healthy first child of a happy young couple. By 3½ weeks of age she thrived, seemed comfortable and well-contained, and had just begun to extend her sleeping periods at night. When Miriam was 4 weeks, her mother fell ill and died of a viral infection within 24 hours. The maternal grandmother immediately took over Miriam's full-time care and soon invested the infant as her own. I began to work with the grandmother a couple of months later. By that time Miriam was at peace and thriving again, but the grandmother described Miriam's immediate response to the upheaval. The baby screamed and fretted almost incessantly, refused food, suffered interference in all bodily functions, and could not be comforted. This state lasted for many days and only gradually diminished. One suspects she experienced a state of vegetative excitation or possibly an interruption in the "going-on-being," caused by the loss of what Winnicott calls the "holding environment" and what

A. Freud terms the auxiliary ego provided by the mothering person. I worked with the grandmother for several years. She was unusually empathic with infants. This seemed to have mitigated even her own initial severe distress so that the child's traumatic response was all the more noteworthy. During her early years Miriam then weathered a number of stresses, and during her fourth year she experienced a near-total loss of her grandmother when the father's new wife insisted on taking her over and placed her in a daycare center. Miriam was deeply distressed but at no point showed a traumatic reaction. The development of drive fusion and ego functions was neither delayed nor impaired.

Danny (Fiedler, 1974), the third child in his family, was 11 months old when he and his father were hospitalized with a virus infection. The father died of it within 48 hours. The mother, distraught and preoccupied with her other more mildly ill children at home, could not visit Danny during his week-long hospital stay during which he underwent many medical procedures. When she came to take him home, he was pale, listless, and did not respond. He no longer walked or crawled, had lost his early speech and intense emotional interest in people and the world around him. He was limp and apathetic and only clung like a little baby. The family moved to a new home, and work with the mother began within a month. With the help of the mother's empathic efforts, Danny resumed crawling at 17 months, which soon turned into heedless hyperactivity and accident-proneness, and he spoke a few words again by nearly 2 years. Testing showed him to be of at least normal intelligence, but his persistent lack of affect and response made him appear mentally retarded.

The therapist's ongoing weekly interviews with the mother continued when Danny entered the Hanna Perkins School at nearly 3 years. His previously constant separation terror had subsided by this time but still reached panic proportions when he thought mother would leave him suddenly; for example, when he momentarily lost sight of her in a store, he screamed in terror to the point of turning blue and lost consciousness. His analysis, begun at age 4, showed that he remembered and missed his father and that his death troubled him in many ways. The real trauma, however, was the temporary loss of the mother at 11 months and some of the medical procedures he endured during her absence at that time; for example, when he was to be photographed, the idea that someone would take his picture reminded him of his X-rays during the early hospitalization and resulted in an episode of terror for him. Although these recurrences of terror states surfaced in barely mitigated form for many years, they were in time supplanted by heightened developmental fears, especially castration anxiety and early superego anxiety. He also began to use passive-into-active repetitions, instinctualized some aspects of the trauma, and linked it with other experiences. This showed itself in his running away, refusal to care for himself, magical denial of masturbatory dangers, and insistence that his mother could cure everything because she was a nurse. Danny's difficulty with drive fusion contributed to particularly harsh, early superego forerunners.

Ruth was 3½ years old when her father was murdered. She learned of this from her mother's frantic, instinctualized account and behavior. The impact was intensified by the mother's chaotic response during the following year and her propensity to externalize her fears, anger, and excitement to everyone, including Ruth, overwhelming them with gruesome details and unrealistic speculations. After a lovingly invested infancy, the child had already suffered repeated overwhelming through sexual and aggressive abuse and, during the months preceding the father's death, she had helplessly witnessed the parents' violent arguments and fights. During the period immediately following the father's death, Ruth seemed to have suffered very frequent states of total overwhelming, suggesting posttraumatic recurrences. These were sometimes ignored and sometimes punished as naughty temper tantrums. There also was evidence that, at least within the year, she overwhelmed others, turning passive into active. Her unfused aggression manifested itself in physical sadistic attacks, especially on younger children, and in self-hurting masturbatory activities.

Ruth's analysis began in her sixth year during her attendance at the Hanna Perkins School. Highly intelligent and verbal, she was plagued by symptoms in all areas of functioning, many fears, extreme ambivalence, and inability to tolerate any increase in stimuli, for example, a change in routine or someone talking to her unexpectedly. Although it was difficult to disentangle to what extent Ruth's earlier experiences affected her response to her father's death and to what extent her integration of its trauma linked them together, some posttraumatic symptoms were understood to relate primarily to the murder: pavor nocturnus, a horror of everything related to violence and death, and recurring episodes of overwhelming fear of annihilation, accompanied by frantic motor discharges and bodily collapse into a fetal position, and by sensations of pain and an expectation of being killed. During the years of analytic work, her pavor nocturnus changed to repetitive nightmares and, later, specific phobic fears at bedtime. Her episodes of trauma recurrence became less frequent and more situation-specific and were mostly limited to transference reactions in the sessions. She also gradually achieved better control of the episodes—first by bringing on the overwhelming when she sensed it coming over her, then by experiencing it mentally without bodily sensations, and still later by being able to withdraw into a closet and calm down when it had barely started. By age 9, almost 6 years after the trauma and 3 years of analysis, Ruth showed evidence of signal anxiety. She could feel the threat of "it's coming" but could prevent feeling or manifesting terror. She coped at those times by asking to be left alone and playing quietly for a while. The contents of the trauma also became integrated in the form of passive-into-active provocations, sadomasochistic masturbation fantasies, and instinctualized aspects of superego, representing murderer and victim internally. Although drive fusion and synthesis were seriously impaired, Ruth could be helped to address and cope with all aspects of mourning the loss of her father through death. Its form, the murder, was the real trauma and has been much harder for her to master.

Jim (Schiff, 1974) was 7¼ years old when he experienced a car accident while driving with his mother, twin, a younger brother, and another mother and her four children. The car hit a bridge abutment and both mothers, Jim's twin, and three of the other family's children were killed. Jim sustained serious head injuries and only recovered consciousness after several weeks. For 3 months he was cared for in a hospital room he shared with his

brother who was casted for limb fractures. He learned of the
deaths there but did not acknowledge them, although his later
analysis revealed that he had clearly remembered the pretraumatic and traumatic events. Jim's initial confusion and hyperactivity were probably organic but persisted after neurological impairment was ruled out. In addition, while he had
been pathologically aggressive, he became quite passive and de-
fenseless in his interactions with others and suffered frequent
spells of sitting motionless, staring and losing touch with the
world so that he failed to respond to what was going on around
him, even to his family's efforts "to get him out of it." These
symptoms were unchanged when he started analysis at age 10,
almost 3 years later, and could then be understood and resolved.

Jim had experienced overwhelming terror and subsequently
heightened anxiety at all levels. Castration fear contributed to
his passivity and hyperactivity. His episodes of apathetic withdrawal ultimately warded off overwhelming sadness. In part
these manifestations were posttraumatic, related to the nature of
the deaths and injuries as well as to the loss of the mother and
unavailability of emotional support and adequate care during
the succeeding period. Jim's analysis revealed, however, that, at
least by that time, his symptoms also had become linked with
earlier separations during which Jim had been aggressively
abused and neglected. These earlier experiences had heightened his developmental anxieties prior to the trauma and
shaped his early defenses, serving especially to ward off extremely helpless feelings of unsafety, sadness, and longing.

DISCUSSION

These vignettes raise rather than answer many questions. The
very selection of the cases and the sequence in which they were
arranged imply that I wish to draw attention to the significance
of developmental factors in our attempts to understand trauma.
Following Freud and A. Freud in recognizing that the causes of
trauma, at any age, depend on the unique individual confluence
of internal and external circumstances, we may yet take it for
granted that the immature ego is more vulnerable to traumatization. Whereas under good enough conditions the auxiliary ego

of the mothering person compensates for the infant's and young child's ego weakness, his very reliance on maternal functioning also increases his vulnerability. He may be traumatized because the mother's auxiliary ego does not function effectively, or because it becomes totally unavailable, or even because the mother actually causes the overwhelming excess of stimulations instead of protecting her child from it. In assessing the developmental factor we therefore have to take into account the interaction of two variables, the developmental status of the child's personality and the nature and availability of the auxiliary ego of the mothering person.

Experience suggests that this two-pronged developmental factor affects not only the initial experience of trauma but the recuperative process. Young children sense this. Regardless of who or what inflicted the trauma, unless the mother is actually absent or emotionally altogether unavailable, they turn to her to avail themselves of her protective and healing ego functions. They cling to her and react to separation from her with renewed annihilation fear or panic. Analytic data show us, time and again, that the child's healing process is greatly facilitated when the mother is not only physically available but emotionally aware of the child's experience, active in assisting him with integration and supportive of his efforts. Unfortunately this applies in reverse as well. Although Miriam was almost too young to view her experience as equivalent to the trauma in a more differentiated personality, it seems likely that the immediate and consistent availability of her grandmother's auxiliary ego favorably affected her subsequent satisfactory progress. Danny's mother was truly helpful and devoted in her assistance to him, but she had been absent for a long time during the traumatic period and was a very different mother when she became available to him once again. Sad, drawn, and burdened by the many demands of her changed life situation, she presented quite a contrast to her earlier happy, smiling self, tackling life with zest and optimism. This had a profound effect on Danny, mitigated but not erased by the mother's, and later the analyst's, acknowledgment and discussion of it. Ruth's mother, though invested in her child, could not fulfill her role as auxiliary ego and was often driven to add new stresses and overstimulation. Even when she could feel with her little girl, she could not help Ruth to contain and integrate the experiences. In part this left Ruth to struggle on her own, in part it led her to identify with the mother's unhelpful ways of coping, for example, it intensified her use of sadomasochistic sexualization and her passive-into-active tendency to overwhelm others. Jim's mother was dead. Although the analyst, from the time of the trauma on, assisted the family in a consultative capacity, it took 3 years before they could provide a measure of physical and emotional parental care. This delayed the start of Jim's analysis and perhaps also contributed to the delay in his recuperative steps. He was still showing the same posttraumatic symptoms.

While wanting to underline how significant a role mothering plays, I am not suggesting that optimal availability of the mother's auxiliary ego cures the effects of trauma or that it is the only deciding factor. We know only too well that mothers cannot prevent all stresses in a child's life and that recuperation from trauma can be impeded by unavoidable further debilitating experiences and no doubt by factors within the child. However, as with bodily traumatic injury, the posttraumatic milieu and protective as well as facilitating nursing care contribute considerably to the recuperative process.

The younger the child, the more total the overwhelming, the less available the mother's auxiliary ego, and the more stressful the posttraumatic period, the slower are the steps in the reparative process. We note this in the general sensitivity to traumatization, the recurrent experiences of annihilation fear or terror/panic instead of progression toward signal anxiety, the damaging impact on all functions which are in the process of development, and especially on integration and drive fusion. The impairment in these latter two areas may cause uneven development even when maturation again gets under way, may interfere with progressive personality growth, and may contribute to chaotic clinical pictures, such as pseudoretardation and atypical or psychotic disturbances (E. Furman, 1956).

The older traumatized child is more likely to be able to "wall off" the trauma in the form of pavor nocturnus, episodes of withdrawal, affect block, and related posttraumatic symptoms. To an extent this protects him from recurrences of traumatic anxiety and helps him to preserve a measure of adaptive functioning until his ego can begin to use defenses and libidinization to assimilate the traumatic event. But whether or how soon such reparative steps are taken again seems to depend in part on the posttraumatic support and experiences.

This division into earlier and later developmental phenomena is not clear-cut. There are overlaps and other significant factors, among them the child's internalization of the mother's ways of auxiliary ego functioning, as was evident in the case of Ruth and as I discussed in greater detail in another context (E. Furman, 1985).

There are also developmental phenomena which are even harder to understand. Traumatized children, especially the younger ones, invariably reexperience the trauma in the transference, with the analyst as the agent who inflicted the trauma. In fact, this is how we usually learn about traumas in child analysis. When I asked several colleagues, among them A. Katan (1973), about their experiences in analyzing adults who had suffered a trauma in childhood, they told me that the patients hardly ever bring the trauma into the transference in this form and that their transference reflects only some aspects or features of it. Does this mean that the transference in childhood operates more strictly under the repetition compulsion? Does it mean that there are different developmental levels in the transference?

Of course, developmental factors do not account for all the many variations of posttraumatic manifestations or of the rate and nature of reparative steps. Nor do I think that the differences can be attributed simply to variations in individual endowment. It seems more likely that other specific factors play a part, either before the trauma or afterward. For example, recurrences of traumatic anxiety are, in some patients, not a sign of difficulty in recuperation but may at certain times point to progress. They sometimes signify that the psychic system has reached a point of transition from pre-ego to ego mechanisms and can begin to admit the anxiety to consciousness as a way of starting to deal with the hitherto unbound traumatic stimuli. Also, some manifestations associated with traumatic injury may stem from different sources. For example, severe damage to integration and drive fusion may be caused by factors other than trauma (E. Furman, 1985).

We also know very little about recovery. A. Freud suggested that complete recovery is impossible, that a vulnerability remains, perhaps unrealized until the individual encounters certain life situations. Miriam's good progress during her early years does not guarantee invulnerability. We would have to follow her analytically throughout her life to gain reliable data. Most cases, followed at least long-term, show that the inner work on a trauma never ceases. Even when the patient achieves signal anxiety in relation to his or her traumatogenic events, the personality continues to expend a great deal of energy on using such signal anxiety to remain on the alert, to differentiate past from present, and to integrate the remnants of the original experience which surface at such times—a form of working through.

This brings us to the role of treatment. Since its historical beginnings, psychoanalysis has been helpful to patients who had suffered a trauma. The very process of tracing a person's earlier traumatic experience and making it available to his consciousness assists him with integrating it, as do many other aspects of the analytic work, not least the transference. However, there are limitations. An analysis can be helpful only within the givens of the patient's own rate and stage of recuperation. When a patient's ego is not ready to assimilate the traumatic event, or when the analysis forces his pace of integration too much, the treatment itself is experienced as a repetition of the traumatic intrusion. This may impede a patient's ability to engage in the analytic work in the first place, or to persist with it when he feels threatened. It may also cause some patients to experience setbacks in the reparative process if they have not been able to protect themselves with sufficient defenses. The analyst's awareness of the patient's precarious integrative capacity and his empathic skill in working with the patient is therefore especially important in these cases, as is an understanding of the steps in the recuperative process and a recognition of the limits of analytic help at certain points.

With children the analyst has an added task, namely, to apprise the parents of the child's psychic state and to enlist and support their functioning as auxiliary egos in relation to the posttraumatic recuperative process—a role that exceeds their usual age-appropriate caring and educational function with the child. The younger the child, the more is it helpful, nay essential, that the parents understand and undertake this role. It is an ongoing round-the-clock job and provides the milieu for the child's effective use of the analysis. With the analyst's support many parents can and do fulfill this need when they are helped to appreciate the reasons for it, just as parents often rally to nurse their child through a bad sickness in cooperation with a caring physician.

Obviously, we know far too little about trauma, but I find that parents, physicians, and professional caretakers know even less. They tend not to appreciate the difference between trauma and stress, between long-term, perhaps lifelong, damage and potentially masterable upset. For example, in my consultations with child life workers in pediatric hospitals I have frequently noted that staff and parents are tempted to regard suggestions about the need for a mother's availability or preparation for procedures as optional frills which, at best, reduce children's unhappiness and, at worst, interfere with "getting on with things." Since prevention is so much easier than cure, especially in regard to trauma, perhaps the child analyst should take part in clarifying these issues with parents and professionals, not only after the trauma when the child needs or is in treatment, but before. Not all but many traumas can be avoided.

SUMMARY

Trauma and attempts at mastering it are metapsychologically differentiated from stress, and clinical manifestations of successive stages in the posttraumatic psychic work are described. Some of these are familiar, others have not been previously recorded. Four case vignettes illustrate the analytic understanding of patients who experienced the parent's death or circumstances related to it as a trauma. All of them raise further questions about trauma and posttraumatic mastery.

BIBLIOGRAPHY

FIEDLER, E. S. (1974). Danny. In Furman (1974), pp. 198–218.
FREUD, A. (1964). Comments on psychic trauma. *W.*, 5:221–241.
FREUD, S. (1920). Beyond the pleasure principle. *S.E.*, 18:7–66.

FURMAN, E. (1956). An ego disturbance in a young child. *Psychoanal. Study Child*, 11:312–335.

—— (1974). *A Child's Parent Dies.* New Haven: Yale Univ. Press.

—— (1984). When is the death of a parent traumatic? Read to the Association for Child Psychoanalysis, London.

—— (1985). On fusion, integration, and feeling good. *Psychoanal. Study Child*, 40: 81–110.

FURMAN, R. A. & KATAN, A. (1969). *The Therapeutic Nursery School.* New York: Int. Univ. Press.

GREENSON, R. R. (1949). The psychology of apathy. *Psychoanal. Q.*, 18:290–302.

KATAN, A. (1973). Children who were raped. *Psychoanal. Study Child*, 28:208–224.

SCHIFF, E. J. (1974). Jim. In Furman (1974), pp. 88–95.

WINNICOTT, D. W. (1960a). The theory of the parent-infant relationship. In *The Maturational Processes and the Facilitating Environment*, pp. 37–55. New York: Int. Univ. Press, 1965.

—— (1960b). Ego distortion in terms of true and false self. Ibid., pp. 140–152.

—— (1962). Ego integration in child development. Ibid., pp. 56–63.

—— (1963a). The development of the capacity for concern. Ibid., pp. 73–82.

—— (1963b). Morals and education. Ibid., pp. 93–105.

—— (1963c). Dependence in infant-care, in child-care, and in the psychoanalytic setting. Ibid., pp. 249–260.

YORKE, C., KENNEDY, H., & WISEBERG, S. (1980). Some clinical and theoretical aspects of two developmental lines. In *The Course of Life*, ed. S. I. Greenspan & G. H. Pollock, pp. 619–637. Washington: U.S. Department of Health and Human Services.

YORKE, C. & WISEBERG, S. (1976). A developmental view of anxiety. *Psychoanal. Study Child*, 31:107–138.

Trauma in Childhood

Signs and Sequelae as Seen in the Analysis of an Adolescent

HANSI KENNEDY, Dip. Psych.

PETER'S ANALYSIS LASTED FOR 6 YEARS AND STARTED AT THE AGE OF 13. Early traumatic and disturbing events played a striking part in his pathology and were vividly reexperienced in treatment. This short paper describes some of these reenactments and gives reasons why the experiences from which they derived might properly be called "traumatic."

In spite of Peter's long and, in many ways, successful analysis, he remained a rather depressed young man, dominated by pervasive feelings of inadequacy and resentment from which he tried to escape by sexual activities. During treatment, his compulsive masturbation, accompanied by sadomasochistic fantasies, and his tendency to enactment, increasingly forced me to think of his disturbance in terms of sexual perversion.

During his masturbatory practices, he needed to create, simultaneously or in quick succession, sexual excitement, pain, and anxiety. He masturbated from early childhood, but in adolescence he enhanced his orgastic pleasure by tying a plastic bag over his head. In this way his fantasy that a female partner was

Codirector of the Anna Freud Centre, London, which is at present supported by the G. G. Bunzl Charitable Foundation, London; The Freud Centenary Fund, London; The Anna Freud Foundation, New York; The New-Land Foundation, Inc., New York; The Leo Oppenheimer and Flora Oppenheimer Haas Trust, New York; and a number of private supporters.

Presented at the International Scientific Colloquium on "Repeating: Enactment and Verbalization in Different Stages of Development" held at the Anna Freud Centre, November 1985.

castrating and suffocating him was given an added dimension of reality.

A connection can readily be made between these sexual fantasies and practices and experiences in his third year of life, when he suffered intermittently from painful infections of the penis. These involved his mother in repeated examinations and manipulations of his genitals. Phimosis eventually required circumcision at 2 years, 8 months. His mother stayed with him in the hospital but could only report his bad reaction to the anesthetic. In analysis Peter claimed to have a memory of mother driving him to the hospital for the operation, but this memory lacked any affective coloring.

There can be no doubt from Peter's analytic material that these events were crucial in the formation of his psychopathology and that, at least retroactively, they were experienced as vengeful attacks and punishments by his mother. By the time he entered analysis, his masturbation conflicts were firmly linked with his feelings about his damaged penis and the conviction that he was an inadequate person in every respect. This narcissistic vulnerability and depleted self-esteem had, of course, earlier roots.

Peter was a disappointment to his mother from the day he was born. She was an inexperienced, anxious, rigid mother who was quite unable to cope with an infant whose behavior failed to match her exact expectations. The pregnancy proceeded according to plan until Peter arrived 12 days too early and had to be extracted by forceps. He cried a great deal during the first few months, which upset his parents' regimental household and lifestyle. He did not feed according to his mother's schedule, and her worry about his poor weight gain and slow physical growth led her "to force food into him." She probably became even less responsive to Peter's needs when she became pregnant, for a second time, when he was only 8 months old. All these circumstances reflect an unsatisfactory early interaction between mother and child, and the inadequate and curtailed symbiotic phase formed the core of Peter's disturbed self and object relationship.

In the second year of life, Peter's interaction with mother was dominated by what she described as "their great battle over toilet training." A battle which started when he was only 1 year old went on until well into his third year of life, when daytime bladder control was finally achieved. Contributory factors to this long delay included a stressful 2-week separation from mother and home at the time of the brother's birth, and the onset, some months later, of the phimosis.

The mother's narcissistic hurt and guilt in relation to Peter's imperfections may well have been compensated by her pleasure and pride in the new baby who seemed to thrive both physically and psychologically. Both parents described this younger brother as more satisfactory in every way. Not surprisingly, Peter's development began to lag, and according to the mother, his younger brother talked before he did. Irrespective of the accuracy of this information, it does suggest that Peter could not express his feelings in words at the time of the circumcision.

The unfavorable comparison which began on the day his brother was born became a bane of Peter's life. He felt that his brother was not only better loved but was superior in every respect. Two years before his referral for treatment, which ostensibly was for learning difficulties in spite of his good intelligence (IQ 120+), Peter had suffered the ultimate humiliation of his younger brother's advance to a class above him at school.

He envied but also idealized this brother, casting him in the role of a genius—a second Einstein—whom he could never emulate. His revengeful hatred of the brother, an ever recurring theme in the analysis, was understood as a displacement of feelings he harbored toward his mother for producing the brother and for favoring him. Later in treatment this also appeared as an oedipal displacement from the father who "possessed" the mother.

I have discussed elsewhere the transference developments in Peter's analysis (1980). They led to a very clever recasting of his pathology in terms of a double identification: with the clever Jews who were nevertheless discriminated against and circumcised, and with the powerful, sadistic, yet morally despicable Nazis. This expressed both the ambivalent investment of self and object and the sadomasochistic object relationship. It provided immense opportunities not only for the development of the analytic process, but also for resistance and stagnation in the analytic work when he used the treatment to gratify his sadomas-

ochism. Even the most careful monitoring of countertransference cannot prevent a sadomasochistic patient from exploiting
the analytic situation for perverse gratification. At all times Peter
worked hard to get himself into a state of sexual excitement
which served to ward off his depressive feeling states.

I hope that this brief overview will provide sufficient background to give perspective to the analytic material which follows.
This is unavoidably selective, but I hope it indicates the significance of Peter's experiences around the phimosis and circumcision.

Both anxiety and guilt helped to make Peter a secretive boy
who, throughout the first year of analysis, deliberately withheld
and distorted material. But at the beginning of treatment the
anxiety was so pervasive that he could hardly communicate verbally. When he talked at all, his speech was difficult to understand and he was reduced to muttering under his breath such
comments as "What is going to happen?" or "I haven't told you
anything about my sins." I felt at the time that he was reacting to
the analytic situation as if it represented the Day of Judgment. In
retrospect it is not difficult to see that the intimacy of the analytic
setting, of being alone in the room with a woman who was immediately cast in the role of dangerous castrator, was both terrifying and seductive. Affectively, it seemed to have revived the
traumatic childhood experiences in the most dramatic way.

In the early weeks of treatment he would silently draw maps of
the London Underground system and respond to any comment
I made by blotting them out. He would do so with such ferocity
that big holes were all that were left on the paper. Thus, while my
attempts to establish contact through verbalization always mobilized fears that I might discover what he was deliberately trying
to keep hidden, his sexual preoccupations were betrayed by his
actions and concomitant affect.

Intense anxiety about his damaged penis was evident from the
way he treated the felt-pens he used for drawing. He often handled them roughly and then anxiously looked at the tips for
damage.

As if to underline his derisive rejection of my cautious and
carefully worded interpretations, he also rejected my felt-pens
and brought his own from home. This led to a strange enact-

ment in the third week of treatment. He selected a red pen and found that the protective cap was stuck so that he could not use it. He began to pull and push the cap with mounting excitement and anxiety. Once or twice he held it out to me, apparently to elicit my participation, but then mistrustfully withdrew it. His face was flushed and his hands were covered with red paint when he finally succeeded in pulling off the cap. He anxiously inspected the tip, hitherto protected, to see if it was damaged; and he disparagingly declared that it was now useless and that his mother would jolly well have to provide a new one. While this material opened up the analytic work on his masturbation conflicts, and his view of the mother as responsible for his damaged penis, the full significance of his enactment in terms of his childhood experiences when his penis was sore and he had difficulty in urinating was recognized only some months later in connection with another, more dramatic, enactment.

Following his brother's visit home from boarding school (week 36) we had an unusually good session. For once Peter seemed in touch with his unhappiness and was able to talk about his anger and resentment with his parents for being interested only in his brother. He complained that the whole weekend was spent in praise of his brother's good examination results and in making plans for his brother's future privileged education. He had experienced all this as a deliberate humiliation and reproach from his parents and throughout the weekend had felt an unwanted outsider in his own family. I had commented on the long-standing nature of such feelings and how they must have contributed to his pervasively low self-esteem. Peter replied that the brother was the cause of all his trouble and that he wished him dead or, better still, that he had never been born. Right at the end of this session it emerged that the weekend had also been the occasion for the celebration of the brother's birthday.

He arrived the next day in a completely different state of mind. He was regressed; his communications were again nonverbal; his nose was blocked by an attack of hayfever, and he was desperate about the discomfort. He considered phoning his mother for advice, but reproachfully demanded instead that I do something about his agony and provide him at least with tissues. This I did. He started to attack his nose in a most sadistic manner. He placed a paper tissue on his lap, leaned over it, and tried to force mucus out of his nose. He pulled, pushed, poked, and blew, using both hands for these manipulations. He was totally self-absorbed in this frenetic activity which went on for quite some time until I intervened. I suggested that his concern about, and vicious treatment of, his nose really referred to his penis and that he might be remembering something of what happened to it when he was a small boy and had phimosis. I tried to put into words some of the discomfort and pain he must have suffered at the time, especially when urinating or when his penis was touched by his mother. Peter listened attentively and smilingly said that I saw sex in everything. But he at once stopped attacking his nose and showed no further signs of discomfort from the hay fever.

Similar material reappeared on many subsequent occasions; it was particularly telling when we explored his compulsive need to masturbate. He explained that every time he failed to ejaculate he would have to try again. As this sometimes happened 10 or 12 times a day, it made his penis so sore that he feared permanent damage. In this way he was also attacking himself, while in his fantasies he was raping a girl.

The equation of ejaculation and urination, as a means of attack on the female object, persisted from his toilet-training battle with mother. This battle was the background to his somatic and psychological experiences at the time of the phimosis and circumcision. This was also the psychological content of enactments during the early months of treatment, when he wanted to use his felt-pens on me, tried to squirt drops at me with his nasal dispenser, and left little pools of water all over the floor of my room. Later, when verbalization replaced acting, he would just threaten to piss on me when he felt he needed to counterattack. There was a mounting excitement and triumph at the height of the attack, but this was at once followed by fear of retaliation. But eventually we learned that an important motive for the attack had been the wish to engage the object—even if it was only in battle.

This sadomasochistic mode of relating was evident in all of Peter's relationships outside the analysis as well. He provoked others to counterattack through his nonverbal attacks and abuse.

With his mother, he still achieved closeness through his body. While she was quite impervious to his psychological needs, she always appeared concerned about his physical ailments and imperfections. The slightest complaint of pains in his neck or back secured the mother's immediate attention, and she would start to massage him. She repeatedly drew attention to a minor impairment in the movement of his left arm for which she gave him physiotherapy. She often dragged him to doctors, e.g., for a verruca which she thought should be excised rather than treated medically as the doctor suggested. There were endless battles about cleanliness and about the need for Peter's hair to be "trimmed" (a term he also used to describe circumcision).

In this way the mother reinforced Peter's castration anxiety, and she communicated her view of him as imperfect. But her physical ministrations sexually excited her adolescent son and in this way she perpetuated and compounded his difficulties. When the doctor suggested prophylactic injections for the hay fever, the mother persuaded him to let her give Peter the course of injections herself. This both excited Peter and increased his anxieties. Although he feared that she might hurt or even kill him, he submitted to her without protest. In the analysis he spoke of using the experience as a stimulus for new variations of his sexual fantasies.

I can see with hindsight that this material was also enacted in the transference, long before the full implications were understood. In the eighth week of treatment he developed a sudden pain in his back and wanted me to do something about it. Instead of exploring with me what the "something" could mean, he quite literally stripped to the waist, ostensibly to see what his mother could have put in his vest to cause the pain.

There can be little doubt that the somatic and psychological experiences occasioned by the phimosis and circumcision were experienced by Peter as abuse and victimization. Child abuse by mothers and medical experiments by Nazi doctors on the sexual organs of concentration camp victims were recurring topics in the analysis. He always emphasized that such brutalities left the victims physically mutilated, mentally retarded, or even dead. He, of course, saw himself both as physically mutilated and mentally retarded.

It would seem that the traumatogenic experiences in his second and third year of life also unleashed massive aggression which his disciplinarian parents met with condemnation, physical beatings, and further assaults and abuse. Peter's "sins" and "guilty crimes," to which he alluded at the beginning of treatment, referred to quite violent, aggressive attacks on animals and children. He "accidentally" killed a kitten; he hit a boy over the head so that he needed six stitches; and he almost drowned a girl in the swimming pool. These episodes must have occurred between the ages of 4 and 8. He was riddled with guilt about these murderous attacks. After his banishment to boarding school, his behavior was reversed. Though, in more subtle ways, he may well have invited sexual attacks and humiliations, he himself soon became the butt and victim of others.

Primitive aggression threatens to destroy the object and the self and mobilizes massive anxiety. It may well be that for Peter the *anesthetic* concretized and dramatized self destruction, death, and suffocation. The mother had told us that Peter reacted badly to the anesthetic, but was unable to remember anything else about the circumcision. It may be speculative to suggest that Peter brought into analysis somatic memories of the panic he experienced when given the anesthetic, but the idea was prompted by the following events.

From time to time Peter froze into a motionless state and sat for several minutes with fixed staring eyes and a masklike facial expression. He would emerge from this trancelike state, either spontaneously or in response to my intervention, only after a violent jerking movement of his head, which was suggestive of a deliberate effort to rid himself of something compelling and terrifying. In discussion various hypotheses were suggested to account for these puzzling episodes. Did they indicate petit mal caused by organic impairment? Did they suggest a kind of hysterical twilight state or even some kind of hallucinatory experience? Did they represent attempts to immobilize his body in order to control sexual excitement and terrifying fantasies?

As soon as Peter's fear of treatment lessened and he could

begin to permit himself to convey his feelings and fantasies, these trancelike states disappeared and an organic basis seemed unlikely. But a defensive "withdrawal into fantasy" in the face of anxiety, or painful affect mobilized by any kind of internal or external impingement, remained. At such times Peter was always difficult to reach.

It is of interest that in the third year of treatment the trancelike state made a brief reappearance in one of the sessions. I noted that it was a dramatization of the early states because by that time Peter's self-observing capacities were sufficiently developed to prevent precipitation into panic. He could also acknowledge what had happened and explore it a little. He recalled the frequency of such panic states in and out of analysis and thought of them collectively as "my madness." He thought now that it was his way of "shutting off" the outside world and concentrating exclusively on a fantasy. I was doubtful whether he really had this degree of voluntary control. We were able to link the heightened state of anxiety in this particular session to a transference fantasy that his sadistic attacks would really destroy me, bring treatment to an end, and leave him totally abandoned. It was this "painful" realization he must have tried to "shut out."

I have always harbored the fantasy that the anesthetic was given with a mask and bottle. If this were so, it would bring the anesthetic experience close to suffocation. This would make sense of Peter's perception of death as suffocation, and his use of a plastic bag, in later adolescence, to support his fantasies of castration and suffocation by a big woman. It is a fact that fantasies of being victimized, passively overwhelmed, and cruelly punished to the point of death were sexually exciting just because the aggression was turned against the self and alleviated guilt.

DISCUSSION

The events surrounding the phimosis, the concomitant interventions, and subsequent operation profoundly affected Peter's development. Self and object representations were crystallized around these experiences, and the relationship locked in a sadomasochistic battle for survival. The perception of his mother as malicious attacker, whose longed-for attention and concern could be attained only by suffering pain and by relinquishing his penis, absorbed, restructured, and organized a whole range of earlier experiences and conflicts.

His unrequited longing to be loved, his envy of the brother as usurper of his rightful place, the dangers stemming from his heightened aggression—nurtured by unmet early needs, forced feeding, and rigid toilet training—all became organized around the experiences engendered by the phimosis and circumcision. The anal phase battle for power and control acquired a particularly potent input from hurting and being hurt and became focused on the penis. The mother became all important as the provider of pain and sexual excitement—a sadistic attacker and seducer—and a powerful model for identification.

All this colored the way Peter came to experience his rivalry with the feared and powerful oedipal father, his highly ambivalent relationship to his brother, his banishment from home at the age of 8, and his relationships to teachers and peers at boarding school. What was so striking in Peter's analysis was the way in which all the avenues pursued analytically ultimately led to the experiences surrounding the circumcision.

How do we conceptualize the nature of such an "organizing experience" (Yorke 1986) which not only shapes what Herzog (1985) has called "the developmental line of personal meaning" but also propels the psychosexual development along a deviant path and generally constricts ego functioning?

Of course, the analysis only gradually and laboriously unraveled the various layers and developmental transformations of Peter's masturbation fantasies and conflicts. But how do we explain the emergence of specific and apparently encapsulated memories, through the most primitive, symbolic, and concretized enactments at the beginning of the analysis?

Do these unconscious enactments of the manipulations of his penis, the difficulties in urinating, and the experiences of the anesthetic reflect the "traumatic" impact of these events? Affectively they were all highly charged with an admixture of excitement, pain, and panic. Are we to interpret them as signs of "trauma" in the classical sense, that they mobilized a degree of affective excitation which overwhelmed vulnerable ego functions; could not be dealt with at the time, became encapsulated as primitive memory structures, until they were reworked and raised to a higher level of integration in the course of the analysis?

There were also some technical implications concerning reconstruction, which arise when working with a patient like Peter. I found it useful to organize *my* reconstructions around the "trauma of the circumcision" because this was most meaningful in terms of Peter's *current* experience. But in the view taken of an intrapsychic "organizing experience," reconstructions of this kind may also be more meaningful in terms of the childhood past. Reconstructions must be intrapsychically meaningful rather than be historically or developmentally accurate.

BIBLIOGRAPHY

HERZOG, J. M. (1985). Early somatic illness and pain. Presented at the Anna Freud Centre Colloquium.

KENNEDY, H. & YORKE, C. (1980). Childhood neurosis v. developmental deviations. *Dialogue: J. Psychoanal. Perspectives*, 4:21–33.

YORKE, C. (1986). Reflections on the problem of psychic trauma. *Psychoanal. Study Child*, 41:221–236.

Reflections on the Problem of Psychic Trauma

CLIFFORD YORKE, F.R.C.Psych., D.P.M.

A SYMPOSIUM ON TRAUMA, ORGANIZED BY THE ASSOCIATION FOR Child Psychoanalysis and held in London in 1984, bore witness to the continuing interest in the subject. Prepared papers by Jules Glenn (1984) and by Edgcumbe and Gavshon (1985) stimulated lively debate; but it was clear from the very active discussions that a number of issues remained unresolved. Twenty years earlier a symposium on the same subject led to an extensive collection of papers edited by Sidney Furst (1967) and did a great deal to map out the ground and clarify some important points. The contributions to this symposium led Anna Freud (1967) to point out that a number of technical terms in psychoanalysis had, in the course of time, suffered a widening use which had blurred meaning to a point at which valuable concepts were lost. She continued:

> We are in the position of witnessing this typical process with regard to the definition of trauma which extends at present from the original notion of the break through the stimulus barrier at one extreme to the notions of the accumulative, the strain, the retrospective, the screen trauma, until it becomes difficult at the other extreme to differentiate between adverse, pathogenic influences in general and trauma in particular [p. 235f.].

Codirector of the Anna Freud Centre, London, which is at present supported by the G. G. Bunzl Charitable Foundation, London; The Freud Centenary Fund, London; The Anna Freud Foundation, New York; The New-Land Foundation, Inc., New York; The Leo Oppenheimer and Flora Oppenheimer Haas Trust, New York; and a number of private supporters.

She added that, like everyone else, she too had tended to use the term *trauma* rather loosely until then, but that she would find it easier to avoid this in the future.

Careful consideration of these papers, including Anna Freud's own contributions, together with subsequent writings on the subject, suggest that this is more easily said than done. There is a repeated difficulty in restricting the definition of trauma to a serviceable theoretical concept that meets clinical needs and experience. This paper makes no such attempt, but argues that, if full benefit is to be derived from the many important contributions made to the subject, it is necessary to draw clear distinctions between three different conditions. Two of these were repeatedly discussed by Freud, namely, *traumatic neurosis* and *traumatic (automatic) anxiety.* The third, which may be called the *post-traumatic neuroticlike state,* requires separate discussion and illustration.

Freud's view of the nature of the *traumatic neurosis* was particularly clearly set out in *Beyond the Pleasure Principle* (1920) in the course of discussion of the significance of the compulsion to repeat. The disturbance arises when the ego is totally unprepared for a "traumatizing" event *of an external kind.* A contemporary example would be that of a car crash coming totally out of the blue, of which the driver had no anticipation and no opportunity for psychic preparation. Freud's view was that, in such conditions, the stimulus barrier broke down and the ego was overwhelmed with a degree of anxiety that it was totally unable to master at the time. The ego was "knocked out" and was temporarily unable to function. This period of loss of functioning follows immediately on impact and continues for a short and slightly variable period. In the current example an observer would see the victim as dazed, and would no doubt refer to him as suffering from "shock." The inference that ego functioning is lost is supported by the fact that the subject retains a clear recollection of the circumstances of the crash, but has no memory for the period immediately following the collision.

The subsequent clinical picture is well known. It is characterized by restlessness and variable but diffuse anxiety. A striking feature is the recurring dream in which the circumstances of the crash are vividly relived. These frightening dreams were, in

Freud's view, not really "dreams" at all in the sense in which these are understood psychoanalytically. They are a vivid reexperience of the disturbing event during sleep, in the course of which the excess excitation, bound by the ego in its attempted restoration of functioning, is fractionally and repeatedly discharged. The traumatic event may also be relived in the form of daydreams or preoccupations during the day.

In the present context, two clinical points must be made about this condition. The first is that even the fully blown picture tends to resolve itself, without treatment, in somewhere around 8 months, although there are exceptions. Even a minor degree of anticipation may allow sufficient preparation for the "shock" to be less pronounced and for recovery to take place within a comparatively short time. The factors which occasionally lead to an extremely protracted result are not always easy to understand. The second and related point is that, if the victim can be invited by the therapist to recollect the trauma over and over again, with appropriate affective discharge, the period during which the condition persists can be materially reduced. In World War II, psychiatrists dealing with traumatic neuroses (as opposed to battle exhaustion) arising in the front line found that chemical abreactions using ether or pentothal restored the victim to normal functioning within something like three weeks. We now know that the abreaction can be carried out without chemical assistance. The traumatic neurosis can therefore be conceptualized in terms of Breuer and Freud's notion of "strangulated affect" (1895) and, indeed, this was explicitly foreshadowed by Freud (1893) and was considered in relation to the abreactive process.

The second condition with which we are concerned is *traumatic (automatic) anxiety*. It is well known that Freud reformulated the theory of anxiety in 1926. Anxiety was no longer initiated by repression; repression was initiated by anxiety. Anxiety functioned as a danger signal seated in the ego that warned of an impending situation of danger. The danger itself was such that, if the ego were unable to mobilize its defenses, it would be overwhelmed and rendered helpless by automatic anxiety in the face of a "traumatic anxiety-situation" (p. 148). The prototype of these danger situations was considered by Freud to be the trauma of birth. Although studies by Spitz (1947) cast considerable doubt on whether birth per se is a trauma at all and emphasized the role of the nurse, midwife, or doctor in initiating the child's "negatively tinged excitation" (1965, p. 38), Freud had been quite clear that these responses were essentially vegetative and preceded the child's capacity to experience psychic anxiety. With the acquisition of this capacity, the child is subject to that form of pervasive psychic excitation which Freud had in mind in speaking of automatic anxiety.

It is this pervasive anxiety which floods the ego when a traumatic anxiety situation is encountered and overwhelms the ego. The sequence of these basic danger situations is familiar. When the very young child is threatened by a degree of pervasive anxiety with which he is unable to deal, and which can only be assuaged by the ministrations of a mother who detects the source of that anxiety, we have the prototype for later fears of annihilation. This is followed by fear of the loss of the object, fear of the loss of the object's love, castration anxiety, and fear of loss of the superego's love (Freud, 1926). Once ego development is sufficiently advanced to take an affective sample of one of these basic danger situations, to experience them in miniature, it can try to bring to bear its resources to ward off the threat and avoid the onset of pervasive (traumatic) anxiety.

Further comment is called for on traumatic anxiety and traumatic neurosis. First, traumatic anxiety is experienced by every child at all stages of development, is very often rapidly reversible, and is, to that extent, *not a traumatizing experience* in the sense of Edgcumbe and Gavshon (1985). Every infant, when his needs are not met, experiences "traumatic" anxiety. Indeed, if this is balanced by a reasonable measure of gratification, so that the balance between pleasure and pain is not seriously disturbed, the frustration is a motivating factor in development. The Garden of Eden offers little incentive for its inhabitants to set out on further explorations.

The situation is quite different in the traumatic neuroses. At first sight, it may appear that this condition shares with traumatic anxiety the state of reduction to helplessness. There are, nevertheless, important differences. When the ego is overwhelmed in the traumatic neurosis, it is not simply flooded with pervasive anxiety. It is totally knocked out by a flood of excitation. What is experienced is not psychic anxiety but somatic vegetative excitation. A fuller account of the developmental factors involved in this process has been given elsewhere (Yorke and Wiseberg, 1977; Yorke et al., 1980), and its relevance for the concept of trauma has been discussed by Furman (1984).

A breach of the stimulus barrier initiates the traumatic neurosis. The question arises of whether or not one can reasonably postulate a protective shield against excessive stimuli from within as well as without. Anna Freud (1967) explicitly said that one could. She took as her starting point Freud's statement that "the essence of a traumatic situation is an experience of helplessness on the part of the ego in the face of accumulation of excitation whether of external or internal origin." Since she considered that this quotation designated the ego as "the central victim in the traumatic event," she argued that "it implies that there exists not one stimulus barrier (against environmental stimuli) but two protective shields against two types of dangers threatening from the inner as well as from the outer world. These include, of course, those occasions where otherwise harmless external happenings are given threatening meaning on the basis of existing internal constellations" (p. 236).

It is important to observe that, in the statement quoted by Anna Freud, Freud was referring to *traumatic situations*—that is, those of *basic danger*. He was not referring to events that precipitate a traumatic neurosis. The one threatens or leads to pervasive anxiety; the other to vegetative excitation and involves a breach of the stimulus barrier. It is unfortunate that "reduction to helplessness" is so often held to characterize the two without the necessary psychoanalytic qualifications which show how different they are.

The fact that this difference is repeatedly overlooked may well spring from Freud's varied uses of the word "trauma" in different contexts and in different circumstances. The problem is in part a historical one and is compounded by the persistence, with fluctuating emphasis, of the preanalytic, traumatic theory of neurosis into later formulations. In this connection, Greenacre's account (1967) of the different meanings of the word "trauma" in succeeding stages of Freud's writings is indispensable. She reminds us, for example, that, in reviewing his work with Breuer, he referred to "traumas" following the most trivial experiences of childhood (Freud, 1906), while, in the *Introductory Lectures* many years later, he compared the traumatic neuroses with the symptom neuroses, and said that, although the two could not be closely compared, even in the latter there was no need to abandon the "traumatic line of approach as being erroneous: it must be possible to fit it in and subsume it somewhere else" (1916–17, p. 276).

It seems possible that considerations of this kind underlie the notion of a second barrier against *internal* stimuli. To avoid further perpetuation of ambiguities, a breakthrough of such a stimulus barrier would have to be distinguished from an untimely penetration of the *repression* barrier. Only two conditions come to mind where the concept of an internal *stimulus* barrier might appear, at first sight, useful: namely, the stage IV nightmare in adults and pavor nocturnus in children. Studies of these conditions, which seem identical in all essentials, indicate that they occur during NREM sleep and are related, not to dream material of the usual kind, but to frightening thoughts which follow the secondary process (Fisher et al., 1970). The well-known result—that the child sits bolt upright in a state of absolute terror and total confusion—may suggest that something analogous to the initial stage of traumatic neurosis has occurred by virtue of an invasion of the barrier from within. Ego functioning is again knocked out. It is during the resulting state of confusion that the individual may be endangered—a patient of my acquaintance who suffered repeatedly from stage IV nightmares once walked, in her disorientation, through a second floor window and seriously injured herself.

Nevertheless, pavor nocturnus and the stage IV nightmare differ in at least two major particulars from the condition resulting from the breach of an *external* stimulus barrier. First, they occur in a state of altered consciousness, when the ego is already vulnerable. Secondly, the result is not a persisting disorder. Even though the substantial impairment of ego functioning may last for many minutes or even longer, once it is over, the child or adult returns to normal health. And while these nocturnal states

require further study, the need for a concept of a second stimulus barrier appears, even in this restricted clinical context, an
open question.

If the part played by the economic factor in all these conditions is taken more fully into account, the strength of the stimulus barrier or, in the case of traumatic anxiety, of other opposing agents, is as important as the strength of the force ranged
against them (A. Freud, 1967). Vulnerability is not evenly dis-
tributed among people; it is well known, for example, that the
level of the pain threshold varies from person to person. One
can certainly encounter cases of psychic shock that stop short of
traumatic neurosis and suggest that any breach of the barrier has
been less than total. It would indeed make nonsense of the concept of a developmental line of anxiety if all gradations between
vegetative excitation, pervasive psychic anxiety, and signal anxiety were held not to exist. While this consideration should certainly be kept in mind in what has been said, it does not invalidate
the usefulness of the distinctions which have been emphasized.
On any developmental line, way stations are still way stations and
cannot be telescoped together.

The third condition to be discussed is what I have called the
posttraumatic neuroticlike state. It may best be considered with the
help of an extended illustration. The patient, a Scotsman in early
middle age, was a businessman with pharmaceutical training. In
the course of analysis, he relived in the transference a fantasy
that his head was inside his mother's bottom and was being con-
stricted by it. The context in which this occurred is of special
interest.

He did not seek help on account of any somatic symptoms. His
initial complaints were of intermittent free-floating anxiety, episodes of mild depressive affect without any specific conscious
content, and difficulties in establishing friendly relationships
with others. He had a girl friend of whom he was somewhat
possessive, but his relationships were otherwise formal and restricted to essential contact.

A few weeks after the start of treatment he expressed a number of fantasies in which I was attacked about the head—first by
unknown persons, then by himself. In these attacks the brain

and skull were seriously damaged. I commented on the growing intensity and frequency of these fantasies. He then told me that, around the age of 4 or 4½, he had been admitted to a hospital for a mastoidectomy, after a good deal of pain. He remembered the stay there as something horrific. Visiting was not allowed, and he had no access to his family. His happiest memory was of greeting his father who came to collect him on discharge.

These concerns dominated the treatment for a considerable time. Fantasies of sadistic violence, in which he viciously attacked my head, appeared again and again in limitless variations. To begin with, these fantasies were not reported with appropriate affect, and although the sadism itself was expressed in the most direct manner, it was accompanied by only the most muted of feeling states.

A sadomasochistic transference expressed the reexperience of the frightening operation in which he was either the victim or the vengeful attacker. I was repeatedly equated with the surgeon who drove knives into his body and mutilated his victim's skull, or who put damaging or dangerous words into his ears. The fantasy that he was the victim of a violent homosexual inter-course, experienced in terms of the chisel and the skull, soon came into awareness and became the subject of protracted working through.

Before long, it became clear that the reexperience of the operation was in no way limited to content of this kind. It had become the overdetermined center of all manner of conflict and anxiety. Almost everything that concerned or disturbed him appeared to have some reference to this one dramatic episode. The anesthesia under which the operation was conducted (in fantasy or reality) played a central role. Episodes of drowsiness occurred in the analytic session; feelings of suffocation appeared with unfailing regularity; fantasies of being overwhelmed by smells, of being smothered and reduced to oblivion, brought repeated distress as the associated affect became more available.

If, as a result of the continuing analytic work, material centered on the operation, the anesthesia and all the circumstances that went with it slowly yielded to a better understanding of the patient's intense conflicts at almost every stage of development, they did so reluctantly and only intermittently. When, for example, positive oedipal material became a central feature of our work, the wish to enter into the body of the analyst and mother slowly achieved direct expression. The childhood nature of the fantasy was graphically illustrated by the "recollection" with which this vignette began. He was standing like a 3-year-old behind his mother's legs with his arms clasped firmly around her thighs. This was immediately followed by the fantasy that, in this position, he would have his head right up his mother's skirts, and in no time at all was pushing it firmly into her bottom. At this point in the session he complained of a headache; and when I relieved him of this with an interpretation of the oppressive force around him, the pain gave way to a *pleasant* and *welcome* anesthesia as the warmth and the smell overcame him.

It is striking how completely the phallic and anal material came together in the patient's childhood fantasies and their current reexperience. The orality, too, was conspicuous. At one time or another, every part instinct or its derivatives achieved some form of expression in the context of the trauma as he remembered it or, perhaps more correctly, fantasized it. Thus, the thoughts of being peacefully put to sleep were linked with the notion of satiation at the breast and resulting contented oblivion; but even this brought to mind fantasies of anesthetic intubation.

Exhibitionism and scopophilia played a considerable part in this man's material. It was repeatedly presented in terms of the hospital experience. Getting undressed was linked in his mind with a fantasy of being stripped naked by the nurse, and getting dressed in terms of being wrapped in hospital gear or in bandages. The nurse repeatedly came to represent the woman who humiliated him, mocked him, and exposed his tiny genitals to view. And, inasmuch as there was always another side to the conflict, she could also represent the protector who clothed him and at times hid him comfortingly from view. The intense ambivalence was manifest in these myriad ways at nearly every stage of treatment. Impulses to urinate and fears of wetting the couch were almost inextricably linked with fears of a scolding for failing to ask for a bedpan. Skin erotism, likewise, was manifest in terms of the many things that were done to his body in preparation for the surgical assault. (In later phases of the analysis all

these manifestations were shown to have far more varied determinants as these were brought into awareness.)

The way in which the analysis repeatedly brought to consciousness apparent manifestations of the surgical trauma may
best be conveyed by some sessional material. I have chosen an
illustration from the fourth year of treatment to give some indication of the persistence of this content and to demonstrate how,
even at this stage in the analysis, it could still play a conspicuous
part in the treatment.

Part of my consulting room had been freshly painted. When
the patient lay on the couch, he expressed his pleasure at the
smell of new paint. He had experienced some feelings of dizziness the previous day, as if his brain were being damaged. He
had a fantasy that he was suffering from a brain disorder, perhaps of an infective kind. It made him very sensitive to what he
called "levels of consciousness."

At his club the previous day, he had found himself feeling
angry with a fellow committee member. This colleague who,
incidentally, was a doctor, always spoke with authority, as if he
knew everything and had a right to be in charge. The conversation was becoming somewhat acrimonious, though he himself
had not expressed his feelings. He looked around the room and
reflected that the building was falling down. They would have to
move. This seemed to add to "the general air of acrimony and
discontent." The hostility seemed too much for him, and he was
somewhat alarmed when the man who assumed so much authority began attacking one of the women members. He realized that
his own feeling was unmistakably a childhood one that brought
back to life quarrels between his parents, in which he was always
the mediator. He wanted to attack his doctor colleague.

We had already, in previous sessions, had occasion to look at
his fantasies of a violent primal scene, in which he intervened
and rescued his mother from the hostile father. No doubt it was
the work we had already done that helped him to say, suddenly
and decisively, "I realize it can't really be about the doctor on the
committee. I have no real quarrel with him. I suppose you're the
one I really want to attack, but *that* makes me feel guilty and
bad." He then observed that he had experienced the unsteadiness, the dizziness of which he had spoken, on leaving the committee meeting.

After acknowledging his comments on the primal scene and his reexperience in terms of myself and my wife, I suggested to him that he must be struck by the way in which so many of his thoughts still took us back to the operation in childhood. The fantasy of neurological or brain damage still returned, and the unsteadiness, presumably, was still linked to the anesthetic experiences. Could it be that, in his fantasy, the attack on his own head and the concomitant anesthesia followed the attack on myself in the form of the committee doctor? Did he perhaps experience this as a retaliation for his own aggression? "Well," he responded, "I *do* have a sense of being unjustifiably hostile to older men. I get angry when I'm not treated as an equal." I suggested that, when he experienced the childhood feeling to which he had referred, he was not treating *himself* as an equal. He was silent for a time.

After some reflection, he said he must annoy his girl friend by repeatedly drifting off in his thoughts whenever she talked to him. He thought this must make her quite angry. He recalled that his mother used to "drift off" whenever he wanted to talk to her, so perhaps he was retaliating for his mother's behavior by doing the same to his girl friend. Some comments about the forthcoming weekend as well as a future holiday brought thoughts of my "drifting away" from him and physically absenting myself in the same way that his mother had done when she had forcibly sent him to the hospital.

For some time, almost any session picked at random would contain *some* reference, however slight or disguised, to the hospital experience although, as the analytic work proceeded, there were longer stretches when any such reference was marginal. And although physical experiences played no part in the discomforts that drove this man to seek treatment, they repeatedly played a part in the analysis. They appeared in bodily sensations, in feelings of impaired consciousness, of unsteadiness, and of transient pain. Although their appearance was not exclusive to the consulting room and affected him elsewhere, and even imposed themselves upon his patterns of sleep, they almost always had transference manifestations. But perhaps the most striking feature of all was that, with rare exceptions, they could be traced to fantasies and reexperiences of the hospital trauma, especially the operation itself.

If, as I believe, this hospital experience can properly be regarded as a trauma, it appears to have attracted to itself, almost
like a magnet, nearly all the major conflicts, expectable or otherwise, which preceded it as well as so many conflicts which must
have followed it. The hospital experience therefore functions as
an organizer (Kennedy, 1986) which structures the patient's disturbances and anxieties and lends them the shape they assume
when they reemerge in analysis. The analytic task in a case such
as this consists in the slow isolation of the trauma from all that
goes before and almost all that follows after. Whether this can
ever be completely accomplished is another matter. However
this may be, it seems justified to call cases of this kind *posttraumatic neuroticlike states.*

Some of these points may be made with greater force in the
light of a treatment session from a comparatively late stage in the
analysis. The patient reported that he was awakened during the
night by his girl friend who was now pregnant. She said she
couldn't sleep on account of a rash that was itching. He looked at
it, could not identify it, gave her some calamine lotion, and went
to sleep. He had a dream in which his feet were sinking into mud.
When he finally extricated himself, the mud was clinging to his
body.

In his associations he recalled that, the day before, he had
been trying to repair a leak in the water tank and, in doing so,
had become very dirty. For some time he had felt very smelly and
dirty for reasons which puzzled him. He reminded me of the
several occasions on which he had already referred to this experience. There was a note of reproach in his voice. He said there
was a bit in the dream which suggested that he had managed to
find a way of dealing with the mud and getting rid of it.

This reminded him that he had been somewhat intrigued by
his girl friend's rash and was determined to find a way to help
her. He was a keen reader of medical literature and always regretted he had not become a doctor. He got hold of some text-
books on dermatology and decided it must be an allergic response. With more detective work and further questioning of his
girl friend he traced the cause of the allergy and dealt with it
successfully. He was proud of his accurate diagnosis and treatment. The cause for the reproachful tone soon became clear. *He*

had got *his* girl friend "out of the mud": why hadn't I solved his problem with the dirty skin in the same effective way he had solved hers?

He turned again to his fascination with rashes. When he examined his girl friend, he had put his ear to her tummy to see if he could feel the baby kicking or hear the heart beat. He couldn't. He had a fleeting fantasy that the child would be *brain damaged*. But he couldn't understand why the rash should make him listen for the child. He also noticed that, right now, he felt very hot as well as sticky.

I said that I wondered if he was recalling some childhood illness of his own in which he was hot because he had a fever, and felt dirty and sticky because he had a rash. Perhaps it was an illness which sometimes led to brain damage. He said, "That's funny. As you were talking I thought of measles. I *did* have German measles—I think at 6 or 7, but I had forgotten about it until now. I was frightened because my mother left me to go out. I heard later that she'd knocked down a child who had to be taken to the hospital with a broken arm." I said, "So this was another illness linked with brain damage and an absent mother who injured a child." This reminded him that he, too, had once broken his leg and had a greenstick fracture of the fibia. He remembered being taken to the hospital lying in the back of the car. He paused, and then went on, "I know I'd also suffered from chicken pox, though I'm not sure when. I had a small cousin whose brain was already damaged and who died from the measles about the same time."

He again thought about the water tank. (Earlier, we had traced part of his interest in water to a childhood fascination with urination, especially in little girls.) Whenever he was hot, he longed for something cool on his skin. He remembered that as a child his favorite book was *The Water Babies* and it was the chimney sweep with the filthy skin who was at the center of the story. He went back to the greenstick fracture. He remembered begging his mother to relieve him of the pain. When he got to the hospital, the anesthetic did just that and it was marvelous.

In the analysis he had already discovered that he liked the smell of new paint; and the pleasant effects of a little alcohol before he went to bed gave him a sense of freedom from disease.

But he only acquired his bedtime habit during analysis, and it was necessary to understand his pleasure in terms of its significance in the transference. It had for some time been progressively easier to link his recurrent experiences with both pleasure and pain and with conflicts of a varied nature deriving from different developmental phases. They were no longer to be understood in the light of an inevitable link with the "traumatic event." The separation of my patient's trauma from other historical aspects of his development allowed him to welcome a whole range of positive experiences and pleasurable activities as well as to understand the many miseries which had occurred independently of the operation or the anesthetic in a new light.

The material from the foregoing session is not, however, primarily reported to emphasize this point. It is the striking illustration of the way in which *later* significant events, conflicts, and experiences were drawn into the trauma that has to be underlined. Glover (1929), in reporting a patient who remembered how he burned his hand when he was about 3½ but had no recollection of a circumcision occurring at the same time, suggested that traumatic memories might have a screening function. Furst (1967) discussed this postulate in underlining the fact that a "screen trauma," like a screen memory, can serve either to cover another, more significant trauma or else can stand for a group or series of traumatic events. A point of this kind has indeed been repeatedly made in the analytic literature and is described, for example, by Anna Freud (1951) and by Kris (1956) in his discussion of strain trauma. What we are dealing with in my adult patient, however, is something more; *future* events are drawn *back* and absorbed into the single trauma long after it occurred.

Hansi Kennedy (1986) described the treatment of an adolescent whose phimosis in early life was the subject of his mother's intrusive ministrations and led at the age of 2 years 8 months to operative treatment. The boy felt deeply that he had never been loved, and the attention given to his penis represented his principal tie to the mother. A leading feature of the analysis was the repetition, in thinly disguised enactments, of the manipulation of his genitals and the painful excitement this engendered in the transference. This dominated the early stages of the treatment, and its sadomasochistic character could be traced long afterward. The author took the view that the boy's protracted experience of the mother's genital attentions and the subsequent operation had a decisive effect on all later development, as well as serving to incorporate all the antecedent conflicts. For this reason, Kennedy refers to the boy's collective experiences as an "organizer" in a sense comparable to my use of the term in connection with my adult patient.

It may rightly be asked what is meant by the term *organizer*. I have the impression that Kennedy's use of the term is, like mine, descriptive. That does not mean that our uses are identical, although, in each instance, we try to convey and identify a pathological process in terms which may be both clinically and theoretically useful. It is true that the presenting clinical pictures are very different, but the events which in each case became such a powerful determinant in shaping the nature and quality of the treatment experience can surely be called *traumatic*.

Summary

Discussion of psychic trauma has been handicapped by colloquial use of the term which broadens its application to a point where it undermines its psychoanalytic usefulness. The problem is compounded by a blurring of distinctions between what can properly be called the *traumatic neurosis* and what is often referred to as *traumatic anxiety*. This sometimes results in hybrid concepts in which earlier and important precisions are lost. Furthermore, it seems possible that our understanding of the trauma concept has not been made easier by the hypothesis of a breakthrough of the *barrier against internal stimuli*—a notion that risks confusion with an untimely breakthrough of the *repression barrier*. This is not to say that the notion should be abandoned without further consideration.

Further thought needs to be given to the *posttraumatic neurotic-like states*. Although these have been understood in terms of trauma as "organizer," this term is used by both Kennedy and myself in a descriptive sense. This does not obviate the necessity for greater metapsychological clarity in the further study of these conditions. That task still lies ahead.

BIBLIOGRAPHY

BREUER, J. & FREUD, S. (1895). Studies on hysteria. *S.E.*, 2.
EDGCUMBE, R. & GAVSHON, A. (1985). Clinical comparisons of traumatic events and reactions. *Bull. Anna Freud Centre*, 8:3–21.
FISHER, C., BYRNE, J., EDWARDS, A., & KAHN, E. (1970). The psychophysiological study of nightmares. *J. Amer. Psychoanal. Assn.*, 18:747–782.
FREUD, A. (1951). Observations on child development. *Psychoanal. Study Child*, 6:18–30.
——— (1967). Comments on trauma. In *Psychic Trauma*, ed. S. S. Furst, pp. 235–245. New York: Basic Books.
FREUD, S. (1893). On the psychical mechanism of hysterical phenomena. *S.E.*, 3:27–39.
——— (1906). My views on the part played by sexuality in the aetiology of the neuroses. *S.E.*, 12:272–279.
——— (1916–17). Introductory lectures on psycho-analysis. *S.E.*, 15 & 16.
——— (1920). Beyond the pleasure principle. *S.E.*, 18:7–64.
——— (1926). Inhibitions, symptoms and anxiety. *S.E.*, 20:77–175.
FURMAN, E. (1984). Contribution to Symposium on Trauma. Association for Child Psychoanalysis, London.
FURST, S. S., ed. (1967). *Psychic Trauma*. New York: Basic Books.
GLENN, J. (1984). Contribution to Symposium on Trauma. Association for Child Psychoanalysis, London.
GLOVER, E. (1929). The screening function of traumatic memories. *Int. J. Psychoanal.*, 10:90–93.
GREENACRE, P. (1967). The influence of infantile trauma on genetic patterns. In *Psychic Trauma*, ed. S. S. Furst, pp. 108–153. New York: Basic Books.
KENNEDY, H. (1986). Trauma in childhood. *Psychoanal. Study Child*, 41:209–219.
KRIS, E. (1956). The recovery of childhood memories in psychoanalysis. *Psychoanal. Study Child*, 11:54–88.
SPITZ, R. A. (1947). *Birth and the First Fifteen Minutes of Life*, 16mm film.
——— (1965). *The First Year of Life*. New York: Int. Univ. Press.
YORKE, C., KENNEDY, H., & WISEBERG, S. (1980). Some clinical and theoretical aspects of two developmental lines. In *The Course of Life*, ed. S. I. Greenspan & G. H. Pollock, 1:619–637. Washington: U.S. Department of Health & Human Services.
YORKE, C. & WISEBERG, S. (1977). A developmental view of anxiety. *Psychoanal. Study Child*, 31:107–135.

DEVELOPMENT

Special Solutions to Phallic-Aggressive Conflicts in Male Twins

STEVEN L. ABLON, M.D., ALEXANDRA M. HARRISON, M.D., ARTHUR F. VALENSTEIN, M.D., AND SANFORD GIFFORD, M.D.

THE BIRTH OF TWINS IS UNUSUAL AND IN THAT SENSE IS AN EXPERI-ment of nature for the study of many aspects of normal and pathological development. The special features of twinship intensify many developmental phenomena, enabling them to be seen in sharper focus. Analyzing adult twins, we saw that manifestations and vicissitudes of phallic aggression, as well as their precursors, were prominent in the analytic material, and they became a major focus in the evolution of the analytic situation and in its outcome.

Our use of the term aggression includes both its pathological, conflict-ridden expressions and its adaptive, sublimated potentialities. As a result of early conflict, normal aggression for adaptive functioning is often inhibited and becomes unavailable in order to nullify sadistic or destructive expressions. Anxiety and unconscious fears that all relationships be subject to a "dog eat dog" paradigm limit the potentiality for assertiveness; and one

Dr. Ablon is a training and supervising analyst at the Boston Psychoanalytic Society and Institute. Dr. Harrison is director of Child Psychiatry Training at the Cambridge Hospital, Cambridge, Mass. Dr. Valenstein is a clinical professor of psychiatry emeritus, at Harvard Medical School. Dr. Gifford is an associate clinical professor of psychiatry at Harvard Medical School.

must always be alert for "who will damage or even destroy whom?" Consequently aggression is not constructively available for the adaptive purposes of living. When the resolution of aggressive conflicts on the preoedipal level is incomplete or distorted, the unfolding of competitive strivings is affected. In our experience phallic strivings frequently undergo unusual compromises in the competitive struggles of twins within the capsule of the twinship.

The exigent sorting out of aggression among twins was pointed out quite clearly by Dorothy Burlingham over 30 years ago. The theme of phallic aggression and its variations, however, including competition, was only one of the many features she so richly described. In this paper we explore in more detail the development of phallic aggression in male twins and its centrality in the analysis of twins. To set the stage for our consideration of the complexities of this subject we begin with the story of Jacob and Esau which, like many myths and legends, highlights man's conflicts and struggles in a dramatic and succinct way.

The story of Jacob and Esau is an epic description of the relationship of male twins. The vicissitudes of phallic aggression and competition are a central motif of the story. When Rebekah conceived, the children "struggled together within her." As the twins grew up, the firstborn, Esau, became a hunter, "a man of the field," while Jacob was quiet, "dwelling in tents." The father, Isaac, loved Esau because he liked to eat the game Esau hunted, but their mother, Rebekah, loved Jacob. One day Esau came in from the field faint with hunger. When Esau asked for some soup, Jacob insisted that Esau first sell him his birthright. Being on the threshold of death, Esau knew his birthright was of no value to him then and he sold it to Jacob. Years later when Isaac was old and his eyesight was failing, Rebekah put Esau's best clothes on Jacob as well as goat skins on his hands and neck so Jacob would seem hairy like Esau. Thinking he was Esau, Isaac gave Jacob his last blessing.

When Esau discovered that Jacob had tricked him out of his father's blessing, he wept, hated his brother, and planned to kill Jacob. But when Rebekah heard about Esau's plan for revenge, she and Isaac sent Jacob away. Jacob was gone 20 years. During this time he married, prospered, and had many sons. When

Jacob returned to his land, he was afraid Esau would attack him and sent gifts ahead in the hope of appeasing Esau. Jacob was left alone, and a stranger wrestled with him until daybreak. When the stranger saw that he could not defeat Jacob, he touched the hollow of his thigh, and Jacob's thigh was put out of joint. Yet Jacob would not let the man go unless he blessed him. Jacob and Esau were reunited and then departed for their own lands.

The story of Jacob and Esau highlights aggression as it enters into the competitive struggle between twins. Like other famous stories, myths, and legends, it expresses in symbolic and metaphorical language our deepest longings and conflicts. In this paper we will explore how the vicissitudes of phallic aggression in male twins are expressed in themes such as competition for the birthright and the wish to be preferred by and to identify with one of the parents. We will examine the significance of shifts between passive and active, feminine and masculine, phallic and receptive, and how these shifts and consolidations are influenced by a complex interplay of constitutional and developmental factors, life events, and internal psychodynamic advances and regressions. And we discuss how the difficulties twins experience in separating, individuating, and pursuing lives independent of each other relate to regression from phallic competitive issues.

After a brief selective review of the literature and research on twins, we present material from the analyses of two adult male patients, one an identical twin and the other a fraternal, opposite-sex twin. In reviewing our clinical material and the story of Jacob and Esau, we highlight patterns of phallic aggression in these twins, solutions to these conflicts arising therefrom, and their implications for the psychoanalysis of twins and nontwins.

SELECTIVE LITERATURE REVIEW

In considering some problems of aggression in twins, we begin with the assumption that although there are no conflicts so unique that they cannot also be detected in siblings and only children, growing up as a twin accentuates certain normal developmental conflicts and reduces the intensity of others. The analysis of a twin provides an opportunity to observe a variety of aggressive conflicts with unusual clarity, whether the twins are identical (Arlow, 1960; Joseph and Tabor, 1961), fraternal (Orr, 1941), or opposite-sex fraternal (Glenn, 1966). As with other analytic studies of twins which tend to emphasize pathology, we must remind outselves that most twins successfully survive their twinship, despite its special advantages and difficulties, and that all psychopathology in twins is not necessarily the result of the twinship (Glenn, 1966; Winestine, 1969).

MUTUAL STIMULATION OF AGGRESSION

The mutual stimulation of aggression has been directly observed by Burlingham (1952, 1963) as a crescendo of self-perpetuating excitement, physically violent and highly sexualized, precipitated by imitative play or competition for objects, so intense and absorbing that the presence of others is virtually excluded. Even though similar phenomena can be seen between any two siblings, the intensity and repetitiousness within twin pairs, either identical or fraternal, commonly lead to a variety of special solutions. One takes the form of a "nonaggression pact," in which intrapair aggression is renounced through a "fantasy of absolute equality." The stronger twin inhibits his superior abilities and allows the weaker but more competitive twin to come abreast or even win. This recalls the mechanism of "retiring in favor of a rival" that Freud (1920) mentions as a possible predisposition to homosexuality in one of his few references to twins. Because competition is heightened between twins, there is a greater likelihood of becoming bound to either the active-aggressive or passive-aggressive position. In addition, the constant togetherness and pleasurable interaction which reinforce the interdependency serve to inhibit aggressive chance-taking within the twinship. To risk assertiveness one against the other means to unsettle the active-passive balance, which is more heavily weighted for twins than in other sibling relationships. Other familiar patterns of resolution include an alliance of the twins (the "gang of two") with the potentiated aggression externalized in "mischief" acted out against others, as in the "Katzenjammer Kids" or Wilhelm Busch's Max and Moritz. Among other patterns are "separate but equal" role assignments in which each twin chooses an area of noncompeting prowess. Hartmann (1934–35) had first pointed out this resolution to intertwin competition in his concept of *Vertretbarkeit,* or interchangeability. This pattern is also represented in the classic twin myth of the Dioscuri, which emphasizes similarity and complementarity in different but related fields (Castor the charioteer and Polydeuces the boxer); the latter was Zeus's son who pleads, when the moral Castor is killed, to share his immortality with his twin by each living on alternate days (Graves, 1955).

INDIVIDUAL DIFFERENCES WITHIN TWIN PAIRS

Individual differences within twin pairs, either in birth order or in size, physical strength, and innate behavior patterns, contribute important elements to the evolution of dominance and submission, and to an emphasis on both unity and similarity as well as highly differentiated and separate identities. However, these innate intrapair differences undergo a continuous modification under the influence of parental attitudes. Parents may see their twins as identical replicas of each other, as separate individuals with contrasting features, or as an undifferentiated unit ("the twins"). Later the twins' own attitudes toward mutual identification or separation-individuation contribute a third element to this complex interaction. This may widen or narrow the influence of major or minor innate differences, denying substantial asymmetries in size or physical health, or magnifying insignificant traits that might pass unnoticed or be taken for granted in a singleton without the constant comparisons that twins experience. The outcome of this process determines the fate of early innate ego tendencies. The twins are seen as the strong and weak, the healthy and sick, the smart and stupid, or (in same-sex twins) as the more masculine and the more feminine.

MODIFICATIONS IN EGO AND SUPEREGO DEVELOPMENT

Every twin, except those separated at birth, grows up with an object tie with his twin, auxiliary in addition to the primary object tie with his mother and father. For both identical and fraternal pairs, this strong object relationship between the two is likely to affect ego and superego development. Ego maturation may be delayed or accelerated by a supplementary object tie, facilitating the twins' separation from the primary attachment to their mother, and yet inhibiting or delaying the resolution of the oedipus complex. In essence, the primary separation from mother is likely to be mitigated or displaced onto a later conflict over separation from the twin, which may occur at a more or less vulnerable period of ego development. Corresponding effects on the superego are more complex but also show both positive and negative features. There may be heightened competitive conflicts involving envy that may connect with well-sublimated concerns about justice and equality, or to litigious and paranoid preoccupations with feeling cheated. Superego deficits may arise individually from projecting guilt for aggression onto the twin, or collectively in both, through a narcissistic immunity to moral scruples derived from their special status as twins ("the psychology of the exception"). Latency period varieties of "twin morality" (strict respect for each other's rights and total indifference to the rights of others) have many sources, as in Burlingham's (1946) concept of "the gang of two" derived from adolescent group formations, or the chronic sense of injustice and outraged innocence when both twins are punished for the deeds of one.

CLINICAL MATERIAL

CASE 1

Mr. A., a 27-year-old businessman and an identical twin, entered analysis because of panic attacks which occurred at night and in which he felt out of control of his thoughts, caught in the grip of one preoccupying idea, as if he were in a "downward spiral." He first experienced the panics on vacations visiting his parents at home during graduate school. During these episodes he would lie in bed and feel his limbs form first a Y and then an X.

A. was the firstborn, had his father's first name, and had always been his mother's favorite. The intimacy between them included his mother's involvement in his childhood encopresis, which she treated with laxatives and occasional enemas. A. was also always slightly ahead of his brother, B., his only sibling, in academic, athletic, and musical competitions.

Early in the analysis Mr. A. learned to identify a variety of his own obsessional defenses and was able to modify his use of isolation of affect and reaction formation, for example, in a way which allowed him greater affective freedom. A more intransigent defense, however, was the retreat from his phallic aggression into passivity and femininity. Again and again in the analytic hour he would become frightened by phallic-aggressive fantasies and feelings, such as in a competition at work, or in a confrontation with a traffic cop, and would pull back into a good little boy or "little girl" role.

Later on, Mr. A. elaborated the metaphor of the X and the Y on several different levels as he struggled to establish himself as a man with his girlfriend. On an oedipal level of the transference, he tried to seduce his woman analyst with his words, becoming more sexually free in his talk with her. He had a dream about a baseball game in which he was "put right back into the game" and although he was "rusty," he "did pretty good things with the ball." He became angry at her husband for having the right to park his car in her driveway, while he had to park his car on the street. In his relationship with his brother, his view of B. as the more successful of the two began to change. Instead of feeling inadequate in relation to B.'s married status, he enjoyed B.'s envy of his "tom at life."

This forward movement, the active phallic or "Y chromosome" part of the metaphor, was balanced by a corresponding retreat into a passive, feminine "X chromosome" position. The back-and-forth movement recalled the description of his moving his limbs back and forth in bed before his panic episode. This defensive position seemed rooted in a residuum of incomplete differentiation from both mother and twin, and seemed to have contributed to later unresolved conflicts in oedipal and adolescent stages of development. He had a dream in which he and his brother were both catchers on the same baseball team: "I went to the manager. There were two of us in that position. I said, 'There are Allanson and Smith ahead of us, so you can drop us both if you want, or we'd be glad to play if you want.'" In response to the challenge, "Play ball!" Mr. A. responded, "We come as a pair." His choice of the passive, feminine role in the twin relationship and his conflict about it were illustrated by another dream. In the dream Mr. A. was angry at his brother for not returning his tie. In association to the dream he recalled a time when he was angry at his brother for not bringing him the sheet music he needed to play his horn at a wedding. He was angry at B. for the "tie" that bound them, and also for taking the tie that represented the one penis shared by both twins in his fantasy. This fantasy was developed further: "I think of B. as him being sharper than I was, a little more aggressive, taking the first step. Once he'd done it, there wasn't any need for me to, really. Maybe I could reap the rewards of his aggression and still stay behind and be the good one."

In the transference neurosis the analyst was the twin and as such represented the two polarities of the twinship—the omnipotent mother twin who nurtured him and was interested in every intimate detail of his life, and the phallic twin who was willing to "take the first step" and keep the penis for him until he should ask for it. In this overdetermined negative oedipal position, A. could remain close to his mother, his twin, and his father, apparently without giving up anything. However, this solution did not allow him to own his manhood and to assert himself with women or at work. After a painful rejection by his girlfriend, who shared many of the features of the analyst in the transference, Mr. A. made a less idealized relationship with a new woman.

Toward the end of the analysis, Mr. A. began to talk about whether, given the hopelessness of his wishes to have the analyst as a lover, he could ever become a man without leaving her. In the same session that he talked about his attachment to the analyst interfering with his making a commitment to a woman, he described an image of being in a lake and the analyst pushing him away from the side and saying, "You can swim!" The metaphor of deep water emerged as a prominent theme. After returning from his summer vacation Mr. A. related an experience: he had been swimming in the ocean and without being aware of it had allowed himself to be passively carried out by the tide. When he realized his situation, he became afraid and called out to a woman he saw standing on the distant shore. She did not respond, apparently unable to hear him over the noise of the waves. He recovered himself and swam back to shore. Shortly thereafter he began to talk about termination and his wish to finish after one more year. In response to the analyst's questions, Mr. A. said that she could not hear because the ocean was too loud and his cries were too weak. "The fear was not of drowning but of collapsing. It's a kind of feeling I have occasionally about life—struggling forever and never being able to rest." He explained that in order to do what he had to do, he must prepare to leave the analyst. He was concerned that he might never do all he had hoped to do with her, but that he had to "break free of the strength of the undertow."

He said, "It's a feeling that it's time to go on, to be on my own, and not to depend on you, a feeling that I won't be completely adult until I'm out of here." In the last week of the analysis he related an experience of going swimming in a lake the weekend before. "I see this as a kind of repeat of the image I've had, stepping off the shallow end of the lake and going to swim in the deep water myself. It's a good deal less fearsome than the ocean, doesn't have an undertow, more manageable. It's like growing up and leaving my mother in order to live a life of my own. I'm going to miss you immensely, and you'll miss me too, but it has to be."

An interesting feature of this analysis was the prominence of the twin in dream material and in the transference. In the transference the twin appeared as a sibling and also as a substitute to or a complement for parental transference figures. In this way the twin as a phallic competitor dominated the representations of the oedipal father, and the powerful preoedipal maternal transference was inextricably linked to the longings for the dyadic relationship of the twinship. Although in the transference Mr. A. recapitulated much which was transparently oedipal, oedipal conflicts were underscored by the conflict created within the twinship between opposite drive derivatives. The split between active and passive, masculine and feminine served as protection against oedipal competition and constituted a defensive stalemate in the separation-individuation process. This stalemate both prevented the merger with his double and made it impossible to separate, since to choose one libidinal position meant to give up the other.

When Mr. A. went home on vacation, he felt pulled into being a special little boy with his mother. Underlying the oedipal threat accompanying this wish was the fear of conversion from Y to X, of regression into an undifferentiated state in which he would lose his penis and become immersed in an oceanic oneness. The threat of this regression provoked his panic attacks. The panics disappeared when Mr. A. re-created the tie to the securing figure, the analyst-twin, the complement of whichever instinctual position Mr. A. assumed.

He was then confronted with the question of whether he could fight with his "twin," i.e., the analyst, in order to own his penis and stay in the relationship. The prospect of such a fight was frightening to him. The other alternatives were to take his penis and go, or to stay and comply. On an oedipal level this dilemma meant to leave home or to stay with mother as a castrated boy. On a preoedipal level it meant escaping or giving in to the regressive pull to merge with the other. Mr. A. chose the first alternative in deciding that he needed to leave the analyst "to become a man."

At termination, Mr. A. had grown significantly in his ability to be a forceful, effective man in his profession. He had made a passionate, tender, less idealized relationship with the new girlfriend and thought happily of marrying her and starting a family. He did maintain, however, a sense of vulnerability about his masculinity and about his autonomy which seemed to represent incomplete resolution of the twin transference.

CASE 2

Mr. C. decided to undertake an analysis when he was 28 years old because he felt unable to enjoy himself, lacked confidence, and was burdened by procrastination. He was the first of the twins to be born and initially was bigger and weighed more than his twin sister. He recalled being told how his sister would cry and be fed first. Then she continued to cry and would be fed again instead of him. Subsequently she became larger and stronger. They fought frequently, and she always won. His sister was more aggressive and "feisty." She would sit on his chest and hold him down. Finally at age 4, when he grew bigger and stronger than his twin sister and could defend himself, she with-

drew and played less with him. Until age 10, they shared a bedroom. At that time he was given a smaller, less attractive room of
his own. He thought he was being punished and the separation
from his twin sister made him very sad. His mother was an active,
controlling woman, while his father was passive, distant, and
competitive. For Mr. C., interactions with his father largely involved competitive intellectual games in which his father defeat-
ed him time after time. Gradually Mr. C. withdrew and was
viewed in his family as a sweet, passive boy.

At the beginning of the analysis Mr. C. explored his wishes for
closeness and his fears in these situations. He felt he needed to
hide his angry, competitive feelings. He thought that these feelings were unacceptable to his twin sister, his parents, and his
analyst, and he felt they made him vulnerable to punishment
and injury. Struggling with these anxieties, Mr. C. retreated
rapidly from an assertive phallic position to a passive anal one.
He thought there was a "dark place" within him with "messy,
rotten feelings" that were potentially explosive and could destroy others and himself. To protect himself from these dangers,
he presented only his passive side and depicted himself as slow,
sweet, and inept. In the analytic situation Mr. C. became passive
and withholding, his associations were less free, and he had
difficulty making connections in the material. In the second year
of analysis Mr. C. brought his analyst an "immense, big, long
dream." He felt enraged that his analyst, like his mother, whom
he used to call to flush his bowel movements down the toilet,
demanded enormous amounts of effort and work of him, but
was never satisfied. It appeared that as a little boy he had felt he
couldn't win his mother's praise with his penis and instead had
attempted to accomplish this with his bowel movements, which
his mother then flushed down the toilet. This frustration again
led to his retreating to being an inept little boy.

At first in the transference Mr. C.'s fear of retaliation for what
he achieved, for his success, was related to his fear of his competitive, castrating father. However, as the analysis progressed,
it became clear that his fear of retaliation was more directly
related to his feelings about sharing with his twin sister. He felt
that he was "dispensable," as if his "twin sister had been brought
into this world to remind me I could be replaced, and I'd lose

everything." In his family and in the transference, if he were to "survive," he seemed to need to be a "lovable koala bear" and not the little boy with murderous and sexual feelings toward his sister and his analyst. In this context Mr. C. imagined that having the last analytic hour in the day made him special. He recalled how prior to his appendectomy at age 6, he had been sick often and at such times felt particularly loved and cared for by his mother. He thought that the surgery was a punishment for the sexual and competitive feelings aroused by his mother's attention.

As the analysis progressed Mr. C. was able to explore how his early struggles with his twin sister about dominance and with his mother about constipation were the root of his persistent feelings that women made him give up his autonomy, assertiveness, and penis. He talked about "not making a splash" with his words in analysis and with his actions in his life. Not procrastinating meant the forbidden incestuous bowel movement would fall into the toilet. He focused on the splash in the toilet and hid from his analyst that he used his penis with his girlfriends, many of whom reminded him of his twin sister. Mr. C. would turn on his side on the couch to hide his penis, thinking that his analyst didn't have one and wanted his, like his twin sister, both to castrate him and to have his penis in the forbidden incestuous act. He thought that to be close to his analyst, he had to be a woman. Not daring to have a penis, he said, "Women have been castrated; they've had it done to them. They are dangerous, and they are yearning to get their penis back."

Mr. C. spoke increasingly of "wanting my birthright." His associations led to Jacob and Esau and Cain and Abel (Cain and analyst). He became more aware of his murderousness toward his twin sister and his analyst, and his guilt as well as his sense of resulting loneliness. He thought his independence, separateness, and phallic assertiveness would be responsible for his sister's death. The theme of "I want it all" became central in the analysis. He said, "The intensity of my fears is related to the intensity of my greed. He became afraid that his analyst would kill him because of all that he had, just as he felt his twin sister would kill him out of jealousy. He told his analyst, "You're jealous of my life; if I win, you've got to lose." His feelings of wanting it all, that two people could not have the same breast, aroused fury and fear in relation to his analyst, and these feelings and the competition were carried forward into the bathroom and into the phallic-oedipal situation. He recalled how, when he was 3 years old, his twin sister had sat on him and how powerless he became. He associated to Amazon women and the Amazon river sweeping away everything in their paths and his conviction that he would never be a force with which to be reckoned. He was frightened of his retributive sadistic fantasies of possessing a penis that was "too big and too hot, that made women writhe in pain, anger, frustration, and excitement." Mr. C. felt tortured, crushed, made to submit in analysis, and he longed to turn the tables, to rip his analyst's arm out of its socket, to take away the analyst's "dearest possessions" and cause him "incalculable pain." At the same time he longed for his analyst to be different from his unavailable, passive, yet competitive father. He wanted his analyst to admire his sports car and his penis, to enjoy his strutting his stuff. As he became more forceful and assertive in his life, he was able to become more intimate, assertive, and passionate with women. He changed to a new career, one he had always longed for but had avoided out of his fear of the prominence and competition involved. Mr. C. wanted his analyst to view him as a young warrior, to admire, support, and promote him and to protect him from his jealous, competitive twin sister.

After 6 years of analysis in the termination phase, Mr. C. had a dream that reflected the strength of his phallic-aggressive conflicts in the context of the twinship and the transference. He dreamed that he was living in a house not too far from his twin sister's house. Hers was smaller but quite similar. He went to take a look at her house. The kitchen was near the top, and he walked up an open staircase on the outside wall. Inside there was a very ornate silver picture frame. It had his mother's initials on it. On one side of the frame were the children, on the other his mother and father. When he left his sister's house, he thought it wasn't so bad or so small. His associations focused on a package he had received in the mail. It had to do with something his uncle had left him in his will. It was a bedroom set that could not be divided. He remembered thinking about his twin sister lately, worrying about her, and feeling he would like to talk with her. He recalled that their birthday was coming up in exactly 2 weeks. He thought of how the laundry put a rip in one of his shirts. How much should he charge them? And yet he shouldn't be greedy. He spoke of how in the dream the picture frame was his but was in his twin sister's house. He wondered whether he really deserved the bigger house? Then he wondered about his penis. How did he get it? Maybe it was his sister's. Maybe it was his. Could it just go away? He wondered that maybe it was not the penis but rather the fancy holes that were of interest. Why did his twin sister actually keep the better room? Was it because of his penis or her hole? What was really desirable? He wondered about the picture on the reverse side of the frame. His mother was on the back side. It was not clear to what extent his father was even in the picture. Perhaps he was wishing that his father would go away. At that point he said that he felt very anxious. He recalled wanting his father's help but not wanting any rivals.

In Mr. C.'s dream, competition was evident on many levels. There was competition for the birthright, the "bedroom set that can't be divided," and greedy feelings involving the staircase, the access to the kitchen and nurturance. There was competition between Mr. C. and his twin sister for who would have the bigger house, the bigger room, the penis, or the fancier genitals. He expressed his oedipal longings to have his mother's picture frame and to put his frame in his twin sister's house. A striking aspect of the analytic material was his retreat from his oedipal wishes to his impression that his sister had both the penis and the better room. Concomitantly, he regressed to anal issues reciprocally with his mother's interest in his backside, as well as to passive longings for his father's and his analyst's help (negative oedipal resolutions).

Subsequently Mr. C. became preoccupied with his elegant sports car. In analysis he thought he was spinning his wheels, grinding away in a little ditch, pointlessly. Before he had been going in leaps and bounds. Now he felt bogged down and stuck. He felt that the analysis was a "monkey on my back, a pain in the rear." He would rather be leaping and bounding ahead in his new, powerful, and highly responsive sports car. At the same time he was embarrassed to possess such a sports car. He really had great potential, but he didn't want to engage it and use it, to let it go full force. He experienced his analyst as his twin sister, "holding him down," keeping him "stuck," having the penis, and giving him a "pain in the ass." If he were truly assertive and phallic, he would risk retaliation and abandonment. As this was analyzed, he described that his sports car was like having "a leopard in the garage, snarling, dangerous, very fast, powerful." Now he couln't resist letting him out a little. He asked himself, "when a car goes into a garage, does it belong to the garage or outside?" He worried whether he could get it back out of the garage or must it remain there, "stuck, lost, confiscated, imprisoned?" He worried that as with his twin sister, if his analyst knew about his sports car, he would want to take it away and keep it locked up in his own garage. He wondered if his analyst had a snow blower in his garage. Perhaps the analyst might be jealous of him, and then he thought of how a snow blower ate up snow and spit it out as a grey soup. He thought it was sad to view the world as a "place of snares and snow blowers."

Mr. C. described how within his situation in the twinship the phallic assignment had to be resolved in a more drastic way. In his competition with his twin, he had come to believe that unambiguously claiming his phallic endowment would invite envy and attack from his twin. He could enjoy the fantasy of what he would like to do with his penis, and even what he could actually do, but he dared not let it out, let it rip, let it fly. He retreated to an anal position in that his penis was hidden in his garage and would have to be pried out of him. He concealed, in effect, he gave up his phallic potency, and subordinated himself to his twin and his analyst in order to avoid retaliative attack and the risk of abandonment. There was a sense that despite analyzing and working through these issues, the analysis should continue indefinitely. In this respect the analytic situation reflected Mr. C.'s powerful tie to his twin sister and to his mother. The regressive and defensive aspects of this tie impeded his struggle toward independence and toward his capacity to become phallic, competitive, and assertive. In fact, though, when the analysis ended, Mr. C. realized that he had emerged as a man in his own right.

DISCUSSION

The developmental course and consolidation of phallic aggression is made more complex by the experience of being a twin, being facilitated in some aspects while being inhibited in other respects. As we studied the analyses of two adult male twins we were impressed by the extent to which these men struggled with their phallic aggression as each attempted to emerge as a man in his own right. Not surprisingly, these developments were markedly influenced by the substrata of preoedipal determinants within the twinship. These analyses illustrate similar patterns but with different vicissitudes. Mr. C.'s emergence as a man in the phallic sense was subverted by his tie to his aggressive sister who early sat on him, dominated him, and put him down. His sister's phallic preponderance impelled him to fall back toward a homosexual position and into an anal retentive preoccupation that hung on for years.

Mr. A.'s access to phallic potentialities was inhibited and he largely retreated from phallic aggression and from a wish for victory over his twin brother. Separation from his twin was inhibited, and instead the mutual interdependency of the twins was accentuated with elements of homosexual surrender. Mr. A. reacted against normative competitive aggression by becoming passive, taking a "castrated," humiliated, and submissive position vis-à-vis his brother. Interestingly, both Mr. A. and Mr. C. were encopretic during childhood. This regression compromised their autonomy and assertiveness, while at the same time it expressed a latent anal stubbornness and aggression. In both cases this lent a special quality to their access to the mother. In their analyses, it became evident that there had been particularly gratifying aspects in a nurturing relationship with the twin. Mr. C. had clung to sharing a room with his twin sister, even though, like his mother, her nurturant qualities were limited. Mr. A.'s mother was more nurturing, and this apparently made it more difficult to relinquish his tie to his twin. In terminating their analyses, both Mr. A. and Mr. C. had to loosen and then give up a transference tie to the mother-twin-analyst, in order to turn their commitment to a woman in an autonomous, phallic, and assertive fashion, consistent with marriage and genitality.

The analytic work with these men elucidated sequential steps in the phallic-oedipal development of male twins. The initial separation from the preoedipal mother was likely to be mitigated by the strength of the tie to the twin. This may have delayed the resolution of the separation-individuation experience from the mother which then further potentiated the pull to union with the twin. Mr. C. recalled the sadness he felt at moving into a separate room from his twin sister when he was 10. Mr. A. pictured himself and his twin as a "couple, a kind of comedy team together." He related how each of them could finish a joke begun by the other. In contrast to this closeness, the need for separation and individuation which was more exigent between twins led to a more forceful competition, stimulated as it was by the constant and unusually intense interactions within the twinship. Furthermore, it may have overdetermined competition with the father, leading to an oedipal situation in twins which was more complex and possibly more psychologically hazardous. In the data from the analyses of both Mr. A. and Mr. C., we were impressed with how competition with the twin appeared more prominent than competition with the father. Mr. A. imagined Mr. B.'s opinion of any new woman he dated. Mr. C., in his dream, competed with his twin sister for "the bigger room, the bigger house, the penis, the fancier genitals." As the enhanced competition became a problem for development and adaptation, it may also have been sublimated in high achievement. Both patients were productive and accomplished.

Identification with the father was influenced by the increased tendency of twins to view themselves in terms of dualisms such as active/passive and masculine/feminine. Taking reciprocal positions not only served to lessen or neutralize the heightened phallic competitiveness between twins, but it also served to resolve the earlier difficulty in differentiation, one twin from the other. This was an important feature of Mr. C.'s fantasy that just as his twin sister had the bigger room, so did the penis belong to her. In a similar way Mr. A. had the fantasy that there was but one penis between the twins, and that rather than risk being "cut off," he would allow his twin to own it: "Maybe I could reap the rewards of his aggression and still stay behind and be the good one." Although aggression and phallic competition were common enough between siblings and in other relationships, in our experience the intensity of the competition within a twinship was impressive, especially as it assumed phallic qualities. In our cases it was clearly associated with a defensive regressive pull to merge in the twin relationship. Regarding the differences between monozygotic and fraternal twins, we agree with Glenn (1966) that dissimilar twins share many of the same tendencies toward mutual identification and difficulties in self-object differentiation seen in generally identical monozygotic twins. This applies to difficulties with phallic aggression as well.

Our observations about phallic-aggressive development in male twins is more or less applicable to the analysis of twins, and also for analytic work in general. First there is the maturational experience of separating from the mother, which overdetermines, by displacement in parallel, the compelling issue of separating from the twin. Then there is the fantasy issue of who possesses the penis which is often seen as singular and indivisible. This can be surprisingly literal, but even more is inclusive of a special phallic potentiality, not only with reference to the twin but also in reference to the father. Finally, twins struggle to secure primary access to the mother, first at the dyadic level, then to gain in the contest for winning out in due course in the triadic-oedipal situation. Notwithstanding, the twin will have to renounce both the dyadic and oedipal claim upon his mother and also upon his twin if he is to realize more mature relationships in the course of time. In a corollary sense, the goal of an analysis of a twin requires that he be able to resolve satisfactorily the transference neurosis and separate from the analyst as well as from his twin. A neurotic resolution of the transference might entail falling back from the oedipal into the dyadic tie to the twin and, in a parallel transference sense, into an unresolved tie to the analyst. The very complexity of the problem of separating may invite a neurotic resolution by way of a defensive regression away from phallic assertiveness both to the dyadic mother-child and twin-twin level.

SUMMARY

We have studied data that emerged in the analyses of male adult twins. As a result we have identified certain patterns of phallic aggression in twins and particular solutions to conflicts arising from this aggression. These patterns are consequent to competition between them for the birthright, the preferred position, and identification with the parent. Solutions to these conflicts include shifts between active and passive, feminine and masculine, and phallic and receptive positions both in the characterological sense and in the phallic-active and the phallic-receptive sense. These shifts often involve an inhibition of phallic aggression and assertiveness by the potentially stronger twin.

Using material from the analyses of two adult male twins, we have illustrated how both analytic patients struggled with conflicts predominantly involving emergence as a man in the phallic direction. The vicissitudes of phallic aggression can be clearly delineated and analyzed by appreciating the intensity of the twin interrelationship and its effect upon the transference. Significant consequences of competition on the emergence of autonomy were illustrated by material from the cases, particularly with respect to the potential for regression into a passive dependent role. Finally, we showed that such observations about the development of phallic aggression and competition in male twins are meaningful and technically useful for the analysis of twins and also for analytic work in general.

BIBLIOGRAPHY

ARLOW, J. A. (1960). Fantasy systems in twins. *Psychoanal. Q.*, 29:175–199.

BURLINGHAM, D. (1946). Twins. *Psychoanal. Study Child*, 2:61–73.

———— (1949). Twins. In *Searchlights on Delinquency*, ed. K. R. Eissler, pp. 284–287. New York: Int. Univ. Press.

———— (1952). *Twins*. New York: Int. Univ. Press.

BURLINGHAM, D. & BARRON, A. T. (1963). A study of identical twins. *Psychoanal. Study Child*, 18:367–423.

FREUD, S. (1920). The psychogenesis of a case of homosexuality in a woman. *S.E.*, 18:145–172.

GLENN, J. (1966). Opposite-sex twins. *J. Amer. Psychoanal. Assn.*, 14:736–759.

GRAVES, R. (1955). *The Greek Myths*. Baltimore: Penguin Books.

HARTMANN, H. (1934–35). Psychiatrische Zwillingsstudien. *Jahrb. Psychiat. Neurol.*, 50 & 51.

JOSEPH, E. D. & TABOR, J. H. (1961). The simultaneous analysis of a pair of identical twins and the twinning reaction. *Psychoanal. Study Child*, 16:275–299.

ORR, D. W. (1941). A psychoanalytic study of a fraternal twin. *Psychoanal. Q.*, 10:284–296.

WINESTINE, M. C. (1969). Twinship and psychological differentiation. *J. Amer. Acad. Child Psychiat.*, 8:436–455.

The Female Oedipus Complex and the Relationship to the Body

M. EGLÉ LAUFER

WOMEN'S LIVES AND THEIR OWN VIEW OF THEMSELVES HAVE changed dramatically over the past 50 years since Freud wrote his last paper on the subject. Moreover, the opposition to Freud's view, voiced by some analysts at that time, has gained support both from analysts and women themselves. Janine Chasseguet-Smirgel (1984) said, "the works of Kestemberg, Galenson, Roiphe . . . have in my view invalidated and discredited the claims of the theory of phallic monism to be regarded any longer as the gospel truth. In fact, it is not simply a question of rejecting this infantile sexual theory as purely defensive, but of drawing the consequences of this rejection for psycho-analytic theory overall. If the girl stands in the first place not for *deficiency,* but primordially for *receptacle,* then our conceptions of psychosexual evolution must change direction or even be reversed, the site of what is most instinctual and animal to the human being must be rediscovered" (p. 169). I think what she is saying here expresses something that we have all been aware of for a long time in our clinical work.

Like Chasseguet, I have, of course, also been impressed by the findings of child and adult analysts who have shown convincingly that the little girl's awareness of her own body is not primarily that of lacking a penis. She has a much earlier awareness of her body as containing an inside space and of the openings in her

Member of the British Psycho-Analytical Society. Staff member of the Brent Consultation Centre and the Centre for Research into Adolescent Breakdown, London.

body, the mouth, anus, and possibly the vagina. I believe, however, that we must now understand how these circumstances relate to the early history of the development of the girl's *relationship* to her own body and how it will shape and determine her future development.

From my own clinical observations of disturbed adolescent girls and women who had experienced a psychotic or depressive breakdown following the birth of their first child, it seemed to me that the conflicts underlying the path toward pathological development were in fact not so different from those described by Freud and others and that it was therefore more a matter of finding a different way of understanding the concepts that Freud had made central to the understanding of pathology. It was for this reason that I have chosen to examine the theme of the castration complex in feminine development which Freud made central to his theory of female development (1931). What I have tried to clarify is that the *significance* of the early, infantile, masturbatory activity and sensory experiences together with their accompanying fantasies, which include the awareness of inner space and of body openings, lies in the relationship that this establishes between the girl and her own body and the extent to which this relationship then facilitates or hinders the child's ability to detach herself from her dependence on the mother. The ongoing *early* oedipal conflict can then be understood as inevitably leading to a later point in development where the awareness of reality—the separation from the mother and the impingement on the child's omnipotent fantasies of the unrivaled role of the father in relation to the mother—*has* to be acknowledged by both the male and female child. With this acknowledgment the child, boy or girl, also has to make an accompanying change in the relation to his or her own body and its contents. The outcome of this change, the resolution of the oedipal conflict, whether it takes on a defensive character, and to what extent this defensive character will affect the child's capacity for the perception of reality will point the way to future pathology or normality (M. Laufer, 1982).

Freud (1905) saw the role of sexuality in mental life as inextricably linked with pathological development and symptom formation. He postulated that there can be no disturbance in mental functioning without an accompanying disturbance in the sexual life of the person. I think we have taken a long time to understand that this is not simply a statement about genital functioning as such—i.e., of orgastic or reproductive capacity. It is a way of saying that in order to remain free of pathology, as adults, we have to be able to experience our bodies as a source of pleasure and instinctual gratification. But although we cannot "give up" the pleasure principle as the source of infantile omnipotence, we must find a way to accommodate external reality so that we can maintain an area of our lives in which the pleasure principle can still reign supreme.

Freud, it seems to me, was the first to recognize the girl's biologically determined, *relative* difficulty in achieving this—relative, that is, to the boy. I believe that girls behave as if they "lacked something," however much they may have been told or been aware that they didn't and that they had other powers or capacities. Penis envy may appear outdated, in our present social climate, but behaviorally the concept still has a validity and the power to shape women's lives. It is for this reason that I have started out on the assumption that although the findings of Klein (1928) Horney (1923), and Jones (1927) must be included in our thinking as well as the change in women's awareness of themselves, the problem is how to include them rather than perpetuating a controversy as to who has the "complete truth."

Similarly, I too have, of course, been aware that the little girl's attachment to her father does not *begin* when she turns away from her relationship to her mother. Clearly, the child has an intense and libidinized relationship to the father before the actual pressure to resolve the oedipal situation becomes imperative. I would see the developmental task or problem more simply: how far can the girl relinquish the libidinal tie to the mother without having to find some symptomatic compromise solution through identification with the father or a masochistic submission to the father. Clinically, in the transference, it has seemed to me more a question of whether the relationship to the father and later to men is allowed into the space the girl has been able to create between herself and her internalized mother, or whether his presence continues to act like an ineffectual shadow in her life that is felt as a threat which comes between her and the internalized mother.

My own conclusions are still changing in the light of my clinical experiences and those of others. These have come from work with adolescent girls who are developmentally faced with the task of changing their relationship to their body from that of the prepubertal child to that of a sexual adult woman, or of pregnant young women where the task is one of changing the relationship to themselves to that of identifying with their own mother's maternal role. In both these situations the pathological, defensive symptomatology which may result demonstrates the genetic history of the earlier development of the relationship to their bodies. What has impressed me most has been the capacity of some women either to deny the reality of the changes taking place in their bodies or their compelling need to physically attack their own bodies or later that of their babies during these critical developmental periods.

In order to explain these pathological phenomena I think we have to take seriously the events in our patients' lives as biological realities and not only as a metaphor that can have interchangeable meanings in fantasy. This makes the issue of the timing and function of the resolution of the oedipal conflict a critical issue. If we regard the resolution of the depressive position as the central issue and hence only see the resolution of the infant's relationship to the breast as central to the therapeutic task, I think we risk entering into the patient's own delusional system when applying it to clinical work with the disturbed adolescent or the psychotic areas of functioning in the adult patient. We then leave them without having made conscious their relationship to their adult sexual body and their internal experience of it. For this reason the timing of the resolution of the oedipal conflict is still central to our controversy.

Yet it seems to me that it would be most helpful if we were to change the emphasis of the argument of whether a so-called "preoedipal period" exists or whether the oedipal situation is there from much earlier—that is, about when the relationship to the parents begins to take on a competitive and triangular meaning to the child—to when does this ongoing conflict *have* to find some resolution. My own answer would be that while the infant or the "preoedipal" child can avoid the task of *resolving* the oedipal conflict for a prolonged period by the creation of its own fantasy and later by masturbatory activity which maintains the infantile omnipotence, this effort has to succumb at some point to the realization of the differences between the sexes. It is the defenses against this awareness which we see as the "psychical rigidity" Freud (1933, p. 134) spoke of in the pathological development of women.

The way I have understood the significance of the earlier phase is that it is the period in which the relationship to the girl's own body becomes established. The decisive factor is the extent to which she is left with a narcissistic libidinal cathexis of her body rather than vulnerable to her self-destructive impulses, because the predominance of a narcissistic cathexis will help her to negotiate possessing a female body and becoming a mother who can enjoy her child's body. Or, as Freud (1933) said, "But the phase of the affectionate pre-Oedipus attachment is the decisive one for a woman's future: during it preparations are made for the acquisition of characteristics with which she will later fulfil her role in the sexual function and perform her invaluable social tasks" (p. 134).

The significance of the oedipus complex in development, and specifically the manner in which it is dissolved in the girl's development by the end of the oedipal period, have been, and still are, the focus for much theoretical disagreement. Central to the past and present controversies has been the idea that Freud created a false view of female development because he was influenced by the idea of the supremacy of the phallus and that he subordinated women to this idea. In fact, it is as if Freud has come to represent what we have learned to recognize—that in society there is, and always has been, a deep unconscious need to idealize the penis into a symbolic phallus and that this need is common to both men and women. But I believe that the framework of the questions that Freud laid down as requiring an answer about the differences he observed in the development of males and females still does help us to understand how such a fantasy can come into being and how it comes to exercise such a dominating influence on the unconscious and on the capacity to live with the reality of one's body.

I will limit myself to three main themes in Freud's formulations which are central to these questions. First, Freud defined the girl's perception of her body as being "castrated" and as-

sumed that the manner in which she dealt with this formed the
basis of her castration complex and determined her future sexual development. Second, I shall describe the nature of the early
attachment to the mother and ask whether it is different from
that of the boy from the beginning, or whether it only takes on a
different course at some later point in development, as suggested to Freud by the observation that girls have a longer period of attachment to the mother than boys; or, putting it another
way, is there something different in this early relationship that
then makes it more difficult for the girl to detach herself from
the mother? Third, I repeat Freud's very fundamental question:
what is it that enables the girl to give up the homosexual object at
all and to make a heterosexual object choice, i.e., to turn from
the mother to the father as a libidinal object? And must this
result, as Helene Deutsch (1930) suggests, in a masochistic libidinal surrender to the father, through turning the acceptance
of castration into the fantasy of the castration wish?

   Although I can no longer accept the description Freud (1925)
gives of the little girl's reaction to the sight of the penis as constituting an actual event that then signals a landmark in her
development,[1] I do believe that something has to occur, optimally as part of a gradual process rather than contained in a
traumatic event, which functions as an organizer of all the earlier
experiences and perceptions and which will lay the foundation
for the way the girl will relate to herself as a *woman* in her adult
life. That is, however much I have come to understand the essential part played by the early experiences in the capacity for normal development, as in the capacity for object relationships and
in the relationship to oneself and one's body, I think that the
manner in which the existing psychic organization of the little
girl reacts to the inevitable demand to see herself as belonging to
the same sex as her mother (and one that differentiates her from
the father) crucially impinges on her previously established narcissistic organization and leads her into a different developmental path from that of the boy, whether it is toward normality or a
more pathological development. To view herself as "not having
a body that enables her to become a man" which is how I under-

---

1. In "Female Sexuality" (1931) Freud himself modifies this view.

stand the term "castrated," irrespective of her awareness of her receptive capacities or of having a vagina, means that at some point in her development she must give up the fantasy of being able to keep her mother's love to herself, because it simultaneously implies an understanding that there exists a longed-for satisfaction which her mother can obtain from the father, *and* that it is one which the girl can never hope to replace (Lampl-de Groot, 1927).

Up to this time, the girl (like the boy) has been able through her masturbatory fantasies and the accompanying sensory experiences to invest her body and its products with the omnipotent power of being both the potential giver of gratification to the mother, or of being able to take over the role of "frustrator" of the mother through the discovered capacity to achieve her own gratification by using her own body. The meaning of these early fantasies of using the body and its products, in the infant's attempts to maintain infantile omnipotence, and as a defense against the primitive anxieties of being destroyed, was investigated by Melanie Klein (1928) who has made an important contribution to our understanding the intensity of the persecutory anxieties that help to attach the girl to her mother. I also think that if the masturbatory experiences help the girl to internalize a positive relationship to her actual body, they will enable her to risk being less dependent on the mother for her survival and gratification, and can then act as a basis on which she is better able to accept her castration with less persecutory anxiety.

The libidinal relationship to the father is initially contained in the fantasy of the overlapping, interchangeable relationship to the images of both mother and father, where the parents (insofar as they then become gradually separated in the child's mind) are experienced as gratifying each other—but initially only through the same means that are available to the child, i.e., through mouth, anus, breast, feces, clitoris, or penis, where the father can be both giver and receiver, as can the child and the mother. In this respect, I cannot see that the girl's awareness of an extra opening, the vagina, adds to the awareness of a difference in her potential role of giving or receiving. Paula Heimann (1952) summarizes this early stage of development of the oedipus complex as "the infant . . . divines that there are physical intimacies between his parents—and in so far recognizes a reality; but he conceives of these intimacies in terms of his own impulses, in other words, his notions are determined by projection and by so much are a gross distortion of reality. The parents do to one another what he himself would like to do" (p. 163). Even if we conceptualize the infant as perceiving the mother as *containing* the father's penis in the early oral relationship (as described by Melanie Klein, 1928), this does not add anything of special significance to the girl's early development of the awareness of herself as female and different from the male, since its significance is the same for both the boy and the girl—that of seeing the mother as the primary object who frustrates the desire for gratification and thus is responsible for the narcissistic injury this inflicts on the infant.

Freud (1931) made it clear that he too was aware of how these early frustrations at the breast constitute a narcissistic injury to the infant's sense of omnipotence, but he still laid stress on the difference between these early and gradual developments of the infant's sense of reality of his own helplessness and the specific nature of the later injury that the lack of a penis evokes in the girl. Melanie Klein's work provides us with details of the destructive fantasies against the mother who not only contains the penis but the babies inside her body which both the boy and the girl feel deprived of in their wish to identify themselves with the mother. But it is the anxiety aroused by the destructive fantasies related to this blow to her omnipotence which the girl, as different from the boy, feels unable to allay through finding a means in the use of her body. Possessing at least the potential of a potent penis, the boy can use it as a defense against the anxiety of his projected fantasies of a devouring, unsatisfied, and envious mother. It is here that Melanie Klein has contributed, for me, to answering Freud's question not only why there is so much aggression exhibited by the girl to the mother, or why she appears to blame the mother for all the deprivation (including the lack of a penis), but to the understanding of how her relative inability to detach herself from the mother, relative (that is) to that of the boy, derives from the anxiety coming from the projection onto her mother of the fantasy of her own dissatisfaction and disappointment. Detaching herself can then only be felt as depriving her mother of her satisfaction.

But I think this view of the girl as needing a penis in order both to feel she can satisfy the mother and to maintain her belief that the mother can still satisfy her own wish for a baby confirms Freud's view that penis *envy*, the wish for the penis, in the girl is an expression of the wish to live out her primary libidinal aim— of giving or being given a baby by the mother, while the fantasy of actually possessing a penis is a secondary pathological structure whose aim is defensive and related to persecutory anxiety (Jones, 1927).

Freud (1931) talked of the girl's "acceptance of castration" as being simultaneous with the time at which the libidinal tie to the mother is given up. Reviewing his description of the options that are then open to the girl, I have found it helpful to make use of my clinical experience of the transference relationship in the analysis of adolescent girls and young adult women. This seems to indicate quite clearly that the libidinal tie to the mother has very often not been given up at all. Sublimatory as well as sexual activities in women are still extremely vulnerable to inhibition and other defenses because of the intense anxiety aroused either by the mother's envy or by the identification with the forbidden possession of the father's penis. Freud also points to this problem in his comment on the high incidence of frigidity in women, which he sees as an inhibition of sexuality. He said (1931), "Indeed, we had to reckon with the possibility that a number of women remain arrested in their original attachment to their mother and never achieve a true change-over towards men" (p. 226).

Further clinical evidence for this view comes from the high incidence of postnatal depression in women after the birth of their first child. This can be understood as the final process of mourning for the loss of the tie to their mother that becoming a mother involves. In addition, it can also be understood as representing an identification with the fantasy of a dissatisfied and depressed mother who has to be kept appeased by the daughter's giving up or inhibiting her own potential satisfaction and enjoyment of having produced her own child. For some women this conflict can become so intense that the reality of the baby has to be disavowed altogether, the relationship to the baby cannot become established, and instead the woman will experience an acute psychotic state with all the subsequent danger of violence either against herself or the baby.

In severely disturbed adolescent girls, what can be observed clinically is how the effort to defend against the still existing libidinal attachment to the mother—which has now the added danger of becoming an incestuous homosexual tie to the mother—can lead to the compelling need to direct aggression against their own body in an attempt to detach themselves from their sexual body and its meaning, as in suicide attempts, self-cutting, anorexia, bulimia, and so on.

Freud describes the outcome of the castration complex as resulting in either an eventual "acceptance of castration" or a setting up of the masculinity complex as an attempt to maintain the "disavowal" of castration. He makes the point that both the boy's and the girl's first reaction to the task of allowing the perception of the "absence of a penis" into their awareness—that is, their first recognition of the difference between male and female—is one of disavowal. But once the girl has accepted herself as being without a penis, i.e., castrated, the most significant difference between the boy and the girl is that in the girl it leads to a repression of her sexuality. He makes it clear that he is here referring specifically to a phallic sexuality—that is, the relation of the girl to her own genitals both as a source of pleasurable experience and as containing her active aims to give her mother satisfaction or a baby—and these have to be repressed because "they have proved totally unrealizable." He continues, however, to say that "the passive [i.e., the receptive] trends have not escaped disappointment either. With the turning-away from the mother clitoral masturbation frequently ceases as well; and often enough when the small girl represses her previous masculinity a considerable portion of her sexual trends in general is permanently injured too. The transition to the father-object is accomplished with the help of the passive trends in so far as they have escaped the catastrophe. The path to the development of femininity now lies open to the girl, to the extent to which it is not restricted by the remains of the pre-Oedipus attachment to her mother which she has surmounted" (p. 239). Later he makes it clear that if the girl is to develop normally, she must take the father as a sexual object in the final stage of her oedipus complex and before its final resolution. I think this view has aroused some of the most intense criticism of the psychoanalytic theory of female sexuality since it lends itself to the equating of the "passive aims" with the idea of "masochism" as if masochism were an essential part of normal female sexuality.

From my clinical observations of adult women who showed a marked masochistic trend in their sexual relations, I would be more inclined to say that if the girl has been able to give up the libidinal attachment to the mother, resulting from the acceptance of herself as castrated, and with it her hatred of the mother, then the passive aims which she uses to maintain a relationship to the father have more of a narcissistic wish attached than the directly sexual wish of castration or penetration. The satisfaction that the girl seeks, I think, is that of still feeling her body valued and desired, even though it now appears to contain only her pregenital passive wishes. But once a libidinal aim is included in the passive, wishful fantasy directed at the father, it must take on a masochistic meaning since the "acceptance of castration" has now taken on a wishful quality and has become a "castration wish." And the "castration wish" then forms the basis for a masochistic fantasy of being castrated by the father through penetration. This occurs only where there is a displacement of the aggression related to the still unbroken tie to the mother and not as a result of detachment from the mother. It represents a compromise in order to keep repressed the existence of the libidinal tie to the mother through the possession of the fantasy penis which the father must take from her, while the hatred of the mother becomes internalized into the superego structure.

Normal latency fantasies for the girl are of being chosen instead of having to choose, of being desired instead of experiencing sexual desire herself. These wishful fantasies, and the wish for a baby, can allow the passive pregenital longings to continue to find expression, without the anxiety of regressive longings for the mother. But I do not see this suppression of sexuality during latency as necessarily leading, as Freud (1931) suggests, to the extinction of the girl's sexuality in her adult life. Rather it seems to me to be an expression of the fantasy depicted in "The Sleeping Beauty" that everybody has to remain asleep, the girl princess as well as her parents the king and queen, until she is discovered and her resistance surmounted by the prince. This fable is not so much a story of passive masochistic surrender to the man, but of the need to control both the parents and her sexuality and her own "prickly" hatred, during latency, in order later to allow the prince to gain entry to the palace and to discover the girl's hidden vagina.

The other alternative is the formation of a masculinity complex. Although Freud comments that if it persists into adulthood, it can lead to a homosexual object choice, it is often confused with penis envy. From a diagnostic point of view a careful distinction must be made between the two. Penis envy and competitive behavior with men express the wish for a penis, while the masculinity complex contains the fantasy of possessing a penis. The distinction marks the difference between normality or neurotic development, even distorted by envy and the need to compete with men, and more severe pathology which may contain a psychotic area at its core. The continued disavowal of castration into adulthood through the construction of a fantasy of a body that includes a penis must distort the relationship with reality to a degree that leaves the woman with the potential for a psychotic breakdown when faced by reality with a challenge to that fantasy, as Freud (1931) points out when he talks of the normal first disavowal by the girl.

A young woman who had retained a fantasy of possessing a penis into young adulthood, for instance, felt consciously free of all anxiety in a satisfactory homosexual relationship, but then felt compelled to break off the relationship when it began to force her to acknowledge that she could neither give nor receive a baby. The initial lack of anxiety about her homosexuality resulted from her ability to gratify the wish to continue to deny castration. The wish for a baby, however, brought with it the anxiety of experiencing a break with the reality of her body in order to maintain the disavowal of castration, and with it the danger of severely damaging attacks on her own body as an expression of her hatred and disappointment in its failure.

I have observed similar transitory paranoid states in adult women who feel dependent on the need to masturbate, where the paranoid reaction becomes comprehensible only when it becomes clear how it relates unconsciously to masturbatory activity and fantasies. I think such evidence in the transference of psychotic anxiety in connection with masturbatory activity must always relate to the fantasy that the body includes a penis and differs from more neurotic anxiety seen in the transference as the fear of the analyst's disgust or contempt. However, it could also be argued that the fantasy of possessing a penis can be used as a defense, without necessarily posing a danger of an underlying psychosis, until the first experience of penetration of the vagina. It is only then that the masculinity complex must finally be given up, if the construction of a psychotic body image is to be avoided and the subsequent pull toward a homosexual object choice. The importance of the first act of penetration is referred to by Freud (1918) when he examines the custom in some primitive societies of allowing the first act of penetration to be carried out by a person other than the prospective husband. He attributes this to a fear of the hostility that is aroused in a woman and becomes directed at the man who carries out the act. He makes it clear that the aggression is related to a fantasy that the act of penetration is a renewed confirmation of lacking a penis.

In discussing female development in terms of the significance of the castration complex, and the special nature of the girl's relationship to her mother, I have said little about the girl's relationship to the father beyond my discomfort at, or perhaps disbelief in, the concept of the girl turning to her father when she has succeeded in detaching herself from the mother, before the final resolution of the oedipus complex. I think, as do many analysts, that there is a much earlier libidinal attachment to the father. The idea of the "oedipus complex" being made up of a constant move between the negative and the positive complex, beginning from the time when the child—boy or girl—first begins to differentiate between himself or herself and the nurturing object, seems more correct nowadays than to assume that there is a sudden shift to the father. However, the basic dependence on the mother as the nurturing object exerts a constant force on the girl, as well as on the boy, to relinquish the libidinal attachment to the father and to put an identification with him in its place—an identification which then allows the child to continue to feel in exclusive possession of the mother. The girl therefore certainly forms much earlier libidinal attachments to her father, but she also has to relinquish them because of her greater anxiety. The final dissolution of the oedipus complex marks the resolution of the conflict between the positive and negative oedipal situation by the giving up of both attachments and maintaining only an "affectionate tie," as Freud (1924) described it for the boy. This then allows the girl to move into latency and to use her identifications with both parents as the basis of her sublimatory activity.

The third possible outcome of the castration complex proposed by Freud consists in a general revulsion from sexuality by the girl. It is to be distinguished from that of the girl who, although also giving up masturbation, still remains sufficiently in touch with her passive wishes with which to turn to the father. The crucial issue for future development would therefore be whether in thus rejecting her own sexuality, the relationship to the father also has to be renounced. A father who is overtly sexual toward his daughter may have to become an "object of revulsion" for the girl because of her need to keep her own sexual feelings repressed. In the normal adolescent girl such an attitude may be revived as her initial reaction to the awareness of the penis in its sexual role, but she can gradually come to relate to the male's penis as she is able to relate more positively toward her own genitals. If the revulsion toward her own sexual body remains too intense, however, the problem of relating to a man's penis can remain unresolved. This may again lay the adolescent girl open either to regressing to the pregenital relationship to the mother or to seeking a homosexual relationship. Although I agree that in the course of normal development a relationship to the father has to become established after the dissolution of the negative oedipal complex, I do not believe that the wish for a baby with which the girl turns to the father has to imply an instinctual wish for gratification. If it does, as I said earlier, I believe it must contain a masochistic fantasy, the aim of which is to deflect and keep repressed the intense violent and sadistic impulses that still tie the girl to the mother.

I now turn to some clinical material of an 18-year-old adolescent girl who began analysis after a severe suicide attempt. Because the relationship to the father had never been established in the early preoedipal period in a way that could then lead to a normal oedipal conflict, the girl remained attached to the mother and had no means of feeling that she could relate to her female sexual body other than as an identification with that of her mother's. This in turn compelled her to attempt to destroy it because of the conflict aroused by her effort to feel that she could be in control of her own body. The castration complex had been resolved by the disavowal of castration and men were seen by her as violent intruders into the fantasy of union of herself with the mother—that is, as a projection which contained her own hatred of the mother.

In a preliminary interview Mary described herself as having "been dead" since the age of 16. It had therefore not been any particular event which finally led to her attempt to kill herself. She said she hated her body and related it to her disgust with her mother's body because her mother suffered from a colonic disorder and she did not want to have to think about her mother's body. She had in fact ceased to have any interest in her own body and its appearance at the age of 16 at the time of her mother's illness. This followed shortly after she had been away from home for the first time, staying with another family. An elderly male relative of that family had kissed her in a sexual way and had frightened and disgusted her. At that time she also gave up seeing a boyfriend with whom she had gone out once, on the grounds that her mother didn't approve of him. From that time onward she retreated into her studies and only went out when accompanied by her mother or her female friends. Her suicide attempt was preceded by a period during which she secretly and compulsively stuffed herself with food; as a result, she then felt disgusted with her own body. It was as if what she had experienced at 16 was the failure of her capacity to allow a man to relate to her body sexually because she had been unable to integrate her own sexual development in any way other than as something disgusting and repelling.

When she was seen at 18 for assessment, she was dressed in a little girl's dress covered over by a coat which she kept on in order to keep her body completely hidden. She knew that her problems were related to her mother; she felt that she either had to allow herself to be completely dominated and "eaten up" by her mother or that by removing herself and becoming independent she would cause her mother to collapse and "to starve." She saw her attempt to kill herself as the only independent action that she had been able to do and that she had felt forced into by her terror and despair at her own helplessness. She used her relationship to her father to feed herself with the fantasy that he preferred her to her mother and that her mother wanted to be rid of her in order to have the father to herself. At these times she felt afraid that her mother was trying to poison her.

In the transference she experienced the analyst both as an intruder into her fantasy in which she was together and united with her mother and her body, while at the same time trying to keep repressed her wish to give in to the analyst and be dominated by her with the fantasy that this would destroy the mother. Her body was used to live out this fantasy in alternately repelling the analyst by silence and secretiveness and later in falling asleep throughout the sessions.

Her first "attempt" at sexual intercourse was initiated by her inviting a man to stay the night in her apartment and then furiously fighting with him when he tried to approach her sexually. The following day she reported triumphantly that she had proved that she could be strong enough to prevent a man from raping her. In this way she succeeded in living out her fantasy that I, the analyst, would love her and that we could remain united as long as she could prevent the act of penetration which would compel us both to acknowledge a man's penis and our own helplessness as castrated women and therefore our hatred of each other.

As long as she could feel strong enough to keep the man's penis outside and from intruding into her own and my reality, we could remain in her fantasy as totally dependent on each other for our needs. Men, she felt, were there only for us to be seen together with so that we appeared normal like other women. Her fear of even that wish was of being seen with a man who might then be the admired one and she would be left out feeling jealous. In this way she expressed her wish to deny the existence of the penis completely, even as something that she could own and use in relation to other women. Only in this way could she feel in control of her own hatred and jealous feelings.

Her sexual life was dominated by the fantasy of being given an enema, as she had once experienced when 4 years old from her mother. This fantasy provided the motivation for making her feel that if she could not control her bodily needs (as in eating), she would have to reject her body altogether, as in killing herself, because of her disgust with it. The predominance of the anus in her mental life could deny both her own vagina and the penis and therefore the sexual difference between male and female. In this way she could continue to see herself as able to satisfy her mother's needs and feel in control of her own needs.

For this girl, the absence of a libidinal relationship to the father meant that even a shift away from the mother by displacement onto the father of the masochistic wish to be castrated was not open to her. When she began analysis, she lived with a constant belief that her parents were about to separate. Mary had already experienced herself as an object of disgust during latency, as was shown in the repeated nightmares she reported having had of being covered by crawling insects or skin diseases making her feel "like a leper, untouchable."

The actual experiences of her infancy could not be established, and thus we did not know how far this relationship to her body was defensive against the terror of an excessive intrusion in infancy or how far it was based on her belief that she had had insufficient bodily care. Probably both were true since her mother presented herself to me as someone who needed to be told how to look after her daughter while at the same time showing me that she would adhere to any instructions I might give in a frightened and rigid way, as if I was a baby book recommending four hourly feedings. She described her daughter as having been terrified of strangers at 8 months and clinging to her mother and rejecting everyone else. This seemed to be repeated within the transference where I was initially treated as a dangerous stranger who could not be identified as a caring object but only as one who came between her and her mother.

This case seems to me to illustrate how the relationship which the girl forms to her own body in the early preoedipal years determines how the oedipus complex is *finally* resolved; in turn, this then shapes the girl's subsequent ability to form a relationship to her own sexual body after puberty.

BIBLIOGRAPHY

CHASSEGUET-SMIRGEL, J. (1984). The femininity of the analyst in professional practice. *Int. J. Psychoanal.*, 65:169–178.
DEUTSCH, H. (1930). The significance of masochism in the mental life of women. *Int. J. Psychoanal.*, 11:48–60.
FREUD, S. (1905). Three essays on the theory of sexuality. *S.E.*, 7:125–243.
—— (1918). The taboo of virginity. *S.E.*, 11:191–208.
—— (1924). The dissolution of the oedipus complex. *S.E.*, 19:173–179.
—— (1925). Some psychical consequences of the anatomical distinction between the sexes. *S.E.*, 19:248–258.
—— (1931). Female sexuality. *S.E.*, 21:223–243.
—— (1933). Feminity. *S.E.*, 22:112–135.
HEIMANN, P. (1952). Certain functions of introjection and projection in early infancy. In *Developments in Psycho-Analysis*, pp. 122–168. London: Hogarth Press.
HORNEY, K. (1923). On the genesis of the castration complex in women. *Int. J. Psychoanal.*, 5:50–65.
JONES, E. (1927). The early development of female sexuality. In *Papers on Psycho-Analysis*, pp. 438–451. London: Bailliere, Tindall & Cox.
KLEIN, M. (1928). Early stages of the oedipus conflict. *Int. J. Psychoanal.*, 9:169–180.
LAMPL-DE GROOT, J. (1927). The evolution of the oedipus complex in women. *Int. J. Psychoanal.*, 9:332–345.
LAUFER, M. (1982). The formation and shaping of the oedipus complex. *Int. J. Psychoanal.*, 63:217–227.
LAUFER, M. & LAUFER, M. E. (1984). *Adolescence and Developmental Breakdown.* New Haven: Yale Univ. Press.
LAUFER, M. E. (1982). Female masturbation in adolescence and the development of the relationship to the body. *Int. J. Psychoanal.*, 63:295–302.

Talking with Toddlers

KERRY KELLY NOVICK

IN THIS PAPER I WILL DESCRIBE SOME CLINICAL WORK WITH A TODdler and her parents to illustrate a somewhat neglected area of preventive intervention. Work with the G. family gave rise to some questions and thoughts regarding the role of speech in early object relations and ego development, and to an attempt to amalgamate puzzling clinical phenomena with psychoanalytic knowledge and recent research in infant development.

Gina, aged 16 months, was brought by her parents for an evaluation because she had been waking in the night crying inconsolably for up to an hour. During these episodes she did not appear to be fully awake; she would not accept comfort from her father at all, did not seem to respond to her mother with recognition, but cried and kicked until she "wore herself out." Needless to say, her parents were also worn out and very distressed by Gina's suffering and their inability to intervene effectively.

Gina's parents were devoted, conscientious, middle-aged schoolteachers who had tried for many years to conceive their own child. They adopted Gina when she was 4 months old and adored her from the first moment, even though she arrived at the airport screaming furiously and refusing a bottle. She cried angrily in the same way when frustrated or in pain thereafter and the parents felt that there was grieving in her tone at such moments. Gina suffered repeated ear infections, which led to her having tubes inserted surgically in her ears at the age of 13 months. Soon thereafter Gina began to have repeated spells of crying at night and displayed signs of lowered frustration toler-

Faculty, Michigan Psychoanalytic Institute, Ann Arbor, Michigan.

ance by banging her head or pulling at her hair when thwarted. She clung to her mother more frequently at times of transition to her familiar babysitters or when her father took his regular turn at childcare. Within 10 days of the outpatient surgery on her ears, Gina developed a bladder infection which was resistant to the first medication tried. This eventually led to a full urinary tract investigation, including catheterization.

By this time, Gina presented the picture of a very angry, willful 15-month-old. When the parents said "no," Gina laughed and defied them. Because all her gross motor milestones had been delayed compared with fine motor and cognitive skills and she was not yet walking, and also, I suspect, because of the helplessness her anger was arousing in her parents, a full neurological workup was done. No organic problems were found and Gina was assessed as functioning well above her age level in fine motor and social/emotional development, and at the 12-month level in gross motor development, which was within normal limits of variation. Gina began to walk between her parents' first phone call to me and our actual appointment; this step seemed quite literally to relieve much of her frustration, and the self-directed aggressive behavior faded out. When I saw her, it was therefore only the night crying which remained as a mysterious and disturbing behavior. The parents reported that her speech, which had been precocious (single words at 8 months, phrases at 1 year), had appeared to diminish as she began walking, but they could accept that this was normal behavior for an infant concentrating on a new developmental task.

Gina was sitting in her mother's lap, pacifier in her mouth, looking around alertly at the pictures in my waiting room when I went to meet them. Safe in her mother's arms, she responded with a shy smile to my greeting and looked with quick responsiveness and pleasure at the pictures I named for her. Gina indicated most definitely her unwillingness to walk with us into the playroom by holding her legs off the floor, but made no protest at Mrs. G. carrying her, and indeed she seemed eager to look around as long as mother held her. Mrs. G. was apologetic that Gina was not more forthcoming but was easily reassured and relieved by my remark that Gina was absolutely right to take her time with a complete stranger.

I will describe the playroom and the toys I had set out, so that we may better assess Gina's subsequent choices. The playroom is fairly large, all carpeted, with a wool hanging patterned with stars on one wall and a shiny mobile of fish hanging in one corner. There are two large cushions on the floor, one covered with smooth cotton, the other with velvety corduroy, as well as a small table and chairs. I had put out a stacking ring toy, a baby doll with a toy bottle, a Fisher-Price bus with little people, and some cloth blocks. Visible on a shelf, but out of Gina's reach, were a rag doll, some hand puppets, and a toy telephone.

Mrs. G. and I sat down on the floor with Gina. At her mother's mild request, Gina carefully put her pacifier into the top of mother's handbag, then checked twice to make sure it was there. She did not ask for it again during the session. Gina watched us each play with the stacking rings, listened while her mother named their colors, then ventured to lean out from mother's lap to put them on their peg. She smiled at our praise and gurgled with laughter when I dumped them off for her to do it again. Over the next few minutes she warmed up gradually and began exploring the space immediately around her mother. She played a peekaboo game with me, hiding behind her mother's back, then disclosing herself with glee. Gina leaned over her mother's shoulder repeatedly to show me her mother's earrings, and was pleased when I responded by showing her mine. She detoured to the baby doll and fed her with the bottle for a while, but returned again and again to show me her mother's earrings. After about seven repetitions, she pointed to her own ears and I said, "Those are Gina's ears, like Mommy's and Mrs. Novick's. Gina does not have earrings. Those are Gina's nice ears; there are Mommy's [I pointed] and here are Mrs. Novick's." Gina led me through the sequence again, then pointed her little index finger and shook it. Mrs. G. exclaimed, "Oh she wants to tell you her poem!"

Gina's 'poem' turned out to be a song with accompanying gestures which is commonly sung in mother-toddler classes and playgroups: "Five little monkeys jumping on the bed, one fell off and bumped his little head, mother called the doctor and the doctor said, 'NO MORE MONKEYS JUMPING ON THE BED!' Four little monkeys . . . etc." The doctor's caveat is accompanied by finger-wagging in the familiar gesture of scolding. Gina made the appropriate gestures as her mother chanted the words, and then she went to the toy shelf and pointed at the toy telephone. Mother assumed she wanted to play calling Grandma, which is a frequent game and real event at home, so the mother held the phone and spoke "talking to Grandma" dialogue. Gina listened patiently, then handed me the phone.

I pretended to call her, said hello, and asked how she was. Gina wagged her finger and handed me the phone again. Then a hypothesis began to crystallize; I tested it by pretending I was calling the doctor to ask how Gina's ears were. I reported from the phone that the doctor said Gina's ears were very nice and very good, that Gina was very nice and very good, and that she had tubes in her ears to take the hurt away. Gina pushed the phone into my hands again and again. Mother's eyes filled with tears as I repeated the doctor dialogue and we both became convinced that Gina had connected her medical difficulties with being a naughty, disobedient girl. I added to the phone conversation that now the hurt was gone, so Gina wouldn't have to wake up crying in the night anymore, and mommy and daddy wouldn't have to call the doctor so worried again. Gina turned to pick up the dolly and feed her once more, then got down on hands and knees, crawled to Mother's handbag for her pacifier, and settled with a sigh against Mother's lap.

When Mr. and Mrs. G. came together with Gina a week later, they reported that the night crying had ceased from that day and had not recurred. In the second session Gina made a beeline for the toy telephone and pushed it eagerly into my hands. After two or three repeitions of the doctor dialogue she turned to the baby doll and fed it tenderly with the toy bottle. Gina offered me a turn with the doll and I took the opportunity to tell a story about how the doll's ears had hurt, like Gina's, and the doll's wee-wee had hurt, like Gina's, but the doctor had said they were lovely ears and wouldn't hurt anymore. I looked at the doll's diapers, smiled a lot, and said the dolly's wee-wee wouldn't hurt anymore either and what a nice wee-wee the dolly had.

I met with the parents for one further session to talk to them about talking to Gina. Both parents had stimulated her intellectually, reading books to her from the beginning, but they had stayed on a concrete, naming level. It had not occurred to them to make causal connections for Gina yet, and certainly not to attempt to link events and feelings. Between the second session with Gina and the parent session, however, both father and mother had made an effort to take the time and trouble to explain things to Gina. They reported with affecting astonishment how much more tractable she had become. In addition to the phenomenological expansion of Gina's cognitive horizons, they were including the crucial element of feelings. In the supermarket they talked with Gina about being tired and how hard it was to wait; they extended their conscientious naming of objects into the realm of intangibles. Their increased joy in their child and Gina's relief made me feel confident of their capacity to manage the subsequent developmental hurdles more easily.

DISCUSSION

The brief clinical contact I described above was gratifying to all concerned, but it raises many questions. The first area to be investigated involves understanding how Gina used what she had available to her to attempt to master overwhelming, probably traumatic, events and sensations. Here I will look at the intellectual development of infants before expressive speech is evident. The second has to do with trying to understand the parents' role in the psychological events I reconstructed, and this introduces the meaning in the parent-child relationship of different stages of the infant's intellectual development.

The current explosion of research on infants includes much investigation of infant learning; over the last 10 years or so this work has moved forward from the constraints of strictly Piagetian or anti-Piagetian studies to include a fuller view of the functioning child as a feeling, thinking, and doing person. Jerome Bruner (1983) provides a creative multifaceted account of the speech development of two little boys, which illuminates both sets of questions posed by Gina's problem and its resolution. Bruner examines particularly the games of the first year— peekaboo, object exchange, and hide-and-seek—as they arise in the context of the mother-child relationship and provide a setting for the development of speech.

Bruner describes the appearance of pointing from the age of 6 months on and notes that the child's ability to comprehend the adult's point preceded his own ability consistently by 1 or 2 months. This is a pattern which recurs in various infant studies; we should keep in mind that Gina and her peers are taking in meaningful material well before they can express similar content communicatively. By 11 to 13 months, the infant becomes capable of "indexicals," which relate a sign to an immediate element of nonlinguistic context; these are the pointing and naming games of the young toddler. Once these are in the repertoire, the infant can move on to relating words to other words. Mr. and Mrs. G. reported that Gina was in this stage by 11 months.

Robert McCall (1979) suggested that "although the predominant character of mental performance changes from stage to stage, mental behavior at every age serves two functions—the acquisition of information and the disposition of the organism to influence the inanimate and animate environment, the latter notion being similar to White's (1959) concept of effectance" (p. 728f.). McCall and his coworkers proposed a description of stages in the developmental function of mental behavior, with major transitions occurring at 2 months, 8 months, 13 months, and 21 months. "The major cognitive event hypothesized to occur at approximately 8 months . . . is the separation of means from ends. . . . At approximately 13 months, stage IV marks the onset of complete sensorimotor decentering. The infant can appreciate the independence of entities in the world and understand that they carry with them their own properties, including their potential to be independent dynamic forces in the environment. . . . This cognition enhances information acquisition and influencing by permitting consensual vocabulary" (1979, p. 729f.).

We know from her parents' report that Gina had been "putting words together" before the medical interventions at 13 months; so she was capable of intellectual manipulation of her experience, but not yet practiced at assigning appropriate meaning to those experiences. Means-end thinking was rapidly being transformed into cause-and-effect hypotheses, but the nature of the connecting links remained obscure. What made Gina put together the specific poem about the monkeys jumping on the bed with her efforts at mastery of invasive procedures? There could be several alternative explanations, some leaning upon the cognitive aspect, in the coincidence of the word "doctor" appearing in Gina's little poem, or upon the experiential aspect of being scolded for defiant toddler behavior and the doctor in the song scolding the disobedient monkeys; perhaps someone affectionately called Gina "a little monkey." A more sophisticated possibility would be using the song as a defense against anxiety aroused by helplessness and aggressive retaliatory impulses in the medical setting. The song was associated with fun with mother and thus stood for completely contrasting affective experience; the reversal defenses are specific to the anal phase, and the thoughts underlying Gina's behavior and symptom may well represent the beginning operation of defense mechanisms. In blaming her own naughtiness for the doctor's intervention, Gina may have been protecting her parents from her hostility; it is not inconceivable that a child this age would have reparative impulses. We have all seen toddlers pat hurt peers or adults consolingly.

Any of these possibilities is plausible, but I feel that they still beg the question of why the *particular* connection was made. I think the answer lies in the direction of multidetermination. It is difficult, perhaps impossible, to know why one thing means more to a baby than another, but it is clear from current research on infancy that cognition cannot be divorced from emotion. The affective life of the child is central to his development in all areas and informs his intellectual development at every point; Anny Katan's (1961) elegant exposition of the role in ego development of the verbalization of feelings is a seminal psychoanalytic statement of this point. The importance of the mother-child relationship has not always been as self-evident to researchers as to parents and so it is still possible to be pleasantly surprised by Bruner's decisive placing of language development in the context of the mutual attention of mother and child. He says, "language acquisition 'begins' before the child utters his first lexico-grammatical speech. It begins when mother and infant create a predictable format of interaction that can serve as a microcosm for communicating and for constituting a shared reality. The transactions that occur in such formats constitute the 'input' from which the child then masters grammar, how to refer and mean, and how to realize his intentions communicatively" (p. 18). I think that Gina chose to make the connections she did because of the multiplicity of links available between the monkey poem and her experiences around doctors, some of which we can describe, others of which are probably inaccessible to us and perhaps to Gina. There are many traceable links: the verbal occurrence of the word doctor, the behavioral sequence of the parents' telephoning in both poem and life, the pain in the head of the monkeys and Gina, scolding going on in life and the poem, physical adventurousness beginning for Gina as it was for the monkeys, etc. There is, however, another kind of multiplicity here—what we may call affective charge. Gina tried to master overwhelming events and sensations; to do this, she brought to bear material loaded with the most powerful affects available to her at the time, all connected to her parents. There was powerful negative charge in the scolding, the pain, the anxiety palpable in the parents' telephone calls to the doctor during the night and the day. On the other hand, great pleasure and gratification accompanied her performance of the poem for her mother; talking to grandma on the phone was a praised activity, while the parents had been urging her positively toward gross motor progression. Berta Bornstein (1935) described a similar condensation of experiences, impulses, and affects in the development of symptoms in a 2½-year-old child and observed how "complicated" was the mental life of a little child.

We must not forget, however, that Gina's efforts to make sense of her experience were taking place invisibly, in thought. She was not communicating the intellectual structure she was creating to her parents because she couldn't talk very much yet, and it didn't occur to them that she might be trying to. Indeed, her heroic mental attempts to master the traumas were failing, and she developed the symptom of night terrors. Luckily, her parents were people who could hear that Gina's crying meant *something,* even if they didn't know what. But this brings us to the second set of questions mentioned above, those involving the meaning in the parent-child relationship of this transitional and momentous phase in the child's mental development.

It is something of a truism that scientists are now demonstrating things about tiny babies that mothers have always known, for example, that infant's facial expressions denote differentiated affects, or that babies recognize their mother's face or voice, etc. It looks as if, at least in the field of infant personality development, science follows life. But when we come to cognitive and language development, common knowledge lags curiously behind scientific observation. Most parents don't assume understanding in their babies or toddlers and few adults advise parents on the basis of babies' capacity for comprehension, whether it be pediatricians helping the frequent management problems of this age group or mothers talking over the toddlers' heads in the supermarket. I think we should be wondering why this should be so in general, just as we wonder why Gina's loving, involved parents never thought to talk to her about anything that was done to her.

Bruner gives us a clue when he says, "One special property of formats involving an infant and an adult is that they are asymmetrical with respect to the knowledge of the partners—one 'knows what's up,' the other does not know or knows less. Insofar as the adult is willing to 'hand over' his knowledge, he can serve in the format as model, scaffold, and monitor until the child achieves requisite mastery" (1983, p. 133). The crux is the adult's willingness or unwillingness to hand over knowledge. We have seen that Gina was well able to think verbally, i.e., that there were specific verbal elements in the theory she built to account for her experiences. But her parents resisted recognition of this capacity for independent intellectual functioning. I think their resistance stemmed in part from the implications of intellectual independence—a child who can think has a separate life. Mr. and Mrs. G. had grappled with adoption and a difficult beginning to build a genuinely close relationship and foster excellent development in Gina. It was not easy for them, nor is it easy for any parent who has enjoyed the bliss of mutuality in the first year to give it up in favor of the uncertain communicative negotiations of the second year. Anny Katan describes how much more difficult it is for parents to guess at the child's feelings than to respond to a pointed finger.

It is not only the independence of the toddler that parents may find difficult to accept and manage; the anal phase brings with it

aggressive impulses and feelings which arouse powerful coun-
terreactions in others. Parents may respond by hostile suppression of the toddler's defiance and rage, which carries with it
suppression of accompanying tendrils of ego growth, or they
may respond with their characteristic defenses against their own
aggressive impulses, which serve equally to blot out perceptions
of what is going on in the child.

Given good-enough parenting and good-enough stimulation,
however, the child with adequate endowment will move inexora-
bly toward thought and speech. Perhaps the "terrible twos" are a
creation of the adult world's resistance to joining and fostering
intellectual mastery of the internal and external environments
by the infant toddling toward autonomy. Gina became happier,
calmer, and "easier to manage" when her parents could see that
she could understand the explanations of the inner and outer
worlds they began to offer her. Gina has shown us that toddlers
will make theories to account for their experiences whatever we
do or don't do. But if we want their theories to reflect our view of
reality and become part of a more sophisticated shared reality
leading to progressive development and enrichment of the parent-child relationship, then we must provide the necessary ingredients and talk to our toddlers.

BIBLIOGRAPHY

BORNSTEIN, B. (1935). Phobia in a two-and-a-half year old. *Psychoanal. Q.*,
4:93–119.
BRUNER, J. (1983). *Child's Talk*. New York: Norton.
KATAN, A. (1961). Some thoughts about the role of verbalization in early child-
hood. *Psychoanal. Study Child*, 16:184–188.
McCALL, R. B. (1979). The development of intellectual functioning in infancy
and the prediction of later IQ. In *Handbook of Infant Development*, ed. J. D.
Osofsky, pp. 707–742. New York: Wiley.
WHITE, R. W. (1959). Motivation reconsidered. *Psychol. Rev.*, 66:297–333.

On the Concept of Mourning in Childhood

Reactions of a 2½-Year-Old Girl to the Death of Her Father

CHRISTINA SEKAER, M.D.
AND SHERI KATZ, M.S.

SUE WAS 28 MONTHS OLD WHEN HER FATHER'S DEATH CONFRONTED her with a loss that her personality development and cognitive skills scarcely allowed her to comprehend. Sue's efforts to deal with her loss will be the focus of this paper and will be discussed with regard to the long-debated issue of whether or not children are capable of mourning (R. Furman, 1964a, 1964b; Wolfenstein, 1966; Nagera, 1970; E. Furman, 1974; Bowlby, 1980). Sekaer (1986) suggested the term "childhood mourning" for the process by which children may work through a loss and proceed with normal development. The notion of childhood mourning emphasizes the differences from adult mourning, while at the same time stressing that decathexis, identification, reality testing, cognitive understanding of death, and other aspects of adult mourning may occur, but in a manner specific to children. Sue's reactions illustrate some of these similarities to and differences from adult mourning.

Christina Sekaer is an assistant attending in psychiatry at St. Luke's Hospital of the St. Luke's–Roosevelt Hospital Center, New York, N.Y.

Sheri Katz is a language and learning specialist at the Fieldston Lower School of the Ethical Culture Schools, N.Y.

SELECTED LITERATURE REVIEW

For adults, Freud (1917) described the work of mourning as dealing with a conflict between the wish to maintain a libidinal tie to the internal representation of the lost object versus the demands of recognizing the reality of the loss. Memories of the lost one are hypercathected and then gradually decathected as the reality of the loss is accepted.

Arguing that children *cannot* mourn, Deutsch (1937) said that a young child's ego lacked the strength and development to tolerate intense pain, and that a child was unable to carry out the work of mourning. Nagera (1970) described the child's need for the parent to aid in his development as too strong to allow decathexis. Wolfenstein (1965, 1966, 1969) believed that decathexis of the internalized parental images as a normal part of adolescence must occur before a person can fully decathect a parent lost to death.

In contrast, Anna Freud (1960) argued that by the age of 2 or 3 a child who has achieved object constancy should be able to comprehend "the external fact" of the loss as well as to effect "the corresponding inner changes." For a child of 2 or older, she said, "the nearer to object constancy, the longer the duration of grief reactions with corresponding approximation to the adult internal process of mourning" (p. 59). Bowlby (1960) stressed the similarity of adult and child reactions to loss, noting that even in the first year of life an infant may experience the "rupture of a key relationship and the consequent intense pain of yearning" (p. 35). Bowlby (1980) discussed the development of the child's cognitive ability to maintain a representation of mother even in her absence, stressing object permanence rather than (libidinal) object constancy.

Robert Furman (1964a, 1964b) wrote that a child of 3 or 4 who has attained the postambivalent phallic phase of object relationships should be capable of "the painful internal decathexis of the lost object that is the essence of mourning" (p. 322). Erna Furman (1974) said that children from the age of 2 years on could attain a sufficient understanding of death and "could apply this concept to the loss of a loved person when realistic and continuous help in understanding facts and feelings was available from surviving love objects" (p. 125).

Lopez and Kliman (1979) describe Diane, bereaved at 19 months, who, with the aid of analysis begun at age 4, "experienced a process that did not in principle differ from what Freud (1917) called the 'work of mourning'" (p. 265). In Diane's analysis fantasies, ideas, and affects stimulated by mother's death were revived and submitted to reality's verdict. Rather than a full decathexis followed by a hiatus before a new attachment was made, libido was withdrawn gradually and shifted to her stepmother, a process facilitated by the analyst.

When considering the prolonged and painful process of remembering and reality testing described by Freud (1917), one must keep in mind whose reality one is referring to. While it seems obvious that whatever mourning or adaptive processes children can carry out must occur within their own experience of the world, this realization is often overlooked. For example, Anna Freud (1960) refers to "the external fact," Erna Furman (1974) to "the concept of death," "the facts," "reality," "understanding," etc., and yet the meaning of these terms as perceived by the child is not made explicit. Thus Erna Furman (1974) discusses Sally, age 4, "who clearly understood and accepted the meaning of death"; later in therapy although "previously realistic about death, she now revealed a confusion . . . asking if [the dead] father was now too big for his clothes" (p. 138). Clearly Sally had not "understood" on adult terms.

Piaget (1927) described a sequence of distinctions made by children about life: the term life is first applied to all activity or motion, then to self-initiated motion, then only to animals and plants. But things that cannot be directly experienced, such as the sun, moon, clouds, and wind, are still credited with life often until well into latency. Bemporad (1978) notes, "The child's concepts are in fact only preconcepts; they are sometimes too general and sometimes too specific . . . reasoning [sometimes] . . . is successful, but only when it does not go far beyond mere memory for past events" (p. 82). A child's restating of adult teaching may not indicate understanding; Erna Furman (1974) reports Susy, a 3-year-old, stating, "mommy is dead, and when you're dead you can't ever come back. That's right, daddy, isn't it?" (p. 51). But how can she "know" that this is final if she is too young yet to conceptualize this fact? A child comprehends permanent loss without higher cognitive functioning to structure events in a context of time, space, and causality, and within a reality which is distorted by wishful fantasy and prelogical animistic thinking. His "mourning," if it occurs, must be done without comprehension of the implications of loss beyond his developmental level.

To compare the inner work following a loss requires consideration of what the concepts of decathexis and identification mean at different ages. Regarding decathexis, writers are generally agreed that when a child does *not* react with pain, it is due either to defenses against such painful work for pathological reasons or to defenses based on an inability to do the work because of age. But when painful reactions *do* occur, not all agree that decathexis is going on.

Wolfenstein (1966) criticizes the use of painful memories as evidence of decathexis, noting that the 6-year-old boy who Robert Furman said "mourned" in fact "painfully missed his mother in many circumstances where formerly she was with him. . . . [But we] can miss and long for someone we still hope to see again" (p. 95). She felt children acknowledge, on the surface, the fact of the death, while on another level they expect the parent to return. Wolfenstein (1966) also described a 10-year-old boy who she said did not mourn but rather transferred his tie from his dead mother to his grandmother without a "protracted sadness or withdrawal into painful preoccupation with memories of the lost object" and without a hiatus before a new attachment was formed (p. 121).

Very young children who are still internalizing parental functions that have not yet become autonomous may lose functions such as speech, walking, and perception (Anna Freud, 1939–45; Erna Furman, 1974). Decathexis, if one is to call it that, of a primary object may entail loss of part of himself. As Nagera (1970) states, "Complete withdrawal of cathexis from the lost object will leave the child in a 'developmental vacuum' unless a suitable substitute object is readily found. . . . [Death] cannot lead to the type of decathexis that will be observed in the case of the adult" (p. 380).

As with "decathexis," the term "identification" differs in meaning according to the age of the child. Jacobson (1954) describes the development from early primitive identifications to "true ego identifications" (p. 43). She notes that primitive identifications "disregard the realistic differences between the self and the object" (p. 46), whereas later identifications alter the child's ego realistically in selective ways. Diane, as described by Lopez and Kliman (1979), reacted to her mother's suicide by developing "global identifications"; for example, she would fall and hurt herself in apparent copying of mother's suicidal leap. With an older child one would not expect such primitive identifications.

Identifications used by children in reaction to death may interfere with growth in that a child's normal development involves identifying with and differentiating himself from his parents. McDevitt (1980) describes identifications used in the resolution of the rapprochement crisis as important for building psychic structure. After the conclusion of rapprochement a bereaved child might be much less vulnerable to regression and loss of structure at least in part due to identifications formed by this age. Winnie, reported by Barnes (1964), might be such a case. Having lost her mother at 2½ years, Winnie was able to go through a "mourning" process at age 3 when assisted by her grandmother. She apparently did not become severely symptomatic after this (though a follow-up is not given).

Splitting of the ego is described as another defensive or pathological process that may occur when mourning is not completed. Wolfenstein (1966) considers it to be common in bereaved children. Freud (1927) describes such a split in the ego of an adult who maintained that his father (dead since he was 2 years old) was still alive and also knew that his father was dead. Nagera (1970) notes that secretly held fantasies of the continued existence of the dead parent are very common in bereaved latency-aged children who also are fully aware of the facts of the death. Splits in the ego prevent decathexis, leave the ego impoverished by the need to maintain such a split, and thus are considered pathological.

Unlike an adult, a bereaved child must deal not only with the immediate loss, but also with the impact of the loss at subsequent stages of his development. It may not be possible to separate reactions to a death from difficulties due to the "developmental vacuum" of a missing parent (Nagera, 1970).

This is not to say that children cannot mourn. For each stage of development one may postulate an optimum degree to which mourning can be accomplished. If this is achieved, one may say that a normal childhood mourning is in progress; if this is *not* achieved, a pathological process may be occurring.

Childhood mourning delineates a process by which children may respond to bereavement and proceed with a relatively normal development. Based on a synthesis of the literature, Sekaer (1986) views this process not as a deficient version of adult mourning, but rather as one unique to the child's capacities. Thus a child needs adult help to understand death and still cannot do so beyond his own developmental level. A child also needs an adult to serve as a focus for his emotional reactions; unlike an adult, he cannot make use of a hiatus in attachment, by withdrawing into himself, in order to work through the loss. Identifications with a dead parent may interfere with identifications occurring as a normal part of a child's development. Full decathexis of the dead may not be possible or necessarily the best goal if a substitute attachment is not available.

In a further discussion of creative processes and transitional phenomena in bereaved children, Sekaer (1986) suggested the term "imaginary parent" to refer to fantasies of the dead parent as still alive; such imaginary parents may be gradually decathected as the child's need for the parent diminishes. Imaginary parents are an example, along with "mourning at a distance" through pets, toys, or fictional characters, of the bereaved child's heightened use of creative channels. Imaginary parents may serve a developmental purpose not unlike a transitional object or an imaginary companion; the fantasied person would "fade away" as no longer needed.

CASE REPORT

We shall discuss a 2½-year-old bereaved child whose reactions appear nonpathological and yet clearly limited by her level of development. Sue S., who had been attending full-time daycare from the age of 3 months, experienced the death of her father at

28 months. The supportive structure of her experience at the daycare center and her therapeutic relationship with a teacher appeared to compensate for some of her mother's unavailability due to the loss. Thus the opportunity developed to observe the reactions of a 2½-year-old girl to the death of her father under circumstances which could facilitate rather than hinder their expression.

DEVELOPMENTAL DATA

Until her father's death Sue's development had proceeded in spite of recurrent tensions in the home. During Sue's early life her mother, while being generally warm and supportive, was occasionally unavailable due to personal preoccupations and physical health issues. Sue's father was also inconsistently available. Nevertheless he was strongly invested in her from the start, proud of her achievements, especially language, and pleased with her femininity. Sue lived with mother, father, and an older sister.

Sue's early development appeared normal in social, cognitive, motor, and emotional areas. At 4 months she sobered to strangers, at 8 months she showed separation anxiety and formed specific attachments to her mother and daycare teacher. A normal recurrence of separation anxiety was noted at 17 months at a time when tensions arose between her parents; for a while Sue avoided her mother when she came for her and turned to strangers. Although this appeared to resolve, at 24 months Sue again showed some signs of difficulty. Tension was again high at home, and Sue often shared her father's bed as her parents stayed apart. For a few weeks Sue showed isolation of affect, narrating anxiety-filled events without feeling; she developed a shallow seductive manner and sought out strangers while being provocative with her teachers. Sue was moved with her age group to the third year classroom, and individual play sessions with one of her new teachers were begun to assist Sue in developing a closer relationship with her.[1] These sessions had been in progress and a closer tie with this special teacher had begun to

1. The special teacher was Sheri Katz. The daycare supervisor was Virginia Flynn.

form when, at 28 months, Sue's father became suddenly ill with a cardiovascular disorder. After a couple of days he was taken to the hospital in a police car. There, following a few days' illness with very poor prognosis, he died. Sue did not visit in the hospital, but did attend the open casket funeral.

REACTIONS TO THE DEATH

After Mr. S.'s death Sue's individual sessions with the special teacher were continued. These sessions did not constitute an analytic experience but rather an enriched extension of her daycare experience. Attempts to arrange for a more intensive analytic therapy were not made because of the lack of more severe or chronic symptom formation. The teacher's role was one of offering nurturance, verbalizing feelings, clarifying cognitive distortions, and encouraging Sue to express thoughts and feelings. Their relationship intensified after the death and became a focus for Sue's concerns about death. Sue used the sessions for fantasy play and expression of feelings often focused on her father. In the classroom she remained invested in the activities and play of the group; when issues about her father arose, she limited herself to more realistic comments and questions. Sue's teacher had a long-standing interest in childhood bereavement (Katz, 1976). Such understanding is helpful to perceive the needs and to tolerate the stress of helping a bereaved child. Assisting a child with concerns and feelings about death can evoke deep feelings about an adult's own prior experiences of loss. For one student teacher, Sue's loss evoked intense memories of her own father's death when she was 5, and led to her starting therapy. More frequently there is denial and inability to observe and sustain the painful responses of the young child (McDonald, 1964).

   Prior to the death, Sue's mother had made use of the daycare and her own weekly sessions with a staff social worker to plan for and then return to school and to discuss difficulties in her relationship with her husband. After the death, Mrs. S. did not hide her sad feelings from Sue, and they talked of the death. Mrs. S. tended not to be tolerant of regressive behavior and instead encouraged Sue's independence. Though empathic with Sue in general, her mother seemed not as available as the teacher to Sue regarding her father's death; for example, several months after the death Mrs. S. expressed surprise that Sue was still upset about it. As is true of bereaved parents in general, Mrs. S.'s struggle to cope with her own grief left her less able to be of help to Sue.

Sue was able to speak about her father's illness and death when they occurred and thereafter. In her sessions and in the class Sue began to show a variety of symptoms. She cried often. She became irritable, aggressive with peers, and clingy with adults. A sleep disturbance developed. Separation anxiety was renewed. These reactions diminished in intensity in the first months after the death. Following these initial reactions Sue continued to show preoccupation and concern with death, illness, and separation, while in other ways she resumed what appeared to be her normal development; she remained tied to her mother while social and cognitive development continued. As a very verbal child Sue received support, understanding, and clarification from her teachers and, to some extent, at home.

But what processes were going on as Sue continued with her life? How could her 2- to 3-year-old mentality deal with the fact of loss? The next part of the paper will deal with a closer examination of some of Sue's reactions between 28 and 36 months as she struggled to comprehend and integrate events.

COGNITION

Sue learned and remembered many facts about her father's death. Yet reality for Sue was subject to distortion according to her wishes, as is typical of primary process thinking. Thus the fact of death (if only as a label for her father's state) remained present in her mind along with its denial. Sue had known that her father was in the hospital and said that he went there to get better. After his death she often announced to familiar and unfamiliar people, "My daddy died." Once when her peers responded to this announcement by echoing in turn, "My daddy died," Sue angrily made the distinction: "My daddy's dead, not yours!" Although she knew this fact, she occasionally asserted the opposite without being disturbed by the contradiction, announcing, "He at work" or "He coming to get me."

Sue's words reflected the irreversible nature of death as she said, "He's sleeping there," pointing to the sky, "He can't get out of the box." Or on another occasion, "He can't come back." However, such comments were sometimes reversed as:

Sue: My daddy, he lay down on my mommy's bed and he sleeping on mommy's bed.

Teacher: Does he sleep on mommy's bed now?

Sue: No, because he went up in the sky and that's why he died.

Teacher: What does he do in the sky?

Sue: He dying.

Teacher: Can he visit you?

Sue (pouting): Not anymore 'cause he died. He died up in the sky. Because he died in the sky. I miss my daddy. I know he comes to my house on Sunday.[2]

Her comment about missing daddy is followed by reassertion that he is alive and will visit. Typical of prelogical thought, she feels no need to integrate her wish with her contradictory knowledge of reality.

In a less affect-laden context Sue seemed to demonstrate more stable awareness of past-present-future, animate-inanimate, and of the irreversibility of death. A boy noticed a dead fish in the tank at the Center, asked why it was dead, and then said it was sick. Sue came in, asked, "The fish is dead? Let me see." She noticed its large open eyes. Her teacher clarified that it could not see anymore now that it was dead. Sue answered, "He can't see. He's dead. Like he dead. Like my daddy dead." They talked about things that the dead fish couldn't do (eat or swim or play with the other fish). Sue said, "He can't come back. Good-bye fish." As the teacher began to wrap it in a paper towel, Sue gently took over, wrapped the fish and put it in the garbage, saying, "There it goes. Away." When the teacher said this fish couldn't swim around anymore with the other fish, Sue went to the fish

---

2. Excerpts are taken from a daily record kept by Sue's special teacher. This record was rewritten in narrative form and parts have been published (Katz and Flynn, 1982).

tank and announced, "Swimming! Look! These fish didn't die." When she saw her mother that afternoon, Sue said, "The fish died, like my daddy died." Sue did not continue to ask about the dead fish. It is possible that her "understanding" of the loss remained in her mind along with some ongoing notion of the fish's continued existence, as was the case for her father. It seems more likely that acceptance of the fish's death was due to a lack of emotional need for the fish to be alive and therefore a lack of continuing concern for it.

At one point, several months after the death, Mrs. S., following her own religious beliefs, spoke of her husband as though he were still present. Sue became quite confused and in class spoke of him as alive. Mrs. S. was advised not to share such ideas with Sue, and Sue's confusion subsided.

Sue's curiosity and need to understand her father's death were evident in her efforts to reason about it. These efforts incorporated ideas she had been told as well as her own experiences and remained limited to her developmental level of thinking. Such reasoning thus included application of memories of previous experiences to the present and transductive reasoning from particular to particular without true deductive or inductive reasoning (Ginsburg and Opper, 1979). What follows are examples of Sue's thinking in several areas.

Sleeping was confused with death for several months. Sue had been told that her father was "sleeping in Heaven." She had seen him and kissed him good-bye in his coffin; she and her sister had played at being dead in a box after the funeral. In the weeks after this she fought sleep; she was fragile and whimpering at naptime and kept her eyes open despite fatigue. Her mother reported that Sue was waking up sobbing in the middle of the night. Sue said of her father, "He awake. No. He sleeping there" and pointed up to the sky. A few weeks later she said, "My daddy is sleeping. My daddy can't get out of the box!" Clarifications on a concrete level were helpful; thus after Sue was several times told of the difference between sleeping and being dead, her sleeping difficulty resolved.

Travel and "far away" are similar preconcepts that for Sue were associated with death. The fear was present that since one died in the sky, another might die in the sky. When her special teacher was leaving on vacation, Sue told her that she was flying away from her, that she wasn't coming back, that she would die like her daddy died; "He went far away." They discussed the difference between a trip on an airplane (a person can return, stays healthy) and dying. Sue said, "My daddy died. I didn't see him for a long, long time." She then asked about herself, "I'm not gonna die?" about the teacher, "You're not gonna die?" and then about each of her classmates in turn, "Doug's not gonna die?" etc.

Certain forms of travel such as taxis and planes were associated with dying. Sue talked about her father riding in cars, taxis, and school buses, and tied these memories closely to thoughts of his death. The memory of a taxi ride with her father maintained a special significance. Sue said, "My daddy went in the car, and me too. He told the taxi to stop." Several days later she told her friend Doug, "My daddy died. Did your daddy die?" Doug answered, "No," and Sue asked, "Did your daddy ride on a school bus?" She then asked her teacher if her daddy had died and whether he had gone in a school bus, adding that her daddy went in a taxi.

Sue's preconception of travel related to death is too general; thus since her father "went in a taxi," she appeared to associate taxis, buses, etc., with death. She reasoned with transductive logic that since he went in a taxi, others who did so might die too. Furthermore, Sue had no grasp of ideas of chance. As Piaget and Inhelder (1951) showed, children at her age (and older) have only a primitive notion of taking turns. She tried to reason within the small number of her peers whether death will occur to each of them. The concept of "chance," the idea that what happened to her father was very unlikely to happen to her mother or to her—that is, "statistically low odds"—could not be called upon as a reassurance. Instead Sue reassured herself concretely.

Sue was particularly confused about the difference between flying in airplanes and going to heaven. At one point without the teachers' knowledge Sue's mother had talked of taking a plane trip with Sue. In daycare Sue said, "I not sick. I not fly up in the sky. Mommy gonna fly up in the sky. Like daddy fly. You not fly up in the sky?" Her teacher talked of having flown in an airplane in the sky during her winter vacation. She explained that she wasn't sick or hurt and that she came back home on another airplane when she was ready, unlike Sue's father who was very sick and died and could not ever return. Sue then said, "I go fly with mommy and daddy. I go on horses with mommy and daddy." They talked about trips she used to take with her mother and father and further clarifications were made. When the teacher explained Sue's confusion to Mrs. S., they were able to continue these discussions at home and Sue's anxiety abated. One must also wonder what "in the sky" meant to Sue. Piaget (1927) quotes a boy of 8: "Is the sky alive?— Yes, because if it were dead, why then it would fall down" (p. 289).

Sue associated medical things with dying and avoided medical play for several weeks after her father's death. She averted her eyes from a stethoscope, saying, "It's not here. Forgot in room. Lost it"; or she tossed it aside. After a few weeks this shifted to a strong interest in playing doctor, as she gave shots and Band-Aids and talked about her father.

One day while reading *Nicki Goes to the Doctor*, she called the instrument a "deathoscope" and then denied feeling afraid of shots "because people don't need shots and daddy didn't need a shot." On another occasion death was associated with a Band-Aid as Sue, her teacher, and a classmate conversed:

Classmate: My mommy died.

Sue: Your mommy not die. My mo—my daddy died.

Teacher: What happened to your daddy?

Sue: He died.

Teacher: How did that happen?

Sue: My daddy had a Band-Aid. My daddy died. My mommy didn't die.

Classmate: My daddy didn't die. He go to work.

That afternoon when the classmate's father came for him, Sue said to him, "See, your daddy not dead."

In part because of her inability to specify causes, Sue seemed to wonder about her ability to precipitate death. On a walk Sue started to pull some ivy vines that another child had just been told not to pull up. A volunteer teacher told her to stop because she was making the plants die. Sue pulled back, looked very frightened, gazed around her at the trees and plants, and asked, "Everything gonna die?" She was then reassured and agreed she had been very scared. The volunteer's comment became quickly generalized, as it touched on a source of anxiety in Sue.

Sue's heightened separation anxiety immediately after the death, and through the ensuing months with her special teacher, indicated fear of further loss. "Because" there was one loss there may be another. Brief separations from her teacher evoked a variety of behaviors from Sue that seemed to be efforts to master this fear. These behaviors did not occur in isolation. Experiences involving separation were linked together by association either with events recognized as similar and/or with the affects involved in these past events. The following incidents illustrate how Sue, when threatened by separation from her teacher, referred either through action or words to specific, past, related experiences.

When her teacher told Sue about a brief trip she was taking, Sue immediately grabbed a child's pacifier and answered in a stream of infantile syllables. She then asked to read a book, *Hop on Pop,* which she had read daily with a temporary summer worker who had left 3 months earlier (when Sue was 25 months.) Sue sang, "Daddy, daddy, happy birthday" and suddenly broke into sobs, asked to join the teacher on her trip, and shook her head "no" in disbelief about reassurances that the teacher would return and that she would be taken care of safely. That afternoon Sue had a difficult time separating from the teacher, throwing herself on the floor, demanding a bottle, and then threatening to "tell daddy." The turning to the remembered book appeared to be an attempt to control her reaction to the threatened separation.

Bemporad (1978) makes the point that for a young child affective experiences are "of the moment" and that moods are not held over time due to the child's lack of inner mental continuity unless the outer circumstances continually provoke certain feelings. Sue did not become depressed in the adult sense. She did not go into a continued, lasting depressive mood. She did, however, remain sensitized to separation experiences and associated memories over time.

In the following example, an incident is remembered and referred to 4 months later. On a walk with her group Sue announced to some porcelain figures in a store window, "My daddy died." Soon after, Sue saw her sister, walking by with her school class. The sister hugged Sue and then left. Sue cried and called for her sister and her daddy. Her temporary caregiver, Anny, picked her up and Sue clung to her neck whimpering. Sue's special teacher who was busy with the others left Sue to calm down with Anny and went on with the rest of the group to the park. As soon as Sue arrived in the park, she stumbled, fell, and ran to her special teacher crying in her arms for a long time. Sue had been upset at being left with Anny.

Sue referred to this incident 4 months later when her teacher was again unavailable. The teacher had just returned from a 4-day illness during which Sue was cared for by her group's second regular teacher, Mary. Sue arrived, saw her special teacher, and asked for Mary. She slapped her special teacher who tried to help her with her coat and let Mary help instead. Her teacher initiated a conversation, saying, "You haven't seen me in a long time." Sue then rushed to her and pulled herself onto her lap. The teacher told her that she must have been angry at her for having been gone for so long, and that Sue must have been worried because she was sick even though she had been told she was getting better. Sue asked if the teacher lay in bed and watched television, if she took medicine, and if she "drank lots of soda to get better." Then Sue said, "I was very mad." The teacher asked at whom, and she said at Anny for picking her up when she saw her sister.

Sue was clearly angry with her teacher for being out sick as she slapped her and turned from her. She talked of a time when she had wanted her teacher and had instead been left with Anny. As she again felt close to her teacher, she shifted the anger to Anny and to the past incident. One may presume that Sue was also angry at her father, but this was not expressed directly.

OBJECT CONSTANCY, SEPARATION-INDIVIDUATION

Sue showed clear evidence of having achieved some degree of (libidinal) object constancy. She often sang or recited to herself phrases "I want mommy" or "daddy" to comfort herself. She remembered specific incidents with painful longing. When Mary was describing her sadness at the death of an uncle to Sue's special teacher, Sue called the two teachers by name and said, "Remember my daddy in the picture? My daddy went far away. My daddy got me an umbrella." Her face fell sadly, and she added, "I saw my daddy in the picture."

The ability to see the other as separate from oneself assists one in modulating the fear that what happened to another person may happen to oneself or mother or specific others. This ability was not fully developed in Sue. Thus when mother returned from visiting father in the hospital, Sue asked, "Are you feeling better mommy?" as though it were mother who was sick. Sue frequently reassured herself, "My daddy died. My mommy didn't die." She also used her peers to compare whose father had died and whose hadn't.

Illness in her mother increased Sue's fears, and with this stress her sense of self merged with her mother as she feared they both would die. Once when mother was ill with a bad cold and her attention was inconsistent to Sue, Sue was very distressed and fearful that her mother's illness would cause them all to die. She showed her teacher scrapes on her face where she had fallen and told her of getting a shot at the doctor's the day before. She then said, "I went in an airplane in the sky with my mommy and daddy. No, I didn't. My daddy died."

Because Sue could not reason in a generalized causal way, she could not clearly comprehend what made people die and therefore could not use even concrete operational logical thought to comprehend as an adult can and to reassure herself that she too would not die or that others would not. Adults with helpful explanations cannot "correct" this logic or raise it to a higher level which must wait for later development.

Thus Sue did not let this unresolved issue rest. In a follow-up visit[3] Sue still feared her mother too would die. Sue used the toilet; when she flushed it, she asked her teacher, "Do it bother

---

3. The daycare center enrolled children only up to the age of 3 years. Sue's special teacher continued to meet with Sue after her move to the new school for a series of weekly follow-up sessions.

you?" and reassured herself, "People don't go down." After a few minutes she began to sing, "Where's my mommy? She died? No, she didn't," and continued, "My mommy didn't die. Only my daddy. Doug's daddy didn't die. He said his mommy died. She didn't. I miss my daddy."

AFFECTIVE REACTIONS

Sue's reactions to her father's death included varied expressions of affect. To integrate affective experiences one must tolerate affect and also limit it so as not to be overwhelmed. Sue did not become overwhelmed and disorganized by her father's death. She did not constrict or omit affect but instead experienced a wide affective range.

A storybook in which a hunter shoots and kills the mother of Babar, the Elephant, became a focus for a variety of feelings and primitive fantasies as Sue would open the book to the page of the shooting on different occasions. Sue usually expressed anger at the hunter, shouting and hitting his picture. But she also slapped the dead mother or slapped at the crying Babar. Sue feared Babar would die: "Babar [was shot], not his mommy." Another time the gun going off was associated with her daddy dying.

Although Sue played out murderous and angry impulses, she did not acknowledge directly anger at her father for dying. For example, Sue excitedly called a policeman the daddy. Then she put down the policeman and picked up the lion and the horse.

Sue: Lion angry at horse. Biting him.

Teacher: Why is the lion so angry with the horse?

Sue: Because he died.

Teacher: The lion is mad that the horse died. Your daddy died too. Are you angry at daddy?

Sue: He awake. No. He sleeping there [pointing to the sky].

Sue picked up the elephant and threw it, saying, "He died." She then threw the horse, "He died." Then two mothers, "She died."

Teacher: They're all dying.

Sue: They awake.

Sue put them away and asked to end the session.

Here the suggestion of anger at her father interrupted the play; Sue had the dolls "die," denied this, and then ended the session. Such direct interpretations were rarely made. Playing out various emotions, especially anger, was encouraged to help her accept and express her own feelings on the level she presented them. It is possible that unspoken feelings, such as anger at her father, could become a focus for later conflict and symptom formation, or for resolution at a later age. For example, Sue's lack of anger directed at her father may represent splitting and idealization of him with the anger displaced to others.

Although Sue often gave in to the impulse to cry, she stressed that she did not cry; e.g., hearing another child cry, she said, "Somebody's crying. I'm not crying. I don't cry." In another example, Sue climbed into the teacher's lap, began to stroke her hair, and said, "You look pretty like a queen. I hold you. You won't cry." She soon asked if the teacher would always stay her teacher when she grew older. The teacher explained that, after Sue left, Sue would have new teachers who would help her and that she could visit the Center. Sue responded, "My daddy can't come for me yet. He at work. I didn't cry home sick. Mommy cried home sick. Daddy at work." Her face fell suddenly and she said, "I never see my daddy."

Sue stressed she didn't cry, mommy cried. Crying must be controlled and is also unpleasant as she reassured her teacher, "You won't cry." Anticipation of separation from the teacher seemed to stir feelings for her father, which she tried to ward off. As Wolfenstein (1966) suggests, children fear that pain or anger "may continue without letup and increase to intolerable intensity" (p. 103). Sue also needed to feel independent and not to regress.

Although Sue stressed not crying and maintaining control, she often cried. In a follow-up session she showed her teacher a bruise on her elbow and said that she fell running but that she didn't cry because she was a big girl. In her play she put lady bugs "in the oven so they got burned up. They not gonna cry." She made a play-doh roller coaster that went fast and said it was not scary. She said that if the teacher thought a roller coaster was scary, she should have held on. She asked, "Did you let go? Was you crying?" That same session she told of pinching her finger in the door and that she didn't cry. The school director noted that in fact Sue had screamed very loudly when she pinched her finger.

In the following example Sue shows her continued need to deny crying while at the same time she is able to label sadness and to articulate a cause. On the sixth follow-up visit Sue was interested in a story about a boy's pet dog who became ill and died in a book entitled *Grownups Cry Too*. Sue renamed the book *Grownups Don't Cry*, asking to see the dog, and saying, "That boy misses his dog. That dog gonna be fine." On the next and final session Sue asked to see "the boy who missed his dog," adding, "Not my dog died." The teacher answered that someone else special to her had died and she said, "My daddy died. That's why I get sad."

PSYCHOSEXUAL DEVELOPMENT

Psychosexually, Sue appeared to be between an anal and an early phallic phase. She had achieved toilet training and did not regress. She struggled to control her impulses and for the most part succeeded. This process of increasing control continued after her father's death along with increased verbalization of affect. For example, Sue used play to express and master ambivalent feelings after an aggressive act. Although biting was not a frequent occurrence for Sue, one day she bit a peer without provocation and announced, "I talk to daddy." She sang lustily, "I bit Larry, da da da da da da," then regressed into a stream of babytalk. She then noted the alligator emblem on her teacher's shirt, put her finger on it, cried "ouch," shook her finger, and told the teacher, "I take your alligator off." She covered it with her palms, "It went away," and then played peekaboo with it under her hand. Sue bit, attributed the urge to bite to the alligator, was herself bitten, and made the alligator come and go.

Sue's play often expressed ambivalence particularly in association with issues of illness and death, as the following examples from play sessions illustrate:

Sue threw a doll, Ernie, then nursed him with a Band-Aid and threw him again. She said, "Ernie, a Band-Aid. My finger hurts," and showed the teacher her finger. She found Ernie, threw him again, and expressed concern that he felt sad. Later she refused to bid Ernie good-bye, saying, "I don't want to kiss him good-bye."

Sue gently put a large doll, Betsy, to sleep saying, "Don't bother my Betsy. She needs a Band-Aid. For everything. You bothering my baby!" (to her teacher). She lifted the phone to say that her teacher was "bothering my Betsy sleep. I asked her not to bother Betsy. Betsy." Then she stomped angrily on Betsy. She pointed a finger at the teacher and said loudly, "You step on her. You did it." Sue then smiled and said, "I'm gonna be a monster."

PRECURSORS OF GUILT

As one would expect at her age, Sue did not express guilt or self-reproach. She did show, however, a transient tendency to fall and hurt herself. This was marked particularly just after her father's death and again just after her move to the new school. That getting hurt had significance is suggested in the following example. Sue picked up the book about Babar, flipped to the page where the hunter shoots Babar's mommy, and said, "The boy had to shoot the hunter." She then turned and scrambled up the back of the couch to a precarious position, leaning out over the back of the couch above the floor. The teacher told her that she had to get down, that she might hurt herself. She answered, "I want to go hurt myself," but came down. The teacher told her she wouldn't let her do things where she could get hurt as she helped her down. Sue then commanded, "Finish that book!" in a stern voice. "Who's shot?" Sue asked, and answered, "Babar, not his mommy." Then Sue closed the book again.

Sue seemed to want the child to be hurt rather than the adult. Self-hurting did not lead to real danger, nor did it become a chronic symptom for Sue. That such behavior was noted occasionally seemed consistent with the view that Sue had many unintegrated feelings, reactions, and unelaborated primitive fantasies.

Other examples reflecting precursors of guilt might include an incident wherein she noted her big teeth in a mirror and commanded to herself, "No biting!" and also her fear "Everything gonna die?" in response to her pulling up a plant.

IDENTIFICATION

Adults and children are often noted to identify with the lost object in a global or partial way, more global reactions occurring when less differentiation from the object has been achieved before the loss. Although Sue feared she would die, she did not seem to identify in a global way with her dead father. That is, she did not act as though she were her father. Instead Sue showed some interest in, or selective identifications with, aspects of her father, consistent with having achieved a more differentiated view of him. Thus she liked beaded necklaces. She commented that she had big eyes like her daddy, and she sang particular songs noting that they were songs he had sung. She also referred to daddy as a "monster daddy" at a time when she was playing "monster" scaring her peers. But none of these were persistent or intense interests.

Discussion

Sue's reactions to her father's death appear consistent with the concept of childhood mourning (Sekaer, 1986) in that Sue reacted to bereavement without developing serious fixations or conflicts, at least at the time, and appeared able to proceed with her development. Sue did not "mourn" like an adult, according to Freud's definition, since reality was tested only on a primitive level. Sue appeared to fit Anna Freud's criteria, but with the following limitations: she "understood" the "external fact" while at the same time maintaining contradictory facts in mind. Death was viewed as a departure: "He went far away . . . in the sky"; although Sue stated, "he can't come back," she did not accept the finality as she complained at 36 months, "I never see my daddy," and said, "He at work. . . . He can't come for me yet." The "fact" that she knew he "died" and "can't get out of the box" did not conflict with her other ideas. She appeared at least transiently to comprehend irreversibility with regard to a fish, but with her father she continued to view death as reversible. The dead cannot "do things," as she agreed the fish could not swim, and yet her daddy (as she said under stress) was "at work" and "can't get out of the box."

Causality was not understood by Sue, and instead with her primitive logic she associated by juxtaposition medical phenomena, forms of transportation, etc. She reacted fearfully to sleep as death. She also could not understand the low statistical likelihood of death at a young age. She had primitive notions of her own power, pulling up a plant and fearing "everything gonna die." Reality testing occurred with adult prompting: "Can he visit you now?" "No because he died." But the reasons for the death continued to be not understood and its irreversibility to be contradicted. Within these cognitive limits, clarifications of some of Sue's concrete confusions were definitely helpful. Thus explaining that sleep did not mean death alleviated her sleep difficulty, and explanations that flying in a plane was not "dying in the sky" resolved her fears about a trip. These explanations did *not* become generalized, nor did they lead to a higher cognitive level of thought.

Nagera (1970) says that the latency child's lack of acceptance of death is due to the child's *need* to keep the tie. The cognitive *inability to comprehend* the finality of death can also account for the split in the acceptance of "facts" of death and the continued belief in life of the lost one. Sue, typical for her prelogical level of thought, maintained many contradictory "facts" and ideas in her mind; this could not truly be called a split in her ego until she reached the level where more integrated thought is present. It is possible that Sue's mother conveyed to Sue some lack of acceptance of the finality of her husband's death and *her* wishes for his return, thereby undermining Sue's reality testing, but this appeared to play a minor role compared to Sue's cognitive limitations. Lopez and Kliman (1979) and Erna Furman (1974) argue that with adult help the "reality" can be understood and accepted. Yet, without follow-up one cannot rule out the existence or development of splits in the ego wherein the expectation of return of the parent is maintained even after such apparent childhood acceptance of "the facts."

The timing of bereavement in childhood is particularly important. Sue's personality development at the time of the death was at a plateau, perhaps more stable than it would have been a few months earlier or later. Sue had apparently achieved resolution of rapprochement. She gave evidence of libidinal object constancy as she talked of both her mother and father in their absence to reassure herself and continued to long for and talk of her father 8 months after his death. Sue had not yet shown evidence of oedipal conflicts at the time of the death. The stability of her personality is evidenced by the fact that she did not regress cognitively nor develop evident fixations on oral or anal levels. Similarly she did not regress along lines of separation-individuation nor deviate toward a less than optimal rapprochement outcome as described by McDevitt. Winnie (Barnes, 1964) appears to have been at a similar stage, whereas Diane (Lopez and Kliman, 1979) at 19 months was much more disrupted by her loss.

Sue did not appear to use identification with her father as a way of maintaining his presence. Though she played at being dead in a box after the funeral, she did not go on to reenact the death as did Lopez and Kliman's patient, who imitated, in jumping and falling, her mother's suicidal leap. Sue did not become confused about sexual identity nor act out being her father in other ways. Instead there were minimal selective imitations and identifications, such as singing songs he had sung or playing monster at a time she spoke of him as a monster. Perhaps there was less need to identify with him because her cognitive abilities did not exclude her maintaining a conscious belief in his existence. Or perhaps Sue as a preoedipal child did not need her father as strongly, being still more tied in with her mother. Sue's identifications with her mother were evident in her internalized controls, in her feminine manner and appearance, and in her play with mothering activities. She seemed to have had less of her personality dependent on identifications with her father. Or it is possible that Sue will identify more with her father in the future, for example, when she goes through the oedipal stage.

According to the Furmans, Anna Freud, and others, Sue should have been capable of decathecting her father. She did not appear to do this in the adult sense of detaching libido from the mental representation of the dead one, at least not fully detaching libido. But she did react affectively and cognitively in a prolonged struggle to deal with the death. One might infer decathexis from her observed sadness and longing for her father and from specific painful memories she described, e.g., "My daddy got me an umbrella." But the pain did not derive from knowledge that he would never return so much as from an awareness of his current absence, "I never see my daddy. . . . My daddy died. I didn't see him for a long, long time." Since she still talked of him as returning, "He at work. He can't come for me yet," she had clearly not gotten rid of the libidinal tie to him and held on to a belief in his continued existence.

Sue did not omit affect as did Deutsch's patients. But a great deal of her affect about the death emerged only in the private play sessions in her relationship to her special teacher. Sue's use of this tie, which intensified after her father's death, does not fit Wolfenstein's description of an "adaptation reaction" because it was not used *instead of* expressing pain over her loss. Sue could not turn inward alone to a preoccupation with thoughts about father as adults do, but was able to express feelings about the loss in the context of this relationship. Left alone, Sue may well have covered up her feelings and "omitted affect." Unlike an adult in grief, Sue needed an adult to share her feelings. It is doubtful that Sue would have worked through her loss with her mother. Her mother was herself bereaved, and thus less available to Sue, and also was inclined to minimize Sue's reactions to the death. Barnes's case omitted affect at 2½ after her mother's death until her grandmother was able to share the affective experience with her; one wonders if Winnie would have gone on to become symptomatic if grandmother had not become available to her. Diane used her transference tie to Lopez as a focus around which to organize her feelings, wishes, and memories about her mother.

If one follows the adult model, one might focus on assisting the child to accept the finality of death and to decathect the dead. If one, like Wolfenstein, views mourning as decathexis of the dead followed by a hiatus and then a recathexis of a new person, one may decide that a transfer of cathexis to another person is not mourning, but only an "adaptation." But if a child is better off avoiding a developmental vacuum, the optimal response for the child may be to transfer the tie to someone else or to maintain the cathexis of the dead one until it can be more slowly withdrawn. Sue did not have a substitute for her father at home onto whom she could transfer cathexis. Maintaining the fantasy of the dead's continued existence may allow the child to go on with crucial steps in development without interfering with reality testing in other areas.

Adults develop conscious and unconscious fantasies that embody and express the meaning of death to them. In normal mourning, realistic causes of death are accepted and irrational or pathological beliefs (e.g., that one's bad wishes caused a death) are given up. In a case cited by Neubauer (1967), "Mommy has killed Daddy . . . by giving him 'doody' to eat" was apparently a precocious formulation by a 2½-year-old. In Sue's play a single clear-cut theme representing the meaning of the death did not emerge. The death was viewed as a separation loss for which no single clear cause was articulated. Instead several possible themes were touched on: her ambivalent play, e.g., with the doll, Betsy, may have been a displacement of her mixed feelings of concern for and anger at her father. Her wish to have "Babar shot, not the mommy" and to hurt herself may have represented some early primitive guilt reactions. Her lack of expression of anger directed at her father may have meant such feelings were being denied or split off and could become a focus for later conflict. Or it may be that the death did not need to take on a pathological meaning based on inner or external conflicts on Sue's part. The fact that she did not become seriously symptomatic in the 8 months following his loss may mean she was reacting to the death in a nonpathological way within the limits for her age. In fact, it is this lack of development of serious or chronic symptoms that seems most comparable to *normal* mourning in an adult. Clearly Sue did react to and struggle to integrate her loss, facilitated by her therapeutic experience with her teacher, and yet without overt signs of pathology.

Children often find their own creative solutions to developmental or traumatic stresses. Infants create transitional objects to assist with separation from mother. Older children create imaginary companions to cope with a variety of stresses. Bereaved children sometimes maintain their dead parent as though still living in fantasy, as an imaginary parent (Sekaer, 1986). Sue readily expressed thoughts about her father as living ("He at work" . . . "My daddy can't come for me yet"). Her talk of father as returning at times and as not coming back at other times can be explained as typical inconsistencies of prelogical thought rather than a fantasy. However, her use of her father in remembered and fantasied roles took several forms. He assuaged loneliness and undid the loss ("I know he comes to my house on Sunday"). She invokes him as a punisher when angry at her teacher ("I'll tell daddy"); here he is also her rescuer helping her deal with the teacher. She spoke of her father as a scary monster who got shot, and seemed to identify with him as she played monster and scared other children. She thought of him as at a distance unable to reach her ("He at work. . . . My daddy can't come for me yet"). While these fragments hardly constitute an integrated fantasy of an imaginary parent, nevertheless they may represent the roots of such a fantasy which could become more integrated as her relationship to this imaginary father develops over time. The fact that she is motivated to think of him in these ways may represent the beginnings of a specifically cathected use of creativity. If Sue is able to use other substitutes along the lines of her special teacher (or a stepfather), she may feel less need for her father and may elaborate fewer fantasies about him, investing instead the substitute.

Children may also mourn at a distance (Wolfenstein, 1966), expressing affect for the dead one displaced onto toys, fictional characters, or pets. Sue appeared to do this in a primitive way through her use of the book about Babar, the Elephant, and with the dolls, Betsy and Ernie, insofar as she played out themes of loss and death with them. Though she certainly was able to express sadness and longing for her father, she seemed able to express more anger and ambivalence with Babar, Betsy, and Ernie, than with her father.

One may argue that the impact of the trauma, for Sue, may still have pathological effects in the future, that the loss may take on other meanings, e.g., as Sue goes through the oedipal stage, and that symptoms may form later. This is a problem inherent in discussion of any childhood trauma (Nagera, 1966). Since the child is growing and developing, any trauma may be reactivated if it resonates with later developmental conflicts even without further traumatic events. If one would call this a delayed pathological response, then one cannot speak of any childhood trauma as resolved until the child is grown. It is possible that analysis would have accomplished more by way of integrating Sue's feelings and fantasies. But perhaps not.

We may consider that Sue went through a childhood mourning with the help of her therapeutic relationship with her teacher to the extent that she resolved her reactions to the death as much as possible for her developmental level. Not all children who lose a parent react in a pathological manner; further studies are needed of bereaved children who do well, with or without therapeutic intervention, and of how they accomplish this.

BIBLIOGRAPHY

BARNES, M. J. (1964). Reactions to the death of a mother. *Psychoanal. Study Child,* 19:334–357.

BEMPORAD, J. R. (1978). A developmental approach to depression in childhood and adolescence. *J. Amer. Acad. Psychoanal.,* 6:325–352.

BOWLBY, J. (1960). Grief and mourning in infancy and early childhood. *Psychoanal. Study Child,* 15:9–52.

———— (1980). *Attachment and Loss.* New York: Basic Books.

DEUTSCH, H. (1937). Absence of grief. *Psychoanal. Q.,* 6:12–22.

FREUD, A. (1939–45). Infants without families. *W.,* 3.

———— (1960). Discussion of Dr. John Bowlby's paper. *Psychoanal. Study Child,* 15:53–62.

FREUD, S. (1917). Mourning and melancholia. *S.E.,* 14:243–258.

———— (1927). Fetishism. *S.E.,* 21:149–57.

FURMAN, E. (1974). *A Child's Parent Dies.* New Haven: Yale Univ. Press.

FURMAN, R. A. (1964a). Death and the young child. *Psychoanal. Study Child,* 19:321–333.

———— (1964b). Death of a six-year-old's mother during his analysis. *Psychoanal. Study Child,* 1:377–397.

GINSBURG, H. & OPPER, S. (1979). *Piaget's Theory of Intellectual Development.* Englewood Cliffs, N.J.: Prentice-Hall.

JACOBSON, E. (1954). The self and the object world. *Psychoanal. Study Child,* 9:75–127.

KATZ, S. (1976). The development of a child's concept of death. Unpublished thesis, New College.

KATZ, S. & FLYNN, V. (1982). A young child's response to death. *Daycare & Early Education,* fall, pp. 22–25.

LOPEZ, T. & KLIMAN, G. W. (1979). Mourning in the analysis of a 4-year-old. *Psychoanal. Study Child,* 34:235–271.

McDEVITT, J. (1980). The role of internalization in the development of object relations during the separation-individuation phase. In *Rapprochement,* ed. R. Lax, S. Bach, & J. A. Burland, pp. 135–150. New York: Aronson.

McDonald, M. (1964). A study of the reaction of nursery school children to the death of a child's mother. *Psychoanal. Study Child,* 19:358–376.

Nagera, H. (1966). *Early Childhood Disturbances, the Infantile Neurosis, and the Adulthood Disturbances.* New York: Int. Univ. Press.

———— (1970). Children's reactions to the death of important objects. *Psychoanal. Study Child,* 25:360–400.

Neubauer, P. B. (1967). Trauma and psychopathology. In *Psychic Trauma,* ed. S. Furst, pp. 85–107. New York: Basic Books.

Piaget, J. (1927). *The Child's Conception of the World.* New York: Littlefield, Adams, 1979.

Piaget, J. & Inhelder, B. (1951). *The Origin of the Idea of Chance in Children.* New York: Norton, 1975.

Sekaer, C. (1986). Toward a definition of childhood mourning (in press).

Winnicott, D. W. (1953). Transitional objects and transitional phenomena. *Int. J. Psychoanal.,* 34:89–97.

Wolfenstein, M. (1965). Death of a parent and death of a president. In *Children and the Death of a President,* ed. M. Wolfenstein & G. W. Kliman, pp. 62–79. New York: Doubleday.

———— (1966). How is mourning possible? *Psychoanal. Study Child,* 21:93–123.

———— (1969). Loss, rage, and repetition. *Psychoanal. Study Child,* 24:432–460.

Denial in Adolescence

Some Paradoxical Aspects
H. SHMUEL ERLICH, Ph.D.

THE QUESTION OF THE CHRONOLOGICAL CLASSIFICATION OF THE mechanisms of defense is an old one. Anna Freud, in her classic monograph (1936), has already touched on it and reached the conclusion that it should probably be left alone. "Instead," she wrote, we should "study in detail the situations which call forth the defensive reactions" (p. 57). This paper is correspondingly not going to advance the untenable proposition that there is in any way an association between the developmental crisis of adolescence and the emergence of the mechanism of denial. Both clinical and developmental experience make it abundantly clear that denial appears in relatively early childhood, although we may assert that the capacity for some differentiation of self from external reality is a prerequisite for its emergence. Once it appears, however, it becomes a constant, if only potential, feature of intrapsychic functioning throughout life.

Following Anna Freud's suggestion, we have actually learned a great deal about the nature of specific defenses by studying the vicissitudes of the situations that called them forth. Why under certain circumstances one prefers a particular defense mechanism to others may shed light on the defense itself. It seems to me that the same process could fruitfully be undertaken in the

Senior lecturer in clinical psychology, Hebrew University of Jerusalem; member, Israel Psychoanalytic Association; faculty, Israel Institute of Psychoanalysis.

Earlier versions of this paper were presented at the International Symposium on Denial, January 1985 in Jerusalem; and at the Yale University Child Study Center, September 1985.

reverse: we may gain a good deal of understanding about a particular situation or phenomenon by studying it through the prism of the defense mechanism employed to handle it. Such a study must rely, of course, on some previous knowledge of the defense in question.

I propose to look at the developmental crisis of adolescence through the operation of denial or disavowal. In doing so, I do not mean for a moment to suggest that adolescence is exclusively under the sway of denial as a defense mechanism, that this is the only or even main defense during the period, or that they are somehow uniquely associated with one another, so that adolescence more than other developmental periods can be characterized by denial. I do not think that such assertions can be proven, nor that they are particularly reasonable. But I do believe that a special fit can be shown to exist between some of the tasks and conflicts faced by the adolescent's ego and the method of handling and resolving conflictual tasks afforded by denial. Furthermore, I believe that the understanding of this fit can greatly enhance and contribute to our understanding of both adolescence and the operation of denial.

Although most clinicians would probably readily agree that compared to other age groups adolescents are no less, and probably even more so, disposed to deny, very little seems to have been written on the specific use or meaning of the utilization of denial in this period. As early as 1957, Jacobson pointed to a linkage between denial and action, or the tendency toward acting out: to the extent that acting out is designed to avoid remembering, it is a form of denial. In a later and much celebrated work, Jacobson (1964) seems to have set the stage for what has been the predominant theme in the adolescent literature, namely, the association of denial in adolescence with the adolescent's need to counteract the experience of his limitations. Internally, the adolescent is pitted between the seductive upheaval of a libidinal id and the iron grip of a sadistic superego, while externally he flaunts his independence of thought and action. Faced with such overwhelming pressures, the adolescent ego resorts to denial and isolation. The adolescent may make a great show of his acceptance, or rejection, or rebelling against various philosophies, views, and patterns of action. In reality, however, "for a long time he may not be able to achieve more than a pretense of independence, maintained with the aid of such denial and isolation mechanisms" (p. 184).

Echoing this theme of the adolescent's resorting to denial as a way of combating his helplessness and limitations, Blos (1963), in speaking about the predilection of some adolescents to taking refuge in the "magic of action and gesture," sees in it a reflection of the adolescent's "need to deny his helplessness through action, to affirm by exaggeration his independence from the archaic omnipotent mother, to counteract the regressive pull to passivity by denying his dependence on reality itself" (1979, p. 259). If the adolescent's efforts to resolve the conflicts presented by the incest taboo and bisexuality should founder, he "protects himself by a stubborn denial of any self-limitation, that grave affront to narcissism" (p. 480).

In a similar vein, Blos sees in the obedient son, who is ready to submit to the omnipotent, idealized good father and to trust in him, an attitude that is not based on anything realistic, and therefore something akin to denial (1979, p. 386). In all of these descriptions denial is associated exclusively with the smallness, weakness, dependence, and vulnerability of the adolescent vis-à-vis the parental figures, or of the adolescent ego faced with limitations to its narcissistic aspirations and in its dealings with unresolved negative oedipal issues.

Let us turn at this point from this brief review of the salient features of the treatment of adolescent denial in the literature to an equally brief examination of the mechanism of denial in and of itself. Freud referred to disavowal in a few telling contexts: in connection with castration anxiety (1923b), particularly as it stems from the recognition of the anatomical differences between the sexes (1925b) and in relation to fetishism (1927b); in discussing religion (1927a) and the pains of living; in studying the commonalities and differences of neurosis and psychosis (1924); and finally, in describing the mechanism of the splitting of the ego (1924, 1936, 1940). Two central characteristics emerge very clearly from Freud's treatment of the subject: (1) the relationship between denial and reality; and (2) the intimate tie between denial and splitting of the ego. I would like to underscore and develop these two aspects, since I see them as intrin-

H. Shmuel Erlich

sically and significantly related both to adolescence and to adolescent denial.

Denial is always in some primary focal relation to an aspect of *external reality*. While the work of denial proceeds from a relation to a segment of external reality, or perhaps even more accurately, from the relation between one's inner experience and a portion or phase of external reality, it must naturally have serious impact and implication for internal reality as well. When we speak of denial or of disavowal,[1] we are referring to that special psychological way by which something that is "really real," so to speak, is really there and we are in a certain relation to it, is rendered psychologically nonexistent, i.e., is nullified by the ego. This is obviously very different from the case of other defenses whose impact is primarily or exclusively on internal reality, and which strive to make all sorts of shifts and alterations only in our inner, psychic reality. Whereas the latter affect what happens at the interface of ego and id, the work of denial proceeds primarily at the level of ego and reality. In this sense, *it has an impact on both internal and external reality: internally,* mostly by affecting the ego's sense of what is real; and *externally,* through an alteration of the veridicality of perceptual processes. The most immediate implication of the recourse to denial is there-

---

1. The relationship between the terms "denial," "disavowal," and "negation" is ambiguous, frequently leading to confusion. One source of this ambiguity has to do with the translation of Freud's German. Freud first used the German *leugnen* in the context of denial, and then substituted for it the allied German form *verleugnen*. Both are usually translated as "to deny." In his paper on "Negation" (1925a) he introduced yet another term, using the German *verneinen,* which is also translatable as "to deny." Throughout the *Standard Edition* the latter is translated as "to negate," whereas *verleugnen* is translated with "to disavow" (see Editor's footnote 1 to Freud, 1923b, p. 143). Clearly, these are linguistically and psychologically overlapping functions to some extent. To the conceptual and linguistic contributions to this ambiguity must be added the geographic one, which is responsible for different preferences that follow a locally established norm. It should be pointed out that in the Index of the *Standard Edition* the term "denial" simply does not appear. This indicates, however, that we attempt to follow their definition and utilization with extra care, so as to minimize confusion and ambiguity. In this paper I follow common usage to the extent that I use "denial" and "disavowal" interchangeably, but maintain the distinction between this process and "negation," which is not included in my discussion.

fore the fact that it places the ego in an extremely hazardous, or at least a highly complex position in regard to reality.

Since reality testing is a *sine qua non*, essential aspect of the ego, the denial of a facet of external reality immediately places a tremendous burden on its continued integrity, and calls into question its ability to maintain its good function. Clearly, such crass handling of reality cannot go unnoticed or uncompensated. Sooner or later, with a greater or lesser degree of psychiatric righteousness, the culprit ego will have to face the music. But we are still left with the question: Why does the ego resort to a defense that endangers its very existence, and how does it manage to survive such a potential self-destruction?

An easy solution to this problem might be found if we could have relegated denial to the period of earliest childhood, when reality testing is still rough and poorly established; or if we could make the assertion that denial operates only in adults undergoing severe regressions, e.g., psychosis, and thus once again to regard denial as characterizing only those states in which ego pathology is both rampant and severe. Quantitative factors may be at work, alongside qualitative ones. Indeed, we speak at times of "blatant denial," referring to those instances where the aspect of reality denied is so preponderant that to deny it would have required a much greater expenditure of psychic energy, or suspension of good reality testing, than to merely ignore some relatively minor or unimportant aspect of reality. This is clearly not the case, however, and would in fact be a misleading way of applying the concept.

In answering our question, two points present themselves. In the first place, far from being involved in repudiating minor or inconsequent aspects of reality, denial is typically called upon precisely when very painful, highly charged, and conflicted issues are at stake. If this is not the case, the ego is far more likely to call upon defenses of lower costs to itself, e.g., displacement, avoidance, negation, or repression. We are probably correct in asserting that the ego is forced to call upon denial when faced with a piece of reality highly regarded by it, but also extremely threatening, and at the same time almost unavoidable by any other means.

Secondly, we must remember that *we may properly speak of denial*

only when and where it coexists with otherwise good reality testing, as
Anna Freud (1936) already established. If this condition were
not observed, we would have to restrict ourselves to speak of
denial only where regression is an accompanying process or
defense. It is, of course, true that we frequently meet with denial
in psychotic and otherwise regressed patients. But it is equally
true, as I am certain everyone has encountered, that we also find
denial in nonpsychotic persons, even if such encounters may be
accompanied by feelings of incredulity or dismay. We may perhaps even hazard making a risky statement in this connection: to
the extent that we do find denial in psychotics, this may be testimony to the fact that some good, more adequate reality testing
may still be preserved. The higher incidence of denial in psy-
chotically regressed populations may indeed not reflect lowered
reality testing per se, but rather something else, which is also
connected with denial, namely, the prerequisite tendency toward splitting of the ego; it is this tendency that is much more
preponderant in these populations, and hence there may be
easier recourse to denial.

We have thus come around to what constitutes the second
characteristic of disavowal, which complements and sheds light
on the first. If denial requires that good reality testing continues
to prevail in the rest of the ego, while a highly charged aspect of
reality is being denied, the implication can be only one: that the
ego has undergone a psychological process we have come to
regard as ubiquitous, namely, it has split or divided itself into
different parts. Thus, some portion of the ego experiences reality in a manner that can be described as being in adequate,
realistic contact with it, while other portions behave and respond
in a highly distorted way, as if whatever is regarded or sensed as
frightening or obnoxious does not really exist at all.

How is all of this related to adolescence and to adolescent
denial? Before we answer this question more directly, let us take
a second look at one of Freud's last papers in which he establishes
the role of the splitting of the ego in the operation of denial. I
refer to "A Disturbance of Memory on the Acropolis" (1936), in
which the octogenerian Freud describes to the 70-year-old Ro-
main Rolland an incident that took place in 1904, when Freud
was 48. On a holiday trip to the Mediterranean seaboard with his

younger brother, they both had a hard time accepting a friend's advice in Trieste that they should not proceed to the island of Corfu, as they had planned, but instead take the boat to Athens. Despite their gloomy mood and indecision, they followed the suggestion. When finally standing on the Acropolis, Freud had the surprising thought: "So all this really *does* exist, just as we learnt at school!" Freud's introspective account goes on to introduce the notion of the splitting of the ego:

> . . . the person who gave expression to the remark was divided . . . from another person who took cognizance of the remark; and both were astonished, though not by the same thing. The first behaved as though he were obliged, *under the impact of an unequivocal observation,* to believe in something *the reality of which had hitherto seemed doubtful.* . . . The second person, on the other hand, was justifiably astonished, because he had been unaware that the real existence of Athens, the Acropolis, and the landscape around it had ever been the object of doubt. What *he had been expecting was rather some expression of delight or admiration* [p. 241; my italics].

Freud's continued analysis of this fragment of experience centers around the feeling that to be given the actual opportunity to see Athens aroused strong feelings of incredulity, regret, and even depression—it was too good to be true! The fulfillment of this long-standing wish actually gave rise to a subjective experience of derealization, which is akin to depersonalization. It asserts that what is perceived is unreal, and aims to defend the ego by disavowing a piece of reality. But the denial is not merely of something in the here and now, but of something made meaningful through its intimate significance within one's past. It is in this connection that Freud's account becomes more eloquent, but also immediately and openly pertinent to adolescence:

> It is not true that in my schooldays I ever doubted the real existence of Athens. I only doubted whether *I should ever see Athens.* It seemed to me beyond the realms of possibility that I should travel so far—that I should 'go such a long way'. This was linked up with the limitations and poverty of our conditions of life in my youth. My longing to travel was no doubt also the expression of a wish to escape from that pressure, like the force which drives so many adolescent children to run away from

home. . . . When first one catches sight of the sea, crosses the
ocean and experiences as realities cities and lands which for so
long had been distant, unattainable things of desire—one feels
oneself like a hero who has performed deeds of improbable
greatness [p. 241 ff.; my italics.]

What is then stirred up, however, by the joy of the fulfillment
of such long-standing childhood dreams is the sense of guilt:

It must be that a sense of guilt was attached to the satisfaction in
having gone such a long way: there was something about it that
was wrong, that from earliest times had been forbidden. It was
something to do with a child's criticism of his father, with the
undervaluation which took place of the overvaluation of earlier
childhood. It seems as though the essence of success was to have
got further than one's father, and as though to excel one's father
was still something forbidden [p. 247].

Freud's personal account is not merely revealing—it strikes
the chords which I believe are the real issues around which
adolescent denial can most cogently be understood and met. For
to view adolescent denial as being couched primarily in weakness
and vulnerability is to distort our understanding of what happens at this crucial developmental crossroads. It is true that a
good deal of adolescent experience centers on issues of vulnerability, and hence of weakness—certainly internal, and to
some extent also on external weakness. And yet such emphasis
seems to miss the picture in some crucial way. The adolescent
arrives at this stage of development slightly out of breath, so to
speak: he has been panting and postponing for so long, in fact,
for all his life. He has deferred burning wishes and aspirations
for genital fulfillment, oedipal strivings, competition for supremacy and primariness, for strength and wisdom, for power,
accuracy, and control through knowledge—for so long, that, for
all he knows, these needs, wishes, fantasies, and aspirations may
indeed be only the myths invented by his elders in order to
subjugate and control him. His experience as a child in the world
of adults, whom he looks up to and wishes to emulate, has been
governed by a highly specific, constantly repeated, implicit injunction, underlying all his encounters with frustration, delay of
gratification, and postponement of self-indulgent fulfillment.

That injunction, clearly etched in his memory, says, "Not now, later—when you grow up." And now he suddenly finds himself standing in disbelief, with a mixture of joy and incredulity, on top of his Acropolis—he has finally arrived, or so it seems.

It seems to be of small wonder that the overwhelming sense of the adolescent should be one of derealization and depersonalization whenever he is faced with the new evidence of his senses— with the reality of his being as big, frequently as powerful, and to his mind certainly as smart as his elders. It is reality that tells him, in no uncertain terms, that the time has come to call in his debts, to collect the long-deferred promises. Reality also tells him that, should he only begin to allow his wishes some expression, he could not really be stopped. The sense of power and strength and the intoxicating nearness of the spoils of victory are almost overwhelming.

What are the obstacles to the adolescent's realization of his potential? A great deal has been written and said on this subject, so I will only briefly allude to the main themes. The most serious obstacles stem from the fact that those early aspirations are intimately tied to the same libidinally invested, infantile figures. The reawakened threats of incest, on the one hand, and the tremendous pulls to passivity and dependency on the other, require renewed and redoubled efforts at separation-individuation (Blos, 1967), as well as a shoring up of the old oedipal renunciations (A. Freud, 1958).

It very quickly becomes painfully obvious to the adolescent that his having arrived at his Acropolis, at the attainment of adultlike physical stature, sexual prowess, and the capacity for truly abstract logical and cognitive manipulations, is not quite what he had hoped for and imagined all through childhood. It is as though an eager guest has arrived too early at a party that hasn't quite started yet, and finds himself detained in the foyer by his embarrassed hosts "for just a little while longer." His forced detention may prove very valuable to him. It actually enables him to proceed with the internal work of modifying and remodeling psychic structure and object relations that are his real ticket to adulthood. Thus, he can gradually develop the capacity to escape the regressive pulls of passive-maternal and negative-oedipal strivings. He may remodel his superego along

milder, more reality-appropriate lines. His renunciation of the
oedipal longings opens the door to extrafamilial relationships in
which fuller expression of drives and wishes will eventually be
possible and even welcome. Through homoerotic, narcissistically invested first love relationships he can integrate his narcissistic
aspirations and strengthen his sense of self sufficiently, so as to
allow for his subsequent embarkation on heterosexual love relationships. Finally, out of these new capacities in both object relations and vis-à-vis his own self, a new sense of identity is shaped
and consolidated so as to be serviceable for times to come.

We can see and appreciate the importance of the adolescent
delay before reaching full adulthood. But to the *adolescent,* the
experience is one in which he must constantly engage in massive
denial. He must deny his *strength,* the reality of much of his
attainments, so as not to face prematurely the full consequences
of what and where he really is. In other words, he must deny the
reality of having arrived at the party, or at the Acropolis, so as to
be able to go on delaying and postponing. But he must equally
vehemently deny the reality of his weakness, stemming from
whatever immaturities still remain and persist in him, on both
the internal and external levels, and hence of his second best or
"not quite making it yet" status. For to fully accept and experience those portions of his reality, external as well as internal, that
are weak and childlike, immediately threatens him with unbearable, if covertly desired, headlong surrender to his longings for
childish passivity, with total capitulation to those forces he
strains to escape.

It is precisely this sense of the admixture of strengths and
weaknesses that arouses in the adolescent incredulity and joy on
the one hand, and tremendous fears and guilt over regressive
wishes on the other. He typically handles this dilemma by splitting his ego, by experiencing and presenting himself as strong,
potent, sexual, and capable on the one hand, while also showing
himself to be weak, small, vulnerable, asexual, and incapable.
This split in his ego enables one part of his self to deny the *real*
existence of the other, and yet for *all* of him to go on and accept
the continued but necessary delay a little bit longer. Subjectively,
the experienced split in the ego gives rise to states in which he
either feels himself to be unreal, as in depersonalization, or ex-

periences his external reality as unreal, as in derealization. Objectively, this process of ego splitting and denial of conflicting portions of his reality is precisely what enables the adolescent to establish the necessary psychological preconditions for the achievement of the moratorium he so much needs in order to consolidate his developmental gains.

While much depends, of course, on a variety of other factors that govern the overall state of ego strength, it is here, in this conflict between his strength and weakness, that we may look for the source of many adolescent experiences of a slightly dissociative nature.

I would like to stress that these dissociative experiences occur by and large at a subclinical level. They are another one of those sources of confusion that make the diagnosis and treatment of adolescent phenomena such a difficult task. We must also recognize that, much as they are a feature of the adolescent's subjective experience, these ego splits and the denials that are grafted onto and made possible by them are not at all easily verbalized or shared by the adolescent. This, of course, is a source of much consternation to the adults interacting with him, as they can never be certain which frame of mind they will find him in, and their response to his denial often ranges from rage to exhaustion.

Implications for Treatment and Clinical Illustration

In the hands of the clinician dealing with and treating adolescents, awareness of these subjective states, of the predilection to splitting, and the constant conflict between weakness and strength, regressive surrender and dangerous triumph, forms a powerful tool. Once he understands these conflicts and the developmental impasses they derive from, he can approach the adolescent much more easily. For as much as the adolescent finds it difficult, if not actually impossible and unthinkable, to verbalize these notions for the adult, he is extremely appreciative and relieved when the adult, or the therapist, takes the lead in verbalizing these conflicts for him. The relief is usually very dramatic and the need to deny will usually subside quite strikingly. When these needs are not verbalized and interpreted, however, we may contribute to a deepening split in the ego, helping the adolescent move in the direction of more of an "as if" personality, or to a deeper consolidation of a "false self." This clearly suggests that we must deal with this issue fairly early and forthrightly in adolescent treatment. A brief clinical vignette follows in order to help demonstrate some of the issues raised here.

Tamar, an 18-year-old, came to see me in the midst of real turmoil and crisis in her life. She had spent the last year and a half forming a group of youngsters who, like herself, were interested in doing their compulsory army service in the special format available to Israeli youth, combining regular army training and service with life and work on a kibbutz. As this group which she put together was not sponsored by one of the political or apolitical youth movements, this required concerted and sustained efforts on her part, and was obviously no mean achievement, and a real tribute to her initiative and leadership. Just before they began their official period at the kibbutz, she had spent time abroad, again feeling socially very successful. She arrived from that experience to the kibbutz feeling like "a new person." Her exuberance continued for several days, until the following incident took place. The counselor attached to their group, several years older and much admired by all the girls, showed some interest in her. He invited her to his room, and when she was there he took hold of her hand. She became very flustered, asked, "What's this supposed to mean?" and when he spelled out more clearly his interest in and attraction to her, she bolted and ran out. Over the next few days she became increasingly restless, tearful, and agitated. She was terribly ashamed of the rest of the group and was unable to work with or join them on social gatherings. Even entering the dining hall became unbearably painful. Several days later she left the kibbutz and the group, and withdrew from the program in a way that clearly burned her bridges behind her. She moved back to her hometown, and shortly thereafter came to see me.

Tamar was a big, vibrant, active, and lively girl. She was also a strikingly sensitive, attractive, thoughtful, and verbal person. The dramatic quality of the events and the emotional upheaval that accompanied them were indicative of an impulsiveness and even a measure of self-directed inner violence and aggression, which soon emerged more openly in depressive affect, a tendency to escape the world and hide under her bedcovers, and even some suicidal ideation. Despite these indications of how seriously upset and buffeted she was, Tamar was and still is very far from being psychotic, schizophrenic, or of borderline pathology. She maintained a firm grip on her object relations throughout, continued to be socially active, to work, and to manifest no deficiencies whatsoever in her overall ego functioning. Her central and repeated question was a puzzlement—how could this have happened to her, of all people?

Space does not permit much elaboration. Let me therefore summarize the answer that began to take shape as we attempted to understand and deal with her puzzlement. Tamar had lost her father early in her childhood, yet she repressed the feelings attached to him, while she also denied some aspects of the reality and meaning of the loss itself. An example of her denial was her inability to accept the fact that her mother was psychologically capable and available, after a time, for relationships with other men. Her proneness to denial was further prominently demonstrated in her revelation of a shameful childhood secret: for about three years, while in the early school grades, she would masturbate quite openly in class. She remained impervious to all requests by her mother and teachers to stop her habit, professing not to understand what they wanted of her, and simultaneously not having any conscious appreciation of the sexual pleasure she was deriving from it. At the same time, however, she was so embarrassed and ashamed that she actually gauged her progress in life by the gradual distancing and disappearing of all those who were privy to her secret and shame. Thus, moving on to high school was an important step in that direction; her trip abroad was another. Finally, her beginning a new life on the kibbutz meant that she was literally on new social and emotional grounds, thoroughly untainted by her past.

Her encounter with sexuality, in the form of the advances made by the counselor, was doubly significant and meaningful. She was suddenly, without warning or adequate preparation, thrust into a sexualized situation, with strong oedipal overtones, in which she was frightened by the upsurge of her own barely repressed wishes. But this was only one part of the story, the more conventionally focused-on part. She had also made valiant efforts to overcome, master, and deny these feelings and wishes so closely linked with her ego passivity and weakness. She saw them as part and parcel of her shame as a small girl, of what she was then unable to contain and hide. Now, she felt, she was finally big, strong, powerful, and successful—"a new person." As this "strong person" she would no longer have to fear those embarrassing and dangerous impulses, nor would she have to experience her passivity and helplessness before them. She had *repressed* her sexual wishes and oedipal longings for her father. But she now *denied* the *meaning* of the subtler forms of the man's attention, or of the situation she would find herself in if she went to his room. Feeling herself strong and invincible, she could not give way to those feelings and wishes that meant she was simultaneously small, desirous, potentially weak, and passive. Quite obviously, then, her sudden confrontation with the same wishes immediately broke down the denial and brought the "weak" and the "strong" persons in her, as it were, to a head-on, impossible conflict.

An important component of working through the dynamics of this conflict centered on her proneness to such denial. This took the form of becoming acquainted with her subjective experience of mild derealization. She would not, even though she could, distinguish clearly and carefully between reality and fantasy, between dreamlike inner states and the actualities of the situations she would find herself in. Once the diffusion of the boundary was pointed out and described, the different subjective experiences became almost immediately familiar to her. She could describe them with some distance, and gradually exercised control over them.

This tendency to ego splitting, with the attendant lowering of reality testing and self-esteem, and heightening of her proclivity to denial, though well circumscribed, was clearly reflected in many later instances. The usual pattern was one in which she would allow herself to enter situations which could not even be described as compromising, of which she had been given ample notice by the man involved, yet she would deny the clear warnings and innuendo, leading to some real unpleasantness and misunderstanding. She would later laughingly comment about the "unreal" nature of these events, saying that these were things that would ordinarily only be seen to happen in movies. She was actually quite taken aback when her little sister presented her with a poem in which she had clearly described her as confusing light and darkness, dreams and reality.

DISCUSSION

My examination of denial and its special position in adolescence has been implicitly couched in developmental issues. I will now reflect on some of the implications inherent in such a developmental approach in order to make these both more explicit and fruitful.

The most fundamental notion may have to do with the integrative nature of developmental processes. This notion, as represented by Anna Freud's developmental lines (1965), implies that the various intrapsychic components of the adolescent's internal makeup and personality, such as drives, ego functions, superego formation, and object relations, to name but the few most salient ones, are regarded as distinct parts of a whole, each undergoing its own maturational and developmental course. It is the metatask of development to achieve the increasingly good integration of these various parts and components. The strains and energic upheavals of this integrative effort can be observed at various nodal points in development, seen as points of developmental disturbance (A. Freud, 1969). This view of development is primarily a hierarchical-integrative one, in which various distinct functions are increasingly brought together in harmony and into a hierarchical order with each other. This is essentially the model introduced by Freud (1905) with regard to the development of the sexual drive and its component instincts. I would add to this model the notion of the dialectics between different developmental stages, implying that each component is also in some antagonism to its own previous source, aim, or object. In adolescence, for example, the various components are also antagonistically related to their earlier, infantile, and/or latency sources. Out of the tension of having to oppose, each component is propelled forward in its own developmental track.

This way of thinking about development brings to mind a horse race, with the various components alluded to serving as the different horses or riders, all bent forward toward some common aim or finishing line, yet some of them racing ahead more rapidly than others, who may lag behind for a time. This metaphor may serve for all developmental periods. But when we apply it to adolescence, a paradox immediately comes to mind, which indeed captures something unique to this developmental stage. For in adolescence we may observe the race to enter into some of its final laps and therefore also its fiercest, most competitive and accelerated phases. At the very same time, however, the adolescent can be seen, and indeed needs to be allowed, to be at a standstill. This need is what is usually referred to as the need of the adolescent for a moratorium, in the service of integrating and harmonizing his developmental achievements. Denial, and the ego splitting it entails, can be seen as an important tool in achieving this adolescent moratorium. It allows the adolescent the respite he requires in order to bring together and integrate his strengths and weaknesses while standing still or marking time. Such a prolonged or momentary "holding off" through denial, as well as other intrapsychic mechanisms, assists the adolescent in preventing either side of him from becoming too dominant prematurely in action or in character formation. An overly keen or rigidly precise insistence on objective reality at this stage may indeed have deleterious effects. The need for denial and its adaptive, developmentally beneficent use may be compared with Winnicott's admonition in reference to the creation of the child's transitional object (1953). The magical and illusory aspects of the toddler's achievement in creating the transitional object fly, in that sense, in the face of good reality testing. Yet too strict an adherence to or insistence on good reality testing robs the child of his creation, to the detriment of the subsequent development of his capacity for fantasy life, imagination, and adequate formation of his sense of self and other.

There are numerous corollaries and manifestations of the inherently paradoxical nature of the adolescent tension between strength and weakness, between underlying helplessness and grandiose omnipotence. One such corollary is the adolescent's preoccupation with and frequently encountered predilection for some form of flirtation with death. In certain instances, when this predilection is coupled with strong longings for maternal reunion on the one hand, and particular qualities of cognitive functioning on the other, it may constitute a serious indication of suicidal tendencies (Erlich, 1978). Denial can be seen to play an important role in this context. In the first place, it is crucially related to the adolescent's weakness, the regressive pull of the powerful longings for union and fusion with the early, mostly preoedipal mother. It enables him, on the one hand, to deny these feelings of yearning for another, long-past state. On the other hand, it makes possible such obvious cognitive errors as are involved in a concrete treatment of one's own continued existence after death. These cognitive errors are at base the reflection of the admixture of more advanced and abstract levels of cognition with more concrete, childish ones. Yet denial plays an important role here, in continuing the split in the ego that makes it in turn possible for two cognitive modes, and the very different ideation attached to each, to continue to exist side by side, in a parallel fashion. The flirtation with death, with its underlying omnipotent underpinnings, constitutes a subtle denial of the adolescent's real strength, and paradoxically also of his weakness, both of which are implied in his realization of his actual flesh-and-blood, finite existence, as well as the libidinal and aggressive implications it entails, in the sense of his actual ability to terminate this existence, again with all its aggressive and libidinal meanings and consequences.

My discussion of the role of denial in adolescent development would be incomplete if I did not examine it also in relation to the recurring process of separation-individuation during adolescence (Blos, 1967) and point to at least some of the many implications. Notably, in both Freud's own journey to the Acropolis as in his reference to "the force which drives so many adolescent children to run away from home," his allusions to "crossing the oceans" and "experiencing as realities cities and lands which for so long had been distant, unattainable things of desire"; as well as in the incidences in our clinical vignette of going abroad, leaving home, and returning there—in all of these the imagery of travel, of moving across space (and time), is very prominent. This is immediately connected with the adolescent's struggle

with his own distance from the family, from the libidinal and
aggressive object relations and internalized objects of the past,
and the establishment of his own autonomy and identity.

There are several levels at which we may note the impact that
the adolescent's need to deny both his strengths and weaknesses
and the ongoing process of his separation-individuation have on
one another. The adolescent's concerns with weakness and wishes for strength are couched in his earlier object relations with
significant others, with whom he compares himself and with
whom he also established deep identificatory processes. In fact,
the comparative process may be viewed as but one aspect of these
deeper, more pervasive identificatory processes. It is important
to bear in mind that such identifications also represent, at another level, residual defensive actions—the resolutions of sexual
and aggressive conflicts permanently structuralized and absorbed by the ego (Freud, 1923a). As such, they are set up in
order to fend off, control, and contain a variety of specific and
nonspecific anxieties. The best model for this process, in terms
of clarity and decisiveness, is the resolution of castration anxiety
over phallic-genital strivings in the course of the oedipal phase
of development and the subsequent identification with the par-
ent(s), resulting in the consolidation of the superego and its
anxiety. Even in terms of this model, it was always important to
emphasize that the identification is with both the active and
passive parents, with both masculinity and femininity, and, in
my terms, with both strength and weakness. As the adolescent
compares himself to the significant others who represent for
him the various aspects of strength and weakness, he is therefore, in the first place, stirring up the old anxieties that such
comparisons evoked in him. But because of his need to separate
and individuate, he is also running the danger of undermining,
as it were, the defensive value of his old identifications. For now
"to be like" the significant other is no longer as acceptable a
solution as it was in childhood. Indeed, "to be like" carries within
itself the implications of a *being* object relation (Erlich and Blatt,
1985), namely, a relation experienced primarily in terms of narcissistic boundlessness and oneness of self and object. Such a
striving for being one with the other obviously runs counter to
the requirements of the separation-individuation process, which
dictates a pull in the opposite direction.

Thus the very processes of intrapsychic identification the adolescent engages in in order to gain his freedom and autonomy arouse, or threaten him with, some of the old anxieties he has sought to escape as a child, such as anxiety over oral-cannibalistic incorporation of the object, anal destructiveness, or castration anxiety over phallic-competitive strivings toward the object. The older, primarily libidinally cathected identifications are challenged and undermined, at least in terms of their defensive functioning, by the newly arrived-at comparisons of self to significant other. On the other hand, the process of individuation of self from other requires that he not allow himself a narcissistic, fusion or merger type identification with the old familial objects. We may find in these constraints some of the forces that are behind the adolescent's need to set up narcissistically based, ego-idealized, new self-comparative processes as such powerful alternatives to the older, libidinally invested identifications. Furthermore, it may also provide an explanation for what makes it necessary for him to remove the arena for such self-comparisons from the old, familial one to newly acquired and narcissistically heavily invested extrafamilial objects.

There is, however, a deeper level to this dilemma. Beyond his need to compare and identify himself, the adolescent is burdened by the need to encompass, shoulder, and internalize the various attributes, contents, and consequences of such identifications into himself. He must, in order to complete the process he embarked on, attribute the strength and weakness he finds and develops to himself and work them into his own newly reestablished ego identity and sense of self (Erickson, 1959). In this sense, he is engaged in a process which leaves him increasingly with only his own self to contend with, as being responsible for both his strengths and weaknesses. This responsibility is, in effect, a newly achieved liberation and loneliness. The adolescent senses the tremendous opportunities and risks of finding himself alone at the apex of his achievement, of standing alone on top of his Acropolis after his long climb up. Denial in this connection is therefore clearly a means for postponing the elaboration of the developmental capacity to be alone (Winnicott, 1958).

We may take another step further here, and take a brief look at the confluence of early object relations, the development of adequate ego functioning, and good reality testing. The very young child experiences reality largely through the interaction with and internalization of object relations with significant adults. His perceptual processes are constantly shaped and influenced by such internalizations, just as much as they play a role in the evolvement of such interactions and relationships. It is through this matrix of dynamic, interactive, internal structuring of both perception (ego functioning) and object relations that the child acquires and establishes his sense of reality, internal and external, as well as his capacity to test and discriminate about reality. There is an inherent connection between, or almost a sameness about, the child's capacity to *know* about himself, about others, and about the real world. One might say, in a sense, that "good reality testing is good other-relating." Whatever the child *knows* about reality implies essentially a knowledge shared and sustained by an object relation with a significant adult. *Knowing* is thus much more than mere cognizing. It can be traced to its libidinal roots, already familiar to us in the Biblical sense of the term.[2]

Thus viewed through the prism of denial, we can see in relief the dynamic struggles between the adolescent's need for separating and individuating, establishing an autonomous sense of self and other, and his need, on the other hand, to rely upon and reintegrate into this new self early object relations around which much of his sense of inner and outer reality had been formed and organized. He must now leave behind much of his old libidinal investment in objects, even though that investment is also a cornerstone of his knowledge about the world and external reality, as well as the more internal, experiential reality of his own self and of others. If he is determined to know more about reality, he must gradually have less recourse to denial, so that his ego can operate more fully and freely in its focal relation to reality, both internal and external. It may now become his new need to know reality as much and as intensely as only he himself can and must know it. This newly reestablished and reintegrated need is, perhaps, also what will now contribute more heavily than most other needs to his eventual gaining of autonomy and self-sufficiency as an adult, contending with the realities of him-

2. "And Adam knew Eve his wife; and she conceived and bore Cain" (Genesis, 4:1). "And Adam knew his wife again; and she bore a son" (Genesis, 4:25).

self and others. This need to know what is "really there" will also be, however, what leads to his being alone with his responsibilities, facing both his guilt over what he knows and his own doubt in it, and doing his best not to take shelter in denial.

SUMMARY

I have reviewed the particular fit between denial and adolescent development and experience. Denial, in my view, directly involves some aspect of external reality, and indirectly also internal reality, and is made possible by a split in the ego. In the adolescent, the real attainment of adultlike possibilities creates an enormous conflict between the need and wish to exercise these new capacities, the anxiety aroused by them, and the fear of equally potent regressive childhood pulls. The adolescent, caught between his real strengths and weaknesses, tends to split his subjective experience, denying through action, gesture, or experience the more disturbing parts at the moment. Denial, in the adolescent contexts pursued here, is evidently closely linked with the developmental paradoxes and fundamental contradictions that make human functioning the complex phenomenon that it is. For the adolescent, denial may be used in the service of integration and forward developmental thrust, but also to achieve moratorium and mark time. It may sustain the adolescent's efforts toward separation from parental figures and standing alone, disavowing the anxieties engendered. But it may also represent the ultimate renunciation of autonomy, of the capacity to know the world in one's own way and on one's own terms. The most extreme form of the latter is found in the regressive relinquishment of the adolescent's capacity to know, passively resigning himself to a distorted and private view of reality, as is the case in the most severe adolescent psychotic pathologies. The correct assessment and handling of each case is the clinician's prerogative and predicament.

BIBLIOGRAPHY

Blos, P. (1963). The concept of acting out in relation to the adolescent process. *J. Amer. Acad. Child Psychiat.*, 2:118–136.

———— (1967). The second individuation process of adolescence. *Psychoanal. Study Child*, 22:162–186.

———— (1979). *The Adolescent Passage*. New York: Int. Univ. Press.

ERIKSON, E. H. (1959). *Identity and the Life Cycle*. Psychol. Issues, monogr. 1. New York: Int. Univ. Press.

ERLICH, H. S. (1978). Adolescent suicide. *Psychoanal. Study Child*, 33:261–277.

ERLICH, H. S. & BLATT, S. J. (1985). Narcissism and object love. *Psychoanal. Study Child*, 40:57–79.

FREUD, A. (1936). *The Ego and the Mechanisms of Defense*. New York: Int. Univ. Press, 1946.

———— (1958). Adolescence. *Psychoanal. Study Child*, 13:255–278.

———— (1965). *Normality and Pathology in Childhood*. New York: Int. Univ. Press.

———— (1969). Adolescence as a developmental disturbance. *W.*, 7:39–47.

FREUD, S. (1905). Three essays on the theory of sexuality. *S.E.*, 7:135–243.

———— (1923a). The ego and the id. *S.E.*, 19:12–66.

———— (1923b). The infantile genital organization. *S.E.*, 19:141–145.

———— (1924). Neurosis and psychosis. *S.E.*, 19:149–153.

———— (1925a). Negation. *S.E.*, 19:235–239.

———— (1925b). Some psychical consequences of the anatomical distinction between the sexes. *S.E.*, 19:248–258.

———— (1927a). The future of an illusion. *S.E.*, 21:5–56.

———— (1927b). Fetishism. *S.E.*, 21:152–157.

———— (1936). A disturbance of memory on the Acropolis. *S.E.*, 22:239–248.

———— (1940). Splitting of the ego in the process of defence. *S.E.*, 23:275–278.

JACOBSON, E. (1957). Denial and repression. *J. Amer. Psychoanal. Assn.*, 5:61–92.

———— (1964). *The Self and the Object World*. New York: Int. Univ. Press.

WINNICOTT, D. W. (1953). Transitional objects and transitional phenomena. In *Collected Papers*, pp. 229–242. New York: Basic Books, 1957.

———— (1958). The capacity to be alone. In *Maturational Processes and the Facilitating Environment*, pp. 29–36. London: Hogarth Press, 1979.

A Paradigm of Development

The Psychoanalysis of an Adolescent
ROBERT M. GLUCKMAN, M.D.

"PSYCHOANALYSIS IS DEVELOPMENT," STATED A PANELIST AT A meeting of the child psychoanalytic association a few years ago, as he was elaborating on a paper about the therapeutic effects of child psychoanalysis. This is neither a new nor controversial idea in classroom psychoanalysis.

While there is much theoretical exposition of this idea in the literature, clinical data usually are confined to a brief example of fragments of analyses. There are very few case presentations demonstrating the clinical unfolding of the process of redevelopment from beginning to end through analysis. To illustrate how psychoanalysis provides the opportunity for a person fixated in his early development to achieve age-appropriate functioning, I present the case of an adolescent boy whose developmental interferences occurred at the preoedipal and oedipal periods, leaving him totally unprepared for the psychological demands of adolescence. The analysis of this youngster, roughly from ages 15 to 18, particularly illuminates the developmental transition from prelatency to adolescence in terms of one of the most crucial tasks of adolescence: the achievement of sexual maturity.

Sigmund Freud (1905) stated that "One of the main tasks of early adolescence is to give infantile sexual life its final normal shape," namely, "the subordination of component instincts to the primacy of the genital zone" (p. 207). Anna Freud (1958)

Associate professor of Clinical Psychiatry, Northwestern University Medical School, Chicago, Ill.; head of Child Psychiatry, Departments of Psychiatry and Pediatrics, Evanston Hospital, Evanston, Ill.

337

added, "Normally the organization of ego and superego alter sufficiently to accommodate the new, mature forms of sexuality. However, in less favorable circumstances, a rigid, immature ego succeeds in inhibiting or distorting sexual maturity" (p. 257). As Kestenberg (1969) puts it, the job of the psychoanalyst is not only to remove obstacles to orderly development, but to ally himself with the progressive developmental forces of a given phase.

This aspect of our unique task as psychoanalysts is so very important because of the intense resistance to progressive change that takes place at each major transition point. As Davidson (1974) points out, "the adolescent phase provides the opportunity for completion of the wish to become a man or woman" (p. 266); but while the pull toward progression is strong, the resistance against that progression—the wish to remain a child—is also very strong. Without the aid of analysis to foment completion of the adolescent developmental process, the pregenitally fixated adolescent undoubtedly will remain a severely handicapped individual. Psychoanalytic treatment can be regarded as effective, Neubauer (1976) points out, when the excluded components of infantile sexuality are brought into his later organization.

Summarizing many contributions to our understanding of adolescent dynamic psychology and the effects of analytic therapy, Laufer (1981) states that the primary function of adolescence is the establishment of the final sexual organization, and that the essential component of adolescent pathology can best be understood as a breakdown in this developmental process.

THE ANALYSIS OF PAUL

Paul D. was initially brought to me, at the age of 12, with the principal complaint of enuresis, which had begun at age 5. The problem had recurred after Paul had trained himself at age 3 (the parents having practiced a laissez-faire attitude). Paul was the second oldest of five children. Mrs. D. had been a teacher, but was now primarily a mother, wife, and housekeeper; his father was an orthopedic surgeon. Both parents had had analytic therapy.

Mrs. D. described the father as a very bright, talented man, capable of very strong loving feelings but also of intense hostility. He was a very energetic man, who went into analysis primarily because of essential hypertension.

The mother described their family life as somewhat hectic, with the father extremely busy and herself quite burdened with the care of the children. His frequent irritability often would precipitate open arguments between the two of them. Mrs. D. was sure the children felt her tension.

Mrs. D. reported that Paul was the only enuretic child in the family, but that she had also been enuretic as a child. Paul also had a disposition toward asthma, usually of allergic cause but occasionally brought on by emotional stress. She reported that he had been quite shy when entering kindergarten, taking weeks to feel comfortable with the group. He began night wetting at this time, although not every night. He slept soundly, often sleeping through the wetting. Over the years various techniques to overcome the problem had been tried, including an electrical buzzer apparatus, all without success.

Paul's behavior and academic adjustment at school were exemplary, as he was a very bright, conscientious boy, making quite high grades. She described him as a very nice boy, quite responsible, but tending to do things alone rather than with a group of friends. He liked to ride his bike and explore new areas. Other boys seemed to like him, and he them, but he had no use for girls. She saw him as not being strongly masculine in his behavior or appearance, as he was slim and wiry and cried easily, due, she thought, to great sensitivity. Mrs. D. was very sure that Paul had no interest in sex and had engaged in no sexual activity of any kind. She had always been quite close to Paul and he had always been strongly attached to her. She remembered his babyhood as having given her quite a bit of pleasure. In fact, he was the only one of her children who appeared in her dreams during her analysis. During Paul's early years his father had been clearly partial to the oldest boy, but the relationship with Paul had improved over the years. However, on the rare occasions when Paul had argued with his father, Dr. D. had become infuriated.

Paul was a large infant with a rather large head, which created a lot of tension in the mother. She breast fed for several months and enjoyed it. He tended to be rather passive in early life, a little slow in crawling and walking, but a fairly early talker. He napped in the afternoons until shortly before entering kindergarten. He had sucked his thumb until age 6. There was much competition with the older child.

In her own upbringing there had been rigid rules, with little opportunity to express herself openly and freely. She had been a timid, insecure child, with many fears, but very dependent on her mother and devoted to her father, an attorney. She appeared as a large-boned, plain-looking, yet attractive woman, matter-of-fact in manner, with little affectation; she seemed to adapt to reality well.

An interview with the father revealed that his early memories of Paul were of a crying child, which irritated him to the point where he would shake Paul fairly hard. He recalled that Paul was frightened of him and usually shied away, but said that recently they had been getting along much better. His wife had been more protective of Paul than the older boy. Like Mrs. D., he saw Paul as a very sensitive child. His main concerns, however, were the asthma and enuresis.

The interview with Paul at age 12 revealed a slender, blond, pale, delicate-looking boy who was anxious and looked younger than his age. He was inhibited in expressing himself spontaneously due to the anxiety. Tears came readily, creating the impression of a child feeling helpless and seeking protection. He identified bed wetting as his main problem, revealing shame in talking about it. He had no idea why this behavior occurred. His anxiety heightened as I probed for early memories. When he expressed jealousy of the younger children, he began to cry openly. Of particular note in this interview was the impression he made of not having reached psychological or physiological pubescence. When asked his preferred age, he said he wanted to be younger, perhaps 10.

I pointed out to the parents that many boys stop bed wetting as the developmental shift into pubescence takes place, and they decided to wait a while longer to see if this would happen.

Two years later, the mother called and said Paul was still enuretic and was not showing any psychological signs of pubescence. He was almost 15 and in the first months of his second year of high school.

An interview with the mother revealed that the wetting still occurred almost nightly and that Paul had developed an attitude of resignation about it. He continued to do extremely well in school, had some male friends, but had not shown the slightest interest in girls. He had a strong interest in craftwork and did fine creative work with metal and wood. He was also very good at repairing things around the house. One change was that he tended to be less tearful and more able to show open anger. He had begun collecting things, mainly coins and stamps. Mrs. D. described him as a very neat, orderly, well-organized boy. He was a violinist in the school orchestra and delivered newspapers. Mrs. D. said Paul was also interested in earning and saving money. He never kissed her anymore or let her kiss him. She saw Paul's relationship with his father as being fairly good at that time. She also reported the parental relationship as being much better.

Paul was again seen for a diagnostic session, but he related in this session as if he had already made a therapeutic commitment, in that he talked of building a private, secret room in the attic just for himself and told of two dreams he recalled from early childhood. The first dream had to do with mistrust of father figures. The second had a similar theme with reference to peers.

In the second hour, he reported his first treatment dream: a pleasant, benign family outing that turned into a dangerous, threatening experience for him. He described great anxiety related to a fear of dogs. He spoke about setting up a communication system with a friend in his attic room. He had difficulty sitting opposite me and so readily accepted continuing the therapy lying on the couch.

The next several hours had mainly to do with Paul's orientation to the analytic situation and process. He intended to reveal early his principal defenses of intellectualization and compulsive repetition. He mentioned that he planned to assume a passive role in relation to male peers.

Anxiety manifested itself in regard to what meaning I would have for him, and he revealed that when little he had sucked his thumb and rubbed his fingers together to experience a smooth pleasant sensation. He talked of conflicted feelings about growing up and hoped that helping him with this problem was one of the purposes of the therapy; he wondered what he would be like after it was all over. He wanted me to know that he had no use for girls and was sure he would never marry. Then he had a fantasy that the only way anyone would ever know he was an adult would be if he disguised himself as an old man.

He wanted me to know, however, that he really did not wish to continue bed wetting and really did want help. He reported a fantasy of exploring new dark houses and dark caves, and associated having a comfortable, pleasant feeling with such thoughts. Such fantasies expressed regressive wishes to return to an earlier protective state. He wondered how I was going to feel toward him when he told me all his thoughts and said he did not like his father to know when he wet.

He reported that his violin teacher had recently died of a heart attack and related that to his own fear of separation and loss. Then his fantasies turned to control and power and concerns about becoming overly dependent on me. This led to his mentioning his asthma for the first time, which was followed by thoughts of being secretive and withholding.

His first thoughts of sex came in the 25th session, as he wondered whether he would ever have any interest. This was followed by memories of his first enuretic experience at age 5. He remembered having worried that his mother would be angry at him and recalled her coming into his room and looking at him and he feeling very frightened. He became more anxious at this point in the analysis and more resistant to coming for his appointments, but he knew he would come because he always did what his parents asked of him, as he feared something might happen if he did not.

As the analysis progressed, Paul spoke of it as having become the center of his life and said that he noticed that he sometimes had hot, prickly feelings during sessions, to which he associated feelings of fear. At times, he described feeling little and weak during sessions, while at other times he fantasized feeling big and strong.

He frequently revealed thinking that I would try to trick him so he would react certain ways or reveal certain thoughts and feelings. To this he associated feeling more dependent on me— in fact, on the whole analytic experience—and having mixed feelings about it. This became an increasing preoccupation. He wondered how much I would worry about him if he missed an appointment, but he also knew he would not do that because of feeling anxious about displeasing me. He then had thoughts that being a teenager was all right, but it interfered with the pleasures derived from earlier, regressive memories.

He began having more fantasies of superpower and rivalry with other patients of mine. He wondered if he were fighting growing up through his bed wetting. This made him think of how afraid of punishment he was if he did not complete assignments of schoolwork. He reported a dream in which his father was very angry at him for shaking ice off trees onto cars. It reminded him of how angry his father had been when he took the father's typewriter to his attic room without asking permission; as a younger child, he had been in constant fear of his father. He felt very anxious in the dream. He again spoke of his growing dependence on me, which frightened him because it meant being weak and helpless. He made the same association to his bed wetting.

In the 59th hour he told of being afraid of losing a finger in a wood shop and recalled having read of a boy whose arm was sheared off but then sewed back on. I told him that when he folded his arms across his chest, he would wheeze for a brief time; his association was that the wheezing also made him feel little and weak. At times, he said, he had the thought that he might wet himself during his sessions, which no doubt would make me very angry. My anger would frighten him so much that he would cry, as he had so many times for various reasons with his mother and father. He had always been afraid he would be spanked when he wet. These memories aroused resentment toward his father, and he thought of ways he could outsmart him. He then realized he had occasionally had such thoughts about me, too.

In the 73rd hour he wondered for the first time if his wetting had more to do with his mother than his father and also if there was any connection between the wetting and his generally passive nature. He had always thought that if he became too aggressive, his father would get angry at him, which was the way I might react if he ever asserted himself by missing an appointment. He then told me that he had become more fearful since he started analysis but compensated for this by thinking of getting rich and powerful. In the 78th hour he recalled a memory of very early childhood (perhaps a screen memory) of waking up crying and being extremely frightened, and his mother coming in but looking very frightening with her red glowing eyes.

Once he came to a session with his pants wet from rain, to which he jokingly associated that he finally had wet the couch. Then he spoke of having felt more than once like crying when he had been anxious in a session but had not let himself do so because of fear I would get very angry at him, as his father had.

In the 84th hour, his curiosity about my private life was expressed through inquiries about what I kept in a closet and under a drape. His anxiety continued to increase in the sessions as he wondered if I were angry at him for having canceled an appointment to go on a weekend trip with his family.

In the 86th hour, he said that while lying on the couch, he had pleasurable tingling sensations that felt like blood rushing into his extremeties. Then he had a sensation that the ceiling was moving toward and away from him, which led to fantasies of punishment and the statement, "but I have never actually had any physical punishment from you." He fantasized someday missing the appointment, but even though I would get angry, I would miss him.

Paul speculated that his enuresis was related to an excessive dependency on his mother, which made him wonder if those same feelings in the analytic situation might not interfere with cessation of the bed wetting. This led to memories of when he was a little child, sucking his thumb and crying a good deal. He again recalled that the first time he wet was the night he saw his mother with the glowing red eyes, but now he remembered that at about that time she told him she was going to have another baby.

He informed me during the next hour that he had fallen off his bike and sprained his wrist. He had not told his father for fear that his father would do something that would hurt him even more. Paul then speculated that if the parents should die, his enuresis might stop, but he would want to continue his analysis anyway, using his inheritance to do so. His father had gotten angry at him again because he broke a lamp at home. He thought of our relationship as like that of father and son. He then wondered about the vacation his family was planning for the summer; he was not sure he wanted to go and wondered what I would be doing during that time.

Shortly thereafter he fell off his bike again when he looked at a girl coming out of my building, while quickly denying that he had had any sexual thoughts or feelings in relation to her. He promptly added that he had a friend who was interested in girls.

In the 104th hour, he had the first conscious thoughts of homosexuality, comparing himself with a boy he referred to as effeminate. Following this, he remarked on seeing the movie *Moll Flanders* on the late show. He said sexual feelings seem to be impossible for him, as he was still too young to experience them. I interpreted his fear of not letting himself have sexual feelings as a way of not letting himself become adolescent. That night he wet the bed again and had the thought that Julie Andrews really seemed to be a mother, not a lover, type of a person to him.

He told of winning an election in English class, but felt more frightened than pleased about "beating" another boy. Then he reported becoming separated from his father and brother in a museum and being afraid of his father getting angry at him. For this same reason, he felt it was so important to please me. He then missed the next hour without canceling. The following session (110th) was the last before my summer vacation. He explained that he had missed the previous hour because he had fallen asleep and had not awakened until it was too late; he felt very anxious about coming today.

In the first hour after vacation, Paul told me that he was building an underground room in the backyard, but did not want his father to know. He then reported a dream he had had while I was on vacation: "There was a large log house with many residents; all were quite anxious, for an old woman in haggard clothes came and set fire to the bushes around the house. I helped put the fire out, and helped chase the old woman away."

In the next hour he told me of having had a dream that he had missed an appointment. He woke up feeling very frightened. He talked of his fear of God, his father, and me. Things were beginning to change for him; he seemed to be feeling better about himself and was having a greater sense of security in the analytic situation, as he did not seem to be afraid of doing something wrong. Then he told me of doing well in gym, but he had had a fantasy of hurting his leg and not being able to use it. I interpreted the castration fears. In a subsequent hour, he entertained the thought that maybe when he grew up he might want to get married and recalled a bet he had made with his father before he began analysis that he would never get married and that he had also proposed the same bet to me earlier. He had a fantasy that if he came for a session and the outer glass door were locked, he would just crash through it. This brought to mind that when he was little, he would get up at night to look for his mother and would find his parents' door closed. I interpreted the regressive wish. He then spoke of not living up to all his own expectations and feeling disappointed in himself.

When he had his 16th birthday, he spoke of now being able to drive a car, which implied being more grown up; yet he was not sure that was what he wanted. Then he revealed that he had always had some fear of the dark and fantasized wolves being in the dark basement of his house.

When his bike was stolen, he anticipated that both his father and I would be angry and disappointed. Later he spoke of thinking of Kim Novak and having a feeling inside of him that he thought could be what sexual feelings are like; but he still felt very uncomfortable in relation to girls and thought of sex as being dirty—and then he suddenly realized he had said the same thing about his wetting.

The next hour he reported a dream of "being in a park with two women when suddenly my pants and underwear disappeared, but I felt okay because I was sure no one had noticed." He had an awful sensation while lying in bed of something running across his chest, which reminded him that at times he would have a numbness in an arm or leg while on my couch. Then he remembered wheezing a little the previous morning and said breaking away from his parents and growing up were very hard.

While looking at an *Esquire* magazine in the waiting room before another session, he felt fearful of my coming out and catching him, to which he associated that in his mind sex was for men, not boys.

Paul reported a change taking place in his fantasies: he had some thoughts about what it would be like to sexually assault a girl whose picture he saw in a magazine. He said he also had been thinking some about going on a date, but that was as far as he could go, because he still felt a great deal of anxiety. I pointed out that apparently it was safer for him to remain a small child, still wetting the bed, than to become a more mature, sexually capable young man. He talked of also being afraid of his aggressive wishes.

He then glorified being single and said being married and having children still had no appeal to him. We talked about the enuresis as one of his defenses against having more mature sexual feelings. He again talked of his fear of being injured and related it to feeling more competitive with me now. Then he said he could see that his wetting was a way of saying he wanted more of his mother's attention. The idea that his father would think he had sexual desires still made him feel very anxious. He wondered what would happen to him if anything happened to me, to which he associated being at the mercy of his father. I interpreted this as his castration fears, after which he had a full-blown anxiety attack in the session, with sweating, sighing, heart palpitations, etc.

The next hour he said that he had not wet for several days but imagined that girls would reject him now because of bad breath. He really did not have much to offer a girl, because he was underdeveloped physically. That night he wet the bed again and thought when first awakening that he was lying on the analytic couch. Then he asked, "What do you want from me anyway?" and related a dream about waiting in line in a house to use the toilet, but never getting there and waking up wet.

He told of playing poker with friends and winning more often now because he was able to be more aggressive in his play than in the past. He was very self-conscious of his body during the session. His father had injured his leg and was incapacitated, and he did not like seeing his father that way. I commented that apparently he still felt better when seeing his father as big and strong, and himself small and weak, and wondered if he did not feel the same way about me. In the next session, he was wheezing and spoke of having the prickly feeling in the session again. Then he recalled that as a child he would feel anger toward his mother because she denied him certain wishes.

He associated fear of the idea of growing up to feelings of fear of his father and me. Although he thought that if he should really become interested in a girl he would be laughed at and ridiculed, he actually was also coming to realize that he was not such a weak person after all; yet he could not bring himself to ask a girl out. He missed his next session because he "forgot." He later explained, however, that he had been more anxious, to which he associated seeming to be closer to understanding something about himself. He had a sensation as if his whole body would explode, which was followed by a fantasy of his father's car smashing into a wall, and the realization that, if it did, he would not have it to use for a date. Suddenly, he imagined that the picture on the wall next to the couch might fall down and he would get cut.

He began driving to school occasionally and offered a girl a ride home, which she accepted. He still thought, however, that his body was small, weak, and not much good, to which he associated that he did not have very mature sexual organs. Then, with mixed feelings, he recalled a game he and his mother had played at bedtime when he was very little. It was called "No Robbers." He did not elaborate but said he had not wet now for 6 nights. Also, he had been thinking more about dating but still felt awfully scared and thought how pleasant being a child was.

He began reporting feelings of excitement when he saw attractive girls at school. He had not wet for about 2 weeks. Then he related having gone on a bike ride with a girl and having found it hard to wait to come in and tell me about it. They had hardly started out, however, when he had a great need to urinate. He talked of feeling envious of boys walking down the school halls with girls.

He got an "800" on the math section of the SAT but did not feel very excited and found it hard to tell his father. To make a big impression, he drove his father's car to the school picnic. Yet, the night after the picnic, he wet the bed again. He associated this to seeing a girl lying on a blanket with another boy. Then he told me that his father had taken him to an interns' party, which so excited him that he wet the bed that night. I interpreted the retreat to wetting as a safety valve to reassure himself that he was not yet an adult, sexual male.

His older brother went on dates and used their father's car. Driving his father's car made Paul feel very important. The next hour he was late, explaining that he had been at the beach looking at the girls but had felt some fear as he thought of the girls' boyfriends. He wet the bed the next 3 Saturday nights, to which he associated that that was the evening he would like to go on a date. He also bought a *Playboy* magazine but felt scared, to which he associated the anxiety he felt when he was reading *Esquire* in the waiting room. He then reported a dream of being on vacation out West. Everyone in the family was there except his mother. When he went to hunt for her in a private airplane, he found her eating lunch in a mountaintop restaurant. Paul felt greatly relieved. He had been giving girls rides home lately, and then thought that his father had come between himself and his mother when he was little. He told me that there was a girl he liked named Frances and thought that I might know her. He continued to be increasingly dissatisfied with his appearance; his clothes were not stylish enough. In an indirect way he asked my permission to date, which I pointed out to him. His thought then was that the girl's father probably would not like him anyway. Nevertheless, he did ask Frances for a date and she accepted, but he was very uncomfortable about doing so, and only told his father just before he left. He missed the next hour, later explaining that he had felt very anxious about coming in for the session. This was the last appointment before my summer vacation.

During the first session after vacation (216th), he told me he had wet the bed the night before vacation. He had had an argument with his father and felt all right about it. He told of a dream in which he was in a bookstore looking at women in a pornographic book, but the book had a children's "golden book" cover on it. He wondered if this meant he was disguising his grown-up interests by looking like a child. He had felt so anxious while driving a couple of girls on school field trips that he got a headache. He contrasted this with a pleasant memory of his mother bathing him when he was little.

He bought some "in style, teenage clothes" and gave up drinking milk but still feared that he might wet, perhaps on the couch.

This gave rise to his saying that he feared he might not be able to function sexually as other boys could. But in the next hour (223rd) he told me that while doing homework, he had become very excited and wet himself, but it was not urine and had been accompanied by a very pleasant feeling. Then he recalled that the same thing had happened not long before when he had taken a college placement exam. He wondered if his father would be angry if he knew what had happened. He felt less afraid of me now and hence could talk about sexual matters more easily, but still felt inferior to other boys. This was followed by fantasies of getting into fights with other boys over girlfriends and even winning, whereas previously he had always been the one who would get beaten up. He had the fantasy of having a confrontation with his father and coming out all right. The thought occurred to him of taking a girl out on a date and her father being angry, which would frighten Paul. Then he said he was not wetting the bed anymore.

He was finding it increasingly hard to believe that he could go through life without making love to a girl. I told Paul I had to cancel a couple of appointments, and he got angry and accused me of being like his father; I, too, was afraid of his becoming a mature, sexual male; but then he began to wheeze. In the next hour, he said that he had gone to a party with a girl named Linda and had a good time, but did wet the bed that night. I interpreted this as regression after having taken an important progressive developmental step. Before the next hour he was reading an *Esquire* in the waiting room and spoke of feeling no need to hide it from me. Then he told me that he had asked Jill out for New Year's Eve, but she was busy; so he had asked Mary, who happily accepted. His association to Jill turning him down was that she considered him an inferior male. His mother might have had the same opinion about him. He then thought how nice it would be to have a girl not only as a lover but also as someone to take care of him. He had felt some fear of Mary's father when he took her out New Year's Eve.

At the beginning of the next hour, he did not want the paper toweling under his head any longer, as it reminded him of a diaper. This led to some fantasies about me: he thought I really did want him to grow up rather than the opposite and even wanted to help him; yet at times he still felt like a child in my office. I interpreted the feelings of safety for him in this. Then he told me that he had gotten more into the spirit of being a senior and, in fact, was printing a paper specially for seniors and also making ribbons for seniors to wear. He told of having made a casual comment in school that he had "had" a girl, Penny, for a couple of hours, meaning he had been with her, but was razzed by other boys for his use of the expression "had her."

When he remarked that he had not missed an appointment for a long time, I wondered if he were warning me. Sure enough, he missed the next hour, later explaining that he just had to do it, as he was feeling too dependent on me. Subsequently, he had a fantasy of being in bed with a girl, but was impotent. This was followed by his telling me that he had ejaculated again recently as he became very excited one day while printing his senior paper. I pointed out that he said this as if he were making a confession and wondered if it was not still easier telling me about his wetting the bed. He agreed, but said he was now in with all the top senior students and that he was feeling competitive with Penny's boyfriend. I noted that practically every girl he had mentioned had a boyfriend and wondered if this weren't a safety factor for him, while re-creating the triangle situation that he also had with his parents.

Paul took Frances out again but had an accident with his father's car, to which he associated not being able to hide his sexual feelings from him anymore. He then thought that maybe he was getting back at his father in this way. I pointed out that he also wrecked his own good time. He came late for his next appointment and said he was reminded of a teacher getting very angry at him because he did not get a paper in on time.

In the 270th hour, Paul spoke of masturbating for the first time, to which he associated thinking of lying in bed with Frances and being masturbated by her, making him feel "real good." This recalled for him what a good feeling it was as a young child to lie close to his mother. Then he associated the pleasure he experienced while masturbating with the pleasant feeling he had when wetting the bed.

He fantasized becoming a wealthy playboy but realized he really did not know how to relate to girls very well. He thought of how anxious he still felt telling me his sexual fantasies about girls. Yet, he raised the question, "What can you really do to me?" Then he had the fantasy that I could turn the couch into an operating table. He also wondered if the Toronado were not too much car for him to drive, just like getting to be as tall as his father was a little scary. However, around this time, he first spoke of the many nice things about his father and remarked that his relationship with him was changing. He thought he probably would not need to be coming to analysis much longer. That thought made him feel sad, however, and he related it to the idea of leaving home. He then told of ways in which he had come to feel identified with me and that I was also becoming like a friend and confidant. He said that for the first time he thought about someday becoming a father. He also was feeling more ashamed of going out for an evening with his parents rather than a girlfriend.

He now had his own razor, whereas he formerly had used his father's. He again missed an hour and said he did not feel upset by it. He had been to a dance the night before and had come home late. Now he had become obsessed with thoughts of being in bed with a nude girl and often masturbated. This led to thoughts that he was becoming too sexual too soon, as he was not really ready yet. Some girls seemed to be more like his mother, so he did not feel anything sexual toward them; yet he feared rejection by them, too. I wondered if he might not have felt rejected by his mother when his younger siblings were born. He said he had felt that way all his life. He then told of the great anxiety he felt about asking a girl to the senior prom. We talked about this as a big step for him, like a developmental coming-out party, a point of no return. He then told of having taken Chris to a school party and having been treated like a man by her father, which made him feel "great." It gave him the courage to put his arm around her during the evening.

He reported having been accepted by the college of his choice and his father taking him out to dinner to celebrate. He noticed that since he stopped wetting, his room was not nearly as neat and orderly as it had been. Also, he had not felt the need to get top grades at school, but, surprisingly, his last grades were better than ever.

He talked of terminating analysis in June but wondered if I would be angry at him for growing up so fast. He expressed fear that everything might fall apart again when he left therapy. Later he told me that he had asked Chris to the prom, but she was not able to go. He did not feel devastated; in fact, he thought that since she was only a sophomore, he ought to ask a senior. He also had a dream of being in a bedroom with Chris, who looked somewhat like a boy, and feeling nothing sexual toward her. His first thought on waking the next morning was that he probably had wet the bed, but he had not. His thoughts then were of how he used to feel afraid of me but did not anymore. In fact, he said, tongue in cheek, it occurred to him that he would spend the rest of his life proving "Freud" wrong. (It was not clear what Freud, his father, and I were wrong about, but he liked the challenge of trying to prove it.)

He asked Jan, a senior, to the prom, and she gladly accepted. His thoughts about going to the dance were that it was important because it would prove he was not a failure. He had fantasies of accompanying me on my summer vacation, but as an equal. He wondered what I would be like as a "regular friend" and not his analyst, but actually I had seemed more like a parent to him. Something seemed to have happened between him and me that caused him to feel much more sure of himself as a sexual male. There seemed to be something in him that he had taken from me and he related it to my appearing like a father to him.

He went to the prom, drove his father's car, and did not have an accident. He reviewed with me what he had been like when he first came to analysis and how different he was now. The next hour was canceled on short notice because of a conflict with graduation. In the following hour he told me how proud his father had been of him. I commented that his graduation was not only from high school but also from being a little boy. He told me that he had gotten a job for the summer. I reminded him that termination day was just one week away and he expressed surprise. Then he told of having had a dream the night before in which he found a baby duckling in his bed; again on awaking he feared he had been enuretic, but he had not.

Paul fantasized that when he left my office after the last session, he would not have any place to go and maybe he would become depressed. Then he had the thought of staying on the couch until his last appointment. In the next hour, he talked of having thoughts of all the realities in our relationship; for example, that he really was taller than I. Then he told of thinking that maybe he would just explode after he left the office on Thursday but really knew no such thing would happen.

In the last hour, I had him sit up facing me and we primarily chatted about the realistic aspects of his life.

DISCUSSION

Paul represents a classical example of a breakdown in the relatively smooth developmental course one might expect of a child growing up in an intact and, to all indications, caring family environment. However, Paul's failure to develop the regulating controls over urinary functions, his developing preoedipal compulsive personality features, compounded by an intense rivalry and fearfulness of his father, set the stage for his neurosis. Pregenital fixations made it difficult for him to master developmental conflicts of the anal-urethral and phallic-oedipal phases. The lack of adequate structural and functional ego and superego development in latency interfered with his readiness for adolescent task mastery, particularly of socialization and genitalization, so that he remained fixated at a pregenital level, with enuresis continuing as his main source of libidinal discharge. When Paul failed to make the developmental transitions of pubescence that most enuretic preadolescents accomplish, the stage was set for further neurotic inhibitions and conflicts.

Through analytic work over a 3½-year period, Paul was able to experience the progression from pregenitality into full-blown adolescence that should have taken place through his natural development. With the analyst as the parental transference object and the psychoanalytic treatment providing an even broader environmental setting, Paul relived and reworked the traumatic aspects of his earlier life. In this way his analysis became his second developmental experience—one fortunately more successful than the first.

Hence, we are able to see by means of a "laboratory" experience that psychoanalytic treatment of children and adolescents

with severe developmental impairments enables the child to resolve earlier developmental maladaptions in which the preference for passivity predisposed the child to symptomatic difficulties (enuresis and the precipitation of asthmatic attacks) as well as
to deviant social development (characterological and behavioral). Throughout the treatment, especially in the analysis of
the transference and in the significance of the analyst as a real
person, the statement that "psychoanalysis is development" is
strikingly demonstrated.

BIBLIOGRAPHY

ABRAMS, S. (1983). Development. *Pschoanal. Study Child*, 38:113–140.
BION, W. (1965). *Transformations*. New York: Basic Books.
CHETHIK, M. & KALTER, N. (1980). Developmental arrest following divorce. *Amer. Acad. Child Psychiat.*, 19:281–288.
DAVIDSON, H. (1974). The role of identification in the analysis of late adoles- cents. *Adol. Psychiat.*, 3:263–270.
EISSLER, K. R. (1958). Notes on problems of technique in the psychoanalytic treatment of adolescents. *Psychoanal. Study Child*, 13:223–254.
EVANS, R. (1976). Development of the treatment alliance in the analysis of an adolescent boy. *Psychoanal. Study Child*, 31:193–224.
FRAIBERG, S. (1955). Some considerations in the introduction of therapy in puberty. *Psychoanal. Study Child*, 10:264–288.
FREUD, A. (1958). Adolescence. *Psychoanal. Study Child*, 13:255–278.
FREUD, S. (1905). Three essays on the theory of sexuality. *S.E.*, 7:125–243.
GELEERD, E. R. (1957). Some aspects of psychoanalytic technique in adoles- cence. *Psychoanal. Study Child*, 12:263–283.
HARLEY, M. (1974). *The Analyst and the Adolescent at Work*. New York: Quad- rangle.
KERNBERG, O. F. (1979). Psychoanalytic psychotherapy with borderline adoles- cents. *Adol. Psychiat.*, 7:294–321.
KESTENBERG, J. S. (1969). Problems of technique of child analysis in relation to the various developmental stages. *Psychoanal. Study Child*, 24:358–383.
LAUFER, M. (1965). Assessment of adolescent disturbances. *Psychoanal. Study Child*, 20:99–123.
––––––– (1976). The central masturbation fantasy. *Psychoanal. Study Child*, 31:297–316.
––––––– (1978). The nature of adolescent pathology and the psychoanalytic process. *Psychoanl. Study Child*, 33:307–322.
––––––– (1981).The psychoanalyst and the adolescent's sexual development. *Psychoanal. Study Child*, 36:181–192.
MILLER, D. (1978). Early adolescence. *Adol. Psychiat.*, 6:434–447.

NEUBAUER, P. B. (1976). *The Process of Child Development.* New York: New American Library.

NOVICK, J. (1976). Termination of treatment in adolescence. *Adol. Psychiat.,* 5:390–412.

WINNICOTT, D. W. (1965). *The Maturational Process and the Facilitating Environment.* New York: Int. Univ. Press.

YORKE, C. (1983). Clinical notes on developmental pathology with borderline adolescents. *Adol. Psychiat.,* 7:294–321.

Reconstruction of Adolescence in Adult Analysis

ROGER L. GOETTSCHE, M.D.

ANNA FREUD (1958) AND JEANNE LAMPL-DE GROOT (1960) SEPARATELY note the lack of attention devoted to adolescent reconstruction in adult analyses both in analytic practice and in the analytic literature. In fact, at a 1979 discussion of analytic reconstruction, only scant reference was made to the need for reconstructive activities to be devoted to adolescence. One may ask why there is a lack of attention to reconstruction of this important developmental phase, particularly since psychoanalysis from the beginning has directed attention to the impact of earlier experience on adult neurosis. One may also ask why analytic attention should be focused on this difficult developmental phase. Excerpts from an analysis in which adolescent reconstruction played an important role in providing a window through which analyst and analysand could begin to piece together the nature of her infantile experience will be presented. These clinical data will support the thesis that analytic reconstruction of adolescent experience (1) can provide a window through which earlier history may be meaningfully approached; (2) develops an increasingly meaningful and convincing sense of the reality of the analysand's neurotic repetitions and psychic contents; and (3) adds an important new dimension in understanding the adult neurosis through the analysis of the new achievement in adolescence of the final sexual organization (Laufer, 1976).

Assistant clinical professor of psychiatry, Yale University School of Medicine; member, Western New England Psychoanalytic Society.

REVIEW OF LITERATURE

From the beginning psychoanalysis has devoted its attention to the understanding of a patient's past as a way to gain insight into the personality structure and function in the present. Freud found that hysterical symptoms could be understood and alleviated by the recovery of memories of past sexual traumatic experience. At first, the recovery of memories of traumatic seduction and the lifting of the infantile amnesia were the goals of psychoanalysis. After Freud revised the seduction theory and postulated the development of infantile sexuality, the early memories of seduction were seen in a new light. This tension between the actuality of what occurred in childhood and how the elaboration of fantasy (associated with the experience) took place in the inner world of the developing child paved the way for the impotance of psychoanalytic reconstruction as an important opportunity and goal of psychoanalysis.

At the same time, Freud never viewed analytic construction as a simple process of memory retrieval. From the beginning, memories themselves were viewed as mental products subject to processes in the mind like dreams, parapraxes, and symptoms. Freud (1899) noted, "The result was a compromise by which the innocent passages emerged in the patient's memory with pathological strength and clarity. The process which we here see at work—conflict, repression, substitution involving a compromise—returns in all psychoneurotic symptoms and gives us the key to understanding their formation" (p. 308). Memories, in a sense, like fantasies and dreams, are themselves made or constructed: "The result of the conflict is therefore that, instead of the mnemic image which would have been justified by the original event, another is produced which has been to some degree associatively *displaced* from the former one" (p. 307). Or: "I can assure you that people often construct such things unconsciously—almost like works of fiction" (p. 315). And importantly, Freud made clear that these products of displacement may be from one time to another: "A screen memory may be described as 'retrogressive' or as having 'pushed forward' according as the one chronological relation or the other holds between the screen and the thing screened-off" (p. 320).

In his papers on technique Freud concerned himself with the nature of transferences and the tension between repetition and memory, repetition in the present and recollections from the past, and the corresponding tension for the analyst of transference as repetition and transference as resistance to recall as well as transference as a manifestation of neurosis. Hence transference is a focus for interpretive work to help the patient become aware and convinced of the nature of his neurotic repetitions. Current controversies in psychoanalysis have elaborated and refined this point of view (Blum, 1979, 1981; Benner, 1979; Gill, 1979). Freud, however, never lost sight of his conviction that transference was best used analytically to enhance recollection and recall via reconstruction: "Just as happens in dreams, the patient regards the products of the awakening of his unconscious impulses as contemporaneous and real; he seeks to put his passions into action without taking any account of the real situation. The doctor tries to compel him to fit these emotional impulses into the nexus of the treatment and of his life-history, to submit them to intellectual consideration and to understand them in the light of their psychical value" (1912, p. 108). He again highlights that analytic work is required not only on transference but on memories as well; with regard to screen memories Freud (1914) says, "In some cases I have had an impression that the familiar childhood amnesia, which is theoretically so important to us, is completely counterbalanced by screen memories. Not only *some* but *all* of what is essential from childhood has been retained in these memories. It is simply a question of knowing how to extract it out of them by analysis. They represent the forgotten years of childhood as adequately as the manifest content of a dream represents the dream-thoughts" (p. 148).

Freud is clear that neurotic repetitions become repetitions in transference and must be traced back to their infantile sources. Repeating *is* the patient's way of remembering and the analytic task is to transform the repetition into verbal recall by way of reconstruction, or what Freud calls "our therapeutic work": "We soon perceive that the transference is itself only a piece of repetition, and that the repetition is a transference of the forgotten past not only on to the doctor but also on to all the other aspects of the current situation. . . . This state of illness is brought, piece

by piece, within the field and range of operation of the treatment, and while the patient experiences it as something real and
contemporary, we have to do our therapeutic work on it, which
consists in a large measure in tracing it back to the past" (1914, p.
151f.).

Freud never loses sight of this analytic goal in his theoretical
developments of technical recommendations. In a late paper
(1937) he likens the work of the analyst to the work of the archaeologist and compares the difficult distinctions that need to
be made as one traces back the course of history, of a society or
of an individual, particularly as it pertains to determining "the
relative age of his finds" (p. 259). What is most important to
Freud at this time is to arrive at constructions that allow a sense
of conviction in the analyst and analysand as to historical truth.
This line of development remains an important guiding light
for subsequent developments in psychoanalysis. Freud says,
"Quite often we do not succeed in bringing the patient to recollect what has been repressed. Instead of that, if the analysis is
carried out correctly, we produce in him an assured conviction
of the truth of the construction which achieves the same
therapeutic result as a recaptured memory" (p. 265f.). Freud is
clear on what the task of the analyst is in this process: "His task
is to make out what has been forgotten from the traces which it
has left behind or, more correctly, to *construct* it" (p. 258f.).

Anna Freud was the first to note the infrequency with which
adolescent experiences are revived and reconstructed in adult
analysis. She felt the memories were available and recounted,
but the affects remained obscured. "These are elusive mood
swings, difficult to revive, which unlike the affective states of
infancy and early childhood seem disinclined to re-emerge and
be relived in connection with the person of the analyst" (p.
260).

Acknowledging Anna Freud's finding, Jeanne Lampl-de
Groot (1960) reported on two analyses in which "a wealth of
adolescent experiences, real events as well as fantasies and impulses, came to the fore with remarkable liveliness and were
accompanied by strong emotions and impulses" (p. 95f.). The
adolescent material emerged in the later phases of analysis (see
also Hurn, 1970). Lampl-de Groot refers to a conversation with
Freud in which he told her of a young woman who cooperated

with analysis and whose childhood development was reconstructed but without therapeutic result until an adolescent trauma was uncovered and the patient was cured.

Harold Blum (1980) reviewed much of the literature and underscored the continuing importance of attention to this aspect of analytic work. He called attention to the need for adolescent as well as latency reconstruction: "Reconstruction, then, has to be upward into latency and adolescence, as well as backward into the earliest developmental stages in order to understand and work through the patient's loss reactions" (p. 45). He felt reconstructive activities were important in developing a sense of conviction as to the historical truth of the patient's life as well as to the validity of the growing awareness of the neurotic repetitions as they became manifest in psychic content. "It is this living quality of reconstruction which also adds a sense of conviction and reality to the requisite analytic work and which differentiates past and present while creating a new past and present. Reconstruction then comes alive not only in the transference, but in the dissolution of the transference. . . . Reconstruction explains what has been continually repeated in the transference and adult neurosis" (p. 49).

Helen Beiser (1984) appropriately summarized much of the thesis of this paper in her recent paper on self analysis. "One other aspect deserves further attention, although it will only be mentioned in this paper. I was struck by the fact that an actual traumatic incident in adolescence gave meaning to an early childhood memory. It was the repressed adolescent happening that allowed the childhood memory to survive, but without appropriate affect. In my self-analysis as well as during formal analysis, it was the feelings related to adolescent incidents that gave new meaning to experiences of early childhood. It could be that analysts have either put too much emphasis on early childhood, or else on the here-and-now, and have missed the powerful impact that adolescence can have on the development of personality and pathological symptoms" (p. 11).

CLINICAL OBSERVATIONS

The following clinical observations are from an analysis where reconstruction of adolescent experience was central and provided the window through which analyst and analysand could view with clarity her infantile experiences.

The patient, Mrs. A., a married woman in her early 30s, came to analysis to understand excessive fears of speaking in public, dependence on others for approval, and a desire to know herself better to assist in her work as a physician. During the analysis she lived in a home close to her parents.

She described her mother as an austere figure—beautiful but prudish, withholding and interested primarily in the educational pursuits of her children, of whom the patient was the oldest. An upper middle-class woman, Mrs. A.'s mother married because she was pregnant with the patient. Her father, a laborer of foreign extraction, was the past and current central figure in her life. He emerged as warm, sensitive, and seductive, though not very ambitious—a romantic man whose loves in life were his daughter, movies, an occasional concert, and romantic music. In her marriage the patient had "repeated" dynamic aspects of the marital relationship of her own parents.

As the analytic treatment unfolded she formed a rather stable transference neurosis of an oedipal nature with the analyst as father. This experience was manifested in the analysis by her bringing a rose on Valentine's Day, by uncharacteristically having a tryst with a man physically resembling the analyst during a business convention, and by seductive comments before and after analytic hours. She wanted to make it clear, in response to feeling frustrated in the analytic situation, that there were many far more accommodating men in her life who could provide the satisfaction she longed for in the analytic situation.

At the beginning of the second year of analysis she dreamed of "sucking and licking two men's penises and going back and forth between the two feeling very good and roused sexually." Her associations concerned fears and desires to be intensely involved with her husband and the analyst. Toward the end of the hour when asked about the two penises, she responded that they looked like breasts. Several weeks of associations to oral concerns followed. She talked about having been in a period of compulsive overeating, which gradually was resolved by interpretations and working through the frustrated maternal transference longings. Behind erotic transference longing there were oral and maternal longings with genetic roots as implied by her recall of screen memories from her early years. These concerned feelings of maternal deprivation at 17 months when her younger brother, preferred by her mother, was born and she was sent away to her grandparents for two weeks. While we had a glimpse of this constellation, it could not yet be reconstructed for the patient with conviction. For this we had to wait for the reconstruction of her adolescent experiences which followed.

In fact, the more persistent and more structured issue at this point in the analysis became her fears and conflicted desires about feeling deeply involved with her husband and analyst/father. The transference neurosis settled and deepened at this level as she and her husband contemplated a possible move to another city where he could get a better job. Initially, she presented this as simply a career decision that her husband was making unilaterally, and that she as a loyal and faithful wife must go along with and support. As time went on, her contribution became clear. First, this city was a place she had urged him to move to prior to starting analysis; this was a position in the marriage she had not changed after she began her analysis. Second, she made remarks to her husband concerning the erotic nature of her transference which were calculated to make him jealous, much as she had dealt with frustrated transference longings in the analysis. Third, throughout this period, she remained indecisive and passive with regard to her husband's intention, in spite of her more characteristic decisiveness in the marraige. She seemed unable to assert her wish to complete her analysis before moving. This inhibition was interpreted as resulting in part from her guilt feelings about the erotic transference; she felt that to tell her husband she wished to stay was tantamount to announcing a forbidden relationship. More importantly this situation left her feeling helplessly caught between two men, one urging a move to another city, the other urging completion of her analytic work, just as she once had felt in great conflict about her husband, urging marriage before she felt ready, and her seductive and desirable father who was reluctant to "bless" her love relationship. I interpreted her desire that I ask her to stay, much as during late adolescence she had wished her father would make explicit his desire that she not marry. At that time, she compromised by the marriage and living close to her father. It appeared as though she would try to repeat this "compromise" in the analysis.

A dream from this phase of the analysis will illustrate her dilemma:

> I was going to a party in the old house; I crossed a rickety bridge over a hill and went up some stairs. There was a group of young men in their 20s and it was scary; they were James Dean types with leather jackets. I was there to see my friend and felt safe with her. Then I went to the bathroom and there was a large room shaped like a pentagon with doors on all the walls and a woman came in and threw a cigarette into the john. I said I don't want to go here and walked out; it was like a public lavatory. Then I went back and it was like there was a party upstairs and a party downstairs and there were some women I didn't know but felt safe with and I said to them, "This is scary, let's get out of here." Then we went out and there was a truck backing up with a large canvas over the back like a wrecker or garbage truck and there was a woman hanging by a rope around her waist and there was all sort of talk about what to do with her, and a woman riding on a sled being towed behind and then the woman hanging fell and died. At the party there was a man who said 17 will get you 20 and that really scared me.

Her associations centered on exciting and dangerous experiences from adolescence and earlier: "17 will get you 20" reminded her of gambling with her husband; "17 will get you 20 chips." She was reminded in particular of experiences when she was between 17 and 20, traveling to another city to visit her boyfriend (now her husband) and associated to the Mann Act forbidding transporting minors across state lines for sexual activities and the desire for me to ask her to stay. She recalled forbidden activities with girlfriends, one of whom was a wealthy Southern girl who was dating a black man and whose jealous father had them followed to the beach by a private detective. This led to the construction of her wish that her father's jealousy would have taken such frank expression. She then associated to exciting and playful games between her and her father that he stopped in her early adolescence; she was angry but felt she shouldn't be because it must have been her fault. Associations to earlier playful experiences with her father followed from the dream element of the woman left hanging.

Not long afterward a dream reverberating with this earlier one was reported:

> My husband and I are in a shopping mall, an indoor place. He has bought me a record and I am going into a music store to return it. Inside it's dirty and dark. I say this record costs $28.50, it's too much money for the record. I get my money back and go downstairs to another store; it's a linen shop with sheets and towels and very bland pale linens are on the shelf. Behind the counter is a Mexican woman making a basket but not in the ordinary way: I think so much for a nice hand-made thing, it's done by machine. My father comes in with a beautiful Chinese woman: I know he's having an affair. I introduce myself to him using my maiden name. She's 21 years old and I say, "Of course not, she has a 17-year-old daughter." She has wrinkles on her face. Next, my husband and I are out on a street and there are children about 10 or 12. The street is dark with three frightening men with leather jackets—hoodlums: they start throwing knives. I turn to my husband, he is just a kid. I run down a cobblestone street to a church and go up the stairs, there's a light at the top. At the right is a cylinder-shaped building and the door is open; two men and a woman come out, they are in the military and I say three boys are chasing us and I don't know what happened to my husband. They give us a telescope and I woke up thinking I would rescue him.

Her associations were to familiar oedipal themes with the recollection of father having had an affair that had provoked a fight between her parents when she was 10. At that time her mother had threatened her father with violence. In her associations to the dream there were allusions to her own preoedipal experience with nice "hand-made things done by machine," when mother fed her with contraptions that freed her up in caring for the new baby boy when she was 17 months old. However, the bulk of associations emerged from the numbers in the dream and her late adolescent experiences; 21 and 17 referred to her ages of meeting her husband followed by her going back and forth from home to where he lived and her subsequent marriage to him. These numbers also brought to mind numbers 17 will get you 20, alluding to her earlier dream and ideas of sexual danger. The telescope was "hoping" to have a glimpse of who would win the fight, she or her husband, analyst or husband; once again she was helpless because of her conflicting attachments.

At this point a new resistance came into sharper focus. She engaged in glib, hostile, belittling, sarcastic attempts to diminish the importance of her feelings about the analysis. Her need to be in control of the analysis where she felt so helpless and out of control increased. Her relationship with me in the transference became one of helpless submission to my authority as she warded off her feelings of defiance. Difficulties in scheduling became something I imposed on her, or she defiantly would announce schedule changes without warning or discussion. Cooperation and mutuality could not be tolerated at this point. For example, she began to consider furthering her education in a town closer to home but at a school that would require a summer internship. Without inquiring about whether this internship would allow her to continue with analysis or without discussing in the analysis the meanings of her impulsive desire to interrupt in some way, she declared her intention to pursue her plans in defiance of analyzing them.

As this resistance unfolded and was interpreted, a deepening regression and involvement in the transference neurosis occurred. During one hour she commented on my tie. She was afraid to express her delight with this particular tie lest I not wear it again. Later in the hour her associations settled on her father's withdrawal during a playful wrestle with her on the couch when she was 12 in which she had said, "You almost killed me." I interpreted that she was fearful of letting me know of the intensity of her passion for me and my tie for fear I would suddenly turn away in horror and disgust as she had felt her father had done.

Weekend and vacation absences became a confirmation for her that I couldn't stand to hear of the intensity of her passion and wanted to turn away from her. In another way, too, she felt her earlier experience was confirmed; after all, her father had chosen to marry and continued to take to bed a woman who was controlled, passionless, and seemed to her to be invulnerable. On one occasion, she had seen my wife: she imagined that she was a woman like Joanne Woodward unlike the Isadora Duncan she perceived herself to be, volatile, passionate, and an excited, exciting dancer. My choice seemed obvious to her: I preferred the more controlled and measured Joanne Woodward to the passionate Isadora.

As this constellation was interpreted her memories of her twelfth and thirteenth years became sharper. She recalled in particular the summer following her father's withdrawal. She could no longer talk to her father and since her mother had long before devoted herself to the love and care of her siblings, she had no one. She felt isolated, alone, rejected, enraged, and suicidal. On one occasion she attempted to suffocate herself, she felt so desperate. It was this summer of despair and depression she had sought to repeat in the analysis. I was bound to turn away from her; she had to follow suit; there had never been a preoedipal mother to turn to for her.

As analysis of these adolescent experiences proceeded, Mrs. A. became more deeply involved in the transference neurosis. Her struggle centered on difficulty tolerating the fullest experience of a passionate involvement in the analysis and in her marriage. She was more comfortable feeling in control, on top, and uninvolved. On the one hand she felt "in over my head," involved well beyond her comfort; yet on the other hand she wished to gain an omnipotent control over these feelings. Involvement with feelings and with people was dangerous; a favorite expression became, "You're born alone, live alone, and die alone." Her adolescent vow to herself after her father's withdrawal echoed once again, "Never will I get so involved with anyone again." She felt her involvement in the analysis threatened her marraige; it frightened her to feel she was repeating her experience with her father so intensely and not only on an intellectual level. At about this time, an opportunity to pursue a professional goal in another city allowed for her to end analysis. In a note following her termination of analysis and move she wrote: "We did a lot of work on understanding my relationship with my seductive father and now I need to learn more about my relation with the nurturing mother."

Discussion

The analysis of this woman's adolescent experience accomplished two important analytic tasks. First, it allowed for the development of a sense of conviction of the actuality of her adolescent experiences and their continuing importance to her. Second, by analysis of the transference and of her adolescent experiences, a window could be opened through which analyst and analysand could together view the vicissitudes of her earlier preoedipal and oedipal development.

In analysis, many levels of development are active and important. While adolescent issues were reconstructed, memories of earlier oedipal and preoedipal phases of development were reactivated. However, when attention is focused on overall themes, the reconstruction of her adolescent development roughly fell into the phase of adolescence as described by Blos (1962). Her late adolescence, characterized by her struggle between her love for her father and her love for her future husband, was revived in the analysis as a struggle between her involvement in the analysis and her continuing involvement with her husband and his career wish to move to another town. Her middle adolescence, characterized in the analysis by hostility, defiance, sarcastic belittlement, and her desire to interrupt the treatment, was resurrected in her struggle for "object removal" or loosening of object ties to her parents as well as the heightened narcissism and narcissistic vulnerability that ensues. Adolescent concerns around autonomy, dependence, independence, and increased involvement in her peer relations could be seen. Most striking, however, was her revival of her early adolescent experience with both father and mother, when suddenly her father turned away from her physically and emotionally at age 12. This was revived in the analysis by her concern that I would not hear her painful, passionate yearnings.

While many (Ritvo, Adatto, Blos) note the difficulty discerning the end of adolescence, particularly in contrast to the physical events that mark its onset, there are events in an individual life that signal nodal points in developmental crises. The finding of a lasting love object and the involvement of pursuing a career can indicate the internal achievement of sexual identity and the stability and maturity of self and object representations as well as an alignment of autonomous ego-centered aspirations with ego ideal and superego development. Ritvo (1976) comments on the end of adolescence in women: "In her sexual life the woman will have established or be well on the way to genital responsiveness in a mutually satisfying relationship. She will be capable of entering into, maintaining, and deriving satisfaction from a lasting and stable relationship, capable of surviving the average expectable stresses of daily living. She will have articulated these with a reality-attuned ego ideal, which will include the image of herself as a mother, as well as her own place in the community in whatever other capacity she has chosen and achieved" (p. 128).

This patient had married, become a mother, and embarked on a serious career. However, her marriage recapitulated her mother's—she chose a man less ambitious than she; though she was sexually responsive and orgasmic, she had an inhibition of her passion and her capacity to tolerate it; there was the neurotic requirement that she have a close proximity to her father in her marriage; her mothering and career work reflected the same ambivalence that characterized her relationship with her mother. Analysis of her inhibitions in adult life showed a contribution from her late adolescent struggles, particularly around her heterosexual object choice. What Freud (1905) said, "Any finding of an object is, in fact, a refinding of it" (p. 222), is particularly useful in understanding this patient. In an attempt to free herself from the incestuous object who she felt had rebuffed her, she found one just like him, even in physical resemblance. This experience was revived in the analysis as feeling helplessly involved, caught between two men, her analyst and her husband. Her anxieties about this experience are well demonstrated in her dreams. While oedipal and pre-oedipal elements are present in both dreams, the drift of her associations was to adolescent manifestations of these struggles that transgressed social acceptability—"the Mann Act," transporting minors across state lines for the purposes of sexual activity. Interpretation of oedipal, incestuous wishes could allow the patient to distance herself from the more pressing, immediate anxieties derived from dangerous, adolescent, sexual feelings and fantasies.

Allowing for the full expression of this anxious adolescent struggle enhanced her conviction about her current neurotic dilemma, particularly for this sophisticated, modern, and liberated patient. In the analysis of her transference neurosis she reexperienced and recalled how her father had responded to her seeking his approval of her marriage by developing a cough, a response of his which had occurred many times before in the patient's view when he was anxious. As a result, she postponed marriage for one year. She renewed and reexperienced that struggle with the analyst as father; nor was it a surprise that she remained living close to her father and interacted with him on a daily basis. This is not to suggest that her attachment to her father was primarily an adolescent phenomenon. It is clear that her current inhibitions were the result of unresolved oedipal attachment, as was her choice of husband. However, her oedipal involvement with her father remained an influential and shaping force through all subsequent phases of development. Analytic attention to the way in which later and particularly adolescent development was affected by her earlier history was also crucial to appreciating the richness and complexity of human psychic development. Connecting oedipal and adolescent conflicts and coping mechanisms enhanced the patient's conviction that the full nature of her struggles could be understood and worked through.

Aspects of the middle phase of her adolescence were also revived in the analysis, manifested by the loosening of object ties and/or object removal, heightened narcissism, and hostile defiance. While these processes are phase-appropriate during adolescence, when revived in the transference, they may complicate and threaten the therapeutic alliance. Specifically, when her need for distancing from the primary incestuous objects was revived and directed toward me, the analytic alliance was challenged by her diminished capacity for viewing me as a new or therapeutic object. On the other hand, when her need for distancing from the primary incestuous objects became directed toward her internal representations of mother and father, the analytic alliance was stronger and less conflicted. Then there was an increased capacity to view me more objectively and new growth occurred. Lampl-de Groot (1960) hypothesizes that this loosening up of ties results in a loosening up of support from the auxiliary ego, ego ideal, and superego functioning of the parents, thus placing the adolescent in an increasingly vulnerable but also potentially positive developmental situation. The patient's recapitulation of this phase almost resulted in an interruption of the analysis, much as adolescents may need at this time to totally reject their parents. While her mother was busy inviting the "socially acceptable" boys over to the house, and joking with and feeding them, unbeknowst to her parents she was actively seducing a lower working-class Mediterranean boy who was more like her father. The importance of peers during this phase was also evident. At this point she "repeated" her adolescent behavior by reviewing her analytic hours with a group of "analytically interested" friends.

The most dramatic reconstruction concerned her father's sudden turning away from her. This constellation of experiences opened the window through which one could begin to appreciate with greater clarity the vicissitudes of her early preoedipal and oedipal development. Blos (1962) delineates the upsurge of bisexuality as the hallmark of early adolescence; he feels this is more often noted in boys than in girls. Blos cites Deutsch (1944) as referring to the onset of psychosis in girls who had lost their friends and could not find compensation in their mothers. Following the withdrawal of father and mother's unavailability, this patient suffered a suicidal depression which she attempted to repeat in her analysis. Most importantly this experience allowed us to begin to reconstruct her earlier experience, including her oedipal situation. When she was 8 months old her mother became pregnant with her younger brother. In the analysis the brother was brought in by referring to his emotional troubles: "He must be schizophrenic." When she was 17 months old he was born. The patient felt that her mother had cast her aside and was enchanted with her son. She was told she was fed by bottle-propping contraptions, as alluded to in the dream. She was also entertained by "contraptions" that held toys in front of her to distract her from missing her mother when the baby was being fed. Having mastered the rapprochement tensions during her phallic-narcisstic phase (Edgcumbe and Burgner, 1975), she turned to her father not only for confirmation of her genital femininity (Tyson, 1982) but also for coping with the lingering maternal yearnings for love, support, and nurture. This intense involvement with the father remained until her twelfth year. His loss was a devastating traumatic blow during her early adolescence.

Revival of adolescence in the analysis of adult patients is crucial not only in understanding earlier experience but also because important new developments occur during adolescence which must be analyzed in order to understand and relieve adult neurosis and personality configuration. Moses Laufer (1976) states clearly that "although the resolution of oedipal conflict means that the main sexual identifications become fixed and that the core of the body image is established at that time, it is only during adolescence that the content of the sexual wishes and the oedipal identifications become integrated into what I believe to be an irreversible sexual identity" (p. 298). Thus my patient's object choice, her struggle to make the choice, her inhibition of sexual feelings reflect the further development of oedipal vicissitudes as they reemerge and become reintegrated during adolescence. It would be erroneous to interpret her inhibition as a result of oedipal experience alone. It was crucial to acknowledge the importance of father's withdrawal during adolescence.

Why is adolescent reconstruction so frequently not addressed by analysts? Anna Freud and Lampl-de Groot note that adolescent memories are quite accessible in adult analysis, but the tempestuous affects from adolescence are rarely revived in full force in the analytic situation. A first important consideration, then, is the inherent nature of the adolescent experiences themselves, tumultuous and tempestuous, with alternating feelings of passion and asceticism, angry defiance and humble obedience, devoted involvement and narcissistic withdrawal, committed idealism and pessimistic disinterest, that remains difficult to resurrect in a sustained and meaningful way in the analytic situation ın order to achieve a reflective perspective and objective distance.

Adolescence is a time of chaos. In early adolescence a still immature ego is weakened by the surge of approaching biological physical and sexual maturity with increasing libidinal and aggressive drive demands. "The developmental tasks of adolescence put stresses on the defensive and adaptive capacities of the ego. Increased independence and removal from the infantile and childhood love objects to the peer generation involve conflict and the psychic pain of separation and loss. The biologically rooted necessity of establishing intimate relationships on the basis of the sexually mature body and integrating it into the personality generates intense and painful conflict in many, if not all, adolescents" (Ritvo, 1984, p. 453). In middle and late adolescence this struggle persists and waivers as a result of the adolescent's need to turn away from the supportive influence of parental and other potentially helpful authority figures. It is no surprise, then, that our adult patients are reluctant to admit to feelings of chaos, of feeling overwhelmed, and of feeling fragmented so recently in their lives. How much safer to ascribe these feelings of ego weakness to the antiquity and helplessness of early childhood.

A second factor is referred to by a number of writers, including Ritvo, Lampl-de Groot, and Laufer, namely, that the revival of oedipal and preoedipal fantasies during adolescence is not a mere repetition, but rather a reappearance of the conflicts at a higher level of ego functioning with a new ego structure, more mature and integrated in some ways and more vulnerable in others. "The necessity to *act upon* the old oedipal and preoedipal fantasies becomes a source of increased anxiety. The nuclear infantile conflicts come up for final resolution, so to speak, with the difference that there is a greater element of reality to conflicts which earlier had existed largely in fantasy" (Ritvo, 1971, p. 247). This "greater element of reality" works on the side of conviction for both analyst and analysand of the validity of the intrapsychic struggles but leads to greater anxiety as they become revived in the analytic situation particularly in the transference.

Lampl-de Groot makes a similar point that the maturity of the motor and sexual apparatus leads to the thoughts of discharge of fantasy constellations that now are more dangerous. A similarly charged atmosphere and intensity and depth of feelings are present too with children, but adolescent genitality is a different psychic experience than infantile sexuality. The adolescent whose sexual constitution has from early on been characterized by fixation on sadomasochistic and polymorphous-perverse features is very likely to react with anxiety, guilt, and withdrawal from the experience or even the prospect of bodily intimacy (Ritvo, 1984). Lampl-de Groot extends this consideration to the inclusion of ego and superego considerations. While there is maturity and development of ego and superego systems, the adolescent's need to turn away from his primary love objects precludes his use of parental ego and superego as auxiliaries and the resultant ego-superego system may be more vulnerable to drive demands. As this is repeated and reexperienced in the analytic situation, the adult analysand may be under the sway of needing to turn away from the analyst and the therapeutic alliance at the time when it is needed most to assist in tolerating the regressive reemergence of adolescent drive elements.

An additional reason for neglecting attention to adolescent reconstruction may well be the notion that the important conflicts arise from the infantile neurotic situation and that their subsequent influence contributes little to the development of neurosis in adult life. Analysis is difficult enough as it is, and many may feel little can be gained from adding new attention to this difficult developmental phase. It is hoped that the clinical data in this communication will help allay this doubt.

It would seem, then, that the greatest reluctance to uncovering adolescent experience in adult analysis derives from the heart of the analytic situation, the transference-countertransference situation itself. Adolescence is just too close to both analyst and analysand. How much more intellectually and emotionally satisfying to look back into the distance of infancy and early childhood where responsibility may be more easily disavowed and where the affects, however powerful and important, were felt a long time ago. Lampl-de Groot (1960) comments: "The interplay between the patient's anxiety to relive his adolescent emotions and conflicts and the analyst's unconscious shyness to bear the adolescent forms of aggression might be one of the causes of the difficulties we encounter in analyzing and working through an adult patient's adolescence" (p. 99). She comments on the reluctance to bear the revival, particularly of adolescent aggressive fantasies toward the analyst. With infantile fantasies, however, the analyst can remain more neutral, almost smile at the helpless child's aggression toward powerful parental images. Thus the analyst is more inclined to follow the patient in his flight toward infancy to escape the patient's criticisms, reproaches, and hostile demands as well as the sensuous libidinal transference offerings. While Lampl-de Groot focuses on transference-countertransference reluctance to analyze the revived adolescent aggressive drive derivatives, the same can be said of adolescent libidinal drive derivatives as outlined by Ritvo (1984). What Ritvo and Lampl-de Groot state is further elaborated in the findings of this report: the revival in the transference of adolescent aggressive and libidinal drive derivatives creates a strong "regressive pull," closer and more powerful with regard to adult experience than the more distant and less palpable infantile experience. It is then understandable that analyst and analysand together would choose to avoid confronting directly these strong and at times chaotic wishes and fantasies.

A final consideration may be related to how an analyst thinks about and conceptualizes his reconstructive activities. Freud (1937) warned us not to take his metaphors too literally; perhaps this warning should be applied to the metaphor of archaeological reconstruction. Here Freud compares analytic "construction" to the archaeologist reconstructing the history of an earlier civilization as a result of uncovering its buried remains. If archaeological activities are too literally applied to the analytic situation, it may lead to the notion of analysis as an activity of working to uncover the buried remains of the infantile neurosis, as if this experience is lying dormant and unchanged, save by decay, in the adult neurotic patient. Eagerness to achieve "the archaeological find" could lead the analyst to treat as unimportant by comparison the repetitions, regressions, and reintegrations of this experience as it takes place over subsequent developmental phases. The notion that the history of the oedipal situation lies beneath the surface, preserved and unchanged save by decay, also flies in the face of other contributions of Freud. Throughout (1899, 1914, 1937), he stresses the dynamic nature of psychic processes: memories themselves are not static like the photographic plate, but subject to displacement, condensation, and other psychic mechanisms. Thus it may not merely be a matter of semantics that Freud refers to construction rather than reconstruction. That is, construction is an active analytic activity, literally making a new version of the analysand's history. From this point of view, analytic construction provides an actively achieved, new version of the analysand's history by making use of the repetitive nature of psychic contents occurring during all phases of development, including adolescence.

In every adult, traits from early childhood to adolescence persist. Adolescent struggles are not more important in understanding an adult neurosis than understanding the vicissitudes of the infantile neurotic situation. They are parts of a complete psychoanalytic treatment. Therefore increased attention is necessary to include the reconstruction of adolescent experience to enhance the clearer understanding of early experience, to provide a window into earlier times, and also to appreciate the developmental contributions unique to this stage, particularly the achievement of the final sexual organization.

BIBLIOGRAPHY

ADATTO, C. P. (1966). On the metamorphosis from adolescence into adulthood. *J. Amer. Psychoanal. Assn.*, 14:485–509.

BEISER, H. R. (1984). An example of self-analysis. *J. Amer. Psychoanal. Assn.*, 32:3–12.

BLOS, P. (1962). *On Adolescence.* Glenco, Ill.: Free Press.

BLUM, H. P. (1979). The curative and creative aspects of insight. *J. Amer. Psychoanal. Assn. Suppl.*, 27:41–70.

———— (1980). The value of reconstruction in adult psychoanalysis. *Int. J. Psychoanal.*, 61:39–52.

———— (1981). Some current and recurrent problems of psychoanalytic technique. *J. Amer. Psychoanal. Assn.*, 29:47–68.

BRENMAN, E. (1980). The value of reconstruction in adult psychoanalysis. *Int. J. Psychoanal.*, 61:39–52.

BRENNER, C. (1979). The analysis of the transference. *J. Amer. Psychoanal. Assn. Suppl.*, 27:263–287.

DEUTSCH, H. (1944). *The Psychology of Women.* New York: Grune & Stratton.

EDGCUMBE, R. & BURGNER, M. (1975). The phallic-narcissistic phase. *Psychoanal. Study Child,* 30:161–180.

FREUD, A. (1936). *The Ego and the Mechanisms of Defense.* New York: Int. Univ. Press.

––––––– (1958). Adolescence. *Psychoanal. Study Child,* 13:255–278.

FREUD, S. (1899). Screen memories. *S.E.,* 3:301–322.

––––––– (1905). Three essays on the theory of sexuality. *S.E.,* 7:125–243.

––––––– (1912). The dynamics of transference. *S.E.,* 12:97–108.

––––––– (1914). Remembering, repeating, and working through. *S.E.,* 12:145–156.

––––––– (1937). Constructions in analysis. *S.E.,* 23:255–269.

GILL, M. M. (1979). The analysis of the transference. *J. Amer. Psychoanal. Assn. Suppl.,* 27:263–287.

HURN, H. T. (1970). Adolescent transference. *J. Amer. Psychoanal. Assn.,* 18:342–357.

LAMPL-DE GROOT, J. (1960). On adolescence. *Psychoanal. Study Child,* 15:95–103.

LAUFER, M. (1976). The central masturbation fantasy, the final sexual organization, and adolescence. *Psychoanal. Study Child,* 31:297–316.

RITVO, S. (1971). Late adolescence. *Psychoanal. Study Child,* 26:241–263.

––––––– (1976). Adolescent to woman. *J. Amer. Psychoanal. Assn. Suppl.,* 24:127–137.

––––––– (1984). The image and uses of the body in psychic conflict. *Psychoanal. Study Child,* 39:449–469.

TYSON, P. (1982). The role of the father in gender identity, urethral eroticism and phallic narcissism. In *Father and Child,* ed. S. H. Cath, A. R. Gruwitt, & J. M. Ross, pp. 175–188. Boston: Little Brown.

Aspects of Identity Development among Nouveaux Religious Patients

MOSHE HALEVI SPERO, M.S.S.W., Ph.D.

> The self of each person is a product of the combination
> of his memory and his will, of the past and the future.
> —AHAD HA-AM (1956, p. 150)

AMONG THE MANY INTERSECTS BETWEEN RELIGION AND CONTEMPO-
rary psychology has been the sustained interest in pathological
versions of religious conversion or penitence (Casey, 1938;
James, 1902; Mann, 1964; Meissner, 1984; Pruyser, 1977), and
the evolution of models which distinguish between normal and
abnormal or maladaptive motives and processes of religious development (Elkind, 1971; McDargh, 1983; Rizzuto, 1979; Stark,
1971). Such models are of great practical importance in view of
growing interest in psychotherapy with persons whose religious
feelings, beliefs, and perceptions play a significant role in their
psychopathology.[1]

Senior lecturer, School of Social Work, Bar-Ilan University, Ramat Gan,
Israel; clinical psychologist, Sarah Herzog Psychiatric Hospital–Ezrat Nishim
Mental Health Center, Jerusalem, Israel.

I am grateful for research stipends provided by the Research Authority of
Bar-Ilan University and the Center for Absorption in the Sciences, Ministry of
Absorption and Immigration, the State of Israel, 1985. I am especially grateful
to Rami Bar-Giora, director, Eliezer Ilan Child Guidance Clinic, Jerusalem, for
his continuing benevolence and supervision.

1. See, e.g., Atwood (1978), Bergman (1953), Knight (1937), McDargh
(1983), Spero (1980, 1983b, 1985b), Stern (1985), Stolorow and Atwood
(1973).

Of increasing interest are individuals who, with or without a period of intense, consciously experienced shame, guilt, or remorse about their previous life-styles and values, and with or without obvious preexisting psychological disorder, become single-mindedly devoted to new religious life-styles and values, either through conversion or by increased commitment to their childhood religion, *and* whose subsequent life-style is enmeshed with various kinds of psychological turmoil. This turmoil ranges from frank psychosis to character disorder to essentially intact personality organization plagued by doubts, insecurities, and various idiosyncracies. Some forms of contemporary cultic religiosity seem plainly pathogenic, judging from the amount of serious psychopathology evidenced so consistently among their devotees, contiguous with the kinds of methods used by such groups to attract and maintain adherents (Halperin, 1983; Maleson, 1981; Pruyser, 1977; Spero, 1983a). In the majority of cases where the religious system to which the individual has become committed cannot itself be deemed pathogenic, the developmentally oriented practitioner wishes to understand whether or not the psychic turmoil seen among the nouveaux religionists is a consequence of preexisting pathology that has managed to express itself in religious form and/or whether there are certain psychological crises inherent in any form of pervasive ideological transformation that impede smooth transition.

In Jewish communities, the nouveaux religious are known as *ba'alei teshuvah* or *hozrim be-teshuvah* (nonreligious Jews who "return in penitence") and *geirim* (converts). Aviad (1983) estimates that at least 12,000 *ba'alei teshuvah* are studying in religious seminaries in Israel; 62% are male, 34% female, 50% American born, 29% Israeli, and 16% from England and the British Commonwealth. These figures do not include individuals who have left seminaries to return to larger societies or older *ba'alei teshuvah* who do not partake of formal seminary education. Statistics for the American Jewish nouveaux religious community are unavailable, but the number is believed to be about 15,000.

Converts to Judaism historically have comprised the smaller percentage of newly religious and, according to some writers, their psychological experiences in identity formation ought to be distinguished from that of the *ba'al teshuvah* (Buber, 1951; Franzblau, 1965). On the one hand, the majority of contemporary *ba'alei teshuvah* come from backgrounds so divorced from Jewish religious practice and belief as to require complete re-education and undergo psychological transformations tantamount to conversion, though obviously conversion ritual is not necessary. On the other hand, there are different levels of prior religious affiliation and knowledge among *ba'alei teshuvah,* some of which permit relatively less radical transformation from old to new identity.

Glanz and Harrison (1978), following Gordon (1974; see Scobie, 1975), differentiate between radical identity change involved in conversion proper and also among *ba'alei teshuvah* who come from essentially negligible religious background and less radical transformations of those individuals who are either strengthening a marginal Jewish identity or returning to a previously rejected Jewish value system. The latter group is better able to build up cumulative levels of new identity, more easily consolidating the old and new universes of discourse (see also Levine, 1983, p. 269). Thus, Glanz and Harrison believe that those *ba'alei teshuvah* who can assume the identity of a yeshivah student are able to fulfill their spiritual quest by "reorganizing their identity around a Jewish component which was typically marginal to them in their youth" (p. 135).

Glanz and Harrison's point is diagnostically useful. Certainly, the conflicts illustrated by the cases presented in this paper cannot be simply generalized across all nouveaux religionists. Yet, not all *ba'alei teshuvah,* certainly not the majority who become religious later in life, adopt identities as yeshivah students. Second, even in instances where the nouveaux religionist has some previous religious background, a large degree of the smoothness of the process of identity change is dependant upon the interaction between the religionist and the specific kind of religious community into which he or she enters. Indeed, there are many subtle components of the experience of identity transformation which the authors did not explore. And yet the authors take note of a major aspect of this transformational process, one which I believe is common to most nouveaux religionists; namely, that "the past to which they return is not their own, but a recreation of a Jewish mythic past" (p. 135). That is, the past in which nouveaux religionists attempt psychologically to locate themselves does not exist in their personal memory. They may wish to believe that their return is a realization of their "true" identity, yet in almost every instance of religious change the individual experiences some conflict between his new self-image and the memory of earlier years in which self-images, self and object representations, and interests seem incompatible with the new. One needs to understand in greater detail this experience of incompatibility between past and present perceptions of self, in relation to the need for continuity within both personal and group identity, and the psychological impact of such feelings.

The identity-related and other clinical problems of *ba'alei teshuvah* have become focal in a slowly developing literature (Aviad, 1983; Donshik, 1979; Littlewood, 1983; Mester and Klein, 1981; Spero, 1980, 1982). I am particularly interested in the sense of absence of past which appears frequently among patients who have become intensely religious in later life. I will propose a psychoanalytic perspective which relates the temporal sense of continuity, a basic ego function, to object relational aspects of the process of religious identity development, arrests in the process, and treatment. Three clinical illustrations drawn from American and Israeli Jewish communities are provided emphasizing the role of absence of past as a motive for religious identification and as a normative but potentially complicating development once the identification process is underway.

THEORETICAL CONSIDERATIONS

THE CRISIS OF PAST

The problems of most seriously disturbed nouveaux religionists predate the formal stages of ideological change and their current difficulties, including apparently theological ones, are in large measure derivatives of earlier psychic conflict. At the same time, it is axiomatic that the repentance or conversion process, whether rapid or gradual in course, is tumultuous

(James, 1902; Ullman, 1982; Wootton and Allen, 1983). Yet the full significance of religious development is not wholly characterized by the psychosexual conflict model (Meissner, 1984). Religious feelings and ideals *qua* ego interests are also expressions of specific configurations and qualities of object aims, subject to vicissitudes of maturing self-structure and identification (Eagel, 1983; Rizzuto, 1979) and cognitive adaptations (Elkind, 1971). In still other instances, religiosity may be an attempt at mastery of conflict, allowing a constructive pathway for some relatively unencumbered instinctual drive or object aim. Some of my recent research suggests additionally that the process of religious transformation often elicits recapitulation of the stages of separation-individuation outlined by Mahler et al. (1975), seen thematically not only in the religionist's personality profile but also in the nature of his relationship with his religious community and in his conceptualization of his deity. We find in corollary that flaws along the lines of the separation-individuation subphases interfere in characteristic fashion with the stages of religious identity development (Spero, 1986). Summing many points of view, we can say that religious change results in disorder primarily when the following factors coexist: (1) preexisting intrapsychic, interpersonal, or family disorder; (2) excessive external manipulation of the devotee's attentional, cognitive, and conative faculties in order to enforce commitment; and (3) sudden and rapid course of value change and identification with the new religious community and other objects.

This last factor serves as the context for understanding the sense of absence of past among nouveaux religious personalities. Suddenness in religious change must be defined as not simply failure to pace the momentum of change, but as the failure to achieve a qualitative state of mind which derives from healthy, methodological skepticism about one's own sincerity, acknowledging persistent doubts and unanswered questions, and carefully considering the quality of one's relationships with former and current values, roles, and identifications. Any change in religious identity must involve an experiential synthesis of the object relational changes which occur across the spectrum of self-structures and identifications in the wake of the adoption of new ego interests. And this includes changes in the sense of temporal continuity or one's sense of past, present, and future.

The basis for the great crisis of the religious return process lies in the transition from the psychic modification or abandonment of old values and identifications and the subsequent restructuring of the self around new religious values and new object relationships. These important tasks, however, are generally experienced rather globally as a sharp break with what one believed or how one behaved previously and the taking up of new beliefs and behaviors. On the one hand, the penitent or convert feels the necessity to abandon the past, to disinherit a devalued and unmaintainable history in order to make way for new identifications and values. Among Jewish persons, it is the past itself which defines the nouveaux religionist as a *ba'al teshuvah,* with its pejorative connotations and implied *arriviste* status, and therefore is experienced as a powerful motive for its own abandonment. On the other hand, the stable (and not largely conscious) elements of personality—including cognitive style, pattern of mind-body interaction, and storehouse of memories and object representations—tend to remain unchanged by superficial reevaluations of the past. Moreover, the nouveaux religionist does not possess immediately an adequate history with new identifications through which to supplant an abandoned or incomplete sense of the past. This results in crisis.

Garber, a convert to Judaism and a psychologist, gives expression to this crisis of absence of past (1979):

> While I studied with conviction, I sometimes felt that I really had no way to go but determinedly ahead since at some point I also knew that the retreat road to the past had been destroyed forever. That is, when the belief structure starts to take shape and when one begins with sincerity to delve into the authentic history of the Jews, the two—the belief structure and a concept of history—eventually meet, and one emerges with a beginning identity as a Jew. From then on, the non-Jewish world, even one's family, is experienced as remote . . . what is lonely in this cognition is the fact that the candidate knows full well what

he has surrendered but knows only uncertainly what is to take
its place [p. 4].

Many newly religious individuals come to the conclusion that
the devalued past has no place in their current life-styles. This
is especially so when they are influenced by the dichotomizing
philosophies of some religious seminaries which seek thus to
balance the students' need to rapidly acquire a great deal of
information and the attraction of contradictory values and information in the nonreligious world. A minority of nouveaux
religionists attempt to retain dialogue with the past, viewing the
process of repentance as a redirection rather than an oblitera-
tion of the past. Presumably, persons in this group benefit from
particularly supportive families and are personally able to synthesize former and present identifications. Nevertheless, it is
inevitable in all cases that intercourse with the past gradually
diminishes and

> ... the contacts with the past which are maintained must be
> psychologically rationalized [p. 110]. ... All *ba'alei teshuvah*
> have broken ties, left friendship circles behind and assumed
> new interests. Even those who guard continuities notice that
> these diminish in force and number. And yet no matter how
> they proceed in adapting, changing, and conforming to the or-
> thodox reality as they see it, and as it is transmitted to them by
> their teachers, *ba'alei teshuvah* remain 'betwixt and be-
> tween.' ... Consciously or unconsciously, gradually or quickly,
> painfully or with ease, it is realized that *teshuvah* [repentance] is
> a major investment demanding a radical break with the past
> [Aviad, 1983, p. 143f.].

THE SENSE OF PAST AND TEMPORAL CONTINUITY

In terms of object relations theory, the mental representations
which comprise the intrapsychic reflection of reality cannot
summarily be divested and invested with loyalty, affective attitudes, relational histories or "pasts," without damaging the
overall integrity of psychic structure. These characteristics tend
to be stable components of the object representation itself, coupled with some complementary representation of the self in re-

lation to the object (Schafer, 1968). Clinical experience certainly confirms that an apparent lack of memory or disenfranchisement of specific aspects of the past does not mean successful or complete blockade of its motivating or organizing power. Rather, the influence of the past persists in the form of psychic structures, attitudes, identifications, and character traits. Thomas et al. (1966) speak of a "time concept" which embodies temporal and object relational functions, providing for the stabilization of self-boundaries and the ability to contemplate changes in the self without the fear of dissolution or fragmentation. With the attempted disavowal of past loyalties and identifications one risks disavowal or distortion of aspects and potentials of the self.

The sense of past emanates from several factors: (1) temporal aspects of the relationships among internal objects (e.g., age, passage of time, rate of speech); (2) significant emotional states that have become alloyed to temporal ones (e.g., anxiety about *anticipation* based on earlier trauma in which the experience of waiting was emotionally significant); (3) object relational or social meanings attendant to certain repetitive patterns in personal, group, or national behavior; and (4) identification with socially provided symbols, language, and even folklore which convey a tradition and perception of continuity. These factors comprise an inner sense that is "active," as Solnit (1984) and others since Freud have observed, in that the past continuously influences one's perception of the present and anticipations for the future. A healthy sense of past allows for the enduring core sameness or constancy of internal objects upon whom the bedrock of current identifications is based, despite concurrent memory-based impressions of these objects as having varying temporal qualities (e.g., an image of one's father which is at once stable but also records simultaneously the impression of his gradual aging). Reisman et al. (1950) termed this the "sense of inner continuity." In other terms, identity includes a sense of sameness with change; "the self-image is maintained . . . by continual redefinement which accompanies comparison and contrast with others" (Greenacre, 1958, p. 614; see also Mahler et al., 1975, p. 116).

SENSE OF PAST AND MEMORY FUNCTION

The sense of past as a force of continuity throughout the various changes in personality depends upon the success of certain early developments in the perception of time and memory functioning. These factors will influence the way in which critical impressions of the past become linking characteristics among current object relations. The young child cannot coordinate temporal intervals between points or moments of relationship (Piaget, 1927). The sense of physical as well as internal, psychological time develops only secondarily to the child's acquisition of concepts such as simultaneity, additivity, further developments in object constancy, and so forth. By about the age of latency, memory and time perception are fully operational (Rees, 1978).

The sense of past is a basic product and anchor of the reality principle (Freud, 1911a). As an integral ego function, there seem to be several perceptual time functions (Ornstein, 1969; Hartocollis, 1976; Terr, 1984), central of which is maintainance of temporal perspective as a kind of balance between the sense of past and future sufficient to "guarantee our continuity of experience across developments in spite of the many ways we change" (Emde, 1983, p. 165; Melges, 1982). The continuity between past and present is particularly important if we view memory not simply as a record of exact replicas of experience—the so-called trace model—but rather as a conceptual or abstract rendition of experience—the schema model (Paul, 1967). Implicit in these conceptual impressions are sensations of time ensconced in affective, ideational, and object representational components which, in their larger relation to time impressions in other schema, provide the sense of continuity between past and present.

Finally, the sense of continuity is fundamentally related to the development of identity. Kernberg, writing of ego identity in the perspective of time (1980), notes that consolidation of ego identity requires coming to terms, in adolescence and again in middle age, not only with the limits of one's personality but also with "repetitive cycles of activation of one's internalized object relations, which are enacted, again and again, as a limited repertoire of 'personal myths'" (p. 127). Included in this process are a heightened experience of the limits of time and reconciliation of "one's knowledge of one's future derived from knowledge about one's past" (p. 128). It is precisely this process which becomes complicated in the case of the nouveaux religionist by a willingness to adopt as one's own a history which has yet to take on personal meaning, and to disconnect oneself from a past which nevertheless remains in some way a persistent foundation in the religionist's personality.

Solnit (1984, p. 630) considers memory of the past a mode of preparation for coping with the present and future, remembering in the service of coping with challenging or threatening events, strengthening the sense of historical continuity and coherency available to the individual:

> No one can feel good, sound, worthwhile about himself if he does not feel coherent. It is an essential need of the maturing person to feel coherent in terms of how to explain his integrity and uniqueness to himself by "knowing" who he is and what his origins were. . . . As the only creatures capable of knowing their past, the story of their lives, human beings use the constructions and reconstructions of the past in valuing themselves, in coping with their present, and in anticipating and influencing their future.

Memories that are difficult to assimilate and organize, or which have been disorganized by attempted rejection or modification, undermine these preparatory and anticipating functions. The nouveaux religionist could very well be said to initially lack "a balance . . . in which there is neither too little nor too much memory" (p. 629).

TEMPORAL PATTERNS AND JEWISH IDENTITY

Individuals, families, and perhaps even nationalities (with respectively less homogeneity) maintain specific types of time schemes. I will illustrate this with the case of Jewish culture since it bears upon all the case vignettes presented here. The religiously observant Jew is influenced by Judaism's time-bound rituals and beliefs, such as the lunar calendar, the seasonal holidays, the weekly Sabbath, and precise daily calculations of various intervals from sunrise to twilight which demarcate periods for prayer, beginnings and ends of festivals and Sabbath, the duration of the menstrual ritual, and so forth. This sense of time is also built upon the perception of intervals, such as between holidays and Sabbaths, menstrual cycles, or regular prayer and study sessions. The Talmud and midrash, for example, instruct the faithful to ennumerate the days of the week in anticipation of Sabbath (*Talmud, Beiza* 22a; *Mekhiltah* to Exodus 20:8), and to ennumerate the months in reference to the month of the Exodus (Nachmanides to Exodus 12:2, 20:8). Heschel (1951) wrote, "Jewish ritual may be characterized as the art of significant forms in time, as *architecture of time*. The main themes of faith lie in the realm of time" (p. 8). Thus, the broad range of experiences such as longing, anticipating, wishing, remembering, planning, and hoping in a strictly observant Jewish life-style can reinforce a stable network of past, present, and future time schemes *in specific relationship to aspects of identity*, imprinted with specific religiocultural connotations. This perception is additionally reinforced by reliance on traditions transmitted intergenerationally, emphasizing practices that have remained relatively unmodified for hundreds of years.

This hypothesis is supported by Zerubavel's (1981) research on *sociotemporal patterns* which involve the temporal rigidification of social situations and activities. Zerubavel argues that such time patterns serve at least three functions: (1) establish group boundaries; (2) facilitate the dichotomization between sacred and profane (e.g., one second before twilight Saturday night is Sabbath while only one second later is a temporal sphere completely bereft of Sabbath restrictions and holiness); and (3) demarcate private/public domains of life (e.g., work schedules and related roles and contexts). All temporal patterns must be integrated and assimilated at an appropriate pace and rhythm. Zerubavel concludes, "The discussion of the symbolic function of calendrical systems indicates that people clearly view time not only as a physio-mathematical entity, but also as an entity which is embued with meaning . . . anchoring the meaning of social acts and situations" (p. xiv).

What occurs in the case of pervasive ideological change such as in the adoption of new religious practices and beliefs? Concurrent with the assumption of new loyalties and identifications the devotee seeks to internalize new objects or modify old objects in relation to new ones whose symbolic and temporal qualities do not yet have counterparts in the complementary new self-image. The nouveaux religious Jew, for example, may now pray 3 times daily and observe Sabbath every 7 days, but initially has no long-term experiential history with the new ways these customs will frame time, and has not yet organized around such temporal frames his perceptual tendencies and interpersonal relations. In the ordinary turn of events, religious observances and related temporal patterns begin to exert their influence from the earliest years of life, serving to organize those aspects of identity and relationships which have to do with religious definitions. This is the stuff of religious individuals' sense of past. Newly religious devotees, however, may succeed with intellectual knowledge about their religion and in emulating external behavior, but in so doing cannot automatically initiate a retroactive modification of the "nonreligious" foundational memories and prior ways of perceiving time. Nor can the nouveaux religionist's idiosyncratic developmental needs or crises be instantaneously rendered in phase with the specific developmental themes implicit in religious beliefs and rituals (Eilberg, 1984). In comparison to new identifications and time patterning, old memories appear to lack some critically important feature. Compared to old identifications and memories, new memories, habits, and loyalties appear tacked on, unrelated in a deep, historically satisfying way—in a continuity providing way—to the entire sense of self.

Experientially, the result is an intense sense of dislocation and "otherness" during interaction with group members and even during private reflection. To the nouveaux religionist, group members appear to share a somehow private history, an almost personal yet exclusive relationship with mythic and folkloristic heroes. Their every movement within the religious community appears infinitely more graceful, versed, and established than one's own. This is the experience of absence of past. It is an experience where although the individual is allowed full access to group symbols, literature, and ritual—unlike the case of social marginality—he remains unable initially fully to share the temporal perceptions or sense of continuity of the group.

Whereas the religious-born simultaneously internalizes both the religious and nonreligious qualities of parents, peers, and environment, developing from his cultural material an illusion of changelessness among his and all earlier generations (Ostow, 1977), the newly religious essentially belies the illusion of changelessness by rejecting his past and seeking new identifications. He must become in relatively later life self-conscious of all of his efforts to do, say, think, and feel the "right" thing, win love and respect, and admit to all sorts of lack of mastery and incoordination. In the wake of this experience is the painful and often contradictory desire to eradicate the past yet also to save it as an anchor to a period of relatively less instability.[2]

The sense of absence of past may result not only from abandonment of undesirable identifications during religious change. There may already exist a sense of disconnection from the past due to developmental failure or weakness in the earliest stages of memory development or the establishment of the earliest identifications. If we distill what is known about the psychological conflicts of many individuals who have been involved in sudden (and even gradual) religious change, consistently one sees incomplete or unsatisfactory resolution of the various tasks and phases of identity development (Gitelson and Reed, 1981; Halperin, 1983; Levin and Zegans, 1974; Levine and Slater, 1976; Maleson, 1981; Pattison, 1980; Stewart, 1967). These range from problems in the most elementary aspects of self-other differentiation to more complex problems of self-esteem, superego functioning, and quality of object relations. Particularly among contemporary adolescents and young adults, fixation at the moratorium stage of identity development may impel the search for new objects. Yet for a variety of reasons, the search

2. In general, Jewish law sought a balance between the *legal* reality of severance of past in conversion—"A convert is like a newborn child" (*Talmud, Yebamot* 22a)—and the *psychological* reality, which features the persistence of past as well as the ambivalent attitude toward the past. The latter is expressed in the Talmudic account of the conversion of Jethro, father-in-law of Moses (*Talmud, Sanhedrin* 94a to Exodus 18:9).

may be for part objects or for objects with whom destructive relationships are conducted. We also know that identity loss or conflict coincides with loss of the sense of location in time and sometimes a compensatory sense of urgency to fill in the resulting gaps in time (Feinstein, 1980).

In cases of incomplete identification with parental objects and early failure to consolidate the self for its journey through time, a stable sense of past does not develop. There is a weakening of the sense of continuity which plays such an important role in ameliorating the ever-present anxiety of separation. This lacunum may impel the search for objects with which to build a sense of past, even a vicarious one, replete with symbols of continuity and a panoply of histories. Factors such as these surely complicate the normative qualities of the sense of absence of past during the process of religious change.

CASE ILLUSTRATIONS

CASE 1

A 23-year-old, unmarried, intellectually superior yeshivah seminarian who had become very orthodox at age 21 sought psychoanalysis due to feelings of depression, indecisiveness, family conflicts, and a mixture of obsessive-compulsive and anxiety symptoms (Spero, 1984). The patient had always lived in a religious neighborhood, although the family remained unreligious despite the father's formally religious early upbringing. The emotional atmosphere of the home was characterized by violent sibling rivalry, dramatic power struggles between the father and his several sons, and periodic marital conflict.

The patient became religious over a period of a few months following an adolescence of intense, fruitless searching. He took a leave of absence from the university (from which he eventually graduated with highest honors during the second year of treatment) and went to Israel to study Judaism. Despite intense discomfort with his new religious peers and mentors and constant feelings of embarrassment about both his irreligious past and the possible inadequacy of all of his current religious beliefs and practices, he excelled in his studies.

Throughout the several months in Israel, he experienced almost constant anxiety and homesickness and after about 10 months returned to America. Despite his parents' overall support, conflict exploded around his new religious preoccupations, especially those which the father suspected, based on his own experience, were not turning out the way Judaism wished.

The patient experienced great difficulty and terrific anxiety in feeling comfortable among his new religious friends, all of whom genuinely liked him. He dreaded that his irreligious past might come up for discussion and that he would be considered forever the *ba'al teshuvah*. He sometimes despised religious Jews who appeared comfortable with their rich family heritages. He felt uncomfortable when teachers and mentors alluded to communal traditions about which he knew nothing or which were based simply upon historic consensus. His inner reaction was always, "Where was I when these customs were accepted?" In discussions, he felt it necessary but altogether a burden to use the "right" jargon or Talmudic citation or vocal intonations, only later to be irritated with and ashamed of himself as he would obsessively review how disingenuous he must have appeared to others.

A conspicuous sign of the patient's ambivalence which persisted until the beginning of the third year of treatment was the feeling that his *yarmulkah* (skullcap) provoked amusement and derision from passersby. He wore it in order to identify with orthodox Judaism, but it also symbolized for him the homosexual, effeminate image he projected onto "those weak, frail, unworldly Talmudic scholars." His former fashionable hair style was not compatible with the large, black, ancient symbol, and so he adopted a closely cropped hair style typical in his yeshivah community. This in turn made him feel naked, childish, and that the *yarmulkah* was "like a woman's hat or a fool's cap, sticking out like my limp, exposed penis!" He viewed his irreligious friends as real males and felt that they considered his *yarmulkah* ridiculous, despite contradictory evidence. He was then plagued with renewed self-doubts that this preoccupation with his irreligious friends' opinion indicated a failure to break with the past.

An interesting chain of associations was produced regarding

the skullcap during the sixth month of treatment. He commented once that his haircut made him feel like a concentration camp inmate. He then recalled that it was a visit to Auschwitz that "lit the first spark" of his religious concerns. He then reflected about this particular choice of expression in the context of the Nazi crematoria. He felt the survival of the Jews was irrefutable proof of God's existence. If God existed, life must be conducted as He demands. This thought generated others which led to the conclusion that he must *immediately* become religious. But then came another obsession: how would he ever be able to modify retroactively all of his past, how could he atone for 19 years of ignorance and sinful acts, not only in his own life but in his parents' as well?

He spoke of many memories of his childhood and adolescence in which no matter what else their content his irreligiosity stood out in marked contrast with what he experienced of himself at present. The very fact that he could not now change these early self representations, he felt, disconnected him from himself. The desire to disconnect himself from the content of these memories (e.g., recollections of sexual escapades), shameful now additionally because of his religious scruples, masked preexisting conflict regarding their content. On the other hand, the desire to reconnect with this past, expressed in the desire to "cleanse" it retroactively, was the result of a healthy wish to consolidate the numerous introjects which prevented complete identity development. In the early stages of treatment, however, the patient would merely have welded these shame-provoking introjects to the current introjects he was adopting from his idealized religious community. In many ways, even the new introjects were hostile or shame-provoking, sending him caroming between painful representations from the past and present.

Further analysis enabled the young man by the end of the first year of treatment to connect this aspect of his religious identity conflict with deeper oedipal neurosis and to confront the memories of shame- and guilt-provoking parental demands which contributed to his own "personal concentration camp horrors" and patricidal wishes. He believed Jews could only endure the Holocaust and continue to believe in God if they ac-

cepted their entire history and destiny. After a bit of intellec-
tualizing, he then realized that if he rejected his past—which he
by now admitted would not be for primarily religious or moral
reasons—then perhaps his relation to his father would be
merely a biological accident, his oedipal burden totally arbitrary, his constant shame now mortifyingly senseless.

Time factors became problematic as he became involved with
seemingly endless and repeated calculations of the daily prayer
schedule, obsessions about different rabbinic rulings on these
matters, and organizing his work and other activities around
prayer and study obligations. He was very disspirited if he
missed prayer with a quorum but also embarrassed if he was
the first man present and certainly if he came late. Although
prayer with a quorum is a desideratum in Jewish law, his anxiety about missing prayer, his manifold preparations not to miss
prayer or to be punctual for study sessions (which have no religiously mandated schedule), expressed the deeper ambivalence about religious commitments as well as the emergent
oedipal anger and preoedipal shame which were becoming
harder and harder to suppress. Holiday times which found the
general community in the throes of festive if harried preparation found the patient oppressed by a mountain of technicalities and jealous of others whom he perceived as easily carrying through with procedures mastered since earliest
childhood. These disturbed qualities toward time-bound observances stemmed in large part from his difficulty in shifting between a perceptual modality where, in his words, "I defined
what I did with time. . . . I created it and I was free to waste it,"
and now, where "time tells me what to do and where to be, and
I have no experience responding to time in this way."
Eventually, the patient was able to appreciate that he of course
had always been responsive to time schedules, only now the
feeling of strangeness or pressure emerged from the constant,
not yet fully accommodated shifting between the old, "secular"
and new, "sacred" time schedule, requiring attention and planning for behaviors formerly automatic; between temporal
schedules that defined two conflicting inner worlds.

In the transference, the patient became hostile and jealous of
me, or idealized my apparently well-known close relationship

with a particular colleague and also with my father. This was a complicating but very useful aspect of the second and third years of analysis.[3] The patient fantasized regularly about the details of the intimate, long past he believed was shared between me and my colleague and father, and particularly my fortune in being able to continue an already established religious tradition. He attempted comparisons between his own family atmosphere on the Sabbath and mine. He spent much time trying to create a valid portrait of what my religious childhood must have looked like. He then felt puny since he could never have a religious past. At the same time, he wavered among various idealizations of extremely orthodox yeshivah personalities, less fundamentalistic and more Zionistic yeshivah types, hasidic types, and finally what he considered the "perfect" type represented by those who could combine devout religiosity and secular knowledge. Characteristically, as each idealization became more intense, the patient became more self-conscious about the fraudulence of his interest in or of his value to the idealized object. He would then find all sorts of clay feet in the reigning ideal, descending into long periods of silence, despair, and identity confusion.

The patient never felt completely at home within the new religious community. He felt as if everyone was watching him begin from scratch, staring at him humiliatingly as he, an adult, underwent stages of behavior and explored levels of knowledge and feeling which they had all long ago experienced as children. His real past was an embarrassment; his present was childish and could not be articulated with adult, manly, perfect ideals; and the new religious past he would eventually have would never contain a sense of religious past begun at birth.

The patient learned, in addition to great amounts of other analytic work, to discover precursors of mature religiosity in his actual past. He was helped to recognize, for example, that inher-

3. Some analysts might consider this too much contamination for analysis to proceed properly. Of course, the patient did not know me personally prior to the analysis. In fact, as long as an individual does not know the analyst personally, any information the patient manages to learn or infer about the analyst simply becomes additional material whose significance must be explored during analysis.

ent in his neurotic attempt to redo his father's past and in his shame for his father's shame, and to become psychologically healthy for his father by proxy, were germinal tendencies that eventually could become autonomous and mature religious fulfillments of the Jewish ethos of filial piety; that his desire for idealized objects was a perhaps pathologically exaggerated expression of a basic drive that could also express itself in healthy love of fellows; or that his spontaneous dissatisfaction at age 16 with teenage drinking bouts was the precursor to the type of self-restraint that eventually flowered into the systematic self-regulation of his orthodox Jewish life-style.

These insights enabled the patient to establish links between his current religiosity and his own personal past rather than to the identities and histories of others. From my perspective, his travail was always simultaneously a religious and object-relational expression (Spero, 1985a). The patient was, of course, involved with problems stemming from faulty self-other differentiation, failures in identification with his parents, and psychosexual conflicts. All of these contributed in some way to his original motivation to become religious and also to the disordered manner in which this religiosity took expression. The relationship with God the patient sought was for a long time only conducted with an intrapsychic image of God, modeled primarily upon interpersonal relations, and not yet with the reality of God, based on experiences which may transcend interpersonal relationships.

CASE 2

A 36-year-old social worker seen in treatment for 4 years provides an illustration of a particular subgroup of nouveaux religionists. This bright young woman was the only child in a home with minimal Jewish affiliations, where the idea but not the practice of Sabbath was known, and little else offered by way of Jewish tradition save the occasional use of Yiddish and rare encounters with moderately religious relatives. She portrayed her father as oafish, though not without pleasant characteristics, who generally slept or preferred the company of rowdy male friends when not working. Mother was without much drive for activities outside of the home, although she struggled successful-

ly to maintain the household, raise her daughter, and minister to
the demands of her husband and his institutionalized mother.

The patient became more committed to formal religious Judaism at age 17 after attending some basic religion courses offered
by a vibrant young rabbi at a local campus organization. By the
time she was 18 years old, she began to travel to a nearby community to attend religion classes at a seminary. She became disinterested in all pursuits save that of becoming a religious teacher,
although she continued attending college classes. At the seminary she became close with one of the teachers and his family. At
20, she accepted an arranged date with a young, sincere, but
rather immature yeshivah student of ordinary abilities, and decided after 8 dates to marry him. Her parents were upset, but
acceded to the marriage on condition that she continue her secular education toward some advanced degree. Within 6 years, the
patient had given birth to a daughter, taken the master's degree
in social work, and was content with her marriage. Shortly after
receiving her degree, she opened a private practice serving by
preference the largely orthodox yeshivah and hasidic community near her home. She had high hopes of dealing successfully
with the expectable resistances of this clientele, confident that
her directive, somewhat educational-homeopathic approach
would be helpful. It soon became clear that she was unprepared
for the gravity of some of her clients' primitive interpersonal
difficulties—she had always believed that religious Jews were
largely immune to severe pathology by virtue of living morally—
and the personal verbal abuse some of her clients directed toward her. Soon she felt ambivalent toward many of her patients,
then toward her professional identity, and then toward her own
religiosity and her husband's way of life. At this juncture she
elected treatment, after percipitously breaking off with almost
all her patients, and with her marriage in disharmony.

The patient stated that she elected treatment due to concern
about some negative feelings toward her husband which she felt
touched upon areas of old conflict in her relationship with her
parents. She also felt that psychoanalysis would enhance her
professional skills. I informed her in the earliest sessions that we
would wish to explore her desire to seek treatment specifically
with me. She was aware that I had a great deal of experience with

religious patients and believed that a religious therapist (readily apparent if only because I wear a *yarmulkah*) would better comprehend her concerns than a nonreligious therapist. These alleged grounds for compatibility expressed by the patient were given immediate attention so as to uncover early resistance to treatment, hidden behind an appeal to religious collegiality (Pruyser, 1977), and to indicate how religious material would be dealt with throughout our work. Following the patient's discussion of her aspirations as a religious therapist and her evaluation of my advantages as a religious analyst, I suggested that she might be searching for a way to protect her religious feelings from her own ambivalence, such as by idealizing the analyst as a perfect combination of religious and secular interests whose sense of religious obligation would magically control overincisive psychological interpretations that might threaten her religious commitment and profession. The patient initially acknowledged this without much difficulty and accepted the challenge of our work.

She then slowly unfolded a history of unrequited efforts to gain her father's affection, to identify with her mother, and, after a seemingly interminable adolescence, to find some meaning in her dreary life. She recognized the nontheological aspects of her interest in her religious mentors and that their families provided her with an auxiliary source of love. She also began to mention feelings regarding time: how slowly it passed in her home, how much she enjoyed the rush every Friday to prepare for Sabbath and somehow always managing to be prepared with only moments to spare, how much time was wasted in her home in contrast to how Judaism filled her day with demands that had real meaning. Until most recently she felt that "every detail of my life made sense because I had some kind of religious thing to do or think about in common with everyone else Jewish, but in this way I also felt cut off from my parents. Whatever I did with my time, I knew they *didn't!*" Her professional studies and clinical experiences with orthodox Jewish patients began to provoke more conflict. "And then came my religious patients, whose life stories, troubling as they were, showed always how they had been religious throughout it all and from their earliest days. Although I had had this feeling earlier, I now became unable to avoid the feeling that everything religious they did just came natural to them, where in contrast I could still feel myself having to think about doing *mizvot* in just the right way. I could never escape the memories of times when I did *not* have these interests or the fact that my parents, the people I come from, do not do these things. I recall learning the *aleph-bet* when I was 18. I felt small and awfully silly sometimes, despite my protested pride in my courageous ability to be a contemporary Rabbi Akiba" (a famous Talmudic sage who became religious at age 40 and sat among the kindergarten children to learn Hebrew). Later she added, "I had no religious memories going back to childhood. Much of the pain came from remembering those primitive levels of religious development—when I made mistakes or silly errors in practice—which basically happened only years or months ago and not when I was 4 or 10 years old when I probably would have repressed it like you or everyone else."

To a degree, the patient compensated for inferiority feelings by relying upon her professional degree to elevate her above the group. At the same time, she identified with a religious group that essentially looked askance at college studies. Her professional identity represented a threat to many of her acquaintances and patients, and in many ways she had begun to internalize their negative reactions to her. She believed that her position of neutrality with her patients—which to judge from her treatment style she neither ideologically or practically safeguarded—would protect her own past from being revealed. At the same time, her exploration of the lives of her patients would give her numerous pasts or aspects of past to repair or relive vicariously. There were no borderline qualities in this overinvestment in others, but rather an unwholesome, neurotic attempt by an undernourished ego to revise, enrich, and repopulate the past in view of the differences between the unsatisfying objects of the past and the idealistically satisfying ones of the present.

She eventually spoke of a stage just prior to her near-complete departure from social work when she noticed herself working hard to convince one of her clients to modify some disautonomous religious mannerisms which included many obsessional tendencies. Later she felt guilty about possibly destroying the client's religiosity. This feeling was rich in transference implications, but also indicated the consequences of identifying with the group's negative view of psychological services. It also masked her jealousy of and anger with this client who the community fully accepted as religious despite his very blatant abnormal behavior, whereas she was forever the newcomer. In borrowing pasts, this sensitive woman had also borrowed the disorganizing aspects of these pasts. The ensuing 3½ years of psychoanalysis were often very painful as she learned gradually to desist attempts to deny or revise the past and to accept the voids created both by preexistent identity-related crises and by the normative aspects of her religious transformation.

During one stage of the transference, she expressed interest in learning my style of intervention, and this was simple enough to clarify in psychodynamic terms. At about the same time, she began to initiate many discussions about Jewish law and esoterica, seeking my opinion on matters of everyday Jewish practice. Her associations to this type of resistance illustrated the desire to prove herself so competent in matters religious as to appear never to have had a stage of lesser skill or knowledge. The lure of the less demanding ways of her irreligious youth also was present. This was interpreted not so much as spiritual weakness as the wish to eliminate guilt elicited by her successful oedipal rebellion, her ambivalent longing for reunion with her parents, and a powerful dissatisfaction with her feminine role and identity preceding her religious transformation. In one interesting fantasy, she imagined devouring so many tomes of Jewish law that she would be considered a modern Beruriah, the brilliant wife of the Talmudic sage Rabbi Meir, famous for her intelligence but excoriated for her contentiousness. The patient was apparantly aware of Beruriah's infamous quality. She then commented that she indeed intended somehow to read every text of Jewish scholarship translated into English. Ironically, the patient sought to prove her worthiness by idealizing an iconoclast female scholar, yet inadvertently acknowledged her dependency upon study aids aids designed specifically for an increasingly large audience of *ba'alei teshuvah*.

In interpreting these idealizing transferences and her various uses of religious material in the service of resistance, I focused on her attempt to discover and identify with my personal solution to the conflict between religious and secular ideals, and to fashion out of her analysis with me a sort of personal religious history. This history began with her rebirth psychologically, spiritually, and professionally through our work, by substituting memories of emotionally significant analytic sessions for disagreeable ones from her childhood, believing she and the analyst shared a private communion whereby she had the unique privilege of receiving a personal revelation from a master (Kehoe and Gutheil, 1984; Lovinger, 1979; Spero, 1981). Eventually this transitional history was surrendered as well. With reduced pressure from earlier identity conflicts and more autonomy in her religious feelings, she was slowly able to form a true identification with both her current religious values and the precursors of religious sensitivities in her own childhood. These precursors represented a *personal* endowment, with early roots linking her as much to her parents as to her current religious peers, serving as a basis for a sense of continuity around which the technicalities of increased formal religious behavior could now be more healthfully built.

CASE 3

This material is drawn from diagnostic and therapeutic interviews with Louis, age 30, and Janette, age 28, a couple in their fourth year of marriage. I will not review the entire treatment but merely illustrate how a particularly recalcitrant nouveaux religionist was helped to recognize his difficulties with absence of past.

Louis became a religious Jew at 28 after being inspired by a hasidic rabbi who lectured at his prayer group. At the same time, his girlfriend Janette, who came from a completely unidentified Jewish home, attempted to share his new interest in traditional Judaism. She remained, however, less enthusiastic than Louis. Louis's father died when Louis was 12 years old and he was never close to his stepfather. This led to friction and in time he grew distant from both his mother and her husband. Louis had been in counseling sporadically during his college years because of feelings of boredom, unhappiness about his growing estrangement from his mother, and a spate of unsatisfying sexual experiences. Janette described her middle-class parents as loving, but very busy with their own interests, raising their children with very little discipline or guidance. Occasionally she felt lonely as an adolescent; her pleasures during this stage were empty and she felt no sense of purpose. These factors motivated her various communal living arrangements during which she met Louis.

Under the tutelage of the hasidic teacher, the couple moved quickly into an emotionally charged and apparently happy devotion, adopting the mannerisms, beliefs, and argot of the group. Louis maintained a small printing shop. The couple's lives began more and more to center about the group, shared Sabbaths and festive meals, and learning and prayer groups. The teacher encouraged them to establish some outside interests, but they had few. Louis preferred mystical, kabbalistic teachings to the more disciplined work of Talmudic study, and enjoyed immensely the evening banter with fellow *ba'alei teshuvah* about hasidic folklore. He fancied himself a hasid of the purest sort, working hard and joyously in God's and his hasidic Rebbeh's service, but also watchful for the attacks and misunderstandings of nonhasidic Jews. I was asked to see Louis after an incident in which he came to blows with a group member who expressed doubt about Louis's concrete interpretation of some legend which spoke of the supernatural powers of the founder of Hasidism. The friend insisted the legend was intended as hyperbole. As the debate became increasingly heated, Louis smacked his fellow across the face.

Psychological testing revealed mixed features: anxiety, depressive themes in some projective material, obsessive compulsivity, but also unimpaired intellectual functioning and no evidence of faulty or even loose reality testing. His object representations as depicted on various tests were not malevolent or bizarre, but poorly articulated or thinly characterized, portraying most often either passive or unplanned activity. The quality of his object relationships was similar, although here an idealizing tendency emerged more clearly. His early memories portrayed the sadness related to death and loneliness and the search for idealized male figures. At the same time, throughout the first open-ended interview, Louis projected a happy state of mind and an attitude of "no complaints."

The strengths that emerged related almost entirely to religious feelings and the sense of confidence he had established in the hasidic Rebbeh and his local teacher. Both Louis and Janette became enlivened when referring to the Rebbeh, whom they had never met personally. His judgment was deemed unimpeachable and was sought for all major decisions. More than once, Louis responded to inquiries about his past by telling me about the miraculous transformations *others* had effected or by referring to tales about the lives of famous *ba'alei teshuvah*. Louis preferred rabbinic legends and myths which portrayed large, happy families, positive and reciprocal relations between sons and fathers. Indeed, he was thirsty for legendary stories about biblical heroes while showing almost no interest in contemporary Jewish history. The moral themes of these stories were less significant for him than the personal details, the wondrous possibilities, the emotions he could project into each and then identify with.

Louis wished to give the appearance of having no conflict between his prereligious and his present life, but this was merely denial. He was among those nouveaux religious who strive to block out memories and identifications of the past. He was markedly uncomfortable about discussing any former interest which he would look down upon currently. He spoke piously of having done repentance for all his old behaviors and interests and as having no need to reflect back on them. He more than once mentioned a rabbinic ban against "forcing" a convert or *ba'al teshuvah* to confront his errant past. I shared with Louis my belief that there may be pain associated with some of the material he chose not to talk about. I avoided pseudo-theological debate by inviting him to explore just how doing repentance changed him. It was not long before significant material began to emerge.

In the third month of treatment a session began with a stormy, transference-based critique of the emotional emptiness and coldness of the therapist-patient relationship compared to the warmth of the Rebbeh-hasid relationship; then a comment that I would not be able to give him something permanent that could bind us to a common root; and then anger that I was hiding my own past from him. In extolling the Rebbeh-hasid encounter,

Louis spoke in idealized terms, telling folklore and apocryphal anecdotes, yet conveyed nothing that really expressed a personally satisfying relationship. He spoke of traditions, but he was not truly at home in any of these. Soon one could detect a subtle sense of frustration with the unspanned gap which separated the lofty, almost superhuman Rebbeh and the very mortal, small, and lonely hasid.

I reviewed this material and noted that on the one hand he felt that the Rebbeh-hasid relationship was ultimate, yet on the other hand he sought a reciprocal relationship with me. It seemed as if a special emptiness or loneliness persisted despite his newfound faith, more deeply expressing the searching of a son for a much beloved father. Louis was quiet for several moments and then commented that for a long time he had been searching for some tangible or intangible thing which he could construe as an expression of a permanent, enduring, and loving link to his father. He thought he experienced this in the Torah and prayers. God had given these to him—or the Rebbeh had assigned him tasks—much as he now recalled his father had given him certain gifts before he was hospitalized. Louis viewed the Torah as an eternal object that automatically made him part of its endless past and present, which he liked to base on the tradition that the souls of Jews of all generations were present at the Sinaitic Revelation. As Louis had earlier commented, "I'm just picking up where my soul left off 3,000 years ago. The details in between don't matter." He then admitted that his deeper struggle with the incomprehensible gap of 3,000 years was another way of expressing the equally incomprehensible and far more painful gap of 18 years since his father's death.

In the next session, Louis expressed with great emotion that he could not handle the vacuum and emptiness since his father's death, or the occasional impression that all of his memories of their past relationship were only a story he had been told. His interest in legends, it appeared, was that they allowed a connection with the past. A common identity could be more easily wrested from or imposed upon the mute mythic heroes than the vastly more complex living personalities around him or the painful, unchangeable memories of his father. The severed identification with his father had left a void, partially filled in with introjects and reconstructions, which themselves stimulated a search for completion.

DISCUSSION

ABSENCE OF PAST AND IDENTITY FORMATION

In the first part of this paper I discussed the genesis of time and memory functioning and the sense of continuity as components of the sense of self. One can also link the development of a sense of the past to the gradual nature of the identification process. We know that children identify with values just as they do with interpersonal objects. This is due partly to a necessary testing process wherein the child stabilizes the inner representation of these values and determines which aspects are absolute, trustworthy, and unambivalent, and which are not. Moreover, social phenomena and values become of interest to children and adults only because there is some parallel between the functions of these institutions and issues that are relevant in personal development. Thus, the overall quality of any internalized value, belief, or object depends upon the opportunities for the internalized representation or structure to mature along with other psychosexual, cognitive, and interpersonal developments.

In the case of religious transformation the nouveaux religious personality must have ample opportunity to stabilize the inner representations of new values and social phenomena, and to allow the ego to align the intrapsychic parallels *between* new and old values *along* the parallel components of individual personality to which such values are attractive. Included in this process is the internalization of new sociotemporal patterns. For the nouveaux religionist there is initially inadequate relationship with a lived, personal, religious history to permit sufficient parallels to emerge between all earlier levels of psychological development and those aspects of religious life which are of particular stimulus value. The sense of absence of past and the perception of discontinuity are not the result simply of lack or suppression of memories, but also are the consequence of temporal skew among intrapsychic structures as these shift slowly into new patterns of coordination.

Erikson (1959, p. 113) notes, "*Identity formation,* finally, begins where the usefulness of identification ends." Complete identity formation calls for the selective repudiation or the mature assimilation of childhood "part" identifications into a single, relatively stable and enduring pattern, including what we call the sense of self, an enduring configuration "established by successive ego syntheses and resyntheses" (p. 116). Erikson's contribution to the present topic will be appreciated if it is accepted that he uses the term identification the way many contemporary writers use the term introjection (following Schafer, 1968). The nouveaux religionist cannot be satisfied merely with achieving a sense of social "fittedness," as Erikson emphasizes (p. 114), for this may represent merely one of the departmentalized identities which human beings find prepared in their communities (see also Lichtenstein, 1977, p. 164). Without a chrono-phenomenological transformation of identity, the nouveaux religionist is prone to take essentially instrumental religious behaviors and distort them into self-contained practices, lacking further objective conformity (Merton, 1957). I have already suggested that in the early stages of religious change, absence of past, denial of past, and the search for a new past dispose toward ahistoric introjections and idealizations, impeding the process of more complete identity formation.

FOLKLORE AS A LINK WITH THE PAST

In each of the illustrations one sees the tendency to study selectively and idealize the personalities or content of folklore and myth in a manner often quite similar to the ways in which such material is perceived by children during early stages of development. There is a preference for legends which feature in concrete terms the downfall of the wicked, reward for the righteous, exaggerated human capacities for goodness or evil, the interminable beneficence of God, and so forth. This use of legend and myth appears to favor the polarization of good and bad self and object representations, the demarcation of positive and negative ego ideals, and the externalization of hated or feared impulses and identifications. These functions are indeed typical of early stages of development, but recur during the upheaval of religious identification in a way which is regressive but also potentially adaptive (Arlow, 1982; Spero, 1982). The gravitation toward particular themes or heroes is partly determined by the needs of the individual.

In the case of increased religious affiliation in later life, the loss or devaluation of past heroes and ideals may be counteracted by cathexis of fantasy heroes which populate religious mythic literature, utilizing this literature as a transition until more realistic, reliable, and psychologically relevant ideals and identifications have been tested and synthesized into permanent structures. The world of myth, to the degree that it lies closer to primary process ideation, allows expression of the individual's more primitive needs and fantastic aspirations, but it also may provide the earliest opportunity for consolidation between the individual's search for continuity and the deeper psychological characteristics and values of the group (Kernberg, 1980). The danger of this use of myth is that it may encourage dissociation and denial, splitting of object representations, and the persistence of concrete interpretations of reality.

SHAME AND ABSENCE OF PAST

The illustrations emphasize the heightened consciousness of self observed in clinical work with nouveaux religionists. In adolescence such self-consciousness is part of the normative crisis, reawakened in the impact of stimuli bearing upon identity formation such as increased commitment to intimacy with a new social group, problems of occupational choice, competitiveness, and new redistribution of object cathexis in order to reestablish psychosocial self-definition.

The nouveaux religionist faces similar stimuli at whatever stage religious change takes place. He or she must sustain the severing of old commitments and establish intimacy with a new social group, reconsider former occupational or educational goals or levels of involvement in favor of the pursuit of religious study, and redefine his previous occupational or educational behavior in the light of new values. The individual will also have to compete with the religious community, with "older" nouveaux religionists, and occasionally even with children and adolescents for recognition of achievement of satisfactory religious knowledge. Throughout, the self that is exposed is being disconnected inwardly and externally from old histories even as it is being cajoled to accept a new identity structure in which it has no past and to engage in relationships for which it has yet to establish structure.

The case illustrations also reveal the powerful impact of feelings of shame, humiliation, and embarrassment, characterized by the classic sense of audience and feelings of being looked through. Most often, shame reactions occur in the context of actual or dreaded mishaps having to do with the practice of new religious behaviors or with the status of *ba'al teshuvah*. In some cases, such as that of the first patient, the shame reactions concerning religious matters and identity are obviously rooted in deeper problems of self-esteem and poor self-other differentiation.

In other instances, there does not seem to be compelling evidence of long-term psychological disorder or poor self development typical of the shame-prone personality, yet shame reactions are also common during developmental crisis and later trauma (Kinston, 1983; Spero, 1984). The upheaval brought about by the rejection of former identifications and the search for new ones results in the acquisition of many introjects, idealizations, and regression of former identifications into introjects. These are experienced as incompletely depersonified presences in whose shadow the self feels exposed, naked, unworthy, or ashamed. Almost every nouveaux religionist is gripped with ambivalent feelings, such as the conflicting wish on the one hand to display newfound in-group characteristics and to behave in such a way as to confirm common history and on the other hand the fear of tripping up, showing ignorance, or experiencing the childlike level of one's knowledge or emotional satisfaction. Shame is most painful when the experience of being caught in one's foiled attempts at display or of being rejected by an ambivalently cathected object (e.g., the new religious community or the one representing rejected values) reverberates among introjected object and self representations.

A PARADOX OF THE RELIGIOUS TRANSFORMATION

The nouveaux religious individual's relationship with his old-new past and subsequent identity-related tasks can be additionally illuminated by comparison to Erikson's (1958) concept of the "chosen young man," the young person who believes he may, in one form or another, change the course of history.

> The chosen young man extends the problem of his identity to the borders of existence in the known universe. . . . He acts as if mankind were starting all over with his own beginning as an individual, conscious of his singularity as well as his humanity. . . . To him, history ends as well as starts with him; others must look to their memories, to legends, or to books to find models for the present and the future in what their predecessors have said and done [p. 261f.].

This concept is related to the sense of special election or destiny expressed by many *ba'alei teshuvah* (Aviad, 1983) and nouveaux religionists of other faiths. Most nouveaux religionists, to be sure, do not believe that the whole of humanity is beginning anew with their personal rebirth, nor do they manifest the intense megalomania of chosen young persons. However, many indeed choose to revise their personal destiny because they feel powerless to change external conditions, reversing and then projecting any insecurities they may have about their own initiatives in the form of a sense of personal election or special destiny. The nouveaux religionist attempts to lessen the disorganizing impact of the experience of absence of past by adopting the notion that his personal past always contained, if only potentially, the germ of his present religious experiences.[4] As I

---

4. See Freud's (1911b) discussion of the delusional way in which Dr. Schreber traced back into former centuries his family's relationship with the Flechsig family: "In just the same way a young man who is newly engaged, and cannot understand how he can have lived so many years without knowing the girl he is now in love with, will insist that he really made her acquaintance at some former time" (p. 58n.). This seems quite similar to what has been observed among *ba'alei teshuvah* who, in order to bridge the gap between their old and new identities, will point to some early religious belief, behavior, or minimal level of religious education and come to view it retroactively as a "constant force" in their subsequent lives. Others will do the same with some early identi-

have shown, however, this notion cannot become fully satisfying until the religionist is better able to distinguish between the fantasied and realistic aspects of this claim.[5]

The issue for the religionist, as for the chosen young man or the adopted child (Brinich, 1980; Novey, 1966), is whether to define oneself in terms of one's own immediate history or to identify with the history of others or to invent new history. Paradoxically, as Erikson aptly puts it, if a man has a sense of historical continuity—a sense of past—which inheres in healthy identity, he does not tend to act historically, for he is satisfied. In order to "make history," or to make one's own history by linking oneself to religious tradition, the searching person will first have to abandon his socially defined, culturally and personally supported identity, and grope for new definitions and history. This process is inherently disorganizing, anxiety-provoking, involves a tremendous sense of loss and dislocation, and disposes toward percipitous allegience to lesser gods and pseudohistories. The positive, enriching, fulfilling, and reunifying aspects of religious change can only come after the gradual relocation of the self along the lines outlined above.

MOVEMENT AMONG PASTS

A key to adjustment among nouveaux religious individuals is the ability to oscillate in and out of and strike balance between twin experiences: the experience of having been nonreligious and a subsequent experience which eventually develops of having never been nonreligious. The latter experience typically emerges rather suddenly, in a very fleeting and often exaggerated man-

---

fication with or idealization of a religious relative or mentor. In all instances, secondary revision will be apparent. At the same time, this phenomenon is to be distinguished from the mature, adaptive attempt to discover what I have termed precursors to religious development, recognized as such after the individual has acquired sufficient psychological sophistication.

5. In still other instances the experience of special election is also a fulfillment of the wish to regain the seat of the oedipal throne. From the technical standpoint, even if both therapist and patient happen to be religious devotees who subscribe to the belief in special election, it can be acknowledged that dynamics such as those described here influence the particular neurotic and even nonneurotic perceptions the patient lends to such beliefs.

ner. An instructive analogy comes from personal experience. As a recent immigrant to Israel from the United States, I often feel like a tourist (with its negative and positive connotations), an American jaunting about in someone else's home, not really a participant in the local laws, preoccupations, daily goings on, and the like. I feel in a sense that everything round about me will occupy my attention for but a second or two; that soon I will leave this all behind me as I *really* belong elsewhere. Then, perhaps just short of simultaneously, I feel like I have been here *forever*, as if I know every nook and cranny of every stone, like a well-known entity in my own right, as if each and every passing bus or fellow pedestrian will in some way prove significant to me in my new life. The two feelings are almost mutually exclusive and typically rotate. Both together, in some synthesized form wherein all aspects of these double identifications can share in a single continuous tempo, contribute to a livable and creative reality. A 34-year-old Israel Air Force pilot who became religious after his tour of duty in a recent war expressed his intuitive understanding of this oscillating process:

> At some moments, there is only Torah and *mitzvot*, only my *kipah*, to the point where I must almost force myself to return my attention to the dials and to remember that *right now I am flying a plane!* Sometimes I forget that I have many good, irreligious friends. Other times, when I am intently involved in some calculations or instrument work, I wonder to myself whether anyone, even the dials, knows that I am a *religious* Jew, or that my world is no longer the same as it was 10 years ago? Often I borrow one feeling to complement the other. . . . It happens that I was taught a Jewish philosophy which accepted the relation between orthodoxy and the religious ideals of having a profession, serving in my country's self-defense, and more. But the reason I did not become crazy, I think, is because I was able to reintroduce my religious self to my "old" self, to realize that the guy who sometimes feels that he only started living 10 years ago is in fact *me*, born 34 years ago.

SUMMARY

The sense of absence of past is one aspect of the complex phenomenology and dynamics of religious identity development, serving both as a motive and a normative but potentially complicating aspect of religious change. The sense of absence of past highlights the need during identity change to transform time and memory patterns as these impact upon transformations in object relationships and interests. This will allow restoration of the sense of continuity initially broken as an outgrowth of change in religiosity and the radical reevaluation of former loyalties, interests, and identifications. These concepts were illustrated with three Jewish nouveaux religionists who were analytic patients, where the role of absence of past and the psychodynamic function of religious legend, ritual, and sociotemporal patterns were readily apparent. Even when psychological disorder is not present, the consolidation of an optimally functioning religious identity requires an apprenticeship with new time perspectives and experimentation with new idealizations—including the ability to oscillate between former and present self-perceptions, the ability to align past and present psychic structures which have become modified in the course of new identifications, and adequate time to synthesize inner needs and their parallel expression in both the mundane and religious realities.

BIBLIOGRAPHY

ADAH HA-AM [ASHER GINZBURG] (1956). *Al Parshat Derakhim,* vol. 1. Jerusalem: Tefuzot.

ARLOW, J. A. (1982). Unconscious fantasy and political movements. In *Judaism and Psychoanalysis,* ed. M. Ostow, pp. 271–282. New York: Ktav.

ATWOOD, G. E. (1978). On the origins and dynamics of messianic salvation fantasies. *Int. Rev. Psychoanal.,* 5:85–96.

AVIAD, J. (1983). *Return to Judaism.* Chicago: Univ. Chicago Press.

BERGMAN, P. (1953). A religious conversion in the course of psychotherapy. *Amer. J. Psychother.,* 12:41–58.

BRINICH, P. M. (1980). Some potential effects of adoption on self and object representations. *Psychoanal. Study Child,* 35:107–133.

BUBER, M. (1951). *Two Types of Faith.* New York: Macmillan.

CASEY, R. P. (1938). The psychoanalytic study of religion. *J. Abnorm. & Soc. Psychol.,* 33:437–452.

DONSHIK, S. (1979). Some psychological aspects of the modern *ba'al teshuvah.* *Intercom,* 18:6–15.

EAGEL, M. (1983). Interests as object relations. In *Empirical Studies of Psychoanalytic Theories,* ed. J. Masling, pp. 159–187. Hillside, N.J.: Analytic Press.

EILBERG, A. (1984). Views of human development in Jewish rituals. *Smith Coll. Stud. Soc. Wk*, 55:1–23.

ELKIND, D. (1971). The origin of religion in the child. *Rev. Relig. Res.*, 12:35–40.

EMDE, R. N. (1983). The prerepresentational self. *Psychoanal. Study Child*, 38:165–192.

ERIKSON, E. H. (1958). *Young Man Luther*. New York: Norton.

———— (1959). *Identity and the Life Cycle*. Psychol. Issues, monogr. 1. New York: Int. Univ. Press.

FEINSTEIN, S. C. (1980). Identity and adjustment disorders of adolescence. In *Comprehensive Textbook of Psychiatry*, ed. I. Kaplan, A. Freedman, & B. Sadock, pp. 2640–2658. Baltimore: William & Wilkins.

FRANZBLAU, A. (1965). Conversion to Judaism. In *Conversion to Judaism*, ed. D. Eichhorn, pp. 67–89. New York: Ktav.

FREUD, S. (1911a). Formulations on the two principles of mental functioning. *S.E.*, 12:213–226.

———— (1911b). Psychoanalytic notes on an autobiographical account of a case of paranoia (dementia paranoides). *S.E.*, 12:12–84.

GARBER, J. (1979). Psychological aspects of religious change. *Intercom*, 18:3–5.

GITELSON, I. & REED, E. J. (1981). Identity status of Jewish youth pre- and post-cult involvement. *J. Jewish Comm. Serv.*, 57:312–320.

GLANZ, D. & HARRISON, M. T. (1978). Varities of identity transformation. *Jew. J. Sociol.*, 20:129–141.

GORDON, D. (1974). The Jesus people. *Urb. Life & Cult.*, 3:159–178.

GREENACRE, P. (1958). Early physical determinants in the development of the sense of identity. *J. Amer. Psychoanal. Assn.*, 6:612–627.

HALPERIN, D., ed. (1983). *Psychodynamic Perspectives on Religion, Sect, and Cult*. Littleton, Mass.: John Wright/P. S. G.

HARTOCOLLIS, P. (1976). On the experience of time and its dynamics. *J. Amer. Psychoanal. Assn.*, 24:363–375.

HESCHEL, A. J. (1951). *The Sabbath*. New York: Farrar, Straus & Giroux.

JAMES, W. (1902). *The Varieties of Religious Experience*. New York: Modern Library.

KEHOE, N. & GUTHEIL, T. (1984). Shared religious belief as resistance in psychotherapy. *Amer. J. Psychother.*, 38:575–589.

KERNBERG, O. F. (1980). *Internal World and External Reality*. New York: Aronson.

KINSTON, W. (1983). A theoretical context for shame. *Int. J. Psychoanal.*, 64:213–226.

KNIGHT, R. P. (1937). Practical and theoretical considerations in the analysis of a minister. *Psychoanal. Rev.*, 24:350–364.

LEVIN, T. M. & ZEGANS, L. (1974). Identity crises and religious conversion. *Brit. J. Med. Psychol.*, 47:73–82.

LEVINE, S. V. (1983). Alienated Jewish youth and religious seminaries. In *Psychodynamic Perspectives on Religion, Sect. and Cult*, ed. D. Halperin. Littleton, Mass.: John Wright/P.S.G.

LEVINE, S. V. & SLATER, N. (1976). Youth and contemporary religious movements. *Canad. Psychiat. Assn. J.*, 21:411–420.

LICHTENSTEIN, H. (1977). *The Dilemma of Human Identity*. New York: Aronson.

LITTLEWOOD, R. (1983). The antinomian hasid. *Brit. J. Med. Psychol.*, 56:67–78.

LOVINGER, R. (1983). Therapeutic strategies with "religious" resistances. *Psychotherapy*, 16:419–427.

McDARGH, J. (1983). *Psychoanalytic Object Relations Theory and the Study of Religion*. Washington: Univ. Press of America.

MAHLER, M. S., PINE, F., & BERGMAN, A. (1975). *The Psychological Birth of the Human Infant*. New York: Basic Books.

MALESON, F. (1981). Dilemmas in the evaluation and management of religious cultists. *Amer. J. Psychiat.*, 138:925–930.

MANN, J. (1964). Clinical and theoretical aspects of religious beliefs. *J. Amer. Psychoanal. Assn.*, 11:160–170.

MEISSNER, W. W. (1984). *Psychoanalysis and Religious Experience*. New York: Brunner/Mazel.

MELGES, F. T. (1982). *Time and Inner Future*. Sumerset, N.J.: John Wiley.

MERTON, R. K. (1957). *Social Theory and Social Structure*. New York: Free Press.

MESTER, R. & KLEIN, H. (1981). The young Jewish revivalist. *Brit. J. Med. Psychol.*, 54:299–306.

NOVEY, S. (1966). Why some patients conduct actual investigations of their biographies. *J. Amer. Psychoanal. Assn.*, 14:376–387.

ORNSTEIN, R. (1969). *On the Experience of Time*. New York: Pelican.

OSTOW, M. (1977). The psychologic determinants of Jewish identity. *Israel Ann. Psychiat. & Rel. Disc.*, 15:313–335.

PATTISON, E. M. (1980). Religious youth cults as alternative social healing networks. *J. Relig. Health*, 19:275–286.

PAUL, L. H. (1967). The concept of schema in memory theory. In *Motives and Thought*, ed. R. R. Holt, pp. 218–258. New York: Int. Univ. Press.

PIAGET, J. (1927). *The Child's Perception of Time*. New York: Ballantine.

PRUYSER, P. (1971). Assessment of the psychiatric patient's religious beliefs in the psychiatric case study. *Bull. Menninger Clin.*, 35:272–291.

——— (1977). The seamy side of current religious beliefs. *Bull. Menninger Clin.*, 41:329–340.

REES, K. (1978). The child's understanding of his past. *Psychoanal. Study Child*, 33:237–259.

REISMAN, D., DENNEY, R., & GLAZER, N. (1950). *The Lonely Crowd*. New Haven: Yale Univ. Press.

RIZZUTO, A.-M. (1979). *The Birth of the Living God*. Chicago: Univ. Chicago Press.

SCHAFER, R. (1968). *Aspects of Internalization*. New York: Int. Univ. Press.

SCOBIE, G. E. W. (1975). *The Psychology of Religion*. London: Batsford.

SOLNIT, A. J. (1984). Preparing. *Psychoanal. Study Child*, 39:613–632.

SPERO, M. H. (1980). The penitent personality type. *J. Psychol. & Judaism*, 4:131–193.

———— (1981). A clinical note on the therapeutic management of "religious" resistances. *J. Jewish Comm. Serv.*, 57:334–341.

———— (1982). The use of folklore as a developmental phenomenon among nouveaux orthodox religionists. *Amer. J. Psychoanal.*, 42:149–158.

———— (1983a). Psychotherapeutic procedures with religious cult devotees. In *Psychodynamic Perspectives on Religion, Sect, and Cult*, ed. D. Halperin, pp. 295–317. Littleton, Mass.: John Wright/P.S.G.

———— (1983b). Religious patients in psychotherapy. *Brit. J. Med. Psychol.*, 56:287–292.

———— (1984). Shame. *Psychoanal. Study Child*, 39:259–282.

———— (1985a). The reality and the image of God in psychotherapy. *Amer. J. Psychother.*, 39:75–85.

———— (1985b). *Psychotherapy of the Religious Patient*. Springfield, Ill.: Charles C. Thomas.

———— (1986). The stages of repentance from an object relations perspective. Bar-Ilan University, unpublished manuscript.

STARK, R. (1971). Psychotherapy and religious commitment. *Rev. Relig. Res.*, 12:165–175.

STERN, E. M. (1985). *Psychotherapy of the Religiously Committed Patient*. New York: Haworth.

STEWART, C. H. (1967). *Adolescent Religion*. New York: Abingdon.

STOLOROW, R. & ATWOOD, G. E. (1973). Messianic projects and early object relations. *Amer. J. Psychoanal.*, 33:213–215.

THE TALMUD, 18 vols., tr. I. Epstein. London: Soncino, 1961.

TERR, L. C. (1984). Time and trauma. *Psychoanal. Study Child*, 39:633–665.

THOMAS, R., EDGCUMBE, R., KENNEDY, H., KAWENOKA, M., & WEITSNER, L. (1966). Comments on some aspects of self and object representation in a group of psychotic children. *Psychoanal. Study Child*, 21:527–580.

ULLMAN, C. (1982). Cognitive and emotional antecedents of religious conversion. *J. Pers. & Soc. Psychol.*, 43:183–192.

WOOTTON, R. & ALLEN, D. (1983). Dramatic religious conversion and schizophrenic decompensation. *J. Relig. & Health*, 22:212–220.

ZERUBAVEL, E. (1981). *Hidden Rhythms*. Chicago: Univ. Chicago Press.

CLINICAL CONTRIBUTIONS

Consequences of Paternal Nurturing

JUDITH FINGERT CHUSED, M.D.

A GREAT DEAL OF ATTENTION HAS BEEN FOCUSED ON THE ONE-parent family. Until recently, custody decisions after divorce almost always favored the mother, whose ability to nurture was seen as biologically determined and gender-related. Histor-ically, the father was viewed as having a relatively insignificant role in early child development, important only as his support of the mother enabled her to respond appropriately to her infant's needs. Then, in 1951, Loewald recognized the father's role in freeing the infant from the early symbiotic relationship with the mother. As Mahler and Gosliner (1955) pointed out, a pro-longed, exclusive, dyadic relationship with the mother can inter-fere with an infant's development of anxiety-free autonomous functioning. When this occurs, the father, perceived as a sepa-rate object by the infant, is tremendously important for the rela-tively stable, unambivalent relationship he can provide. But even without pathology in the mother-infant dyad, the father's loving support is valuable; first, when the infant struggles with differ-entiation from mother and later, during the rapprochement phase, when the child becomes anxious over the limitations of his and his mother's powers. Until recently, however, the infant's perception of father as separate was thought to be dependent on the early father-infant relationship being different from the in-fant's relationship with his mother.

Vice-chairman, Department of Psychiatry, National Children's Hospital of the District of Columbia; associate clinical professor, George Washington Uni-versity School of Medicine; and training and supervising analyst, Washington Psychoanalytic Institute.

The primary preoedipal dyad has always been conceptualized as infant and mother or infant and mother-surrogate; when the mother was absent or depriving through her own psychopathology, the child was considered at risk for serious emotional and cognitive difficulties. And though it has been recognized that there is a tremendous range in the degree of ego impairment and strength in individuals with a history of an unavailable mother, the influence of the father, as a force mitigating the effect of maternal deprivation, has never been fully examined.

In 1975 Abelin described an infant in whom a symbioticlike relationship developed with both father and mother, with a low-keyness in the absence of either and evidence of psychological refueling from both. Further infant research demonstrated that "infants are attached from the earliest age to both parents" (Lamb, 1980, p. 42). Most recently, Pruett (1983, 1985) observed that the "nurturing instinct" is not confined to females and that children for whom the father was the primary dyadic object developed extremely well in terms of ego functions and object relatedness during the first 4 to 6 years (in fact, during infancy, the children studied seemed more active and curious and less prone to pathological separation or stranger anxiety than infants whose primary dyadic relationship was with the mother).

As fathers become comfortable with their wish to be actively involved in parenting, we are seeing more families in which the father is the primary nurturing figure. In addition, as paternal parenting becomes more acceptable culturally, there is an increasing number of families in which the father is the sole parent.

What the long-term effect of primary nurturing (or sole parenting) by fathers will be is not yet known. Until recently there had been no studies of children of primary nurturing fathers in either the analytic or child development literature, and as yet there are still no observational data about these children's resolution of the oedipal phase or about their later personality structure.

We all know instances in which a nurturing man, married to a woman unable to mother, provided some or most of the primary nurturing for his children, even though the mother remained in the home. In these cases, however, documentation of the specific influence of paternal nurturing is difficult. Only when the mother either died or abandoned the family is the father's role as caregiver clear. But then the child's development reflects *both* the influence of the father and the loss of the mother—and usually, in analytic discussions, it is the loss that is focused on. Nonetheless, it is possible, without minimizing the importance of the loss of the mother, to learn a great deal about the effects of paternal nurturance from cases of father one-parent families, particularly when clinical data are integrated with the observational data that are now being collected. For example, Field (1978) demonstrated that some of the differences between maternal and paternal handling of infants disappear when the father is the primary rather than the secondary caretaker. Of course, these are behavioral data, and they do not reflect the psychic reality that is being created within the infant's mind. For that information, we have to rely on retrospective reconstructions from analyses. Although such reconstructions are not accurate portrayals of the internal reality of the young child, they do provide us with clues as to how early events were perceived and integrated into the developing psychic structure. Thus, in an attempt to explore the intrapsychic effects of paternal nurturing, I present some material from the analysis of a young woman, whose father was a major caretaker throughout her life and the only parent present from age 2½ to 4 years.

The mother was physically present during the patient's earliest years. The patient's core gender identity was solidly female, and she also had a number of character traits that reflected an identification with the mother. However, even during the first 2 years, while the mother was home and in good health, the father provided much of the physical caretaking, and the patient's early dyadic experience was retained intrapsychically in terms of *him*. This is not to say that the mother did not nurture—only that what she provided was fused in the patient's memories of early object relationships with the internal object representation of the father. Her intrapsychic experience thus was different from that described by Mahler (1961); that is, with substitute caretakers "although the mother may be less involved in the actual care of the infant, her image seems to attract so much cathexis that it often, but not always, becomes the cardinal object representation" (p. 334). This patient perceived her father as the primary nurturing figure. But, in addition, he was the primary oedipal object. How this colored the patient's perception of herself, her fantasies, and the specifics of the unconscious conflicts and symptoms which led to her analysis is the subject of this paper.

CLINICAL DATA

B., a successful lawyer, began analysis at age 30 because of depression, severe difficulties in her relationships with men, and the overwhelming feeling that she had to provide for everyone in her life—that no one ever took care of her. B. felt such enormous internal pressure to be a "good girl," to be what she thought others wanted her to be, that she was "living a rented life." She would become guilty with minimal stimulus; however, she also was a master at inducing guilt in others. During the evaluation, although she recognized her need for treatment, she said that if I would not see her myself, the experience of rejection would keep her from going to another therapist.

Her history began with her maternal grandfather who immigrated to the United States in the early 1900s and created a family business, which became the center of the emotional and financial life of his extended family. B. was the older daughter of the grandfather's only daughter; she had a sister 6 years younger. Her mother was self-centered, physically cold, and undemonstrative. B.'s first clear memory of her was from age 4—the mother coming home from the hospital and telling B. that she did not like to be touched. Mother had a rule and a reason for everything; this was burdensome but also comforting to B., who wanted to believe that nothing need be left to chance. In contrast, B.'s father was openly affectionate with her throughout her early years and, by temperament, was the more nurturing, available parent. He worked in the business started by the mother's father, but because he was a son-in-law, his position was not as high as the two biological sons' (the mother's brothers) and his enormous energies were invested instead in his community and in his children. From B.'s first months of life, he changed her diaper, gave her a morning and evening bottle, put her to bed at night, and ministered to her assorted hurts.

When B. was 2½, her mother developed a severe respiratory ailment. For the next 18 months, while the mother was in and out of the hospital, all care was provided by the father, with the maternal grandmother babysitting in emergencies. As the father had a flexible work schedule, he was able to be more available than many fathers in a similar situation. The mother's illness was successfully treated, but shortly after her return home she became pregnant and then developed epilepsy, which lead to further hospitalizations. Although the epilepsy was eventually controlled with medication, the patient was witness to a number of grand mal seizures for which no explanation was given. B. remembered having periods of severe anxiety, lasting for several hours, during which she was frightened that her mother was dying. Her mother refused to openly acknowledge her disorder; and her complaints, her need for two daily naps during which B. had to be silent, left B. feeling somehow responsible for the seizures. In addition, during the pregnancy and the mother's subsequent illness, the once loving father became withdrawn and irritable, with frequent angry outbursts. Nonetheless, he remained actively involved in the home, caring both for mother and his two daughters.

When B. was 6, her mother returned to live at home full time. At that time mother remarked that her extremely happy, outgoing, and somewhat mischievous daughter had become a quiet, somber child, asking, "Where has the chatterbox gone?" For the remaining years of childhood the patient was shy and withdrawn.

During adolescence, B. became increasingly anxious. She began to have frequent arguments with her father, which occasionally escalated into physical struggles, and which would cease only if B. "hysterically" cried and screamed. At the same time she was frightened of displeasing her parents and quite obsessional about schoolwork. When she was 15, a school counselor recommended therapy for her, but her parents refused to consider it.

After high school, she went to college, where she had her first serious relationship with a man. Throughout the several years of this relationship her boyfriend was physically abusive and unfaithful, and the patient suffered continually from feelings of uncertainty and fears of abandonment, developing both phobic and obsessional symptoms in an effort to contain her anxiety.

After college, B. complied with her father's wishes, earned a teacher's certificate, and taught high school for 2 years. However, she thoroughly disliked teaching, so went to law school, and then joined a private law firm. Once there, in spite of indications of success (promotions, praise for her briefs and her performance as a litigator), she continually worried about her acceptability to superiors. In addition, she believed her becoming a lawyer was confusing and irritating to her father, for though it was something he would have wanted for a son (who then would not have had to humble himself in the family business), he had made it clear that he felt girls should be teachers and housewives, not professionals. It was paradoxical that this man who permitted himself to take on the nurturing role usually associated with women still subscribed to the sexual role definitions of his culture.

While in law school, B. broke up with her college boyfriend and, after several brief romances, began a liaison which continued for many years. This relationship also became quite painful, with the man continually critical of her and verbally abusive. He found fault with her hair, her clothes, her friends; even her cat annoyed him. In addition, he felt uncomfortable with all sexual activity, except fellatio, and even this he would permit infrequently (less than once a month). The patient, who had always felt proud of her sexual responsiveness, felt sexually rejected and deprived of an important part of her life. Nonetheless, she was unable to separate from him.

Several years before she began analysis, B. began an affair with a married man, who had "fallen in love" with her. But he also became withdrawn and critical after the relationship became sexual. This last unsuccessful relationship plus a good friend's death from cancer brought B. to treatment "to learn how to live before I die."

B. and I worked together in analysis for 4½ years. A marked agitation, present during the evaluation, was even more prominent on the couch, where she literally wrung her hands as she talked. She began the first session by listing all the people who abused her: her mother, her father, her boyfriend, her boss, her best friend from high school, who always borrowed money and never repaid it—only her cat could be counted on. Her father was the worst; he was completely self-centered, uninterested in her work or in her as a person—for him she existed only to get married and have the grandchildren that he craved. She insisted that he had never really cared about her; that he was a cruel, angry man.

As B. presented her past history during these early months, it was filled with instances of injuries received, gratuitous insults, and repeated experiences of rejection. She spoke as if resigned to these hurts, perceiving them as inevitable and herself as powerless to change events.

At first, her continuous, never-ending complaining was amusing and only mildly irritating. But as my irritation began "leaking out" in the tone of my interventions, I recognized that with me as with others she was setting up a situation in which she could feel injured. She spoke of a need to perform for me; to bring me gifts of work achievements, symptom improvement, jokes. She worried she was repeating herself, was boring me. As with her boss, her friends, and her family, so it was now with me: every exchange was an opportunity for her to feel injured, to overreact with excessive compliance, and to become overwhelmed by the feeling that she was unloved and unlovable. Nothing she could do was enough. Now when I indicated we would have to end an hour, her response was, "It doesn't matter, what I'm saying isn't important."

Basically, the sessions were spent demonstrating her continual suffering at the hands of another, with the other being more and more me. For example, she was fearful of going to work after one hour because she had to choose an associate to take to a trial in Chicago and anticipated that no one would want to go with her. She associated to a co-worker who had recently married; that made her sad—she guessed she'd never marry, that she was a "dried-up prune" just like her cousin said. She'd probably spend the rest of her life never having sex, lying stiff in bed so she wouldn't touch her boyfriend and have to feel him pull away.

She felt bad complaining; she knew I felt all she did was complain. But what could she do, even though I didn't say so, she knew I thought she was unreasonable, that she wanted too much. Why didn't I say so, why didn't I tell her how awful, how hopeless she was? At this point her message was clear: I had judged her and found her wanting, and was not interested in helping her.

Then, slowly, there was a shift in her associations with an increasing number being to situations in which being a woman (or a girl) was the cause of her unhappiness. She felt her promotion would have happened sooner had she been male; that she would have more authority in court had she been male; she would have become a partner in her grandfather's business if she had been born a boy; she could have made up a minyan if she were male; and on and on, including the bitter statement that her parents had really wanted a boy and were disappointed in her from the beginning. She began to talk openly about how much easier life would have been if she were male, and though she did not consciously want a phallus, a dream about masturbating with a banana and being encouraged by her parents to eat it led to the thought of having a penis inside her and the association that if her boyfriend had had sex with her regularly, she wouldn't have minded being a girl "because then his penis would be mine." Her pain when her boyfriend rejected her was enormous, and she felt devastated when she was unable to arouse him sexually. She said getting him to be nice to her was as hard as getting her father to be nice to her, getting her father to acknowledge that it was okay to be a girl.

During this period she idealized me, spoke as if I had the perfect marriage, with a husband who was both supportive and gentle. She wondered, what did she do wrong, why did she always fight with men? She had the thought that as a little girl I had learned how to be the kind of woman men liked, but when she was little no one had time to teach her anything. It was as if I had the knowledge of how to get a man (or the power a man had), but was keeping it from her just as her "mother-father" had. I say "mother-father" because from her associations and her transference perception of me at this point it was not clear which parent she felt was responsible for her difficulties. Unlike patients whose mothers are the primary nurturing object, this patient rarely blamed her mother for her distress. And when she railed at me for what I did not give her, it did not feel like the complaining, the regressive defense against oedipal rivalry, that I am accustomed to experiencing with female patients. Instead, there was a sense of injustice—and a sadness (almost a kind of mourning) that she had to be a woman with all a woman's impulses and feelings when being a man would have been so much easier. Sexually, it was so hard being a woman; she could masturbate, but then she was alone. For her, the joke "The difference between herpes and love is that herpes is forever!" told it all. There was no man she could count on.

Gradually, B.'s complaining about her unresponsive boyfriend decreased, and she began to question what she derived from his being so unresponsive. At the same time she recognized that she frequently perceived me as much more unavailable than I really was. For B., the sexually unresponsive boyfriend, the unfeeling psychiatrist, had been evidence that something was wrong with her—permitting her to hold onto the fantasy that if she could just find out how to be "better," if she could just learn how to turn her boyfriend on, how to make me like her, then she could have what men had by being men; then she could have the unlimited power of the phallus. In essence, her hope that she could one day change her boyfriend and make him sexually responsive enabled her to maintain the fantasy that one day she would possess this power.

Over the past 40 years a vast literature on the psychology of women and the multiple meanings of the phallus, both developmentally and symbolically, has appeared, as Freud's ideas have been scrutinized and amended. There have been reports of the penis as breast, penis as baby, as well as articles claiming that penis envy is a male chauvinist's construction and does not really exist in women (Karme, 1981; and the articles in Blum, 1976). At this point, however, it seems more important to understand the fantasy contained within B.'s internal representation of the penis than to discuss what is normal or abnormal in women. B. imagined the penis to have magical properties which, if possessed, would provide her with complete gratification in every modality. It was as if the penis had become a symbolic representation, intrapsychically, of a mystical preambivalent stage of life, perhaps equivalent to what other patients (and psychoanalytic theoreticians) fantasize about when they speak of the all-gratifying breast. B. spoke as if she believed (or wished) that if she had a penis, all the guilt, the vulnerability, and the pain of loss that she had experienced would never have occurred. It was as if the penis was a talisman, having the power to protect her from harm. B. spoke repeatedly of her mother's withholding "things" (a Chinese chest, a pearl ring that had been the grandmother's), and how mean her father was for not standing up for her, for not making her mother give her these things. And yet, when I once asked her what made these things so important, she said very sadly, "They're not really important, they wouldn't have made me a boy."

During the analysis of another patient, a teenager whose father had assumed custody when she was 14, but who had been "father and mother both" for many years before that, a similar perception of the penis emerged. Quite graphically this patient dreamed and talked about the "giftie" she had expected to get from analysis—something little, that she could hold in her hand, that would grow bigger or smaller at her behest, and that she could hold onto forever.

B.'s idealization of men and the phallus was multidetermined. In her home, men were everything; they were healthy, loving, strong. Women were damaged; they got what they wanted, but only if they were sick, and then only because with their complaining they made people take care of them. She felt that I saw her only because she was sick—it was the same with her father, he took care of her mother only because he had to. Only men could have relationships with each other that were equal and sharing. In this way B. attempted to diminish the significance of her father's attachment to her mother. Thus her idealization of men not only reflected her idealization of the penis as symbolic of the nurturing experience, it also served to deny the importance of the mother as an oedipal rival. For B. was clearly rivalrous with her mother over the father's attention. This became evident to her in association to the loss of her married lover's attention and the abrupt change in his behavior once their relationship became sexual. She had experienced his disinterest as a repetition of the sudden loss of her father's open affection when she was 5 (at which time the mother had become pregnant and then ill again). The emotional loss of father at the very time when she felt most excited (and secure) in being "Daddy's little girl" had left her feeling abandoned, and exposed as inadequate and powerless. In an attempt to deal with her rivalry and her loss, B. tried to deny that the mother had anything of value in her relationship with father. But this required that B. had to repress the memory of the pleasure *she* had had with her father.

Later in the analysis she revealed her fantasy that her married lover had impregnated his wife after he ended their affair. What had made the fantasy so painful, she said, was that *she* had wanted to have his children, that she always felt she would be a good mother, better than his wife, better than her own mother, really.

When she talked of her ex-lover, she became extremely obsessional, ruminating over everything she had said, searching through each exchange and every interaction they had had to try and find what she had done wrong, what had driven him away. Her obsessing seemed, in part, an attempt to drive me away, have me lose interest in what she was saying. I pointed out that she was trying to do to me what she seemed to believe she had done to him, adding that she made it sound as if she were completely responsible for his leaving. Her response was, "It always feels that way; even when I was little, every time my father got mad, I thought, 'Oh, what did I do now.'" What became clear was that it was easier for her to feel responsible and guilty about her father's withdrawal than to feel helpless, powerless to change him. She remembered when the walks with him before dinner, "to work up an appetite" had stopped after her mother developed epilepsy, and how angry she had been, sometimes wishing her mother would die. She thought how different her feelings were from those in the Dylan Thomas poem "Do Not Go Gentle into That Good Night" in which he showed so much love for his dying mother. She was amazed to learn that the poem had been written to his father, questioning, "Could anyone love a father that much?"

In the transference, too, there was evidence of the positive oedipal rivalry that had contributed to her guilt, her fear of loss through retaliation. She was gleeful when a psychiatrist-friend scoffed at one of my interpretations. And when she began to have intercourse with a new boyfriend, she imagined I was jealous of her. One day, after she saw the movie *Rear Window,* she associated to a black and white dress her mother wore (similar to Grace Kelly's) and to a memory of her mother and father going to a party while she stayed home with her grandmother. She recalled their affectionate interchange and her own intense jealousy, her thought of cutting up her mother's dress to make doll clothes. The next hour she reported a dream in which she had been shopping with a friend; the dress the friend picked was ugly. Then she was with her current boyfriend, and as they walked past some colanders in the store, he asked if she wanted one. Her association to the colanders was that they were leaky, like a baby; she thought of her boyfriend asking her, if they got married, would she want a baby. The friend's dress made her think of Grace Kelly's dress and her mother's, except it was a different color, maybe red. I pointed out that I had worn a red dress the preceding day. Reluctantly, she said she didn't like that dress—I looked old in it, too old to have a baby. Although previously she had envied my home (where I have my office), husband, and children, now I seemed like someone divorced or separated, unable to get a man. I said it sounded to me that if she got a man or a baby, I'd be without one. She agreed, adding that she had always thought that her mother had been jealous of her and had used her sickness to get father's attention back. As she saw it, her wish to do away with her mother had led not only to the loss of mother but also to the loss of the intensely positive relationship with father and the arrival of the not very desirable younger sister. The respiratory illness, pregnancy, and epilepsy were fused temporally in her mind; she felt as if her wish to remove her mother from the home had backfired and she was the one who was hurt. She speculated that perhaps it was only after her father became preoccupied with her mother's illness and somewhat impatient in his child care, that she had come to believe that he would really prefer her to be a boy (an idea that was supported by her grandfather's statements that her participation in the family business and family religion were limited by her being a girl).

As she talked, we saw that being a boy was the solution for a number of conflicts: in the fantasized asexual relationship between her father and herself as his son, they could be friends forever. As she would no longer be a rival with her mother for the father's affection, she would feel no guilt for her mother's illness. Finally, as a boy, she would become more important to the mother herself who, in her devotion to the idealized grandfather and obvious pleasure in the father's attention, clearly preferred men. Her sexual feelings themselves would be different—more direct and easier to satisfy.

Because of the specific events in her life during the oedipal period—the withdrawal of her nurturing father when her mother's illness and pregnancy were complicated by epilepsy—the patient had come to perceive her own genital impulses as extremely dangerous, leading to the loss of both mother and father. She felt that as a woman, she was vulnerable to abandonment in a way that a man would never be. And not only was she convinced that her father would have preferred her to be like him; in the analysis, too, she felt that I found her inadequate and was disappointed in her for failing to live up to my expectations.

For many months her envy and jealousy of men took over the transference; perceiving me as if I were a powerful man, she began to use her suffering to "get" me. In response to my clarifications and interpretations, she would continue her litany of suffering, as if to say, "Your words are of no value." When I pointed out how she tried to limit my words by hearing them as worthless or critical and that she gave me only two choices—being a fool or a bully—her rivalry became more open and her criticism of me more direct (no longer did she apologize for being disturbed by my dog's barking). Instead, the very process of analyzing became a battleground. For example, after she did a successful piece of self analysis, during which time I was completely silent, she said, "Tell me, Dr. Chused: was that as good for *you* as it was for *me?*" For the moment, she was the sexually competent child and I was the helpless, impotent father.

Her rivalry felt very much like that of male patients—aimed primarily at denigrating my professional competence. It was as if we were men and she was determined to best me; being a good litigator, this was often not too difficult for her. Only gradually was she able to give up the gratification in her attacks on me and examine her rivalry in terms of an identification and rivalry with her father and the residual feelings that her mother would have been much more available, had she been a son.

Complaints about her parents' unavailability and critical attitude shifted to complaints about me. Occasionally she would be humorous as when I wondered about her agitation and fearful expression at the beginning of each hour, and she said, "But you're the red queen, soon to say, 'Off with her head!' " Most of the time, however, she was deadly serious about the hostility she perceived in me. Although this transference perception contained a projection of her own aggression, more important was its use as a defense against an awareness of the very positive, gratifying, and nurturing qualities of the analysis (the constancy, the listening, and remembering). These she had no control over, and the longing they created in her as well as the memories this longing evoked made her feel truly and painfully helpless.

Slowly and with a great deal of genuine suffering, she began to re-create through association the early relationships she had had with her parents. She noted that she no longer heard the piano playing during her hours and imagined I had asked my son to stop because I was working. This reminded her of how quiet she had to be after her mother got sick. It had not always been that way; she remembered being silly when she made cookies with her, adding, "I guess I wouldn't have dared to be so mischievous when I was little if I hadn't felt loved." But most of all it was father who was remembered.

The memories of her father did not return comfortably; rather they welled up, in association to my interpreting the defensive nature of her perception of me as hurtful. For prior to this point in the analysis, although she had been told that her father had assumed almost total care of her while the mother was hospitalized, her only conscious memories of him were of a withdrawn and often angry man. She had come to the analysis convinced he had never been available to her, with no memory of the early years together.

There were multiple determinants for this massive repression of the memory of the positive dyadic relationship with her father. One was her reluctance to reexperience the pain of that loss. The loss of the mother at age 2½ *was* important, but the nurturing provided by the mother was fused in her memories with that from the father, and that latter loss was devastating. By repressing the very positive early years with father, she could believe that she had not lost anything—that she had had nothing to lose. But an equally important determinant for the repression was her oedipal rivalry and guilt which, by extension, led to guilt over the close preoedipal relationship she had had with her father. The mother's relationship with the father was not dissimilar in appearance to the father's relationship with his very young daughter. He nurtured and coddled the mother, checked on her when she napped, and worried over her diet and her health. I suspect that in the eyes of the oedipal child, the similarity between her father's relationship with her mother and her own early one with him contributed to the extension of guilt back to the earlier period.

When the mother returned to reclaim the father, B. repressed her longing and defended against her helpless frustration and rage by becoming the compliant model child, turning the pain that she was experiencing passively into one that was under her control. Her masochistic suffering served as a compromise formation, and in its defensive function permitted her to repress her early memories, her longing for her father, and her aggressive impulses toward her mother. But the consequence of this behavior was that it had left her without sufficient accessible support, without any *conscious* internal object representation from which to draw sustenance. Although B.'s relationships with men were quite masochistic and thus recapitulated the "false memory" of her relationship with her father, there was no evidence, either in the content of her associations or in the transference, of an erotic gratification in her suffering. Instead, her masochism seemed to serve primarily as a defense against the experience of true vulnerability. Of course, there was hidden gratification in the pain that she inflicted on herself, for through it she literally (through the guilt she provoked) and symbolically made others suffer and at the same time became the despised center of their universe as she had once imagined herself the beloved center of her father's world. This we addressed in the analysis, with some diminution in her investment in suffering. It was the focus on the defensive aspect of the suffering, however, that was most productive. And over time, she became able to see that the fear that I would throw her out was incompatible with her awareness that I was listening to what she was saying.

A most moving sequence then occurred in the analysis. As she became able to acknowledge, first the support she felt from the analytic situation, and then the interest and concern she felt from my listening and remembering, she became flooded with tremendous feelings of sadness for the father she had lost. It was as if she remembered him, their relationship, the wonderful stories he told of his childhood in Germany, only to be able to mourn. "Where had he gone; what had she done to make him so angry?" To realize that his anger was not because of her but because of his helplessness to do anything about his wife's multiple illnesses and hospitalizations, to realize that he cared so much about her mother, at first only made the pain greater.

Her growth from the modification of ego functioning that led to the recovery of early memories and associated mourning was considerable. Not only did her depression, sense of worthlessness, and defensive masochism disappear, but also she became able to respond to a genuinely loving, sexual man. It was as if once the analysis enabled her to work through some of the conflicts over her oedipal impulses, she was able to reclaim the object relationship with her father which had served as the foundation for the positive self representation, the self-esteem, and the self-confidence that had been so evident in her early years and that had leaked through in the courtroom, with clients, and in the "secret" expectations she had of me. Her growing awareness of the discrepancy between her conscious low self-assessment and the sense of self reflected in her behavior also helped her see the "as-if" quality of her suffering.

There had been serious consequences for B. from the repression of the early nurturing relationship with her father that had accompanied the repression of her later, more dangerous, oedipal fantasies. In essence, she lost the conscious memory of a benevolent object. That the father had been a "good enough mother" during separation-individuation was apparent in her solid sense of object constancy, the comfortable integration and autonomy of her ego functions, and her ability to make commitments in relationships. But a benevolent other is essential not only for the movement through separation-individuation, but also throughout development, as the superego, the ego ideal, and the self image emerge out of the integration of experience, what the individual brings to an experience, and the resultant perception of and internalization of the experience. B. had deprived herself of a benevolent object representation in her defense against her oedipal guilt. And in her need to maintain her defensive position, what she had done with her father's love, she did with others'. In order for her to maintain the repression of the very positive aspects of this relationship, she denied the supportive aspects of all relationships. She truly felt unloved and unlovable. Her sense of worthlessness was not only defensive, it was also based on the repeated experience of abuse and loss that she had created for herself.

One can examine the specifics of B.'s development from a number of different perspectives. For example, her mother's chronic illness clearly colored B.'s perception of herself as a woman and contributed to her choice of a masochistic defense. However, even this partial identification with the "sick" mother was modified by the influence of the father's nurturing and the resultant identification with him.

SUMMARY

1. When mothering is inadequate or provided only intermittently, a dyadic relationship with father can provide the continuity and the nurturance that is necessary for the successful navigation of infancy and early childhood, including the phases of separation-individuation. B.'s experience supports Pruett's hypothesis, based on observational data, that fathers can function as mothers during the early years of development. Thus B.'s wish: "I want to be as good a mother as my father was."

2. B.'s positive oedipal impulses were extremely conflictual for her not only because of the mother's illness and prolonged absence from home, but also because of the intensity of the early relationship with father. The positive dyadic experience with father, which was essential during her preoedipal years (given her mother's unavailability), contributed to B.'s difficulty with the oedipal phase.

3. When B. repressed her oedipal longings for her father, she also found it necessary to repress her preoedipal attachment to him, for the guilt and anxiety experienced in the triadic relationship were experienced, retroactively, in the dyadic relationship as well.[1]

4. The repression of the early dyadic experience with father left B. without any conscious internal representation of a benevolent other. The loss of this positive early relationship from her "permissible" conscious memories contributed, in turn, to the harshness of her superego, her narcissistic vulnerability to the responses of others, her low self-esteem, and her feelings of despair.

5. B.'s need to maintain the repression of this positive relationship led to a masochistic perception of every relationship.

6. Another consequence of B.'s early relationship with her father was her intense attachment to the men in her life and her overwhelming fear of loss of the sexual object. Genital pleasure and vulnerability to sexual rejection are present in many women, but the unusual intensity of B.'s was similar to that described in women (Tessman, 1980) whose relationship with their fathers compensated for inadequacies in their mothering.[2]

7. Finally, B.'s idealization of men, both for their phallic powers and for their ability to be warm and giving, was related to her experience with her father. She looked to men, not women, for nurturance and in her fantasies about the penis endowed it with magical, protective powers. For her, possession of the penis promised complete gratification without pain, a return to the fantasized union with an all-giving object.

There is a factor that must be considered in this reconstruction of the effect of early paternal nurturing on a female child. Today paternal involvement in infant care is more and more common. When the patient I have discussed was a young child, it

1. I wonder if, perhaps, for many women with a less than optimal relationship with mother and father providing some or much of the early nurturing, there is a tendency to repress the memory of the positive experience with father because of guilt over oedipal fantasies and wishes. If so, this may contribute to the prevalence of masochistic character traits in women.

2. This may be due to an enhancement of the genital experience with gender-specific preverbal memories of the dyadic relationship with the father.

was still unusual for fathers to be significantly involved in child care. And though B.'s father's assumption of the nurturing role was in part determined by his wife's illness, one must wonder what there was in his character structure that made him willing to assume this role. It may be that his behavior was motivated, in part, by an unconscious feminine identification and a rivalry with his own mother (Leonard, 1966; Burlingham, 1973).

I am left with a number of questions about the psychological consequences of fathers functioning as mothers. B. had a need to defend against an awareness of the positive dyadic relationship with her father because of the enormity of her oedipal guilt. Given the universal nature of oedipal fantasies, is this the consequence of the father one-parent family for the female child? For B., the nurturing preoedipal object and the oedipal object were one (as it is for most males). Only, in her case, because of guilt over the mother's illnesses, which extended throughout the oedipal phase, her need to render unconscious the positive experiences with father was great. Her experience could be compared to that of males who as children either lived alone with their mothers or had fathers who were unavailable. During analysis many of these men reveal a tremendous fear of entrapment that makes intimacy difficult, as the fear of engulfment that accompanies the wish for reunion with the preoedipal/oedipal mother contaminates later heterosexual relationships. On the surface, this was not B.'s problem, for her major heterosexual involvements were quite long-lasting. However, the sadomasochistic cast of these relationships and her behavior in the analysis made it clear that intimacy was tolerable only with the distancing, the separation, that fighting and pain provide. B.'s experience should also be compared with that of children in mother one-parent families as summarized by Neubauer (1960). For her as for them, "When a parent is absent, there is an absence of oedipal reality. The absent parent becomes endowed with magical power either to gratify or punish; aggression against him, and the remaining parent as well, becomes repressed" (p. 308).

I have not discussed the male child in a father one-parent family. I have analyzed only one such child, and this boy had a very different response to his father being both nurturer and oedipal rival—specifically, a tremendous fear of loss of the father through rivalry and a resultant strong feminine identification and negative oedipal attachment. But here again, it was not only the traumatic loss of the mother that rendered the infantile wishes and fantasies so conflictual and pathogenic. For dyadic "possession" of the father, so essential for ego development in the absence of the mother, can also contribute to later intrapsychic conflict in the male child. But this is a topic for future clinical explorations, as we try to understand the consequences of fathers functioning as mothers.

BIBLIOGRAPHY

ABELIN, E. L. (1975). Some further observations and comments on the earliest role of the father. *Int. J. Psychoanal.*, 56:293–302.

BLUM, H. P., ed. (1976). Female psychology. *J. Amer. Psychoanal. Assn. Suppl.*, 24.

BURLINGHAM, D. (1973). The preoedipal infant-father relationship. *Psychoanal. Study Child*, 28:23–47.

FIELD, T. (1978). Interactional behavior of primary versus secondary caretaker fathers. *Develpm. Psychol.*, 14:83–184.

KARME, L. (1981). A clinical report of penis envy. *J. Amer. Psychoanal. Assn.*, 29:427–446.

LAMB, M. (1980). Observational studies in the family setting. In *The Father-Infant Relationship*, ed. F. Pederson, pp. 21–43. New York: Praeger.

LEONARD, M. R. (1966). Fathers and daughters. *Int. J. Psychoanal.*, 47:325–334.

LOEWALD, H. W. (1951). Ego and reality. *Int. J. Psychoanal.*, 32:10–18.

MAHLER, M. S. (1961). On sadness and grief in infancy and childhood. *Psychoanal. Study Child*, 16:332–351.

MAHLER, M. S. & GOSLINER, B. (1955). On symbiotic psychosis. *Psychoanal. Study Child*, 10:195–212.

NEUBAUER, P. B. (1960). The one-parent child and his oedipal development. *Psychoanal. Study Child*, 15:286–309.

PRUETT, K. D. (1983). Infants of primary nurturing fathers. *Psychoanal. Study Child*, 38:257–277.

——— (1985). Oedipal configurations in young father-raised children. *Psychoanal. Study Child*, 40:435–456.

TESSMAN, L. H. (1980). A note on the father's contribution to the daughter's way of loving and working. In *Father and Child*, ed. S. Cath, A. Gurwitt, & J. M. Ross, pp. 219–230. Boston: Little Brown.

The Analyst, His Theory, and the Psychoanalytic Process

MYRON R. HURWITZ, M.D.

MY INTENTION IN THIS PAPER IS TO STIMULATE DISCUSSION AND curiosity with regard to the nature of the impact of the person of the analyst and his theory on the ongoing process and outcome of an analysis. If the person of the analyst and his choice of theory do have important effects, then these factors require our careful attention and raise questions about issues of analyzability and comparability of analytic results (Bachrach, 1983). Recent articles in the literature have stressed the importance of accumulating data and substantiating basic psychoanalytic evidence in our efforts to deepen our understanding of psychoanalytic process (Kaplan, 1981; Stoller, 1982). My personal experience in analysis with two analysts, who had different styles and different theoretical perspectives, sparked my interest in this subject and will be offered as data for consideration along with observations from differing points of view which have appeared in the literature.

In 1897 Freud wrote to Fliess, "I no longer believe in my neurotica" and gave as one of his principal reasons "the certain discovery that there are no indications of reality in the unconscious so that one cannot distinguish between the truth and fiction that is cathected with affect" (p. 260). With his discovery of the power of unconscious fantasy and *internal* reality, Freud introduced a new richness and complexity to our understanding of human experience. He used this discovery to explain the

Assistant clinical professor of psychiatry, University of Connecticut Health Center School of Medicine; member, Western New England Institute for Psychoanalysis.

premature termination of treatment in the case of Dora while at
the same time introducing the concept of transference as a crucial aspect of the psychoanalytic relationship:

> What are transferences? They are new editions or facsimiles of
> the impulses and phantasies which are aroused and made con-
> scious during the progress of the analysis . . . they replace some
> earlier person by the person of the physician . . . a whole series
> of psychological experiences are revived, not as belonging to the
> past, but as applying to the person of the physician at the pre-
> sent moment . . . they may even become conscious, *by cleverly
> taking advantage of some real peculiarity* in the physician's person
> or circumstances and attaching themselves to that. Trans-
> ference is the one thing the presence of which has to be detected
> almost without assistance and with only the slightest clues to go
> upon, *while at the same time the risk of making arbitrary inferences has
> to be avoided* [1905, p. 116; my italics].

The transference interpretation is generally viewed as the ultimate operative factor, the "mutative agent" (Strachey, 1934) in
the therapeutic action of psychoanalysis. While this point of view
is not uniformly accepted, the development, understanding,
and clarification of transference and the transference neurosis
have become generally well-accepted propositions. We are less
clear about how to include the reality of the person of the analyst
and his theory in our formulations.

Analysts come in a variety of physical and psychological pack-
ages. There are an increasing variety of theoretical models from
which the clinician can choose in his attempts to comprehend
and interpret the events which unfold during the course of an
analysis. He may be a Kleinian or a Freudian. He may focus on
impulse-defense constellations, object relations, separation-individuation issues, the vicissitudes of narcissism, oedipal or preoedipal issues. There are many overlapping areas, and it is clear
that clinicians vary widely in their application of these models.
Rangell refers to this situation as diversity within unity (Panel,
1984). This unity of assumptions of psychoanalysis seems well
spelled out by Joseph (1979) who feels that the therapeutic benefits derived from a diversity of theoretical and technical approaches rest on the fact that each deals with some portion of the
individual's unconscious life and starts a ripple effect which then

leads to a wide range of readjustment. "There is no one truth . . . [but] a multitude of truths" (p. 78). The implication is that the therapeutic benefits derived are similar. I do not believe that this is necessarily so and hope the evidence I offer will support my point of view.

The various manifestations of transferences are often described in the literature as if they resided statically in the patient. Technical directives (Freud, 1912a; Greenacre, 1954; Arlow, 1979; Brenner, 1976, 1979) to the analyst are given "to ensure that what emerges into the patient's consciousness is as far as possible endogenously determined; that is, that the thoughts, feelings, fantasies, etc., that the patient perceives represent derivatives of the persistent pressure of his unconscious conflicts" (Arlow, 1979, p. 193). On the other hand, others (Freud, 1937; Fenichel, 1941; A. Freud, 1954; Leavy, 1980; Loewald, 1960, 1971; Racker, 1957; Stone, 1981; Blum, 1981; Dewald, 1982) have written of a more complex interaction between analyst and analysand. They do not minimize "transference" but include the reality of the analyst in their understanding of the process in a variety of ways.

Greenacre (1954) said of the psychoanalytic situation, "If two people are repeatedly alone together, some sort of emotional bond will develop between them" (p. 627). I believe this is a generally accepted proposition. It is from this point on that various observers begin to differ. How is the development of that bond best understood? What influences the development of that bond? What is the nature of the bond? It is also from this point on that we face a major complication in the development and evaluation of theory. I would propose that the theoretical choices that a clinician makes immediately have an effect not only on his understanding of the bond but also on the bond that will develop. "Different psychoanalysts with different theories can construct quite different analysands out of what began as the same patient and confirm their theories in the process" (Michels, 1981). Since psychoanalytic theory is derived from and then tested in the clinical situation, an understanding of this reciprocal relationship is especially important.

Gaining this understanding is a highly complex task. The assumption of a theoretical position is not a simple matter of se-

lecting a "scientific truth." Particularly in psychoanalysis, the
selection of theory represents more personal truth, and must
have important connections to the personality, character, personal and professional life experience of the analyst. "The idea
that we could think out a theory of the structure and functioning of the personality without its having any relation to the
structure and functioning of our own personality should be a
self-evident impossibility" (Guntrip, 1975, p. 156). A choice between alternate ways of practicing science also represents a value system, an ideology, and to one degree or another has irrational elements (Kuhn, 1962; Rothstein, 1980). Thus we are
immediately faced with the fact that in the psychoanalytic situation, we are not simply dealing with the impact of different
theoretical propositions in an isolated way but in combination
with the impact of the person of the analyst on the analysand
which in part the analyst's theoretical stand represents.
Fenichel (1941) noted that "different analysts act differently
and these differences influence the behavior of patients and
the personality of the therapist influences the transference" (p.
72). The complications that arise have to do with how does
one—indeed, can one—separate personality from theory.
Knowledge changes our perceptions and responses (Modell,
1976; Kanzer, 1979a, 1979b). Changes in our responses lead to
changes in our patient's responses. Behaviors of the analyst
which serve as a stimulus to behavior in the analysand (Greenson, 1967) may well trigger responses which the analyst views as
supporting or failing to support his or another's theoretical
position. He may account for these reactions on the basis of
theory when it would be more accurate to view them as related
to the direct impact of his personality.

Other than Guntrip's 1975 paper on his experience of analysis with Fairbairn and Winnicott and Moser's 1974 book in
which he only briefly describes various attempts in analysis
which failed, I am unaware of other articles in the literature in
which analysts reflect on their personal experiences in analysis
with different analysts of different persuasions. Perhaps this is
because of what Fleming and Benedek (1966) refer to as the
seemingly forbidden activity of objectively examining our own
experiences. Be that as it may, every analyst uses his own expe-

rience in analysis as an important aspect of his own developing notions of analytic theory and process. Anecdotes about formative experience in one's own analysis frequently surface between analysts in discussion and are frequently used as data to support a clinical viewpoint or resolve a clinical dilemma.

In sharing aspects of my experiences in analysis, I recognize that it is impossible to do justice to the complexity of any analytic experience, especially one's own. In some small measure, however, I hope to be able to capture and reconstruct my reactions to each of my analysts. In these descriptions, inevitably a great deal more is presented than can be discussed (and much is of course left out). I hope that this does not distract or detract from the primary focus of the paper. I would also like to emphasize that both men maintained an analytic stance. When I speak of emotional openness or guardedness, for example, I am referring to a sense that I had that was not clearly related to overt behaviors or attitudes on their part.

THE ANALYSES

After being accepted into the Western New England Institute for Psychoanalysis, I started my training with Dr. X. He became my training analyst by dint of being the one of two training analysts who had time available and with whom I was able to work out a schedule. I should mention that at that time I was five years postresidency and considered myself reasonably knowledgeable as a psychoanalytically oriented psychotherapist. I felt that so long as there was no major incompatibility, my analytic experience with any competent analyst would be relatively the same. Though there were many difficult times, the analysis overall seemed to me to progress satisfactorily and, in the spring of 1978, a termination date was set by mutual agreement for mid-December. Following the summer break, I received word from the secretary that Dr. X was ill and would not be able to resume work immediately. Shortly thereafter, I received a letter from him saying that I had no doubt heard of his serious illness and suggesting that I continue my analysis with another analyst, as the time that he might return was uncertain. I wrote back to him and told him that I wished to

wait for his return. He agreed "if this met with the approval of
the Education Committee." It was by chance, in a discussion
with a member of the Committee on another matter and asking
about Dr. X, that I learned that he was terminally ill with cancer. He died about a week later.

I present this background to emphasize that to this point I
had been well satisfied with my analysis and found it to be a
helpful and valuable experience. I flirted with the idea of not
continuing. Enraged, sad, and in retrospect somewhat in a state
of shock, I was now faced with choosing another analyst. A
classmate mentioned that Dr. Y might have time available. He
did, we met and began our work together shortly thereafter. I
was not familiar with the publications of either of my analysts at
the time we started our work together. I did attend a clinical
seminar during my fifth year of analysis, taught by Dr. X. Before going on to describe my actual experiences, I think two
important questions must be addressed: the first, what was the
contribution of my prior analysis and in what way did that affect my second analysis; and second, what was the impact under
which the second analysis was undertaken (that is, following the
death of my first analyst).

The analysis with Dr. X contributed significantly to my ability
to associate freely. Superego inhibitions and externalizations
were greatly reduced but not eliminated by a long shot. Various
character defenses were familiar to me and my tolerance for
unwanted feelings and fantasies had greatly increased, along
with my capacity for intimacy. Though I was very familiar with
them, I think I had been able to do relatively little to integrate
my competitiveness, defiance, and rebelliousness. The second
question is more difficult to answer. I was highly ambivalent
about continuing my analysis and had been looking forward to
the freedom that termination represented with regard to time,
money, and the approaching completion of my analytic training. On the other hand, I knew I had more work to do. I continued my analysis with Dr. Y with a sense of resignation. I felt
that I had no real choice. My rage at Dr. X was enhanced by his
death and continued into my second analysis, for some time
serving to hide similar feelings toward Dr. Y.

ANALYSIS WITH DR. X

From the beginning, I found the experience to be anxiety-provoking. Dr. X seemed cool and aloof, self-consciously stand-offish (as I felt he should be). I was uneasy with what I sensed to be an air of impatience about him. Very quickly I developed the sense that I was under the scrutiny of a very stern man, a man of conviction, not to be messed with. My associations were to an orthodox rabbi who terrified me as a child. At the end of the first month, just before the end of the session, he said he had a present for me, and I remember feeling puzzled and a bit embarrassed by the rising pleasurable expectation that was stirred. "What could he have for me?" The session ended and, with a bit of a teasing smile, he handed me his bill. I laughed. I enjoyed the joke but also felt angry and humiliated. The joke was on me. The next day I paid the bill, my check in an envelope just as his bill had been. I handed him the envelope and then on to the couch. My thoughts continued on in association to the check that I had just handed him. It was larger than my mortgage payment. The dream of a home of my own, of being head of my own household, and a successful analysis seemed similar. There were similar hopes and similar anxieties. I was aware of feeling angry and resentful about the price on the one hand and yet a sense of pleasurable anticipation and curiosity on the other. Suddenly, Dr. X said, "What's with the envelope?" Dr. X's question caught me offguard and for the moment I didn't even know what envelope he was talking about. I felt challenged and accused. "Your bill was in an envelope," I shot back defensively, a tide of fear and rage building. "I put the bill in an envelope because some people prefer to have the bill sent," he said, somewhat defensively, I thought. I exploded. He wasn't going to lay any of that stuff on me! He hadn't asked me anything about what I wanted him to do with the bill while on the couch. On the contrary, he had sandbagged me—just about shoved the bill into my hand. As my rage subsided and my attack tapered off, there was a moment of silence. I recovered. It felt good somehow that I had felt that free to express my rage, but I also was a bit embarrassed and ashamed at such a display.

Still I felt that he had been intrusive and wondered why he asked me about the envelope. What was he wondering about? At the same time, I wondered why it was that I had gotten so angry about it. A silence followed. I began to feel annoyed and anxious again. "Why did you feel you had to take the bill?" he asked. He sounded sarcastic and condescending. I did not feel that I could answer him. I had taken it automatically without thinking. I told him that he sounded sarcastic and condescending. It seemed to me that here was a man who was always going to have to be right.

During the first three years of analysis, there were many similar incidents. It was not often that I felt understood or felt that I really understood Dr. X. More often than not I was surprised or shocked or somehow thrown off balance by his interventions. This was interpreted and accepted by me as evidence of resistance at work. Whenever I found myself disagreeing, feeling misunderstood, etc., I was frustrated by my reactions and by his, which was most often silence. Dr. X's interpretations often sounded to me as pronouncements. I would feel fired at, and I often responded with defensive rage and defiance. This was interpreted with an eye to my oedipal strivings, jealousy, and competitiveness, my wish to defeat the powerful father; to accept his interpretations was for me a humiliating submission. At the same time, Dr. X interpreted my defiance itself as a provocation to be beaten which I wanted in order to relieve my guilt stimulated by my patricidal wishes. I wanted him out of the way because he represented my father who was represented in my conscience. I believed that if I could get him out of the way, I would then be free to pursue my libidinal wishes without fear, but the murderous wishes themselves led to guilt, fear of retaliation, and conflict. I often thought I was angry with Dr. X in response to his frustrating and infuriating ways.

While there was a sense that Dr. X's observations had some relevance, they did not seem to me to address enough of what was troubling me directly. As I became more familiar with some of Mahler's work and Kohut's work, there was a resonance with what I sensed to be important issues having to do with separation, recognition, and the maintenance of self-esteem. These were the aspects of the analysis that seemed to be missing. Dr. X viewed my introducing these issues as an attempt to evade directly confronting my oedipal conflicts. During one session, I recall lying on the couch attempting to put into words something that I was feeling. An image gradually formed of my mother standing at the sink preoccupied, and my trying to get her attention. She looked very sad. Suddenly, I felt I understood an aspect of my childhood that had a connection with a constellation of feelings that I carried within me as an adult. My father had been in the service and overseas when I was between 4 to 7 years old. I had never recognized before that not only did I miss him, but also that my mother had been quite depressed at that time and (oedipal longings not an unimportant element) not as available as I would have wished her to have been. At that moment, I was feeling sad for that little boy that was me and sad for my mother. I had never thought before of what that situation must have been like for her or for me. I think, in retrospect, I was feeling like that same little boy on the couch. Dr. X's response was: "So you didn't appreciate the freedom that your mother gave you." I felt confused, nailed again, ungrateful. It seemed so in some way. That was part of what was troubling. Because of her preoccupation, I did have a great deal of freedom and yet that seemed to twist the meaning of what seemed to me to be most important in what I was understanding. I began to feel more confident in my thoughts that there was something specific about Dr. X and my working with him that I was reacting to. I told Dr. X that I was more and more certain that this was so; there was something about his style of delivery, his theory, his tone of voice, perhaps his appearance, that seemed to play an important part in my reactions to him. "You'd respond that way no matter who was in this chair," was Dr. X's reply. "You don't think it has anything to do with you?" I asked. "Nothing," he replied. In retrospect, this represented a turning point in the analysis. I accepted and began to identify with his statement. I also accepted that these responses represented the ongoing evidence of the frustration of a variety of infantile longings and my unwillingness to accept that frustration or to reject or renounce those longings.

Some time in the fifth year of the analysis, we were going through a difficult time and Dr. X raised the possibility of my seeing another analyst. If what he said earlier was so, that it wasn't him, I couldn't see how seeing another analyst would help. I was determined to work my feelings out with him if possible. Deep within me, the fear that I might be unanalyzable began to grow. He agreed to continue our work together. While I continued to feel that Dr. X did not seem to understand certain issues in my life (which began to seem much less important), I struggled against but then began to accept deep feelings of affection and appreciation for him. Over the last year or so of the analysis, I developed a much greater sense of my inner life and fantasies. The constant stirrings of angry competitive feelings and frustrations that I continued to experience were identifed as ongoing evidence of the strength of my rivalrous oedipal struggle against my father. There was no credence given to the possibility that anything in his behavior or attitude was a contribution or stimulating factor. I believe in retrospect that Dr. X took this stand in order to avoid any possibility of diluting my understanding of the intrapsychic components of my reactions. As I began to express warm, appreciative feelings, these were often interpreted as attempts to seduce him, to avoid my defiance, competitiveness, and rage. One day I was feeling particularly close to Dr. X, much less threatened by him than usual. I commented on this feeling and the accompanying sense that at that moment I felt I could say anything to him or face anything in myself. "Do you know why you feel that?" he asked. "No," I said. "Because the hour's up," he said. We laughed together. Yet again, deep within me, I felt hurt. The message was clear. I wasn't so brave, so trusting. I was just a lot of hot air. The only reason I felt that way was because I was about to escape.

When I talked about my reactions to this joke, I felt chided for my sensitivity. My reaction to this itself was interesting. I agreed. I felt that I was "too sensitive." I heard the chiding as a call to grow up, to not be "such a little boy." Rather than understanding and integrating my hurt and vulnerability, I attempted to master them by suppressing them.

During the summer break that was to have preceded my last three months of analysis, I was very excited about the adventure that I had been on and was very much looking forward to completing the journey with Dr. X. I wanted him to be proud of me. I wanted to tell him of my appreciation for his time and effort and patience. The sense was of a shared, successful adventure, but those expressions were not to be. My last letter to Dr. X in which I wished to tell him these things was returned to me unopened, having reached him when he was already too ill to read it.

ANALYSIS WITH DR. Y

My analysis with Dr. Y was ushered in by a dream of being chased through a building that I thought was a synagogue by a Nazi soldier (remember the rabbi). I hated the sense of depicting Dr. Y as a Nazi and told him about it only with difficulty. The dream was filled with terror. One association was my fear that I might experience in this analysis the same sense of persecution which I experienced most particularly in the beginning of my first analysis. Gradually I recognized that my experience with Dr. Y was very different from the experience with Dr. X. He was not as aloof, distant, or guarded. I did not experience his interpretations as pronouncements at all. He offered them as possibilities for me to consider. He did not read my mind or tell me what I was doing. Rather than being disruptive, his comments were more often organizing, serving to increase my awareness of something that I had not been quite aware of previously. I felt that I was able to relate to them. If I did disagree, or if I had a sense that he was somewhat off the mark, I felt listened to and felt that my response was being considered as additional information—not necessarily as resistance. If I did not understand a statement, Dr. Y attempted to restate what he meant, and often this proved helpful. This was in stark contrast to Dr. X's silence in such situations. The result of these differences was a degree of relaxation and freedom from anxiety on the couch that I did not experience, nor did I know was possible to experience, with Dr. X. I do not mean to imply that I was without anxiety. Indeed, I would from time to time still be quite anxious. My rage, competitiveness, and defiance had certainly not gone away, but with Dr. Y these responses were both quantitatively and qualitatively different, more clearly related to idiosyncratic interpretations on my part, and I almost never felt as if they were stimulated directly by him or breached my ability to cope with them. (Cer-

tainly the experience of analysis with Dr. X played an important
part in helping me to be better able to identify these feelings and
to tolerate and manage them.)

One day as I got onto the couch, Dr. Y asked me why I smiled
at him when I came in, "as if we were friends." I felt an immediate, terrifying, sinking feeling in the pit of my stomach. I felt that
he was saying that we weren't friends. I had had similar experiences with Dr. X, resulting in feeling overwhelmed by a sense of
catastrophe, from which it would take me several days to recover. Dr. Y seemed to sense my reaction and, before I said
anything, he went on to say, "I am not saying that we aren't
friends." I felt caught—supported in a way that allowed me to
reflect on the intensity of my reaction, and allowed me to begin
to analyze it, rather than just struggling to manage the feelings.
His intervention also triggered strong feelings of appreciation
for his sensitivity.

It is interesting how much more difficult it is for me to re-
create instances with Dr. Y that would serve as data. Dr. X
seemed uncomfortable with direct expressions of closeness and
guarded himself very carefully. Dr. Y was much more open. It
seemed to me that I could feel more of what was going on in him
and that this was very important in helping me to understand
how not to drown in my own reactions. He did not seem to close
off in response to me. There was a sense that my reactions were
accepted as they were. These were my reactions, and it was the
origins and meanings of these reactions that were important for
me to understand. This was in contrast to having my reactions
given an entirely different meaning.

Dr. Y seemed much more attuned to preoedipal and narcissistic issues, and to have these now included in my analysis
allowed me to work through sources of anxiety and to uncover
early, quite primitive fantasies that had previously been unavailable or only partially understood on an oedipal level. The fuller
understanding and experience of the contribution of preoedipal
longings and fantasies added a sense of stability, depth, and
richness which had been absent up to that point. The following
examples may help to clarify what I am attempting to describe.

There were two memories that came up repeatedly in both
analyses. The first was an early memory dating to about age 4,

just after my mother and I moved with my father to a small house on the army post where he was stationed just prior to going overseas. The memory was of my playing outside by myself and three boys going by in the field behind the house and calling to me, asking if I wanted some candy. I was excited and pleased and ran to them. They pushed me down, went off laughing, and I returned to the house crying. This was repeated over the next two days. The memory was troubling because I couldn't understand why I kept responding to their offer. Why was I so naïve? Dr. X's interpretation on one level revolved around guilt and my need for punishment; I sensed that my father was going overseas and the pleasure of oedipal triumph stimulated so much guilt that I needed to get myself punished. A second interpretation had to do with the desire for the candy as representing unfulfilled and unremitting oedipal longings and the pushing down representing the oedipal defeat which I refused to accept. The first interpretation always left me cold. The second I was able to relate to; it seemed helpful but in some way incomplete.

When this memory came up in my analysis with Dr. Y, together with my ongoing sense of frustration that there was something important in that memory that I still did not understand, he said, "Perhaps you were lonely." My response to this interpretation was to be flooded with memories of that time, and along with those memories, I recalled an awful sense of loneliness which I had repressed. The sense of incomplete understanding was gone and instead was replaced with an understanding of a long period of loneliness in my early life.

The second memory related to age 8 after my father had returned from overseas and we were living in a house near the army base where my father was stationed and shortly after my sister was born. The memory was of watching my mother tend to my sister in the bassinet. Dr. X's interpretation focused on regressive responses to the castration anxiety stimulated by the situation. I understood and appreciated his interpretation intellectually, but I did not really feel any greater understanding. It led to few other associations. Attempts to understand my resistance to this interpretation focused on the strength of my castration anxiety, my defiance, and my feeling that whatever it was that had happened to my sister, I was going to make sure it did not happen to me.

Dr. Y listened to the same material and said, "Perhaps you thought that it was love," referring to my observing my mother's ministrations to my sister. The experience in response to this interpretation was very similar to what I described with the first memory—first a sudden recovery of many memories related to that time, and a much fuller emotional sense of that memory; of my jealously, my rivalry, my love, my longing, and my loneliness—also a memory of how games played out with playmates were related to that experience.

In both instances, associations to these memories centered around feelings of abandonment which, once worked through, opened the way for additional and fuller understanding of these same memories on an oedipal level. It is interesting to note that each analyst made similar interpretations to the same material, but addressed these interpretations to different levels.

Discussion

I shall confine my discussion to two main points: the transferences stimulated, and process and theory.

TRANSFERENCES STIMULATED

The transferences stimulated in response to Dr. X were primarily those of the severe rabbi, the persecutory, vengeful, powerful, oedipal father, admired, feared, hated, loved, but kept at a distance. Superego projections were almost constant. Dr. X's physical appearance was close enough to my father's to have been a stimulus in this direction. Dr. X's style and theoretical stance were also important triggers. His stand that pre-oedipal conflicts and loving feelings for him (the father) were primarily a regressive avoidance to the central oedipal struggle, was, I think, oversimplified, limited the effectiveness of my analysis with him in dealing with these issues, and was an additional source of frustration. His style limited the maternal transference to a sense of being teased. What is, I think, most important to note in all of this is that my reactions would have been interpreted by Dr. X as confirming his theoretical point of view, as I understand it.

My identification with Dr. X was very much an identification with the aggressor with a high titre of ambivalence (Meissner, 1979). I began to note a change in my style of doing therapy and analysis in which there was an uncomfortable tendency to repeated actively what I felt I was experiencing passively. I had become the dutiful son of the tyrannical father and the transmission to the next generation was under way. The sense that I have alluded to of something missing in my relationship with Dr. X was complicated and related to his personal style and his attitudes toward preoedipal issues which served to reinforce my own defensive splitting of these issues from the transferences already mentioned.

The transference responses to Dr. Y were far more complex. The persecutory oedipal father was very much there, but less insistently stimulated. There was also a loving, idealized father and maternal grandfather who served as ego ideal, guides, and models for identification. Above all, there were the complex maternal transferences—the mother who carried me in her womb, who suffered to give me life, loving and supporting, disappointing and castrating, always longed for but never quite available. It is important to note that Dr. Y's appearance and habits also played a role in the transferences stimulated. Dr. Y was short, as was my mother and as was my maternal grandfather. Dr. Y smoked and drank coffee, both of which were passions of my mother and my maternal grandfather during my early years. Dr. Y's style was less intrusive, his theoretical stance more open, broader, and less stimulating of defiant and provocative stances on my part. He offered a perspective that provided a depth and texture to my understanding that went beyond a schematic outline, and his personal availability allowed for a more mature identification (Meissner, 1979). In my transference responses to him and my sense of what happened in my analysis with him, Dr. Y would find, I think, confirmation of his theoretical formulations. Over time, I became aware of changes in my own style of analyzing which were congruent with my sense of what was occurring between Dr. Y and myself.

In describing what goes on in the analyst in framing or coming to an interpretation, Arlow (1979) focuses on the following process: "The timbre of the voice, the rate of speech, the metaphoric expressions, and the configuration of the material transmit meaning beyond that contained in verbal speech alone. All of these are perceived sometimes subliminally and elaborated and conceptualized unconsciously, i.e., intuitively" (p. 201). He says of the various functions of the psychoanalytic situation: "Foremost . . . is to ensure that what emerges into the patient's consciousness is as far as possible endogenously determined, i.e., that the thoughts, fantasies, feelings, etc., that the patient perceives represent derivatives of the persistent pressure of his unconscious conflicts. The analyst . . . may be viewed as presiding over an operative field, observing and eventually influencing a dynamically unstable equilibrium" (p. 193f).

Arlow's description of the psychoanalytic situation and the role of the analyst in this situation represent the point of view in analytic tradition which has as its ideal the "myth" of the impersonal analyst (Little, 1951). No allowance is made for a process going on in the patient that is very similar to that described as going on in the analyst, a process that potentially allows the patient to learn a great deal about his analyst. If the analyst takes Arlow's position, there would seem to be no respectable place for the analysand's reactions to the real, consciously and unconsciously, preceived aspects of the analyst in the analytic situation. Brenner (1976, 1979) takes a similar position in regard to the reality of the analyst and the concept of the therapeutic alliance. He maintains that he sees no advantage to such concepts and feels that all of the patient's reactions should be viewed as transferences and analyzed. Certainly *all* of an individual's responses have relevance to his individual makeup, personal life history, and resultant personality structure. In this sense, all of his responses certainly have endogenous determinants. However, to my mind, this does not make all such responses transferences. Taken to its extreme to make my point, Brenner's view apparently sees no advantage to differentiating a patient's responding to his analyst as if he were being rude when the analyst is not, from an appropriate response to a rude analyst.

If the analyst's theoretical point of view excludes the reality of his personal impact on the process or, at the least, places a high value on his having no personal impact by being a perfect mirror, he is not likely to include this factor in his considerations. For all intents and purposes, it does not exist for that analyst. Such a position does not seem to include a here and a now. As Greenson and Wexler (1969) put it, "if there is a present, . . . we are told little . . . about what to do with it. Surely, we are not to hope it will go away" (p. 28). I believe that the analyst who conducts his analysis as though he were presiding over an operational field in fact will carry on an analysis that does exclude and keep the analysand from learning much about him consciously and does frustrate the analysand in his search beneath the surface (Loewald, 1970). Being aloof, however, does not mean not having an impact on the analysand's reactions. This stance can introduce a iatrogenic element into the analysis which paradoxically such an attitude was intended to avoid. Stone (1967, 1981) has written extensively on his views of such a situation and what he refers to as "spurious iatrogenic regressions" (1981, p. 5) which he feels can be instigated by excessively guarded analysts. My impression is that analysts who take this view—and I believe Dr. X was such an analyst—value insight above all else and tend to view the cognitive analysis of oedipal conflict to be *the* sign of a successful analysis. They view the possibility of there being nonverbal components to the effectiveness of analysis to be nonanalytic.

The attitude of aloofness can be traced to Freud's (1912b) advice to the analyst to adopt a stance of emotional coldness akin to what Freud viewed to be the attitude of a surgeon toward his patients, who "concentrates his mental forces on the single aim of performing the operation as skilfully as possible" (p. 115). "The resolution of the transference . . . —one of the main tasks of the treatment—is made more difficult by an intimate attitude on the doctor's part. . . . The doctor should be opaque to his patients and, like a mirror, should show them nothing but what is shown to him" (p. 118). Fenichel (1941) felt that the notion of the analyst as a mirror was misunderstood. He stressed that the patient should always be able to count on what he referred to as the humanness of the analyst and that it was only important for the analyst "not to join in the game" (p. 72). "The analyst is no more to be permitted to isolate analysis from life than is the patient who misuses lying on the analytic couch for the same purpose" (p. 74).

I believe that Fenichel was right—that in the surgeon analogy Freud meant that the analyst should not avoid introducing something painful if necessary for cure and should avoid becoming overly involved with his patients. In his recommendation of opacity, Freud intended only to warn against the analyst's trading intimacies with his patients and sharing with them details of his own life. Fenichel's point can be supported even more clearly in some of Freud's later writings (1933, 1937). Be that as it may, there have been two opposing groups of analysts with regard to their interpretation of this technical paper and its implementations in their own work. Freud's (1912b) recommendation that anyone wishing to practice analysis should himself be analyzed has undoubtedly played a role in perpetuating these differences, as the next generation of analysts integrate their own analytic experiences and potentially identify with the attitudes of their own analysts.

Earlier I mentioned Greenacre's (1954) statement that if two people are alone together, some sort of emotional bond will develop between them. She traces this tendency to "the original mother-infant quasi-union of the first months of life" (p. 628). She views this as the basic or most primitive transference. While I disagree with her use of transference in this regard, certainly the nature of the bond which develops and which has to be understood cannot be seen as simply the unfolding of a prepackaged closed-system method of relating in the analysand (or in the baby). Mothers, in their care of infants, can be loving or distant, soothing or exciting, frustrating or gratifying. Infants can feel loved or abandoned, soothed or excited, frustrated or gratified. What happens depends on a complicated interaction between infant and mother and the greater or lesser extent to which each member of the dyad responds to or fails to respond to, feels responded to or fails to feel responded to. Infant observation research suggests that this process begins immediately after birth (Emde, 1981). Loewald (1970) sees psychological development and psychic structure as evolving out of an undifferentiated mother-child matrix. I believe that a similar process goes on in the analytic situation and at a level that is initially out of the awareness of the analysand and potentially the analyst as well. The question is in what way can we recognize those interactions that contribute to and perhaps determine the nature and quality of the transference neurosis? In addition to the superficial characteristics of the analyst (Greenson, 1967), and the circumstances under which the analysis is undertaken, the meaning of the analysand, of being an analyst, of the analytic situation, and the meaning of the act of interpretation itself to the analyst can all contribute to responses in the analysand (Loewald, 1970). These factors work subliminally along the lines suggested by Silverman (1978)—constantly serving to fuel the unconscious fantasies, being a chronic salve or irritant until recognized. For example, in my own analytic experience, Dr. X's appearance, tone of voice, and style constantly served to activate painful fantasies of being judged and found wanting. Dr. Y's habit of smoking and drinking coffee, combined with his style, served to foster a feeling of safety and relaxation. The full impact of these characteristics was recognized only as a postanalytic development. Such factors greatly complicate the analytic task and can easily escape notice. Still, "the analytic situation must offer [the patient] . . . an opportunity for experiencing in depth *both* the realistic and the unrealistic aspects of his dealing with objects" (Greenson and Wexler, 1969, p. 38).

Friedman (1969) states that there is a need for a real congruence between patient and analyst as a foundation for the hope that then allows the patient to ally himself with the analyst. Freud himself (1912b) described affectionate feelings for the analyst as an acceptable part of the transference which persists (i.e., not analyzed) and is the vehicle for success in psychoanalysis. In 1937 Freud said that "not every good relation between an analyst and his subject during and after analysis was to be regarded as a transference; there were also friendly relations which were based on reality which proved to be viable" (p. 222). Anna Freud (1954) felt that "we should leave room somewhere for the realization that analyst and patient are two real people of equal adult status in a *real* personal relationship to one another" (p. 618). These observations suggest still another Scylla and Charybdis to be added to the list of conundrums in the analytic situation. If in some way the analyst or the analytic situation is too similar to the already internalized relationships and situations in the patient's life, clarification of those particular internal components will be most difficult and may be impossible (Bibring, 1936; Greenacre, 1959). If, however, there is not enough with which to identify for the analysand, the project is stalled at the outset. It is the area between these extremes that seems to represent the optimum "fit" which serves well as the foundation for ongoing analytic work. It seems to be just this fit that experienced therapists look for in seeking a therapist for themselves (Grunebaum, 1981).

The diagnosis of some adverse aspect to the patient-therapist fit is complicated. There is no way for the analyst to know unless the patient tells him. Because it is so often subliminal in nature, it is not often detected by the patient. Even if it is detected, it may be near impossible for the analysand to communicate. Greenson and Wexler (1969) comment on the difficulty an analysand may have in communicating something negative that he feels to be *real* about the analyst. Even if the patient is able to communicate it, the analyst had no reliable way of differentiating such a perception from transference illusion. The tenacity of such a reaction may be the most consistent objective clue.

Positive responses triggered by such situations may be even more unlikely to be analyzed, as powerful resistance to their recognition and delineation may exist in both analyst and analysand. In addition to the obvious resistances, Stein (1981) states that the role "of the positive, overtly nonerotic transference in maintaining a powerful resistance, not only to the resolution of inhibitions, but also to the analytic exploration of hidden springs of defiance and revenge" is obscure (p. 876).

All of the above touches on what we all know—that to separate neurotic distortion from "reality" is a most complicated task. As I have mentioned, all of our responses have relevance to our individual personality structure. It is vitally important for the analysis, however, to differentiate those reactions of the analysand to the real, consciously or unconsciously perceived aspects of the analyst, from those responses of the analysand to inner stimuli, and which, to a much greater extent, make use of various externalizations. These latter responses represent a much higher degree of reality distortion and, to my mind, represent the clearest manifestations of transference. It is only after the reality of certain aspects of the analyst have been clarified and accepted that the transference use of these characteristics by the analysand can be demonstrated. The impact on the analysis that I believe such a clarification can make centers on the strengthening or undermining of the analysand's capacity to test reality, to trust the analyst, to temper both the analyst and the analysand's grandiosity, and to aid in lifting repressions. I believe the results of such clarifications are related to Nunberg's (1951) observation that conscious perceptions of the ego must be sanctioned by the superego in order to acquire the quality of full, uncontested reality. It may be that for some time the analyst serves as the sanctioning agent in any analysis.

Racker (1957) has written an excellent paper focusing particularly on the importance of the analyst's being aware of his own reactions to the analysand and the impact of these reactions on the patient. He describes the analytic situation in this regard as follows:

> It is an interaction between two personalities, in both of which the ego is under pressure from the id, the superego, and the external world; each personality has its internal and external dependencies, anxieties, and pathological defenses; each is also a child with its internal parents; and each of these whole personalities—that of the analysand and the analyst—responds to every event of the analytic situation . . . there also exist differences and one of these is in 'objectivity'. The analyst's objectivity consists mainly in a certain attitude toward his own subjectivity and countertransferences. . . . True objectivity is based on a form of internal division that enables the analyst to make himself (his own countertransference and subjectivity) an object of his continuous observation and analysis [p. 308f.].

It is just this ability that we hope will develop in the analysand. He then goes on to describe what he views to be the two neurotic extremes. One he refers to as "obsessive" or ideal objectivity which he feels leads to the repressive blocking of subjectivity in an attempt to fulfill the "mythic ideal of the analyst without anxiety or anger." The other extreme Racker refers to as "drowning" in the countertransference in which the analyst himself makes little differentiation between his subjective responses and how these may be translated into the realities of the patient and the patient's inner world (p. 315).

PROCESS AND THEORY

I will limit my discussion to a consideration of two alternatives in theoretical choice and ask the following question: what happens in the analyses of patients whose analysts focus on oedipal conflicts as primary to neurosogenesis and interpret preoedipal factors as defensive regressions, as compared to the analyses of patients whose analysts include preoedipal and perverbal factors as potentially important to neurosogenesis in their own right? I have described significant qualitative differences in my two analyses. It was as a result of my second analysis that I came to view my sense of "something missing" in my first analysis not as neurotic oedipal longing but as a failure to include and be able to accept earlier more archaic issues. In reviewing the literature, I found seemingly similar experiences reported from different vantage points.

Guntrip's (1975) account of his analyses with Fairbairn and Winnicott struck a resonant chord. Guntrip describes Fairbairn as being an essentially nonrelating mirror analyst, a technical interpreter who consistently stayed at an oedipal level. He describes Winnicott as more spontaneous, more intuitive, and more willing to engage in a personal relationship, much more in touch with and able to organize archaic experience. As an example of the differences, he describes the interpretations offered him in response to a certain aspect of his behavior in sessions, namely that he was constantly active and couldn't tolerate gaps of silence. Fairbairn interpreted this behavior as an expression of oedipal rivalry, as Guntrip's attempt to take the analysis out of Fairbairn's hands and to do the job himself, "to steal his father's penis" (p. 152). Winnicott said something different, feeling that there was a relationship between this behavior and the death of his younger brother when Guntrip was 3½ years old: "You can't take your ongoing being for granted. You're afraid to stop acting, talking or being awake. You feel you might die in a gap like Percy. . . . [Mother] couldn't save Percy or you. You're bound to fear I can't keep you alive. . . . You know about 'being active' but not about 'just growing, just breathing' while you sleep, without your having to do anything about it" (p. 152). After this interpretation, Guntrip was better able to tolerate the silences. For Guntrip, the second interpretation had more impact than the first and I think it makes sense that it should. Fairbairn's seems to me to be based in part on his "countertransference" to Guntrip's behavior from which he extrapolated notions of oedipal rivalry. Winnicott's interpretation, on the other hand, is so poignant because it seems so directly to address this man's unique history, and conveys an understanding of the complex feelings that such a tragic situation might stir in a young child. It is not burdened by theory. It addresses very early and primitive developmental concerns, perhaps preverbal. It organizes them. It puts them into words, helping in this way to master them (Loewald, 1970). As Freud (1933) said, "it is truly a matter of conceptions—that is to say, of introducing the right abstract ideas, whose applicaton to the raw material of observation will produce order and clarity in it" (p. 81).

Kramer (1979) reports the unique chance experience of supervising two analysts with different theoretical attitudes and empathic abilities in the treatment of the same patient. Interestingly, an aspect of this patient's behavior was similar to what Guntrip describes of himself. The first analyst interpreted the patient's need to keep him at a distance, to talk constantly, and to interpret her own dreams, either on an oedipal level or as resistance to oedipal material. He disagreed with Kramer's suggestion that issues of separation and individuation and the need to avoid an intrusive mother might have been more important determinants of this behavior. The patient broke off treatment after the analyst's second vacation. She did, however, seek treatment with a second analyst, who, by chance, also sought supervision with Kramer. The second analyst had more empathic understanding of the patient's need to demonstrate and maintain her autonomy. With this ability and his knowledge of the issues of separation-individuation and their transference manifestations, he was able to be appropriately available without being intrusive. This approach gradually allowed for the development of a full analytic experience with this patient.

Kohut (1979) describes two analyses done at different times in his own career with the same patient. The first analysis was conducted along what he felt to be classical lines but proved to be not sufficiently complete. When the patient returned for his second analysis, Kohut had already increased his sensitivity to certain preoedipal issues, organized by him into "self psychology." The second analysis led to a more favorable, complete, and lasting result. Wallerstein (1981), in discussing this paper, raised the question as to "how much the more substantial and enduring result that eventuated from the second analysis . . . was a matter of newer and better theory and how much a matter of better empathy, guided . . . by the enlarged perspectives for understanding that derived from the conceptual additions of the psychology of the self" (p. 393). In discussing the concept of selfobject and preoedipal object as it appears in Kohut's paper, Coen (1981) raised the question, "Is the problem with our theories or with ourselves? Is it that because of incomplete analysis or relative lack of resolution of certain preoedipal issues, many analysts have avoided or have been unable to maintain an analytic stance toward their patients' preoedipal material? Or is it that our understanding of development prior to the oedipal phase, and our theory, has not been sufficiently clear for us to analyze satisfactorily derivatives of preoedipal issues in our adult patients?" (p. 397). I will return to Coen's question at the conclusion of my paper. For the purposes of my discussion at this point, however, I wish to emphasize that regardless of the specifics of theoretical formulation, it was the absence of adequate attention to preoedipal issues that in each of the preceding instances was missing in the first analysis and the addition of which significantly enhanced the second.

Gedo (1980) reviewed two books, one of which describes analyses conducted in accord with Kohut's theory (Goldberg, 1978) and the other reviews analyses conducted along more traditional lines (Firestein, 1978). The outcome of the analyses conducted along "traditional lines" were uniformly disappointing; that is, in follow-up studies, the patients were left with a host of residual difficulties and discomforts. The work in these analyses focused on the derivatives of the oedipus complex. More archaic manifestations were viewed as defenses against oedipal anxieties. The outcome of those analyses conducted along the lines of

Kohut's theory produced important improvements in tension regulation and reorganization of behavior in a more coherent manner. Gedo did not feel, however, that the improvement noted could in fact be accounted for by Kohut's theory and that these analyses were incomplete in that they neglected more advanced sectors of the personality. In these analyses, the focus was more on the dyadic model (preoedipal) and the elucidation of narcissistic transferences and idealizations of the analyst which were often unanalyzed. Gedo summarizes the results of the traditional analyses as follows: "elucidation of oedipal conflicts without working through their developmental antecedents leaves patients with a variety of adaptive deficits and severe subjective discomforts" (p. 382). These findings are consistent with the previous papers in my discussion, and my own experience.

Finally, in his introduction to a panel on the "Technical Consequences of Object Relations Theory" (1980), Ernst Ticho related that in his experience with patients who came for a second analysis, where they complain that they can understand themselves but not apply the knowledge, important early object relations were either not perceived by or not communicated to the patient by their first analyst.

Summary

I have presented a personal case report and related aspects of the literature to call attention to a consideration of the impact of the personality of the analyst and his theory on psychoanalytic process. A long tradition emphasizing the neutrality of the analyst has served to obscure the interpersonal elements that are a part of any human interaction, and has interfered with our integrating these considerations into clinical theory. Just as different parents raise different children, different analysts produce different analysands. It is important that in our ongoing study of the psychoanalytic process, the nature of the differences between analysts be included, attended to, and investigated with the aim of deepening our understanding and broadening our theoretical perspective.

Now, I return to Coen's (1981) question: "Is the problem with our theories or ourselves?" Theory can serve well as a guide but not as a master. We are a long way from having a secure and tidy body of knowledge, yet the theory we do have available can provide a solid base from which we can continue to explore. Problems can arise when rather than live with a degree of uncertainty, ambiguity, or complexity, we apply theory inappropriately and with a degree of authority that inhibits curiosity and further investigation. It is important that our theory avoid overly rigid conceptual models that lead to caricatures rather than portraits of what it is to be human. To do this, it helps to have in mind a variety of schemas consistent with our deepening understanding of human development (Lichtenberg, 1979) in combination with a sensitivity and alertness to the uniqueness of individual experience.

> To find a good parent at the start is the basis of psychic health. In its lack, to find a genuine 'good object' in one's analyst is both a transference experience and a real life experience. In analysis as in real life, all relationships have a subtly dual nature. All through life we take into ourselves both good and bad figures who either strengthen or disturb us, and it is the same in psychoanalytic therapy: it is the meeting and interacting of two real people in all its complex possibilities [Guntrip, 1975, p. 156].

BIBLIOGRAPHY

ARLOW, J. A. (1979). The genesis of interpretation. *J. Amer. Psychoanal. Assn. Suppl.*, 27:193–206.

BACHRACH, H. M. (1983). On the concept of analyzability. *Psychoanal. Q.*, 52:180–204.

BIBRING, G. L. (1936). A contribution to the subject of transference resistance. *Int. J. Psychoanal.*, 17:181–189.

BLUM, H. P. (1981). Some current and recurrent problems of psychoanalytic technique. *J. Amer. Psychoanal. Assn.*, 29:47–68.

BRENNER, C. (1976). *Psychoanalytic Technique and Psychic Conflict.* New York: Int. Univ. Press.

—— (1979). Working alliance, therapeutic alliance and transference. *J. Amer. Psychoanal. Assn. Suppl.*, 27:137–157.

COEN, S. J. (1981). Notes on the concept of selfobject and preoedipal object. *J. Amer. Psychoanal. Assn.*, 29:395–411.

DEWALD, P. (1982). Elements of change and cure in psychoanalysis. *Arch. Gen. Psychiat.*, 40:89–95.

EMDE, R. N. (1981). Changing models of infancy and the nature of early development. *J. Amer. Psychoanal. Assn.*, 29:179–219.

FENICHEL, O. (1941). *Problems of Psychoanalytic Technique*. Albany: Psychoanalytic Quarterly.

FIRESTEIN, S. (1978). *Termination in Psychoanalysis*. New York: Int. Univ. Press.

FLEMING, J. & BENEDEK, T. (1966). *Psychoanalytic Supervision*. New York: Grune & Stratton.

FREUD, A. (1954). Discussion of 'The widening scope of indications for psychoanalysis.' *J. Amer. Psychoanal. Assn.*, 2:607–620.

FREUD, S. (1897). Extracts from the Fliess papers, Letter 69. *S.E.*, 1:259–260.

‾‾‾‾‾ (1905). Fragments of an analysis of a case of hysteria. *S.E.*, 7:3–122.

‾‾‾‾‾ (1912a). The dynamics of transference. *S.E.*, 12:97–108.

‾‾‾‾‾ (1912b). Recommendation to physicians practising psycho-analysis. *S.E.*, 12:109–120.

‾‾‾‾‾ (1933). New introductory lectures on psycho-analysis. *S.E.*, 22:3–182.

‾‾‾‾‾ (1937). Analysis terminable and interminable. *S.E.*, 23:209–253.

FRIEDMAN, L. (1969). The therapeutic alliance. *Int. J. Psychoanal.*, 50:139–154.

GEDO, J. E. (1980). Reflections on some current controversies in psychoanalysis. *J. Amer. Psychoanal. Assn.*, 28:363–383.

GOLDBERG, A., ed. (1978). *The Psychology of the Self*. New York: Int. Univ. Press.

GREENACRE, P. (1954). The role of transference. In *Emotional Growth*, 2:627–640. New York: Int. Univ. Press, 1971.

‾‾‾‾‾ (1959). Certain technical problems in the transference relationship. Ibid., 2:651–669.

GREENSON, R. R. (1967). *The Technique and Practice of Psychoanalysis*. New York: Int. Univ. Press.

GREENSON, R. R. & WEXLER, M. (1969). The non-transference relationship in the psycho-analytic situation. *Int. J. Psychoanal.*, 50:27–39.

GRUNEBAUM, H. (1981). A good therapist is hard to find. Psychotherapy Symposium, Cambridge Hospital.

GUNTRIP, H. (1975). My experience of analysis with Fairbairn and Winnicott. *Int. Rev. Psychoanal.*, 2:145–156.

JOSEPH, E. (1979). Comments on the therapeutic action of psychoanalysis. *J. Amer. Psychoanal. Assn. Suppl.*, 27:71–79.

KANZER, M. (1979a). Object relations theory. *J. Amer. Psychoanal. Assn.*, 27:313–325.

‾‾‾‾‾ (1979b). Developments in psychoanalytic technique. *J. Amer. Psychoanal. Assn. Suppl.*, 27:327–374.

KAPLAN, A. H. (1981). From discovery to validation. *J. Amer. Psychoanal. Assn.*, 29:3–26.

KOHUT, H. (1979). The two analyses of Mr. Z. *Int. J. Psychoanal.*, 60:3–27.

KRAMER, S. (1979). The technical significance and application of Mahler's separation-individuation theory. *J. Amer. Psychoanal. Assn. Suppl.*, 27:241–262.

KUHN, T. S. (1962). *The Structure of Scientific Revolutions*. Chicago: Univ. Chicago Press, 1970.

LEAVY, S. A. (1980). *The Psychoanalytic Dialogue*. New Haven: Yale Univ. Press.

LICHTENBERG, J. D. (1979). Factors in the development of the sense of the object. *J. Amer. Psychoanal. Assn.*, 27:375–386.

LITTLE, M. (1951). Countertransference and the patient's response to it. *Int. J. Psychoanal.*, 32:32–40.

LOEWALD, H. W. (1960). On the therapeutic action of psychoanalysis. *Int. J. Psychoanal.*, 41:16–33.

———— (1970). Psychoanalytic theory and the psychoanalytic process. In *Papers on Psychoanalysis*, pp. 277–301. New Haven: Yale Univ. Press, 1980.

———— (1971). The transference neurosis. *J. Amer. Psychoanal. Assn.*, 19:54–66.

MEISSNER, W. W. (1979). Internalization and object relations. *J. Amer. Psychoanal. Assn.*, 27:345–359.

MICHELS, R. (1981). Psychoanalytic theory and psychoanalytic practice. Read at the Western New England Psychoanalytic Society.

MODEL, A. H. (1976). "The holding environment" and the therapeutic action of psychoanalysis. *J. Amer. Psychoanal. Assn.*, 24:285–308.

MOSER, T. (1974). *Years of Apprenticeship on the Couch.* New York: Urizen Books.

NUNBERG, H. (1951). Transference and reality. *Int. J. Psychoanal.*, 32:1–9.

PANEL (1980). Technical consequences of object relations theory. A. D. Richards, reporter. *J. Amer. Psychoanal. Assn.*, 28:385–395.

———— (1984). The relation between psychoanalytic theory and psychoanalytic technique. A. D. Richards, reporter. *J. Amer. Psychoanal. Assn.*, 32:587–602.

RACKER, H. (1957). The meaning and uses of countertransference. *Psychoanal. Q.*, 26:303–357.

ROTHSTEIN, A. (1980). Psychoanalytic paradigms and their narcissistic investment. *J. Amer. Psychoanal. Assn.*, 28:385–395.

SILVERMAN, L. (1978). The unconscious fantasy as therapeutic agent in psychoanalytic treatment. Read at the Western New England Psychoanalytic Society.

STEIN, M. H. (1981). The unobjectable part of the transference. *J. Amer. Psychoanal. Assn.*, 29:869–892.

STOLLER, R. (1982). Introduction to the new ego. *Psychoanal. & Contemp. Thought.*, 5:501–548.

STONE, L. (1967). The psychoanalytic situation and transference. *J. Amer. Psychoanal. Assn.*, 15:3–57.

———— (1981). Notes on the noninterpretive elements in the psychoanalytic situation and process. *J. Amer. Psychoanal. Assn.*, 29:89–118.

STRACHEY, J. (1934). The nature of the therapeutic action of psychoanalysis. *Int. J. Psychoanal.*, 5:127–159.

WALLERSTEIN, R. S. (1981). The bipolar self. *J. Amer. Psychoanal. Assn.*, 29:377–394.

The Development of Sexual Identity in Homosexual Men

RICHARD A. ISAY, M.D.

IN THIS PAPER I WILL DRAW ON MY CLINICAL WORK TO DISCUSS SOME of the developmental issues in the lives of men who are homosexual that lead to the acquisition of their sexual identity, and to the healthy consolidation and integration during adolescence and adulthood of this identity as part of a positive self-image. My intention is to contribute to our further understanding of homosexual men in general; and specifically I discuss some issues which may act as guidelines in our assessment of their development. By presenting the outline of a normal developmental pathway for the establishment of a positive identity, I am hoping that we will be better able to conceptualize some of the impediments that may interfere with the formation of a gay man's positive self-image and with the full and gratifying expression of his sexuality. In viewing identity formation as a lifelong process that commences in early childhood, I hope to provide a framework for understanding why any attempt to change his sexuality, whether explicitly stated or implicitly guiding the therapy, will inevitably be injurious to a homosexual man's self-esteem.

Analysts view normalcy as a never-obtainable ideal (Offer and Sabshin, 1966). Freud (1937) felt that the distinction between a "normal" mental life and an "abnormal" one was only a matter of degree: "Every normal person, in fact, is only normal on the average. His ego approximates to that of the psychotic in some

Clinical associate professor of psychiatry, Cornell Medical College; faculty, Columbia Center for Psychoanalytic Training and Research.

part or other and to a greater or lesser extent" (p. 235). Jones (1931) wrote that the normal mind does not exist, and Eissler (1960) wrote that "health is a fictitious concept in the psychic stratum." When speaking from the point of view of intrapsychic conflict and the balance of intrapsychic structures, most analysts agree that we are all relatively neurotic and that there is no such thing as a "normal" person.[1]

Although I am aware that in theory analysts do not feel that adaptation should be at the expense of "critical aspects of the internal world" (Abrams, 1979, p. 829), when it comes to our patients acting in the world, psychoanalysts and other dynamically oriented therapists generally tend to be governed by social values and social morality and by the concept of instinctual renunciation as the price of being civilized (Freud, 1927). "Acting out" has a pejorative ring in our literature, and those who consistently act out their impulses are traditionally viewed as not being good analysands (A. Freud, 1968). All homosexuals are viewed as abnormal not only because of social bias (Isay, 1985) and because of the theoretical perspective that maintains they have failed to meet the developmental task of achieving heterosexuality (Isay, 1986), but because they are viewed as acting out sexual impulses rather than containing them, and therefore as not having sublimated their sexuality for the sake of social adaptation.

In this paper "healthy" and "normal" are used interchangeably. By these terms I am referring to the homosexual man's potential to have a well-integrated personality (Klein, 1960); that is, a personality in which there is reasonable intrapsychic harmony so that he may feel positively about his personal identity as a homosexual and may work and live without significant hindrance from intrapsychic conflict.

I am defining as homosexual men who have a predominant erotic preference for others of the same sex; i.e., those whose sexual fantasies are either almost entirely or are exclusively directed toward others of the same sex. Most homosexuals do engage in sexual activity. However, one need not do so to be

---

1. For a review of the analytic views of health and normality, see Hartmann (1939) and Abrams (1979).

homosexual because of the inhibition of sexual behavior due to societal pressures or intrapsychic conflict. There are also those men who may be homosexual but are unaware of their sexual fantasies because of the repression, suppression, or denial of these fantasies. There are also men who are homosexual who are conscious of their homoerotic fantasies, arousal patterns, and even behavior, but cannot acknowledge their homosexuality because of censorious social and intrapsychic pressures. In adults, the homoerotic preference can usually be recollected as being present from the latency years, preadolescence, or from early adolescence (ages 8 to 13), and sometimes even earlier. There are, of course, heterosexual males who for developmental reasons (some adolescents), for opportunistic motives (some delinquents), for situational reasons (some prison inmates), or to defend against anxiety may engage in homosexual behavior for varying periods of time and not be homosexual (Isay, 1986).

The Experience of Being Different

Each of the 40 gay men whom I have seen in psychoanalysis or analytically oriented therapy has reported that starting from about age 4 he experienced that he was "different" from his peers. Being different is described as having been more sensitive than other boys, crying more easily, having one's feelings hurt more easily, having more aesthetic interests than other young boys; i.e., enjoying nature and music, "soft" rather than "hard" objects, and being drawn to other "sensitive" boys, girls, and adults. They felt less aggressive than others of their age and did not enjoy participating in athletics and other "rough and tumble" activities (Friedman and Stern, 1980; Green, 1979; Bell et al., 1981). These differences make these children feel like outsiders in relation to their peers and often to their family as well. The extensive longitudinal studies by Green (1979, 1985) and by Zuger (1978, 1984) corroborate earlier studies by Saghir and Robbins (1973) that demonstrate a high incidence of adult homosexuality among children who display effeminate behavior in childhood. These studies suggest that gender identity disorders and cross-gender behavior in childhood are good indicators of the later development of homosexuality, but it is unclear from these studies what proportion of adult homosexuals have gender disorders in adulthood. In my smaller clinical sample I have found that many of the same characteristics described in these studies of effeminate boys, except for the cross-dressing, are recollected by gay men whom I do not consider to have gender identity disorders; i.e., they experience and perceive themselves as men and not women. I have not observed a qualitative distinction in the early experiences described by those men who as adults are more conventionally masculine and those whose behavior and appearance are more conventionally feminine. However, a closer and quantitative evaluation that is not readily afforded in a clinical setting may reveal some distinctions in early behavior between these groups of gay men.[2]

Part of the experience described by these men as being "different" from their peers appears to have been the perception of same-sex fantasies and early homoerotic arousal patterns. The childhood feeling of being different, consistently acknowledged by gay men, may be unconsciously used as a screen for these earlier repressed childhood memories of sexual arousal by others of the same sex. Although childhood fantasies may be recalled by the adult, like the heterosexual's childhood sexual fantasies, they are most often reconstructed as they manifest themselves in the transference and other current relationships. I will briefly describe three men who illustrate how the child's actual experience of being different from peers in the early latency years may act as a screen for these early sexual feelings.

Alan was a 32-year-old, masculine-appearing, somewhat tight and rigid but handsome man with a small, neat mustache. He initially entered psychotherapy because of feelings of loneliness, dysphoria, anxiety, and dissatisfaction with the quality of his relationships. He seemed moderately depressed and distressed over the breakup during the previous month of a year-long relationship. He had no apparent conflict over his homosex-

2. In my clinical sample, I would consider only one man to have had a gender identity disorder as an adult. He had been a cross-dresser as a child. My experience is, in general, with highly functioning professional men who tend to be masculine in appearance and behavior and to be integrated into heterosexual vocational settings. It may be that my sample is skewed and that these men have less gender disturbances than gay men in the general population.

uality, easily speaking in the initial sessions of his attraction to other men but also of his difficulties in feeling close to them. He had had a 5-year relationship with one man that was "tempestuous" and described as sexually one-sided. He had had a similar experience during a more recent relationship in which he had felt too much in the role of pursuer. Being the pursuer in some relationships made him feel sexually alive and more attracted to his lovers than when he was pursued. However, being the pursuer also made him feel unloved and unlovable.

Early in therapy he spontaneously recollected having felt different from his peers during his childhood. He described this in part as "not liking to hit people or rough stuff. I was more sensitive. I never liked being demanding. I liked playing the piano." He believed that his sense of inadequacy derived from feeling like a perpetual outsider. Peer recognition in adolescence, occurring readily because of his intelligence, good looks, and muscularity, could not enhance his self-esteem. "I never could understand why I was selected for the honor society. When I was chosen, I thought they were talking about someone else and not me."

Alan's father was described as somewhat distant, a man of few words and fewer feelings. His work was viewed by the patient and his mother as being demeaning, although he always earned a reasonable living. His mother was described as clinging, depressed, and needy, but the dominant force in this family in which Alan was favored by both parents over a brother 2 years older. In his artistic and musical interests he perceived himself as being like his mother. His acquiescence, nondemandingness, passivity, and emotional distance were seen as being more like his father.

Early in treatment the transference took the form of indifference toward the therapist, which suggested a need to deny my importance to him. As our work progressed, he met and moved in with a new lover, who was comfortably open in his expression of affection and tenderness toward the patient. He became somewhat less frightened of his feelings within the transference and more open and giving in this new relationship. It was during this period of gradually increasing comfort with the showing of his sexual feelings that he recalled sexual fantasies from when he

was 4 that were centered on muscular comic-book heroes. Many
of his therapy hours dealt with a longing for the father he perceived as being weak. He also recollected that from about 9 he
began to notice his interest in and attention to other boys in his
class. During the course of therapy, as his childhood sexual feelings became more accessible, he became less preoccupied with
feelings of being "different" and less critical of his sexual fantasies and feelings in the present. It seemed likely from our
work, especially from the nature of the transference, that these
early sources of sexual interest and excitement were displacements from and expressions of his repressed sexual feelings
toward his father.

Another patient, Benjamin, entered analysis because of very
low self-esteem, severe dysphoria, discontent with his work and
with his life in general. He readily acknowledged that he was
homosexual, but, unlike Alan, in the earliest hours he wished he
were not. His fears of closeness to men were intense. His mother
was described as intrusive and cloying; his father as gruff and
harsh but always available. He had felt different as a child—in
fact, he could not recall ever feeling any other way. He described
having had no interest in sports but being interested in artistic
and musical endeavors. He did not enjoy playing with either
girls or boys of his own age, and felt isolated and lonely.

During the first months of his analysis he could not recall or
had suppressed the memory of any sexual experiences before
college. By the second year he was able to speak of such sexual
experiences that had occurred when he was 12, when he went to
the West Village and was picked up by a college student who
"taught" him to masturbate. Forays to the West Village continued throughout his adolescence. His typical masturbation
fantasies were of being picked up by a dark, muscular man and
being dominated by him. One aspect of the evolving transference over several years was first the defense against, and then
manifestations of, and finally expressions of the wish to be dominated and sexually penetrated by me. This was accompanied by
recollections of feelings of great warmth and comfort lying in
bed with his father on weekend mornings while he was being
told stories, then of some vague childhood memories of sexual
thoughts about his father and about other boys his age. These

recollections date from about age 4, when he also began to feel he was different from his peers. As was true of Alan, his preoccupation with being different as a child mitigated considerably as these early childhood sexual feelings were recollected.

Another patient, Carl, was a slender and clean-shaven young man who entered treatment while still in college. His analysis continued for 6 years with one brief interruption that occurred between the end of college and the start of graduate school. He entered therapy initially because of low self-esteem and an inability to form meaningful relationships. His sexual activity had largely been confined to the bathroom of the college library and to the stalls of pornographic bookstores. His mother had been extremely attentive until the birth of his younger sibling when he was abruptly sent to prenursery school at 3½ years. She was always ambitious for Carl, and he felt like an extension of her. His father, perceived as being demeaned by her and as having been unsuccessful, was also seen as warm, kind, and loving.

Carl said he felt estranged from other boys throughout his childhood. Like the men described previously, he had had no interest in athletic activities, enjoyed nature, and felt he was more sensitive than his peers. He, like the others, believed these early feelings contributed to his current poor self-image and low self-esteem.

Again, like Alan and Benjamin, Carl initially felt indifferent to me, yet he also seemed devoted to our work and rarely missed an appointment. Throughout the first years he articulated and stressed that he was not attracted to "older men in their 40s," feeling they were "lecherous" and would take advantage of him. He had intense anxiety about being the recipient of anal sex and was often too tight to permit anal penetration, especially if he felt affection for his sexual partner. He was mainly attracted to passive, androgynous-appearing young men, but had masturbation fantasies of powerful black men with large penises.

The very slowly evolving sexual transference was manifested largely in dreams of being passively dominated by me. As these wishes became clearer to him, he also began to have vague recollection of sexual feelings toward other boys in the early years of grade school. The deeply repressed and conflicted wishes to be dominated and penetrated by older men became clear from dreams and the transference, although no childhood attraction to his father was directly recollected. These repressed wishes appeared to stem from early childhood and to encompass the period in which he described his experiences of being different from other children.

To summarize, it has become clear from my analytic and psychotherapeutic work with many adult homosexual men that homoerotic fantasies are often present from the ages of 3, 4, or 5 years. I conceptualize this period as being analogous to the oedipal stage of heterosexual boys, except that the primary sexual object in these homosexual men appears to be their fathers. I do not see evidence either in the nature of the transference or in the nature of the sexual object choice of these men of a defensive shift in erotic interest from their mothers to their fathers. The experience of being different that may exist concurrently with or occur somewhat later than the homoerotic fantasies commences during the early periods of peer socialization. This experience appears to include a preconscious perception of same-sex fantasies.

The period of childhood homoerotic sexual attachment to the father with the derivative fantasies and sexual arousal pattern is the first stage in the acquisition of a homosexual identity. The experience of being different and, in fact, of being an outsider in relation to peers (Bell et al., 1981), often becomes a screen for conflicted sexual feelings. Both the guilt around early homoerotic fantasies and the experience of being different from peers may contribute to the low self-esteem and negative self-percepts of many gay men.

I now turn to the stage of consolidation of a homosexual identity in adolescence and then to some of the developmental impediments that may hinder the healthy consolidation and continuing integration in adulthood of a homosexual orientation as part of a positive identity.

CONSOLIDATION OF SEXUAL IDENTITY

Alan, at the age of 32, was open about his sexuality, and he had acknowledged that he was homosexual during his first year of graduate school. As I mentioned before, this man had little difficulty in recollecting that he had same-sex fantasies and feelings from the age of 4. Fantasies and attraction for classmates continued throughout grade school and high school without abating, but also without his having had any sexual experience. He had been very popular with his peers in high school because of a combination of masculine appearance, intelligence, sensitivity, and good looks. Though he had always felt like an outsider, like most adolescents he cultivated and appreciated peer-group recognition. In order to "fit in" he dated one girl steadily throughout high school, but he was so apprehensive that she might want sex that he would have diarrhea before dates. Because they never did have sex, she broke off the relationship after several years. Throughout this period he continued to deny that he was homosexual.

In college his closest friend was gay. This friend had wanted to have sex with Alan, but, although the attraction was mutual, Alan still could not associate this attraction with a sexuality that was unacceptable to him. "It was okay for him, but not for me. I was a liberal before I knew I was gay." It was in his first year of graduate school, when he was 23, that he fell in love and then suddenly recognized and acknowledged to himself that he was homosexual. After that recognition he had a sexual relationship with a man for the first time. He has been relatively and appropriately open about his sexuality since then.

Alan's experience was similar to that described by others who acknowledged their sexual orientation after a relatively sudden and dramatic breakthrough of barriers of denial and repression. This "aha" experience, caused by the coming together of a long-established sexual arousal pattern with a sexual object, feels like the pieces of an old puzzle falling into place. "Until then I had felt I could never fall in love, that I had no sexual feelings, and that they weren't what they should be." A sense of relief, well-being, and "rightness" follow. This experience is similar to what occasionally happens in analysis or psychotherapy following an interpretation that may have been made many times before and is, at last, cognitively and affectively comprehended.

In the gay man this experience signifies both the conscious recognition of his sexuality and the beginning of its acceptance as part of his identity. The process of recognition and the beginning integration are expectable and normal occurrences in the development of gay men during late adolescence, although the experience is not always as dramatic as with Alan. The initial stage of consolidation of sexuality does not often occur as early in adolescence as it does in heterosexual boys because of the internalized social constraints and prohibitions confronting the homosexual that cause him to suppress and deny his sexuality with greater vigor. Alan's development in this regard was essentially normal. The delay in acknowledging his sexual orientation until age 23 and his degree of denial in the face of early, conscious, sexual fantasies were attributable to the adolescent wish for peer recognition and to the fear that he would fall out of favor with his parents if he were gay.

I will illustrate the process of recognition and the beginning integration of the homosexual orientation with the experience of another man seen in a 2-year analysis following a lengthy previous analysis. With this man the acceptance and consolidation of his sexuality were delayed long beyond late adolescence because of both severe external, social conflicts and internal conflicts.

Donald was in his late 30s before he was able to acknowledge his homosexuality. He had been aware of exclusive homoerotic fantasies since early childhood with arousal by other boys in his class in grade school. Although it is always difficult to assess patient reports of a previous analysis, he perceived that there had been an unconscious collaboration between his previous analyst and himself around a shared need for the patient not to be homosexual. His analyst attempted over many years to analyze the always present homosexuality as a defense against conflicted, competitive, and heterosexual wishes and did not analyze the transference aspects of his unsuccessful and painful attempts at heterosexuality, stemming from his need to be perceived by his analyst, like his parents, as a "good" boy. Donald married during this first analysis, a marriage that lasted 3 years, followed by a divorce and the termination of this first treatment.

After completion of that analysis Donald unconsciously felt released from the confinement of his transference need to please his analyst, and within one month he had an anonymous homosexual encounter, followed by the "click" of recognition of his sexuality and an enormous feeling of relief. For the first time in his life he felt "sexual, vital, and alive." The low self-esteem and depression that had plagued him for many years began to lift spontaneously. The further analytic work was focused by the patient on his feelings of rage about the first analyst, of which there were childhood antecedents, on the previously unanalyzed transference need to please, and on the genetic and developmental origins of the early homosexual arousal patterns. This analytic process further contributed to the integration of his sexuality as part of his identity, mitigating the image he had of himself of being bad, which in part derived from the misunderstood, unrecognized, disowned sexual impulses. A recent two-session follow-up 3 years after termination revealed that he had been involved for the past several years in a gratifying relationship with another man.

Not all homosexual men "come out" to themselves with the suddenness and unexpected great relief experienced by the two men just described. In those who have less need for peer recognition than Alan and less hunger for parental love than Donald, there may be a healthy recognition and integration that occur more gradually with less suppression and denial of their sexuality during adolescence.

Edward, for example, sought therapy for some depression and general dysphoria as he was about to enter graduate school. The depression in large measure was associated with difficulties in dealing with rage at his father who left the family when the patient was 7. His relationship with his mother, described as an intelligent, warm, and loving woman, was generally good, as it was with his stepfather and siblings. He matter-of-factly acknowledged his sexuality during our first hour when he spoke of his relationships and of looking for, but not yet being able to find, the "right man." Like every gay man, he had periods of regret, confusion, and even despair at times about his sexuality, but there was no ambiguity in his mind about the nature of this sexuality.

His first recollected sexual experience was at the age of 8 when he was fondled by an older man. He was uncertain how this occurred, but he felt that he had been a reluctant accomplice in an event remembered with considerable anxiety and guilt. This memory had the qualities of condensation, clarity, and affective investment of a screen memory, but, while I am certain the event did occur, it is still unclear to me if it was also used as a screen for earlier sexual memories.

At age 12 Edward became aware of his attraction to some of his teachers whom he had identified as being gay. He recognized a strong wish to be close to them, although not specifically to be sexual with them. His adolescent masturbation fantasies were of a man lying on top of him, making him feel submissive and cared for. He traveled abroad when he was 15 and had his first mutual sexual contact with a man working in a hotel. It was in his second year of college that he acknowledged he was homosexual, and this occurred in a conversation with a friend. There was no rush of relief following this recognition, as was true of the two previous men, for the acknowledgment of the sexuality had previously been at a preconscious level and the process of integration had been going on over the preceding years of early and middle adolescence. What self-esteem problems this young man had stemmed much less from the early experience of being an outsider or from a conflicted sexual identity than from his identification with an ambivalently viewed father and the injury sustained by the early separation from him.

Edward had acknowledged his sexual orientation more gradually and earlier than either Alan or Donald. His more nourishing maternal environment enabled him to rely less on peer and social conformity in adolescence for self-esteem enhancement and this made it less necessary for him to please in order to feel lovable. As Erikson wrote (1959, p. 39), such a maternal environment "assures the child that it is good to be alive in the particular social coordinates in which he happens to find himself."

The development of the homosexual identity can be, as we have seen, a gradual one beginning in childhood with the acquisition of and the preconscious or conscious recognition of same-sex fantasies and same-sex attraction. There is increasing consolidation of this sexuality with the preponderance of homoerotic masturbation fantasies and sexual arousal patterns during adolescence. There usually is some homosexual activity during this developmental period. But, because of the perception of a "different" sexual orientation, the sense of shame due to perceived social intolerance in general, and to adolescent peer intolerance of homosexuality specifically, there may be surprisingly little overt sexual activity in many normal homosexual adolescents.

When there is sexual activity, it can be distinguished from the homosexual activity of heterosexual boys. It has less of the experimental, accidental, and playful quality of the homosexual activity of heterosexual adolescents. The sexual activity feels "for real," because it usually has a strong affective component, either a passionate feeling of being in love or a longing for love with the sexual partner. This is more like the initial sexual encounters of heterosexual adolescents with girls than the sexual play of these adolescent boys with other boys. Heterosexual boys may, of course, have powerful "crushes" on idealized older men or peers, but these are not usually sexually acted on. When they are, a strong bisexual or homosexual orientation is almost certainly present (Fraiberg, 1961). The heterosexual activity of homosexual adolescents usually has the quality of experimentation similar to the heterosexual boy's homosexual activity, and it is usually accompanied by a good deal of anxiety.

The powerful peer and social pressure during adolescence often delays the conscious recognition and acceptance of a homosexual orientation until late adolescence or early adulthood, even in gay men who seem otherwise to have a positive image of themselves. The conscious recognition and subsequent continuing integration of the homosexuality lead to enhanced self-esteem, to a greater sense of well-being, to a greater capacity to love more confidently both in sexual relationships and friendships with both men and women, and, usually, to increased productivity.

The integration of one's homosexuality into a cohesive and positive self-image is part of the normal development of a healthy homosexual man. However, not all men who are homosexual are able to accept their sexuality. My clinical experience suggests that early developmental problems related to the maternal relationship may interfere with this normal process. Illustratively, I return to Benjamin who, it may be recalled, entered analysis because of extremely low self-esteem. He searched for men who could dominate him and, as an early adolescent, had had frequent homosexual experiences in the West Village. Such extensive sexual experience, as I have indicated before, is not customary in early adolescence. He entered analysis after seeking an extended consultation from another analyst who, he knew by reputation, attempted to change homosexuals to heterosexuals. Though he left this man after a few consultations, he sought help both from him and then from me to alter his sexuality which he believed accounted for his low self-esteem and depression. In his initial interview with me he spoke of his sexuality as though it were a foreign appendage that he would like to have excised. He was very fearful that his homosexuality would be discovered at work, and he would go out of his way not to associate with other gay men.

Benjamin appeared driven to have sex frequently. He could not tolerate the anxiety generated by being alone and feeling separated from his mother. In his nightly forays into dangerous areas of the city, he would have sex indiscriminately with hustlers and drug abusers, at times jeopardizing his property, physical well-being, and, of course, his health.

The intense masochism and the narcissistic injuries that determined the manner in which Benjamin selected his partners and expressed his sexuality were also determinants of the difficulty he had in accepting himself as a homosexual man. His mother, he felt, perceived him as an extension of herself and never conveyed to him a sense of his separateness. Because he had an unconscious perception of, and strongly identified with, her hatred of him, he had little capacity to feel lovable or to accept any aspects of himself without either compensatory inflation or intense hatred. His sexuality, known to his father but secret to his mother, became a focus and displacement of aspects of himself that made him feel hated and hateful. He had no capacity to sustain a sense of himself as a good person in a society that was inimical to and censorious of his sexuality.

Carl was another man who sought analysis because of his low self-esteem. Unlike Benjamin, he had some concern about his inability to form meaningful relationships and some wish to improve this aspect of his life. Carl had a few incidental sexual experiences in his last 2 years of high school, and in college he mainly had anonymous sex or one-night stands that continued during the early years of his analysis. He seemed invariably attracted to men who would not like him or, if they did, he would not be attracted to them or drive them away. He had little or no interest in girls, but he did date occasionally in college in order to please his mother, who spoke often to him about her wish for grandchildren. He readily acknowledged his homosexuality in the early interviews, but also spoke of how he hated himself for being gay. During his analysis he would occasionally speak of going to "one of those shrinks" who would change him. This would occur after feeling particularly close to me and threatened by both the closeness and well-defended sexual feelings. Early in analysis, in school or work situations, like Benjamin, he tended to avoid being seen with other gay men.

Carl's low self-esteem appeared to be associated with his early relationship with his mother. Like Benjamin's mother, she appeared to treat him as an extension of herself, and conveyed in many ways that her goals and gratifications were to be accomplished through his achievements and that his failures and unhappiness would result in her disappointment. Having little sense of himself as a separate person or of his own goals, he was very dependent on peer and social approval for self-esteem regulation, and censorious social attitudes toward his homosexuality weighed heavily on him. Although there was no suggestion that Carl's aggression toward his mother was a primary determinant of his sexual orientation, both this aggression and his masochism played a large role in the manner in which he expressed his homosexuality and the tenuous quality of his relationships. His feelings about his sexuality acted as a displacement from other sources of self-hatred, especially of his rage toward his ambivalently viewed mother. The binding relationship with an impaired and hostile mother, which filled him with rage and self-hatred, eventuated in a profound difficulty in permitting himself any pleasurable sexual activity in the context of a gratifying, loving relationship. As in Benjamin's case, sex was masochistically tinged, contributing to the feeling that his sexual orientation was bad and dirty, and to his failure to integrate it as part of a positive identity.

As Carl's self-image improved through the recognition of the early humiliations and rejections that contributed to his feeling

unlovable, the quality of his object relations also improved. He
was able to have two sustained relationships with people who
cared about him. These more nourishing relations in turn enhanced his self-esteem and his image of himself as a gay man.

With both Benjamin and Carl one aspect of the transference
in the middle of their analyses was a concern: if I was accepting
of them and did not appear to have any intention of converting
their homosexuality to heterosexuality, I must also be homosexual. I therefore became a degraded and denegrated object like
themselves. This important aspect of the transference was a defense against an early, conflicted, erotic attachment to their fathers and a reflection of their later perception and experience of
them. As the conflicts about their sexuality became better analyzed, and the inhibitions to having more gratifying relationships were lifted, both men became better able to experience
themselves and the analyst in a less deprecatory manner, leading
in the later stages of our work to the less inhibited and less
defended expression of the wish for closeness and love both
inside and outside of their analyses.

I will present one further illustration of the delay and disruption in the process of the consolidation of homosexual identity
formation. Fred, whom I initially saw during his first year of
college when he was 17, had left a previous therapist when he
began to encourage him to date women and appeared hostile to
his being homosexual. Fred had experienced the feeling of
being different, along with a conscious perception of early homoerotic fantasy and arousal and the clear memory of homosexual fantasy, from age 9. His masturbation fantasy was exclusively
homosexual. When he initially consulted me, he had no question
about his sexual orientation, although he was fearful of having
sexual contact with or experiencing any emotional closeness to
another boy. We both considered this to be a neurotic inhibition
that was interfering with his sexual expression and therefore
with his capacity to consolidate his identity as a homosexual.

Fred was concerned about the intensity of his homosexual
arousal at college. He felt attracted to many boys, most of whom
were openly gay. This made him particularly anxious because of
the possibility that there would be a mutual attraction and the
potential for consummation of his desire. He was inhibited from

expressing this desire, and if he were "cruised," he refused to return the gaze. In his second year of therapy he fell in love with a classmate and had a brief sexual experience, which he enjoyed, but he found himself so "embarrassed" when he saw his new friend that he could not maintain the relationship. His sexual life became exclusively one of solitary masturbation with increasing pot smoking in an effort to dull his sexual excitement and his self-consciousness about it.

Fred's sexual inhibition stemmed from a fear of humiliation that, by and large, derived from his mother's expressed ambivalence toward him and his father. The constantly chaotic relationship between his mother and father and her denigration of his father made his love and erotic attachment to his father a source of humiliation and shame. Out of rage at both parents and self-protection, Fred became intent on not exposing himself to his mother's humiliating rejection by refusing to become attached to another man and by rejecting any man's interest in him with dismissive contempt. For Benjamin and Carl, the severe narcissistic injury that occurred from their experience of being little more than extensions of their mothers, along with the perception of their mothers' ambivalence and their own rage turned against themselves, neurotically distorted the erotic attachment to their fathers and made emotional intimacy with other men terrifying. The inability to have gratifying relationships kept each of these men from having a positive identity as a homosexual man. Injured self-esteem, fears of intimacy, and the inability to accept their homosexual orientation or to express it in a manner that is emotionally fulfilling appeared to go together in each of these three men.

INTEGRATION OF SEXUAL IDENTITY

The development of sexual identity as a homosexual man is, of course, lifelong. The acquisition of the sexual orientation occurs in childhood, as does the beginning of sexual identity formation, with the feeling of being different and the preconscious recognition of same-sex fantasies. Consolidation occurs during late adolescence and early adulthood with the expression of sexuality motivated by the surge of sexual needs. However, continuing integration of the sexual identity occurs throughout adulthood by both sexual and social relationships with other homosexual men and with varying degrees of involvement in gay social networks (Troiden, 1979).

The process of coming out to other gay men usually leads to "homosocialization," by which I refer to nonsexual contacts with other gay men either within or outside of an established gay community. This aspect of the life of the homosexual man has received little attention from psychoanalysts. Some have stated that "social acceptance" increases the difficulty any homosexual has in being motivated for treatment by reducing the feeling that he is "ill," and should therefore be discouraged because it is not in his interest (Socarides, 1963). Others are quoted as stating that the issue of narcissism is more pervasive in the "sociosexual than in the sexual homosexual groups," and that investment in the homosexual world compensates for maternal deprivation and is an expression of rage (Panel, 1977, p. 190). In the social-psychological literature, there are those who argue the opposite position; namely, that a nearly exclusive association with other gay men is a necessary component of the consolidation of the normal identity as a homosexual (Cass, 1979).

None of these positions conforms to my clinical experience. There are homosexual men with a relatively healthy and comfortable acceptance of their homosexual orientation who do not have extensive, social, gay networks. The degree and nature of involvement in the gay community usually are determined by social and vocational needs, by marital status, and by the availability of other gay men (Weinberg and Williams, 1974, p. 11). The support provided by having many gay friends or by living in a gay community, when this is available, may be unnecessary for those, for example, who receive adequate gratification from social and vocational activities within the heterosexual community. It is also easier for a homosexual man in our society to be integrated into a heterosexual community when he is not coupled and has not "come out." Those who are coupled generally find it more comfortable and better for the stability of the relationship to have the support and relatively unprejudiced structure offered by a gay community or a network of gay friends.

The freedom to be homosocial may also be related to one's

having less need for support from heterosexually oriented peer and social organizations; therefore, it is often indicative of the healthy acceptance of one's sexual orientation and of the self-assurance that precludes the necessity for continued traditional sources of support. Likewise, extensive homosocial involvement may also be suggestive of a rageful need to reject conventional sources of support (Panel, 1977). However, as I have indicated in my descriptions of the nonsexual gay relationships of Benjamin, Carl, and Fred, there was a connection between their poor self-esteem, the inability to have a positive image of their sexuality, and their need to avoid contact with other gay men. As their self-esteem improved through the analysis of early conflict, especially around the problematic relations with their mothers, the transference evolved into one of less self-imposed distance and homosocial contacts increased extensively. For these men homosociability further increased the acceptance of their sexuality and enhanced their feeling of self-worth. In the cases of Alan and Edward, whose self-esteem had not been severely disturbed by early conflict, there was always a capacity for and interest in nonsexual social relationships with other gay men. Insofar as availability and other obligations permit, homosocial relationships are necessary for the continuing consolidation and integration of identity, and the capacity for such relationships is a sign of a relatively positive self-regard. Conversely, the inability or unwillingness to have such relationships suggests impaired self-esteem.

DISCUSSION

It would be inaccurate to conclude from what I have written that all homosexual men who engage in random sexual encounters are beset by neurotic difficulties and that only those who have sustained relationships are "healthy." The selection of multiple partners is best understood as being determined by a number of interactive issues that include social as well as dynamic factors. For example, anonymous sexual activity in public restrooms is more likely to be carried out by homosexual men who cannot risk discovery and disclosure and who are well integrated into a heterosexual community by virtue of religious affiliation, marriage, and vocation (Humphreys, 1972) than by those integrated into a gay subculture. For the same reasons such men may not have a sustained relationship, even though they may be capable or even desirous of having one. The expression of defiance of antihomosexual attitudes (Altman, 1973), the lack of legal and social sanctions of homosexual relationships, the absence of children to bind these relationships, and the availability of partners are some of the other social factors that may play a role in the selection and nature of sexual partners. Foucault (1982–83) was possibly also correct when he wrote that interdictions of our society foster furtive, random, sexual encounters. Furthermore, there is evidence to suggest that biological factors related to male sexuality play a role in the nature of the homosexual man's sexual activity. Human males in general are more promiscuous than females if left to their own devices and when there are opportunities for such behavior. "This is the history of his anthropoid ancestors and this is the history of unrestrained human males everywhere" (Kinsey et al., 1948, p. 589). The human male in general is less object-directed than the human female, who appears to be less interested in variations of partners (Ford and Beach, 1951).

By pointing out these social and biological issues I am not minimizing the importance of the intrapsychic factors that motivate different types of sexual behavior in all human beings. Nor am I underestimating the difficulties some gay men may have in maintaining sustained long-term relationships, which may be caused by these same social as well as by dynamic factors.[3] I do believe, however, that to view the sexual behavior of homosexual men as being unconnected to an external social reality leads to simplistic, unifactorial, dynamic explanations of such behavior (see, e.g., Calef and Weinshel, 1984). In the homosexual man

---

3. Homosexuals cannot be stereotyped with regard to either the nature or the frequency of their sexual behavior. Sustained relationships are more extensive than generally believed (Bell and Weinberg, 1978; McWhirter and Mattison, 1984), and the view that all homosexuals are promiscuous, fueled by the AIDS epidemic, is a pernicious stereotype prominently directed against all minority groups who are feared because of their differences. This includes not only gays, but blacks, Puerto Ricans, and Jews as well, the latter association having been particularly prominent during the Nazi era.

social factors interact with, help to shape, and even modify intra-psychic forces based on early developmental factors. Under-standing and attending to such issues provide the analyst or dynamic therapist with a more complete explanation of any sex-ual behavior. Understanding some of the developmental issues that confront every gay man in the acquisition, consolidation, and integration of his identity will add to, deepen, and enhance the therapist's understanding of his patients' lives.

SUMMARY

I have outlined three broad stages in homosexual identity for-mation: a childhood acquisition stage, the consolidation stage of adolescence and early adulthood, and the integration stage of adulthood. The stage of acquisition is characterized by same-sex fantasies and impulses in early childhood. Memories of these early arousal patterns may be repressed, but do become more accessible through the analysis of the indirect memories that are manifested in the transference and in the choice of sexual ob-jects. They may, of course, also be directly recalled. The experi-ences during early peer socialization of being "different" appear to include the preconscious recognition of same-sex arousal. Other recollected aspects of being different from peers may act as a screen for these repressed sexual memories.

The consolidation and integration of the homosexual orienta-tion appear to be enhanced by a warm and loving mother who permits the child to have an accepting image of himself and of his father. Those homosexual men who have been used by their mothers as narcissistic extensions of themselves and who have unconsciously perceived their mothers' ambivalence toward them tend to have more masochistic tendencies and poorer self-images due to their early narcissistic injuries. They feel greater need for social conformity because of their reliance on peer and social approval for self-esteem maintenance. They are more likely to despise their homosexuality as they do other aspects of themselves, to avoid the companionship of other homosexual men, and to fear intimacy with them. The negative perception of their sexuality is manifested in and reinforced by the ungratify-ing nature of these relationships.

The expression of the homosexual orientation in late adolescence or early adulthood within the context of warm sexual relationships and the capacity to form loving sustained relationships later in adulthood enhance the consolidation and integration of the sexuality as part of a positive identity. This process continues throughout adulthood both through loving relationships, and, insofar as one's social needs permit, through sustaining nonsexual relationships with other gay men.

BIBLIOGRAPHY

ABRAMS, S. (1979). The psychoanalytic normalities. *J. Amer. Psychoanal. Assn.*, 27:821–835.
ALTMAN, D. (1973). *Homosexual.* New York: Avon Books.
BELL, A. P. & WEINBERG, M. S. (1978). *Homosexualities.* New York: Simon & Schuster.
BELL, A. P., WEINBERG, M. S., & HAMMERSMITH, S. K. (1981). *Sexual Preference.* Bloomington: Indiana Univ. Press.
CALEF, V. & WEINSHEL, E. (1984). Anxiety and the restitutive function of homosexual cruising. *Int. J. Psychoanal.*, 65:45–53.
CASS, V. C. (1979). Homosexual identity formation. *J. Homosexual.*, 4:219–235.
EISSLER, K. R. (1960). The efficient soldier. In *Psychoanal. Study Soc.*, 1:39–97. New York: Int. Univ. Press.
ERIKSON, E. H. (1959). *Identity and the Life Cycle.* Psychol. Issues, monogr. 1. New York: Int. Univ. Press.
FORD, C. S. & BEACH, F. A. (1951). *Patterns of Sexual Behavior.* New York: Harper.
FOUCAULT, M. (1982–83). An interview with Michael Foucault. *Salmagundi*, 58–59:10–24.
FRAIBERG, S. (1961). Homosexual conflicts. In *Adolescents,* ed. S. Lorand & H. I. Schneer, pp. 78–112. New York: Paul B. Hoeber.
FREUD, A. (1968). Acting out. *Int. J. Psychoanal.*, 49:165–170.
FREUD, S. (1927). Civilization and its discontents. *S.E.*, 21:3–145.
——— (1937). Analysis terminable and interminable. *S.E.*, 28:211–253.
FRIEDMAN, R. C. & STERN, L. O. (1980). Juvenile aggressivity and sissiness in homosexual and heterosexual males. *J. Acad. Psychoanal.*, 8:427–440.
GREEN, R. (1979). Childhood cross-gender behavior and subsequent sexual preference. *Amer. J. Psychiat.*, 36:106–108.
——— (1985). Gender identity in childhood and later sexual orientation. *Amer. J. Psychiat.*, 142:339–341.
HARTMANN, H. (1939). Psychoanalysis and the concept of health. In *Essays on Ego Psychology*, pp. 1–18. New York: Int. Univ. Press, 1964.
HUMPHREYS, L. (1972). *Out of the Closets.* Englewood Cliffs, N.J.: Prentice-Hall.

Isay, R. A. (1985). On the analytic therapy of homosexual men. *Psychoanal. Study Child,* 40:235–254.

——— (1986). Homosexuality in homosexual and heterosexual men. In *The Psychology of Men,* ed. G. Fogel, F. Lane, & R. Liebert. New York: Basic Books, pp. 277–299.

Jones, E. (1931). The concept of a normal mind. In *Papers on Psycho-Analysis,* pp. 201–216. Baltimore: Williams & Wilkins, 1948.

Kinsey, A. C., Pomeroy, W. B., & Martin, C. E. (1948). *Sexual Behavior in the Human Male.* Philadelphia: Saunders.

Klein, M. (1960). On mental health. *Brit. J. Med. Psychol.,* 33:237–247.

McWhirter, D. P. & Mattison, A. M. (1984). *The Male Couple.* Englewood Cliffs, N.J.: Prentice-Hall.

Offer, D. & Sabshin, M. (1966). *Normality.* New York: Basic Books.

Panel (1977). The Psychoanalytic treatment of male homosexuality. E. C. Payne, reporter, *J. Amer. Psychoanal. Assn.,* 25:183–199.

Saghir, M. T. & Robins, E. (1973). *Male and Female Homosexuality.* Baltimore: Williams & Wilkins.

Socarides, C. W. (1963). The *New York Times,* December 17, p. 33.

Troiden, R. R. (1979). Becoming homosexual. *Psychiatry,* 42:362–373.

Weinberg, M. S. & Williams, C. J. (1974). *Male Homosexuals.* New York: Oxford Univ. Press.

Zuger, B. (1978). Effeminate behavior in boys from childhood. *Comprehen. Psychiat.,* 19:363–369.

——— (1984). Early effeminate behavior in boys. *J. Nerv. Ment. Dis.,* 172:90–96.

Steps in Self Development

RENA HRUSHOVSKI MOSES, Ph.D. and RAFAEL MOSES, M.D.

SYLIA WAS 7 YEARS OLD WHEN I (THE THERAPIST) FIRST MET HER IN Haifa. She had lived in an alien world from the very beginning of her life. At age 3 weeks she had arrived at the children's home— one of hundreds of babies. She stayed there for 4 years. Reports from the home indicate that she had an especially retarded development in all areas. Physically, she was very small and skinny. Mentally, her understanding was quite limited, as was her ability to express herself. Emotionally, she lived in isolation, refusing to play with other children. She would move her body rhythmically, especially before falling asleep. She took every opportunity to carry away whatever happened to come into her hands. She would hide whatever she could in her pockets. She was afraid of heights: when she was lifted up, she would scream in terror. She was also afraid of people, of buses, of activities. Toward the end of her stay in the children's home, she began to show more interest in her surroundings and started to talk more fluently.

Her mother was said to have suffered from epilepsy and a paralyzed leg. Two operations were said to have stopped her fits, but the paralysis remained. She walked with a limp. The social worker at that time described her as a rigid character, given to emotional outbursts and strange behavior. She had shown no interest in Sylia since her birth. On the rare occasions when she went to visit Sylia in the home, she seemed more interested in

Training and supervising analysts, Israel Psychoanalytic Institute.

This paper is based on a Ph.D. dissertation at the Wright Institute under the supervision of Drs. Nevitt Sanford and Mervin Freedman.

491

herself than in her daughter: thus, on one occasion, she had brought a lollipop for Sylia but ate it herself.

The father had worked as an unskilled laborer in the fruit and vegetable market. Occasionally, he would get drunk. The social worker described him as aggressive and cruel. He, too, showed no interest in his daughter.

When Sylia was 4 years old, she was given to a foster family, with whom she stayed for another 4 years. After her first year, she was referred through the social worker to the child guidance clinic because of aggressiveness, truancy, sleep disturbances, and bed wetting. Concurrently, Sylia did not participate in the activities of her kindergarten. She masturbated excessively and had no contact with the teacher or the children.

The clinic examination showed Sylia to be suffering from a primary personality disorder. Psychotherapy was recommended. She had to wait for a year to begin treatment with me. The hope that her continuing in kindergarten during that year would improve her condition proved futile. I saw her first for 3 years from 7 to 10 years of age, usually twice a week. I then stopped working for a year, after which I resumed treatment with Sylia for 3 more years. Treatment was terminated when she was 15 years old.

Sylia maintained contact with me by writing about every 2 months. From the age of 14, Sylia rented a room from a cleaning woman at the children's home. Sylia worked at different jobs, e.g., in a laundry or caring for old people. Thus she partially earned her living. She was given some money for rent from the Welfare Ministry. At age 18, Sylia married. She had met her husband, a fitter, at a club. It was a love match. Sylia is now 30 years old; she has 2 children.

Beginning with the treatment and going on to the last interview with her held when she was 26, we would divide her development into several phases. This division is based on the treatment of which detailed notes were kept. Detailed notes were also made about all subsequent contacts, as well as information gleaned from many sources with whom Sylia had been in contact throughout her life.

PHASE 1: 7 TO 9 YEARS

Failure of the facilitating environment resulted in developmental deficits in her personality. In treatment, Sylia was extremely flighty and restless. When she saw clay, she would cut it into pieces; she mixed all the paints together messily and endlessly. Her capacity for postponement of impulse gratification was minimal. When the time of the therapy hour was due to end, Sylia would repetitively wash her hands, even though I repeatedly told her that time was up. When the daughter of the foster family came to pick her up, Sylia reacted to being hurried by saying that the foster sister was not the teacher here. She came close to me and whispered into my ear: "Maybe some day I'll give you a kiss."

In the first period of treatment, much in her behavior could not be understood. Most of the time she was on the go. I would follow her, carrying things she overloaded herself with, opening doors for her or otherwise being helpful. I allowed myself to be used as a "need-satisfying object" for her. As Winnicott (1958) says, "What matters to the patient is not the accuracy of the interpretation so much as the willingness of the analyst to help, the analyst's capacity to identify with the patient and so to believe in what is needed and to meet the need as soon as the need is indicated verbally or in non-verbal or pre-verbal language" (p. 122). Anna Freud (1965) explained when this was appropriate: "Where the libido defect is due to severe early deprivation in object relations, interpretation of the transferred repetition has no therapeutic results. Instead, the child may answer to the intimacy of the analyst-patient relationship. . . . [On] the basis of this new and different emotional experience, the child may move forward to a more appropriate level of libido development" (p. 231).

As our therapeutic meetings continued, a long period ensued when Sylia consistently sought oral gratifications, either directly for herself or through feeding the dolls. It turned out that this 7-year-old girl was smoking cigarettes which she stole. To help her sublimate these needs, I introduced chocolate cigarettes and provided a nursing bottle. Now Sylia would begin the hour by feeding the doll with the nursing bottle. Soon, however, she would switch the bottle to her own mouth. While drinking, she had an inward gaze, as though she were repeating experiences from long ago. Yet it also seemed as though she were now living new experiences which she had missed at that time.

She poured tea into the nursing bottle, drinking first with the nipple, later without it, smiling all the while. We would both have some cookies which I brought. I had to hold these for her, so she could take bites from them from my hand—when she was not too busy painting or doing something else. It seemed that in this way direct narcissistic gratifications gradually built up early self feelings.

The contact with me at this time was mainly through ordering me around. Sylia was happy to be the ruler and master. "Lisa [the therapist] obeys me," she told her foster mother, as she enjoyed the feeling of being an omnipotent queen. It was hard for her to leave at the end of the hour. Often, I had to take her firmly by the hand and accompany her part of the way home. But there were times when even this was not effective. "I didn't come here just to go home again," she would shout furiously. Then, before I could anticipate what she would do, she began pulling toys from the shelves and littering the floor. For me, these fits of narcissistic rage were hard to tolerate and to control. Sometimes she left, cursing in her native tongue (Persian). She would take toys with her for the return of which I pleaded in vain. Sylia's demands and her greed kept growing: she wanted more time, more toys, more food, more sweets. Melanie Klein (1932) said of this behavior that the small girl "needs these 'good' things to protect her against the 'bad' ones, and to establish a kind of equilibrium inside her" (p. 284).

Sylia thus transmitted the omnipotent feeling of a baby whose mother was always available to her. She needed me for building up her self-esteem, for containing her immense aggression and just managing not to break down under it, but also for mirroring her manifold needs.

Sylia's fear of being alone with me was remarkable. During the first months of therapy she avoided being alone with me by opening the door to the playroom, by being constantly on the go, by doing, running, busying herself without evident rhyme or reason. She would come to me as to the owner of a playroom and not to a person with whom she sought to establish a relationship. Her difficulty in remembering my name was striking. Sylia often came on days when she had no appointment to ask if her appointment was that day. When she found out that it was only 3 days later, she said to her foster mother, "Right that I am going for treatment after I go to sleep and get up, go to sleep and get up, go to sleep and get up?" A few months later, she came to one session, saying cheerfully that she already knew that my name was Lisa.

One day Sylia was wearing a new red coat. It was the first time that she had a new item of clothing. I said how pretty she looked and asked who had given her the coat. Disconcerted, she said her foster mother. Confused, she added that she had two mothers. I could see how bewildered she was about her family relationships. In many ways, I tried to grapple with her identity problems to help her build a more cohesive sense of self and mute or diminish her states of fragmentation. I explained that the mother who had given birth to her had not been able to take care of her because she had been ill. I added that she had been at a babies' home for 4 years. There, her foster mother had chosen her as a foster daughter. I was not at all sure that Sylia understood what I had been saying. I was not even sure that she had been listening. Sylia went on playing in our room, without further comment or question.

Sylia's identity problems were not surprising, given the very real external confusion about who she was. When talking to her social worker and her teacher, I discovered that Sylia was actually known by three different family names: her mother's maiden name, her foster family's name, and her biological father's name. Since the father's surname appeared on Sylia's birth certificate, I suggested that it be used consistently by all concerned.

In order to further increase Sylia's sense of identity, I encouraged the foster mother to celebrate Sylia's birthday for the first time in Sylia's life. To my disappointment and astonishment, Sylia's eighth birthday was not perceived by her as joyful. It was difficult for her to accept presents from those she often felt hostile to—I could not tell if it was due to greed or shame or ambivalent feelings. Sylia showed severe anxiety and guilt.

Once, after being intensely angry at an intrusion by an outside boy, she left the session to go into the courtyard to collect dry plants and stones. Suddenly, pointing at a rock, she fearfully asked if "she" would pursue her. In response to my question, Sylia said, "The grandmother there." I interpreted her inner fear that there was a bad grandmother outside, waiting to punish her. Clearly afraid, she took my hand and pulled me back into the treatment room—something she did very rarely indeed. Attempts on my part to ask more about her fears and fantasies were met by stonewalling, or by orders that I perform different services for her.

Now came a period of repeated questions, all pregnant with many meanings. "How are people run over? How are people treated who have had an accident? Is a foot put in a plaster cast after an accident? Does God see everything and punish those who are bad? Do people who slander others go to hell? That's what children told me." Part of her interest was related to a home for handicapped children situated close to the child guidance clinic where I saw her. I explained to Sylia that children often feared that their anger could cause terrible results. She might well have had such fears of being punished, especially after showing her angry feelings toward me; and even more so, since her foster mother had fallen and broken her leg after an argument with Sylia. Guilt feelings from different sources seemed thus to be involved and intermixed. Later in the same hour Sylia asked in a faltering voice, "How did it happen that my mother became sick?" This was the first time that she had approached the subject of her biological mother's illness directly. In the following hours, she expressed some fragments of fears about her biological mother's illness, and her conflicting feelings related to that illness. "She is limping, she is sick, poor woman. That's why I was thrown out," she exclaimed. "She is wonderful. When she gets well, she'll come and visit me."

One of the terrifying thoughts which Sylia brought up frequently was that it had been Sylia's fault that the mother had become sick. Sylia had apparently been told that her mother became sick and had an operation after Sylia's birth; and that this was what had brought about a paralysis. I told her as authoritatively as I could that she had had no part in her mother's illness; but Sylia would not accept this. Sylia seemed to be talking with inner voices which shut out my words. She asked seemingly nonsensical questions: "Why do birds peck? Why do lizards bite?" In such hours, she would pour much water on the table, then brush it with soap. She enjoyed the foam dropping on the floor and repeated this action over and over. Once, after Sylia had suggested that I be her baby, she fed me and herself with instant pudding. As we ate, she seemed to be telling me a fairy tale: "My mother was a mother who gave no food to her children." As if having realized that she had violated an inner norm, requiring her to say only good things of her mother, she added, "If I meet her in the street, I'll give her a kiss."

At about this time, Sylia's foster parents announced that they could no longer take care of her. In the treatment, Sylia became more aggressive for some weeks, expressing her bitter disappointment in games of shooting. Finally, another family was found, and Sylia seemed pleased with them. There was some improvement both in her behavior and in her studies. Gradually, she seemed to be building up tension-regulating structures. She was able to accept the need for order and for silence and discipline. Now, at age 8, she began for the first time to learn to read. Indirectly, she expressed some of her feelings about the move from one family to another. Coming late to an hour once, she had run all the way. To my comment that she was afraid I might leave her as had her mother and foster mother, she replied, "Right. A mother can leave, but not you." After a pause, as though fumbling for an explanation, she added, "You are an aunt." Some time later, as if out of the blue, Sylia asked me whether I beat my children. "Sometimes, my [current] mother beats me," she added quickly. "Her husband tells her not to, but she does it anyway. He likes me better than she does." "Why does she beat you?" I asked. "I was making trouble," she said sternly, "beatings aren't given for nothing, you know!" She had switched sides again, as she did so often: now she was identifying with the parent's educational function; or was it with the aggressor?

At the end of this phase, when Sylia was close to 10 years old, I took a year off from work after my daughter was born. We tried to work through some of Sylia's feelings of rage and envy, as well as her wishing to be my baby. During that year Sylia was seen by an experienced social worker.

PHASE 2: 10 TO 12 YEARS

When I returned, Sylia was transferred to a boarding school. The recent foster family had not been willing to keep Sylia for several reasons. One such reason related to a sexual seduction by a man in their neighborhood to which she responded, however guiltily.

A new stage in her therapy began at this time. The little trust which Sylia had established, along with other progress, seemed to have been lost as a result of the recent moves: new families, new therapists, new teachers. Disappointments and rejections, real as well as fantasied, increased her need for care and warmth. In her therapy sessions, she wanted to be fed and always requested more food: always more than she was given at first. I fed her, accompanying her feeding with different words, with which I intended to convey what I knew and understood of both her experiences and the wishes aroused in her in the babies' home in which she had grown up earlier. Three years later, Sylia wanted to feed her sister's baby. She mashed a banana and put the spoon into the baby's mouth. She remembered how I had once done the same for her, and said, "At first, I was scared of you, of your face. I didn't know what you want from me, and feared you would harm me. Then one day you took me on your lap and fed me the banana and apple sauce. Then I understood—do you remember?—that you wouldn't harm me, that you meant well. I wasn't afraid anymore and stopped running away. I shall always remember it, even when I am 18 years old."

"Yes, I remember," I told her, "I remember very well."

"I was terribly glad you came to visit me," she said.

"Where did I visit you?" I asked, astonished.

"In the baby home," she said, as though my nurturing her when she was 11 years old had been her first nursing experience; or as if I had, in her mind, become the nurse who took care of her as a baby.

This was a regressive period in Sylia's therapy. Longings for warmth never fulfilled before together with different sexual wishes—reinforced perhaps by the many external changes— seemed to come together in Sylia's cravings to be nurtured by me. While previously regressive trends had been more iso-lated—baby talk, crawling, drinking from the nursing bottle— regression was now experienced more wholeheartedly, as if at last she was being provided with experiences missed in early infancy.

"Mash the bananas," said Sylia, when she saw me coming in, loaded with the fruit she had asked for. Turning her sorrowful gaze on me, she pleaded, "Take me on your lap. Feed me, please!" For a moment I hesitated. Should I take this big girl on my lap like a baby, gratifying her infantile impulses? Or would it perhaps be wiser to interpret her wishes instead? On second thought I consented, realizing that such strong urges were better satisfied in the therapy hours than acted out to her detriment outside.

"Mash the bananas, cut the pear into small pieces, chop up the plums, peel the apples; the peel looks like green excrement; and make some applesauce." I needed to overcome feelings of dis-comfort in putting Sylia on my knees. Once she opened her mouth widely, however, eagerly pointing at the dishes she want-ed to be fed with, I totally forgot her chronological age, and just treated her as she wanted to be treated. Often she would say, "It's so tasty. Always bring me this kind of food." Sylia never forgot to dictate the list of fruits for the next session at the end of an hour. Though she knew that the budget for this was limited, she would become furious if an item was missing. She would throw down the plate like an angry baby whose food had become distasteful. After a while she would look at me, seeking for-giveness. When I pointed out that her anger was that of a baby whose wishes were not fulfilled, she was relieved.

This way of feeding her went on for several weeks. I felt that the experience would be a fuller one if the feeding could be accompanied by words which expressed feelings which she had had when an infant, and which she was now reexperiencing. While she leaned passively against me, eyes closed, enjoying being fed, I talked about how she had been a baby in the huge baby home; how a nurse she had liked had given her a milk bottle, how she had wanted to be held close, to be fed and cud-dled more; and how she had always felt that she had never gotten enough because she was one of hundreds of babies. "Tell me more," she said, hanging on my lips as if wanting to swallow and digest not only my food but also my words—which seemed to echo experiences from those early years. What I did, after some hesitation, was expressed by Ekstein (1966) as he talked about symbolic action: "Symbolic action . . . derives its primary effectiveness not from content but from the soothing tone of a therapist's voice, the repetitive rhythm, the continuity of words, the predictability of voice, words, and rhythm. These can readily be understood as interpretation via a symbolic act modeled after the mother's lullaby to the very young child" (p. 155). Thus "primitive transferences are evoked or maintained, which can serve as the foundation for new and more mature identifica-tions. . . . It is by the continual repetition of such experiences that the secondary process can emerge and extend its domi-nance" (p. 121). It must be clear that the therapeutic activity described facilitated the process of the gradually emerging, gradually more cohesive self, along with a decreased sense of omnipotence, and an increased self-esteem. Equally, we can see how gradually there is a shift toward a more healthily integrated self.

Phase 3: 12 to 14 Years

Sylia wanted a chest of drawers of her own. Failing that, she insisted on having a key to one drawer in the playroom. Since a lock was not possible under the circumstances, her response was to take a corner of the playroom and, during one hour, to build a house of her own. She insisted that nobody invade it. Having begun to implement her plan, she was full of ideas of how to furnish her tiny "house." At the entrance, she placed a toy piano which served as a doorbell. Once she had moved in a few of her favorite toys, there was room only for Sylia herself in the small space left over. She delegated to me the task of finding places for the various objects removed from the corner which her house now "occupied." There was a light in the corner, and Sylia an-nounced the beginning of each hour by turning the light on.

Soon the house became a stage for Sylia. She began to produce scenes from different periods of her life. These reflected memories, fantasies, and choked-off feelings which had never been expressed before. Sylia took the role of her maternal grandmother who had everything she needed: a small, cozy place, food, light, sweets. She wanted me to join in blaming the "lazy mother" who took care neither of her husband nor of the baby, "the poor thing." The drunken father, interested only in his alcoholic beverages, would toss the baby into the air, neglecting both the child and the grandmother. "The baby was dumped in the street," she said. Then, speaking to the child, she said, "Poor thing, I don't have any money to give you. Soon I'll be dead—and then, what will you do?!" Turning back to her husband (me), her voice boomed: "You really are crazy! Go and look after your wife, so she won't have to go begging from other people in the streets." Lowering her voice, she spoke to the baby again, softly, "Poor baby, now you've spilled hot milk on yourself. Do you have a heart in your chest there? Can you feel the pain?" Sylia continued to berate the husband—qua grandmother—then would soothe the baby and argue with the mother.

Her loud voice was heard all over the clinic. Staff members would come to listen outside the door, then leave. Sylia heard or noticed nothing, she was totally absorbed in her play. Finally, I had to interrupt Sylia to announce the end of the session. She looked at me, unbelieving. "Time eats itself up," she said, "or are you lying to me?" Twice a week, for several months, Sylia vividly brought up feelings and fantasies from her past. Her passionate expressiveness, richer than ever before in vocabulary and idiom, seemed to flow straight from the unconscious.

So much was going on that I hardly had time to intervene or interpret. The role assigned to me was to sit on the "revolving" stage, absorb the unique atmosphere, and enact the various roles. Each hour felt like a volcanic eruption. At the end of the session there would be a few more flames leaping up here and there, remnants of hot lava—and gradually everything would subside. Out of Sylia's burning fire from within—carefully concealed by Sylia as she displaced her aggressiveness onto others—grew a common experience for both of us: we could look at it and work on it. Throughout all this, Sylia was turning what had been passively experienced into active mastery. From victim she turned into stage producer and actor. In these episodes, she documented that despite repeated bouts of deprivation and loss, her drives had been banked but not quenched and could be revitalized.

For her twelfth birthday party, I went to the institution at which she lived. Two of us from the clinic were the only guests who appeared, although all her relatives had been invited. Sylia was physically well-developed and looked beautiful no matter how shabby her dress seemed. She danced gracefully and sang in harmony with the others. When Sylia invited me into her room, I was surprised—though I had known she was clean and orderly—how neatly everything was arranged in her drawers. She took out a small bundle of letters and postcards fastened with a clip. These were the letter and cards she had received in her lifetime; she treated them with loving care. They were her private treasure. "Once I waited eagerly to get sweets," she said "now I live to get letters!"

All the girls went out of the institution for the Passover holidays. Sylia asked me to try and persuade her biological mother to have her for the first evening. The answer came immediately in the form of a well-known proverb: "Who will be for me, if I cannot be for myself? Since you must know, I'll tell you: We're going to Tel Aviv from Haifa—and we don't need anybody tailing us!" When we were left alone, Sylia took hold of my hand, and cried quietly, talking about her mother's being mean, being sick in her heart and in her mind. She recovered from the blow after being helped to express her feelings.

Sylia asked many questions about her parents, their divorce, the father's drinking and gambling, the mother's illness—was it cancer? Cancer and crabs—synonymous in Hebrew—were confused in her mind. She wondered about her brother and half-sister. How could her brother be a municipal inspector and gamble on card games at the same time? Soon she asked me to bring milk, pudding, and other foodstuffs for our next hour. As if sensing my reluctance to return to a further period of cooking and eating, she said, "Only this time!" She came to the hour in a good mood, and explained, "It's not that I want to go back to my childhood. I want to cook so I can show that I can be a mother!

Not like that mother of mine! There are good mothers who cook and make cakes, who have patience with their children. That's the kind of mother I want to become! I'll be a patient mother, but I won't spoil my children so they will then boss me around."

PHASE 4: 14 TO 15 YEARS

Sylia brought a storybook about a paralyzed boy which became very central for her. She felt his vulnerability when he was being pitied. It triggered yearnings for a caring uncle like the boy had. She relived her hopes that her mother might be operated on and be well again. To the next session, she brought a story, which she read to me:

> A Composition for Lisa
> by Sylia
>
> How would I wish my life to be?
>
> I wish my mother would become healthy, would love me and not disappoint me each time I see her. One reason that I want to leave the institution is that I want to get far far away from my mother. I don't like her! Because she is sick, she takes out all her anger on me. I am very disappointed. That's why I want to study far away from her; when I am near her I can't concentrate. I think about her, I try to understand—but I can't understand her. Nor can I cure her. She is not like the boy in the story who gets healthy in the end. It is true that my mother is paralyzed— but it's with her mind that something is wrong. This is the end of my composition. It's a very sad composition; it moves the heart only of those who know me.
>
> From Sylia—who is a coward about her mother.

Soon she was able to say about the boy in the storybook, "Yes, I am like him. I have a kind of paralysis inside. It's my mother. I keep thinking of her, though I want terribly to separate myself from her." Sylia again talked about leaving the institution, the city, her mother. I interpreted her wish to distance herself from her mother, adding, "But it's difficult to go away. It is as if your mother is inside you. When you were angry at her, you said that you wanted to eat her up, to swallow her. Little children really think they can do that. They think taking in food is like taking in their mother." "I wouldn't even want to taste her," Sylia reacted with disgust. Yet her facial expression showed the idea did not seem that distant, though it might sound far-fetched to some. I continued, "It may be a comforting feeling to have your mother inside you, all the same." I remembered her fear of becoming an orphan, which had come up immediately after her cannibalistic fantasy. Even as I spoke, I could see Sylia's face changing. All of a sudden she was in agony—as if choking. She gasped, "She doesn't want to get out," she pointed at her throat, "she's strangling me." Her voice sank to a bare whisper, "She's strangling me from within—like a cancer." We were now able to connect this powerful fantasy which had been buried alive in her to the signs she had given of her fear of, but also her interest in, cancer during recent months. Verbalizing this fantasy—the cancer strangling her from within—and beginning to understand it seemed to help Sylia to eject, as it were, the primitively incorporated object. Thus she became more independent of her mother, and freer to identify with me.

Sylia now began to act the role of the psychologist with other girls in the institution. With them and occasionally in role play with me, she would be the psychologist and I a girl.

Sylia: Why do you curse so much?

I: Because. . . .

Sylia: There must be some reason. Did somebody hurt your feelings?

I: I do it without thinking, it just happens.

Sylia: It's automatic? Yes, it goes off like a Katyusha [Russian rocket]. I was just like that. But it irritates others, it makes a bad impression. The girls pay you back. . . . You ought to think before you act.

I: I can't help it.

Sylia: You should rely more on your self. If you really want to, you can be a good girl.

Gradually Sylia stopped playing the psychologist. She became more active in actually helping one of the counselors in her work with the younger girls. Her vocational choice at this time was to become a counselor. There were signs of a general shift in Sylia's attitudes toward the girls. Whereas previously she had been centered mainly on herself, viewing the reality from her personal point of view, she now became more perceptive of external reality and more open. There was more sharing and friendliness. It was a sign of the increased differentiation between Sylia's self and her object that her empathy now increased. She wanted to take care of her sister's new baby, and enjoyed doing so. Yet she was still very much tied to wanting to avoid the mistakes her mother had made. "I'll never put my children in an institution, even if I have hundreds of them," she said. This brought her back to her mother. Finally, she said, "I want to become a detective!" "What is the first mystery you will solve?" I asked. "To find out why I did not have a loving mother," she replied.

It was decided to find a place where Sylia could work close to a mature adult. She would rent a room in the apartment of a cleaning woman of the institution. Sylia was quite attached to her. Sylia was pleased about the decision and felt like a graduate student who was leaving home to live on her own, finishing school and setting out to work. This seemed a good time to inform Sylia of my plan to go abroad for a year or two in 3 months' time. Sylia expressed some anger. The fear of being abandoned which had been triggered by similar occasions in the past seemed less apparent now.

Sylia had changed dramatically in many respects. It was 7 years since I had begun working with her, and she was now able to cope with frustrations, and had learned to satisfy her inner needs in socially constructive and even creative ways. She no longer was full of fears. She clearly showed improved mastery of her anxiety. Her progressive capabilities far outweighed her regressive patterns. I went to visit her in her new home, and she said, "I know now that I will never be like my mother!" The separation was gradual and manageable.

SUBSEQUENT CONTACTS

Two months later, Sylia wrote me as follows:

> Dear Lisa,
> I got your letter and was glad to read what you wrote. How are you? How do you feel? I am very well. How is life in America? I have a story that is similar to what happened between the two of us. It's called "I was saved by a Miracle."

The Story

In a certain family, there was a mute and mentally retarded boy. He had a psychologist whose name was Lisa. She wanted very much to help that poor boy whose name was Benny. She took him to all kinds of parks and showed him all kinds of nice things. She was giving him treatment twice a week for a year. Slowly, slowly the boy got better. One day, all of a sudden, when the boy woke up, he could hear and talk. He called out loudly, "Mother, mother, I can talk, I want to talk." His mother wondered who was talking to her. Then she saw that it was her boy. She hugged him and kissed him, saying, "You are saved. It's a miracle, my son." "I am saved by a miracle," shouted the boy excitedly, "where is my Lisa?" Suddenly somebody knocked at the door. Lisa came in. She was very surprised about the boy. The father came and wanted to give Lisa a lot of money, because she had saved Benny. But Lisa said, "Keep the money for the boy when he grows up." The boy said, "Lisa, take the money, it's yours." So she took it. Lisa wanted to go to America. Then the boy started to cry and said, "You want to leave me. I am attached to you. Why do you want to go? Why?" He gave her a present and Lisa flew far away in a plane. After a year she returned to the house of the child. She knocked at the door. "Yes, come in!" she heard a voice saying. "Does Mrs. Rubin live here? Where is the boy Benny?" she asked. "I am Benny," said the boy, "Who are you?" "I am Lisa who went to America," she said. Then they started to meet again, they are still meeting now. I too want you to come back to me the way you came back to Benny. Write me a long letter.

Sylia

I was away for 2 years. The news that reached me directly and indirectly indicated that Sylia worked steadily in a hospital laundry, continued to live with Sarah, and adjusted well. Just before I returned, Sylia wrote to tell me that after knowing a Moroccan boy, 23 years old, for 2 months, she became engaged. He was working as a carpenter and "owned an apartment." When I returned, Sylia called me fairly soon and came for an unexpected visit with her fiancé to my home! She came to see me several times at my consulting room, declaring that she didn't want to come to a child guidance clinic any more. Concurrently, Sarah was seen by the director of the clinic. There was tension between Sylia and Sarah about Sylia's smoking, her staying overnight with her fiancé, and a more direct invasion of her privacy by Sarah's children. It was the violations of Sylia's privacy inherent in all three areas which were most aggravating to her. After three meetings, tensions subsided and we could withdraw once more from each other. The treatment now seemed ended in a more formal way.

Three years later I met a social worker who worked in the area where Sylia lived. She had known Sylia previously and knew of her treatment with me. Sylia was now 22 years old, married, and the mother of a 1-year-old son. I visited the family and found her to function well as a mother. Much of her conversation centered on her biological father, who had died just before the birth of Sylia's son—named after him. I could sense from how she spoke that a much better relationship had been established between Sylia and her father. It was important to her to restore the positive aspect of his image in her eyes. She was warm to the boy, taking care of him calmly, while at the same time talking with me, also in a relaxed way. She could tell him to wait while she was busy with me, yet did not do this in a rejecting or angry way. The house was clean and orderly; neighbors dropped in. She showed a sense of humor and an ability to distance herself from her shortcomings as a child in talking with me about him and herself. Sylia told me openly and frankly about events of the interim period, with insight into some of her feeling responses and an ability to communicate very meaningfully with me. "It was my fate in life which made me more understanding," she said.

I saw Sylia three more times. First, I visited her in the hospital after the birth of her daughter, and later at home. I was again impressed with how much she seemed at peace with herself, and with her happiness as a wife and mother. I felt that I was talking to a mature woman. My last visit was when Sylia was 26 years old. In a meeting with both Sylia's husband and her brother, I was most impressed with Sylia's ability to handle an emotionally complex situation. She correctly pointed out to her brother that he was patronizing her husband; and nondefensively pointed out that the husband needed time to get to be where the brother already was. She seemed to be in touch with her feelings, to be a separate person from those around her. She allowed her husband a separateness even in areas where she disagreed, e.g., playing cards. Much of her work involved helping people or taking care of them; she also earned good money in the process. Thus they were used by the municipality as a foster family. Her need to take care of others seemed concurrently to fulfill a need to achieve respectability and status; and also to be gratified by the "good" things she gave to those for whom she now cared—in contrast to how she had been treated as a child. These tendencies interfered with her ability to be flexible vis-à-vis those whom she took care of, which included not only her children but also her husband. Thus, the need for reparation seemed at times to interfere with her ability to be warm and giving; and to make her more rigid than she was most of the time. It is probable that such trends came to the fore when Sylia regressed in response to a variety of stresses.

DISCUSSION

What psychological disorder did Sylia suffer from? Clearly, it was more than a neurotic disturbance. Yet it seemed less than a psychotic disorder, though she did once during a treatment hour appear to hallucinate her grandmother. Perhaps Winnicott (1965) would have termed her a schizophrenic, when he said: "the individual's maturational processes (including all that is inherited) require a facilitating environment, especially in the very early stages. Failure of the facilitating environment results in developmental faults in the individual's personality development and in the establishment of the individual's self, and the result is called schizophrenia" (p. 135).

When treatment was offered to Sylia, she was diagnosed as a "primary behavior disorder" at age 6: "The impression is of a girl who is functioning on a somewhat lower level than her age. She finds it difficult to understand her relationship with people around her. There is a disturbance in her thought processes, and in her concept of time. She is perplexed by the reality which she begins to reveal. There are first signs that she is turning her considerable aggressiveness inwards and thus has an inclination to depression." The diagnostic category of primary behavior disorder is more or less equivalent to that of a severe character disorder in an adult.

When Sylia was first seen, she was suffering from gross cognitive and motor disturbances, archaic fears, and flooding by instinctual stimuli. In the area of object relations, Sylia had no attachments to other children at all; with adults, she adapted quickly to new foster families, but did not seem to develop a firm affective relationship. She did, however, show separation reactions when rejected by a foster family. Although Sylia yearned deeply for her mother and her father, she could not be said to have maintained a constant, stable, and emotional relationship with her mother or with other relatives. In all these areas, Sylia's development was faulty. There was no object constancy apparent.

In response to Sylia's needs, I found myself behaving in ways which fit in with Balint's description (1968) of patients with a basic fault: "Apart from being a 'need-recognizing', and perhaps a need-satisfying object, the analyst must also be a 'need-understanding' object" (p. 181). What are the needs, why are they as they are, what makes them fluctuate? The decision to respond to Sylia's regressive needs in the very special feeding situation was taken on the basis of therapeutic considerations. In fact, the therapist had to overcome an inner reluctance to go along with Sylia's demands. She also had to stop to consider whether the encouragement of such regressive behavior might not lead Sylia to deeper regression. The consistently empathic and accepting understanding of Sylia's needs and of her archaic states, as it turned out, came to be experienced by Sylia as a facilitating medium: the developmental processes of the ego and the self seemed to be reinstated. Slowly, a gradual self-demarcation from those around her took place. In many ways, Sylia treated her therapist as an auxiliary ego (or a self-object? Bene, 1977). When she staged parts of her past on a make-believe stage in the playroom, Sylia instructed her therapist to play different roles and to act them out in specific ways. The therapist felt she was acting at Sylia's behest. Sylia related that at times, as she spoke with others, she would hear the therapist's voice speak from within her. Later, when she was playing the psychologist, she had already established more of a border between her and her therapist, and had internalized some of the latter's qualities in a fuller and more consistent way. We understand these processes as a combination of imitation and identification, with the former changing gradually into the latter.

In looking at the development of Sylia over the period reported on, several questions arise. What allowed her to improve so dramatically? Was there a basic readiness at the beginning to respond to treatment? Did Sylia have hidden strengths which emerged during the treatment? If so, could we in retrospect identify some of them? Or were there special ingredients in the therapeutic relationship which allowed her to so respond? How was it that a relationship of twice 50 minutes a week came to be more decisive for Sylia than all her other frustrating love objects?

We believe that Sylia was one of those patients who have a surprising ability to make use of what is offered in therapy. She had a very strong need to express her inner frustrations, tensions, and vulnerabilities, her hurts and angers, her fantasies—a need which came to the surface once a meaningful, permissive, yet holding relationship had been established. Such a need must also be considered as a strength. Sylia seemed to us to have had a particular ability to be authentic. What she said was very close to what she felt. Thus, her feelings could indeed be expressed fairly directly and fully. Her wish to dominate was probably related not only to the narcissistic need to be "a queen" or to have an audience. We believe it was also a reparative act vis-à-vis those past experiences in which she was bossed around, humiliated, and not taken into account. Such reparation, then, came to have a special meaning to her. Furthermore, we can assume that in a girl with such a readiness to express her innermost feelings, hurts, and fantasies, and to act out a reparative scenario coming from within, the relationship in which this was to occur, the therapeutic relationship, would also assume an additional importance. It is also possible that Sylia was ready to begin therapy as she came to the child guidance clinic, whereas at other times of her life—earlier or later—she might have been less ready to utilize what was offered to her. But such a "readiness for therapy," while it may be assumed, is still speculative.

What was the damage to Sylia as she came for treatment? Sylia had not established a single important relationship in which she could communicate—not in her foster families, not in kindergarten or in the first years of school, and not with any members of her biological family. There was a distinct resistance to opening up verbal communication with others. This was clearly communicated by her older sister who was very anxious to establish such communication. In her first contacts with the therapist, Sylia related to the toys and ignored the therapist at first. She was overactive, played a great deal—all apparently in order to avoid talking to the therapist. She seemed afraid to come closer, afraid to trust her. We understand this to mean that some readiness to establish an affective relationship did exist in Sylia, perhaps encapsulated, to be freed by the special conditions of the psychotherapeutic relationship. Gradually, her feelings of guilt and anger could be expressed and enacted in the ways described. Even after Sylia had been in treatment for almost 2 years, when the foster family felt they could tolerate her no longer, Sylia's teachers and her social worker who tried to find a new foster family in fact gave up on her. They thought that twice-a-week therapy was not enough for this highly disturbed child. Psychiatric hospitalization was seriously considered. Finally a case conference led to the decision that the emotional importance of the therapy seemed to warrant continuation.

The guilt over causing her mother's illnesses was a major topic for her. Sylia's remarkably strong tendency to hold on to her mother's image in some way, and not give up on her, was perhaps connected to her guilt feelings. But there must also be some innate strength in this. For Sylia, it was an achievement—related to individuation and separation—when she could give up searching for her mother and hoping to obtain from her what she had been deprived of as a young child.

Another way of formulating this would be to say that her early distrust in therapy was a sign of ego strength (Solnit, 1986). For Sylia, the enactment of her conflicts in the dramatic ways described, served for her to channel her archaic fears and fantasies, as did some of the stories she read, relived, and invented. Her vitality and humor may also have played a role.

A further factor in helping her develop as well as she did, we think, was the quite extensive period of psychotherapy—and even more the period of contact with her psychotherapist. It spanned a number of developmental epochs. During this time, her therapist was available for her as a helper, as support, as a holding environment, as an auxiliary ego, as a trial love object, as someone to identify with. In the different developmental periods, she could bring to her therapy different problems related to the developmental themes which were in the foreground; to express them, to obtain support, and to work them through.

Stolorow's paradigm (1983) emphasized the importance of empathy when he said, "Structuralization of the nuclear self is enabled by repeated experiences of being understood by the therapist, and the evolving perception of the therapist as a progressively more differentiated empathically inquiring object." Searles (1965) expressed something similar when he felt that his "own achievement of an integrated view of the patient, towards whom I have previously been responding upon two or more quite distinct and conflictual levels, is a prelude to the patient's own improved integration" (p. 343). Stolorow (1983) further stated, "The repeated empathic interpretations of the patient's experiences of optimal frustration result in a process of fractionalized withdrawal of narcissistic cathexis from the object and a concomitant replacement of these cathexes in the gradual formation of a psychic structure which now exercises the function which heretofore had been performed by the object" (p. 293). This may not be totally different from the cardinal importance of the nursing activities for a schizophrenic patient (Searles, 1965, p. 540).

We believe that the case of Sylia demonstrates dramatically that some children with major developmental damage present us with a remarkable ability to utilize the therapeutic help offered them. What exactly goes into such an ability and how it can be understood and used in the assessment of children who come for treatment seems to us to be a subject worthy of further study.

BIBLIOGRAPHY

BALINT, M. (1968). *The Basic Fault.* London: Tavistock.
BENE, A. (1977). Jack and Jill. Presented to the British and Israeli Psychoanalytic Societies.
EKSTEIN, R. (1965). *Children of Time and Space.* New York: Appleton.
FREUD, A. (1965). *Normality and Pathology in Childhood.* New York: Int. Univ. Press.
KERNBERG, O. F. (1979). *Borderline States and Pathological Narcissism.* New York: Aronson.

KLEIN, M. (1932). *The Psycho-Analysis of Children.* New York: Grove Press, 1960.

KOHUT, H. (1977). *The Restoration of the Self.* New York: Int. Univ. Press.

SANFORD, N. (1976). *The Disorders of the Self and Their Treatment.* New York: Atherton.

SEARLES, H. F. (1965). *Collected Papers on Schizophrenia and Related Subjects.* New York: Int. Univ. Press.

SOLNIT, A. J. (1986). Personal communication.

STOLOROW, R. D. (1983). Self psychology. In *Reflections on Self Psychology,* ed. J. D. Lichtenberg, pp. 287–296. Hillsdale, N. J.: Analytic Press.

WINNICOTT, D. W. (1958). Child analysis in the latency period. In *The Maturational Processes and the Facilitating Environment,* pp. 115–123. New York: Int. Univ. Press, 1965.

_____ (1959–64). Classification. Ibid., pp. 124–139.

Transitory Symptom Formation in the Analysis of an Obsessional Character

RICHARD L. MUNICH, M.D.

> Fear in an individual is provoked either by the great-
> ness of a danger or by the cessation of emotional
> ties . . . ; the latter is the case of neurotic fear or anxiety.
> [FREUD, 1921, p. 97]

ALTHOUGH VARIOUS ASPECTS OF SYMPTOM FORMATION ARE WELL documented in psychoanalytic literature, there is relatively little written about it during the course of analytic treatment. The literature which does address this issue focuses mainly on transitory symptoms during the course of an hour or several hours (Ferenczi, 1912; Isakower, 1938; Pious, 1961; Luborsky, 1967; Luborsky and Auerbach, 1969), the ebb and flow of psychosomatic ailments and conversion symptoms (Dunbar, 1938; Bergler, 1946; Bettelheim and Sylvester, 1949; Glover, 1955; Hendrick, 1958), the occurrence of symptomatic acts and acting out (Glover, 1924), or on the reappearance of old symptoms during the terminal phase (Schilder, 1938; Rosenblatt, 1963; Miller, 1965). Most of these authors relate the onset of symptoms in the course of treatment to the emergence or interpretation of significant unconscious material, but data from actual cases are

Director of the Division for Extended Treatment Services at the New York Hospital–Cornell Medical Center, Westchester Division, and associate professor of clinical psychiatry of Cornell University Medical College. The author wishes to acknowledge the help of Stanley Leavy, M.D., Ann Appelbaum, M.D., and Darius Ornston, M.D., who offered assistance in the preparation of this manuscript.

sparse. Freud (1918) refers to the onset of transitory symptoms three times in his account of the analysis of the Wolf-Man, but the symptoms are neither described nor accounted for dynamically other than a note about their relation to interpretation. Fenichel (1945) reports the development of a compulsion neurosis in the course of the treatment of a latency-age child, but he does not give case material, nor does he explicate its relationship to the treatment.

This essay will document the onset of a compulsion and trace its relationship to the transference in the course of the analysis of an obsessional man. This patient did not seek treatment for any symptom; rather, he was referred for various difficulties which included diffuse anxiety and depression, marital separation, low self-esteem, and work inhibition. An identifiable symptom developed and was resolved under the influence of a regressive transference neurosis. The development of the symptom, a compulsion, served to clarify underlying dynamic features. I will describe the evolution of the symptom in three separate phases: early in the analysis, lasting for a month; in the middle phase for about two years; and two brief and dramatic reappearances during termination. Material associated with separation and loss coincided with a classical pattern of neurotic symptom formation each time the compulsion appeared. I think that this coincidence accounts for the transitory nature of the symptom in an otherwise well-compensated neurotic character structure.

Background Data

Mr. R. entered his 5-year analysis at age 28, separated from his wife of 4 years and in his third year of graduate school. His complaint of being "stuck" in his life meant that he felt unable to terminate his marriage even though his wife had left him to be with another man, nor could he proceed with work on his dissertation in spite of an outstanding academic record and considerable support from advisors.

The patient described his mother as weird, childlike, tense, and overstimulating when he was young. She gave him frequent enemas and chased him while he hid frightened in a closet. He reported that she became helpless and naïvely seductive as he grew older. Mr. R. felt distant from his father, a quiet and fastidious man, who spent his spare time in solitary gardening. The only thing they ever did together was occasional hunting. The parents, who had their children late in life, worked long hours together. The patient remembered being lonely as a child, spending much time in solitary play. He described an intensely charged relationship with his provocative, teasing, and promiscuous sister, 2½ years his junior. He had a homosexual affair with an older neighbor at ages 10 and 11 in which he played the active role in fellatio, but he was otherwise celibate until his senior year in college.

His father had a large bowel resection and colostomy resulting in impotence when Mr. R. was 12. From mid-adolescence and through his adult life, Mr. R. had recurring diarrhea and pruritus ani which often led him to anal manipulation with salves and suppositories.

Mr. R. did extremely well in college and the first part of graduate school. He and his wife had a "satisfactory" sexual relationship for the year preceding their marriage when Mr. R. was 24, but soon after the marriage she became reluctant to have intercourse. Their relationship gradually deteriorated over the next 4 years; and for the 2 years prior to the analysis, the patient's only sexual outlet had been masturbation. The father died during Mr. R.'s brief psychotherapy, about a year prior to the onset of the analysis, but Mr. R. had not mourned for him.

HISTORY OF THE SYMPTOM IN THE ANALYSIS

FIRST APPEARANCE OF THE SYMPTOM

The analysis proceeded without difficulty from the beginning. The patient's principal defenses were elaborate dreams for which he expected commensurate interpretations; and he maintained distance from the analysis and from his own feelings by means of a highly intellectualized and verbose rhetorical style. This style became even more lofty and arid when he began to describe a passionate affair into which he was drawn by an old girlfriend after 6 months of analysis. The sexual behavior was uncharacteristic of his past history, and was an especially stim-

ulating and frightening contrast to the celibacy of the previous 2
years. During the early part of this affair, he developed the
compulsion to return to his apartment shortly after he left for
work in the morning to make sure his gas stove was turned off.
Although he did not seem particularly disturbed by the symptom at this time, he reported that he had never done anything
like it before, adding ironically that he had not expected to get
worse in the analysis.

In the beginning phase, Mr. R. was deferential and compliant,
addressing the analyst in the tone and manner that one might
use with an esteemed professor. His dreams revealed not only a
homoerotic component to his feelings but also a strong element
of mocking competitiveness in which I was portrayed as a ridiculous and banal figure, usually saying and doing rather ludicrous
things. At the same time, material emerged about his father's
absence and Mr. R.'s futile efforts to establish contact with him
during childhood. By the time of the onset of the symptom, Mr.
R. had shifted from politely listening to the analyst's remarks
and continuing with his monologue to uncritical acceptance. In
this phase, interpretation of the symptom as the wish to turn off
both his anger at his girlfriend's sexual demands and fear of his
own sexual responsiveness led to the end of the affair and remis-
sion of the symptom within a month of its onset. Neither the
symptom nor the stove was mentioned again for 2 years.

SECOND APPEARANCE OF THE SYMPTOM

As the work intensified over the next 2 years, analysis of the, by
then, firmly established homosexual transference began in earnest. By this time, the issue of competition with the analyst was
overt, and there were forthright complaints about the analytic
process. His language was more ordinary, less formal, and more
personal. As a second masochistic, but sexually liberating affair
diminished in intensity, Mr. R. appreciated that he was left with
many sexual feelings of transference. He spoke as if his attachment to me were driving him into a sinful, lusting chase after
women. To avoid the chasing made him aware of his passive
longings for me, a situation that was exciting but also shameful
and intolerable to him. Violent and aggressive thoughts and

fantasies appeared as defenses against the vulnerability he now felt and the bisexuality which had, by this time, become explicit. The patient reported that the compulsion to return home to check that the stove was off had begun again. Associations to a dream in which he and his father were chasing escaped rabbits and another in which he was cutting out his lover's rib, which became his own rib, led, by allusion to the story of Adam and Eve, to interpretation of the patient's wish to have his father inside him and even have his child.

Mr. R.'s initial response to this interpretation of sexual yearnings for his father was anger at me and an intensification of the stove compulsion so that he was often returning home several times after getting halfway to work to make sure the stove was turned off. Sometimes, before leaving, he would check it as many as 10 times. Perhaps related to my intervention when the symptom first appeared, in the patient's mind this activity was mostly connected with anger. Not only did he fear that his house would burn down (also a childhood preoccupation), but he also had fantasies of blowing me away with his shotgun for not helping more with controlling the intense feelings and supporting his rapidly deteriorating reaction formations. At the same time, he pleaded with me to stop making him feel the way he did, and complained more seriously this time that the cure was worse than the disease.

As the months progressed, Mr. R. continued to be preoccupied with the symptom. He reported that when he looked, he could see that the stove was turned off; but he was not convinced. He would tell himself it was off, then leave; but when out the door, he began thinking it was still on. He tried to remember similar preoccupations in childhood which might have predisposed him to compulsions, but he could only describe mildly obsessional character traits such as attention to detail, excessive cleanliness, and overpreparation for classes. These efforts at remembering did, however, lead the patient to the first mourning (in 4 years) of his father and an intense yearning for closeness with me, including the fear of and wish for anal penetration by the analyst. He felt as if his anus were constantly on fire. With shame, he spoke of the pleasure he obtained from defecation, the application of creams and salves, and the insertion of anal suppositories. However, the material was not limited to passive homosexual feelings and wishes. A couple of days before he was to deliver a lecture for his boss, for example, Mr. R. reported a dream fragment in which he was in his father's bed viewing the fireplace, and then being asked to leave by his mother who had invited him. The analysis of these competitive strivings and subsequent disappointments led with great anxiety to fears of fragmentation, dismemberment, and castration. At the same time, he feared that by really opening up and giving vent to his feelings, he would either destroy the analyst or drive him away and then be utterly alone.

Following the emergence and interpretation of these themes, complaints about, and material related to, the symptom diminished over the next 14 months. On a couple of occasions, he even made it to work having forgotten to check and felt pleased with himself when he remembered his forgetting. The theme of turning things off appeared to be displaced during this time onto the intense wish to become a hermit and live a life of celibacy. At this point, the compulsion could at least be modified in intensity by sexual abstinence. Analytic material suggested that he had temporarily identified himself with his impotent father (and the analyst who Mr. R. felt was incapable of helping) as a compromise between the sadistic superego and his instinctual pressures for gratification. This compromise was represented in part by the patient's report that although he no longer had to return to his apartment, he could not yet convince himself the stove was off. He referred to his fear of the basement in his childhood home, specifically the pounding of the gas furnace as it lit, memories of solitary play, and fantasies of sexual conquest in front of a wood-burning stove in the back kitchen, and these led to further memories of the fireplace in his parents' bedroom where he and his sister had slept. Violent fantasies reappeared, specifically of his hunting down, catching, dismembering, and castrating a rapist in the park. But finally, he spoke of his attraction to female buttocks and his long-standing and secret wish to make love from behind.

The anal dialogue resumed. He feared being broken into and robbed of his anger by the analyst, calling it his trump card. He revealed his wish to hold onto his feces and mold them, protesting that if he let all the shit out, he would really be empty. He discussed the fastidiousness of his father and his mother's indiscriminate flatulence. He recounted movingly how burdened his father was by his colostomy: the terror of spillage, the hours his father spent in solitary care of it (memories of which were revived in analyzing a dream in which his father was playing solitaire—his favorite card game), and his father's humiliation when gas would escape and stomal accidents would occur in public or with clients. Mr. R. revealed his close identification with his father's shame and humiliation and his own fascination with the stump. The family fear of the colostomy bag's exploding was mirrored in the patient's fear of humiliating himself by covering those close to him with fecal material. He dreamed of defecating in his pants, and the analysis was interpreted as enema. This led to more material associated with anal masturbation; and in conjunction with the pressure to defecate during an hour, his unconscious wish to soil those around him was interpreted.

Following these revelations and interpretations and approximately 2 years after the symptom's second exacerbation, Mr. R. dreamed of the last analytic appointment. In the last segment of his dream, he awakened to find that overnight visitors at his apartment left the place in shambles. At the same time, he asked himself how he could leave the apartment in such a mess. His impulse was to take the whole morning to clean it up. I remarked that the question reminded me of his earlier efforts to make sure the stove was off before he left each morning. Mr. R. quickly responded that the compulsion had essentially stopped. Each morning, he continued, he checked the stove once, really well, and then left easily. Now, when he looked at the knob and it said "off," he not only could keep the picture of that in his mind, but he also knew it was off. Although the connection had not been made in the analysis, it was now clear, as with many compulsive symptoms, that returning home to check the stove was an effort to undo and control the now conscious, aggressive impulse to soil. The symptom's intense, repetitive, and ritualized form also suggested an erotic component to the impulse; that is, it was not just the identification with father that had to be defended against, but the underlying gratifications which such identification signified (i.e., homosexuality, anal stimulation, and the wish to have a baby).

THIRD APPEARANCE OF THE SYMPTOM

In the 7-month termination phase of the analysis, the symptom reappeared on two mornings. Shortly after deciding to terminate, he began to question me angrily about why I had let him decide to go, felt increasing anxiety about how well things were going with his new girlfriend of several months, H., and even accused people, especially me, of manipulating him into accepting the offer of a fellowship and leaving his comfortable niche. He had a return of violent dreams—this time about mutilating women, especially after sleeping in a room next to H.'s on a weekend retreat. On the morning after returning, he checked and double-checked the stove for the first time in months and concluded that termination meant I would no longer be around to help him modulate his passions.

Events and material leading up to and following the second reappearance of the compulsion in the terminal phase were connected more with the maternal aspects of the transference than had been apparent before. In fact, Mr. R.'s first allusions to termination preceded and, to a certain degree, defended against the growing awareness and intensity of the maternal transference, a transference with erotic as well as aggressive components. Somewhat earlier, his love for and gratitude toward me had taken the form of a wish for "a love that does not have to ask" and was reinforced by associations to his mother in a dream in which he was seduced by an older woman. But frightened about his decision to terminate and angry at me for appearing to manipulate him and throw him out, the patient regressed again to anal material. Frequent bouts of diarrhea and pruritus ani were reported. Not only was Mr. R. upset that he was not made clean and perfect by the analysis; but by permitting termination, I was threatening the patient's important and defensive use of withholding. And withholding was vitally important to the patient in controlling his anger as well as maintaining contact—not only with inner feelings and feces, but also with external objects, especially his mother.

Anger toward me now reached great intensity and was accompanied by several dreams in which fire imagery was prominent. In one, a figure representing me lends the patient a lighter which ignites an explosion resulting in the loss of a finger. And in another, his hometown is in flames and he is between his naked mother and sister on a bed, the latter trying to stick a penis in him. In the dream, he becomes furious at his mother for interfering and tells her to return to his father. Associating to this dream led to childhood memories of seeing his mother nude and fantasies of having intercourse with her from behind. At the same time in the hour, he began shaking and felt as if he were about to explode, a feeling localized mainly in his lower abdomen. This conjunction of fire imagery, somatic explosiveness, and the prominence of anal-erotic and sadistic themes in the context of intensely ambivalent feelings in the transference was finally identified as a critical aspect of his compulsion to make sure the stove was off.

In the meantime, the patient had been speaking for the first time in the analysis of two kinds of masturbation and masturbatory fantasies: one pleasurable kind in which he was simply preparing to or actually making love with H.; and a gray and feelingless, mechanized ritual, usually performed while on the toilet. Fantasies associated with the latter had been vague; but in an hour shortly before he was to lead a graduate colloquium, he felt his penis quivering and reported the wish to be held and comforted by me. The next day, he announced feeling tense; probably, he continued, as a result of having to talk about masturbating the night before, with its associated fantasy of discovering that H. was a virgin, and taking delight in causing her pleasure and pain. But his thoughts had shifted to his anus which had been raw and burning for a few days, and then to me, what to say to me at the last session, and, finally, conscious fantasies of mutual anal intercourse. The next morning he felt furious at me, contemplated suicide briefly and, not only triple-checked the stove before leaving, but returned home again to check it one more time. Although it was clear to Mr. R. at this point that the compulsion was closely related to waxing and waning sexual feelings in the transference, his anger at me continued unabated. He felt the analyst, for whom he cared a great deal, was inviting him to do something that would destroy him.

Subsequent hours were filled with more fire imagery and fury at having to terminate the analysis. He wanted to separate and maintain contact simultaneously, much as he had tried to do by keeping his mother with him in the bathroom as a very young child. Following interpretation of this connection, his anger abruptly focused on his mother. He spoke of her apparent need for him, her tears when he came to her with a problem, and her helplessness just below the surface. He felt he had never had a mother. He dreamed of giving some family jewels to either H. or me, even though his mother actively *objected to the gift*. Initially, this gift appeared to be genital: Can I be a man and give to H., or must I submit yet again to father and give "the family jewels" to the analyst?

This interpretation was incomplete, however, and the anger and anxiety about termination continued. He connected his feelings about H. with me by reporting that he was "shrinking from lovemaking with her like I'm shrinking from the last day in here." Even though H. was making no demands of any sort on him, he complained of women's infinite demandingness. There were many hours in which he felt empty, alone and scared, preoccupied with breasts, breast imagery, and his own monstrous neediness. Then, in a series of dramatic hours, he moved from the demands of women in general, to his mother's demands, and finally her demands (by frequent enemas) that he produce on the toilet. All that he could produce upset him, so he held on. But did it upset only him? After material in which he recounted his mother's squeamishness about bathroom smells, her ritualistic match-lighting after her own defecation, and her refusal to use any other than her own bathroom at home, no matter where she was, he was able to remember vividly his mother's disgust with feces. This also, then, became the gift mother objected to and as a result of which she left him. What complicated matters so much was that their togetherness in the bathroom was, he repeated several times, "the highlight of attention from her." The hours were filled with anger, paranoia about intruders from the outside, and despairing suicidal thoughts. It was clear that the patient was intensely ambivalent about ridding himself of the maternal introject who sat with him at the toilet, stimulated him to produce something he found pleasurable and terrifying, but which she found disgusting. In his infantile thoughts, it mattered little, when she left the bathroom, whether it was because he had finished his work and produced what was asked for, or because she could not tolerate what he had done. Maternal disgust and abandonment became the externalization and gratification of his unconscious and grandiose wish to soil the world.

New components were now added to the meaning of his inability to finish his dissertation and his fear that women (especially now, the idealized H.) would leave him once they knew what he was really like. His masochistic need to submit to feminine demands defended him against his intolerable rage toward women, especially mother, and palliated his unconscious sense of guilt for that rage and its sources. But the masochistic need also kept his identification with mother alive, as well as giving the "returning home" aspect of the compulsion additional meaning. It also contributed to his painful identification with his father's anxiety about his colostomy. In the analysis, insofar as his unconscious wish to maintain the ambivalent contact with his mother and contaminate the environment with his anal contents was exposed, he had felt manipulated and abandoned. This was easily related to his general pattern of withholding and his difficulties with terminating the analysis specifically.

Termination then proceeded without difficulty or drama. Shortly before the last hour, Mr. R. mentioned in passing that the stove no longer was a problem: "I look, but there is no more checking. I seem to be able to keep the picture of its being off in my head."

DISCUSSION

Details of this case provide support for psychoanalytic hypotheses about the etiology and mechanism of obsessive-compulsive symptomatology: specifically the role of regression from oedipal conflict to a level of anal organization, bisexuality, an ambivalent dependence on a sadistic superego, the central importance of anal-erotic and anal-sadistic trends, developmental conflicts and interference during toilet training, and the use of reaction formations, isolation of affect, and undoing as primary defensive operations (Freud, 1908, 1909, 1912, 1913, 1926; Fenichel, 1945; Sandler and Joffee, 1965; Nagera, 1966).

Whereas most of the literature focuses on a regression from phallic themes and aggressive impulses in the development of such symptoms, this analysis suggests that the timing of each onset and the content of the material at those times also served to defend against material associated with separation and loss. That is, the development of the compulsion to make sure his stove was off not only represented a regression from the passive homosexual wishes and castration anxiety induced by the transference neurosis, but the repeated leaving and returning home aspects of the symptom also defended against the affect associated with the parental deprivation of his early life, maternal abandonment at the toilet, the loss of his father just prior to the onset of his analysis, and termination of various relationships during the analysis. Thus, the returning home aspect of the symptom corresponds to the separation reactions during the rapprochement crisis described by Mahler et al. (1975). According to these authors, the toddler of 18 to 21 months finds it necessary during this crisis to keep the mother in sight, to cling to her, or to return frequently in an effort to reassure himself of her presence and her love. Mahler et al. describe problems with the process of leave-taking itself, indecision reminiscent of obsessive-compulsive neurosis, partial internalization of parental attitudes, and, in more serious cases, coercive behavior and splitting of the object world consistent with a borderline transference in adults. The intensity of the rapprochement crisis is heightened if the parents, like Mr. R.'s, are actually unavailable or inappropriately intrusive and overstimulating.

The traumatic effects of overstimulation during this period have also been documented by Greenacre (1952) with respect to repeated enemas, and by Blum (1979) and Shengold (1967) with respect to the primal scene. A combination of heightened sexual and aggressive feelings with a threatened loss played a part in each of the three onsets of the symptom described in this case. In the first instance, the onset occurred in conjunction with the libidinous demands of a sexual affair, a developing homosexual transference, and the absence and loss of his father. The second onset was closely related to an intensification of and beginning working through of the homosexual transference, grief and mourning associated with the father's death, and termination of a year-long affair. And the third onset was in the context of the loss of the analyst and a frankly oedipal situation which elucidated pathogenic aspects of the maternal transference. It is hypothesized that the onset of the symptom is related to this duality: the interdependence of sexual and aggressive feelings with loss in the psychological life of the patient; while its diminution related to their interpretation.

Ferenczi (1912) first described transitory symptoms arising during the analytic work. He attributed their appearance to "representations, in symptom form, of unconscious feeling and thought-excitations which the analysis has stirred up from their inactivity . . . and brought near to the threshold of consciousness" (p. 195). Included in his list of transitory symptom constructions are conversions, obsessional phenomena, hallucinations, illusionary deceptions, character regressions, and expressive displacements. Not only do the transitory symptom formations offer the patient the experience of "conviction" to add to the relevance of the psychical material afforded through free associations, but Ferenczi also asserted that they offer a point of attack for dealing with strong resistances as well as providing information about symptom formation.

Alexander (1923) wrote that these "transitory artificial products of the neurosis are especially seen and in a pronounced form in the analysis of neurotic characters" (p. 11). The patients, he continues, have no symptoms, but their impulsive and compulsive behavior is integral to their lives. This was certainly the case with the patient in this report. His life was, in a sense, "turned off," while all his actions served to reinforce his being "stuck." In this way, he kept his sensitive conscience clear of the sequelae of his instinctual tendencies. The analytic work deprived him of the possibility of gratifying these tendencies and opened the way for the emergence, sometimes via symptoms, of repressed material which could then be examined and interpreted.

Sharpe (1930) noted that one might expect the emerging of fresh symptoms after any interpretation of id wishes. She attributed this to the necessity for repentance, self-castigation, and mourning; furthermore, there may be long periods of these alternating phases, "first the obsessional symptoms in full swing and then grief and self-condemnation" (p. 89). She concludes that the value of this process lies in the fact that the obsession is now in the analysis and that the analyst and the analytic situation have become increasingly important dynamic factors. The analysis then has the opportunity to make the anxiety bearable to the weakened ego, and "this means the possibility of breaking up the organized system in which the unconscious hostile impulses are being constantly cancelled out" (p. 91). Bergler (1946) confirms the view that the constant ebb and flow of symptoms in progressive stages of analysis is completely characteristic of the analytic destruction of the neurosis. Other authors (Dunbar, 1938; Bettelheim and Sylvester, 1949; Kubie, 1950; Glover, 1955; Hendrick, 1958) suggest that variation in the symptom picture is the first sign of progress in the analysis. All agree that transitory symptom formation is related to a changing relationship between drive derivatives and defenses against it.

An added dimension is provided for transitory symptom formation by three writers who postulate a special condition for its development. In trying to understand the transitory occurrences of a "nadir" state in a borderline schizophrenic patient, Pious (1961) hypothesizes a situation in which his patient experiences various degrees of deprivation which led to an "emptying" and then a restitutional "focusing." It was during the focusing phase that symptomatic behavior of all kinds would appear— even at times, the presumably obsessive-compulsive psychoneurosis with which his patient had entered analysis. "As a hypothesis, I suggest that a psychological deprivation, the nature of which is complex and very individually determined, reaches the equivalent of a threshold quantity, at which point the nadir occurs" (p. 52). It is the gradual internalization of the analyst during treatment which serves to protect the patient from his vulnerability to deprivation by increasing the threshold.

Miller (1965) wrote about the return of symptoms in the terminal phase of analysis. He postulates a twofold function for this transitory reappearance: first, it represents evidence of insufficient working through of the symptom; and second, this insufficiency allows the symptom to find a regressive foothold in infantile fantasies of omnipotence in which there is an intimate connection with separation anxiety.

The most thoroughly studied transitory symptom in a given hour is that associated with momentary forgetting (Luborsky, 1967). Momentary forgetting occurs when three factors coincide: (1) when a conscious thought makes contact or associates to derivatives of a "repressed drive-organized complex of thoughts" (p. 215). The derivative is then momentarily forgotten in order to defend against the emergence of the repressed material. (2) Insofar as there is anxiety in the moment, it is related to becoming aware of the thought in the context of the transference. (3) The process is augmented by a somewhat altered state of consciousness which detracts from the attention paid to immediately preceding and succeeding thoughts. Munich (1977) has related this third factor to the appearance of transitory depersonalized states in an adolescent. The congruence of these three factors accounts for the breach in the defensive structure, while the subsequent recovery of the thought seems equivalent to the formation of a symptom. This equivalence exists insofar as the patient focuses his attention (perhaps like Pious's patient) on the recovery of the lost thought, the time involved allows the patient "some distance and isolation from the immediately threatening thoughts so that the recovered thought is likely to be a derivative, toned-down version of the originally emerging threatening thought and therefore accessible to awareness" (p. 216; italics omitted).

In a later article with Auerbach (1969), Luborsky added episodic stomach pain and migraine headache to his symptom-context method of analyzing transitory symptoms. This work confirmed the earlier hypothesis about the requirements for transitory symptom formation: a particular kind of immediately adjacent thought in the context of a larger background state. Direct reference to the therapist was present with patients for whom momentary forgetting and headache were the transitory symptoms.

It is clear from the literature that most writers consider transitory symptom formation as primarily a more visible and graphic example of typical symptom construction; furthermore, whatever instability of the psychic structures a transitory symptom may indicate, that instability results from the vicissitudes of the analytic situation, especially the transference. The classical view of symptom formation posits stress, conflict, and regression as prerequisites to the process, while the symptom itself is often a symbolic representation and substitute and/or distorted gratification of the wish mobilized by the stressful conflict (Freud, 1912, 1926; Waelder, 1930; Arlow, 1963; Panel, 1963).

When Mr. R.'s symptom first appeared, the early stage of the analysis and the brevity of its duration made it difficult to ascertain the relative contribution of the various stresses he was experiencing. The uncharacteristically rapid and full sexual behavior in combination with his increased use of stylized language in describing his new affair suggested anxiety about heterosexual contact in addition to concern about revealing it to me. This oedipal configuration paralleled his early marital situation, just prior to the end of sexual relations with his wife. Once the analysis began, instead of stopping his sexual behavior, he developed the compulsion, thus turning something else off. Material related to the transference suggested that he might also be in flight from increasing homosexual impulses, while the repeated references to his deceased father heightened this possibility. The possibly correct and probably premature interpretation of his fear and anger about the sexuality and its demands brought an end to both the affair and the symptom. It was as if he heard the interpretation as a paternal prohibition against his activities, a prohibition which sided with and confirmed the presence of a harshly sadistic component of his superego. At the same time, and insofar as he heard the interpretation as an injunction, the impulsiveness with which he entered into the sexual arrangement also called forth the absent father in the form of the analytic intervention.

At the first onset of the symptom, it seems reasonable to postulate stress from the instinctual demands associated with his oedipal conflict, a regression to an earlier level of organization, and formation of a ritualized compromise formation. In a sense, the rapid disappearance of the symptom following its interpretation was symptomatic itself, and most certainly related to the transference. But subsequent developments made it important to note the presence of material related to the father's absence.

Although the second and more prolonged onset of the compulsion was clearly associated with a regression from negative oedipal issues, it was heralded by the separation from the second girlfriend and accompanied by the first mourning of the father. This mourning not only included grief over his death, but also brought from repression the sadness and anger associated with Mr. R.'s lack of contact with him as a child. Furthermore, substantial progress was made in understanding the meaning of the symptom as an identification with his father, especially around the latter's fastidiousness and later colostomy and impotence, while the emerging of aggressive fantasies revealed its anal-erotic and anal-sadistic origins. The conjunction of sexual curiosity and exploration with very early play around the stove in the back kitchen, childhood fears of the gas furnace in the basement, and preoccupations with the destruction of his home by fire, the connection of fire and fire imagery with sexual desire in the parental bedroom, familial concerns about escaping gas and stomal accidents, mother's indiscriminate flatulence and ritualistic match-lighting after defecation, and the patient's anal sensations of burning condensed and focused in the wish to check and inhibit his gas stove.

The symptom's modulation by sexual abstinence suggested that the deterioration of the sexual aspect of marriage, the cooling off of his affairs, and his preoccupation with celibacy were all in the service of relieving his castration anxiety. The sexual abstinence and conscious fantasies of celibacy also served to augment his identification with the impotent and absent father. Although interpretation of his castration anxiety, as well as his passive homosexual wishes, served to diminish the intensity of the symptom somewhat, its overdetermination and deeper roots required further work. Finally, the analysis of these themes in the context of the transference led to the unconscious and conflicted masturbatory fantasy of destructively inundating all around him with fecal material. Interpreting this material meant taking cognizance of the hostile and aggressive affects which were so prominent during this phase of the analysis. What made matters so intense were the anticipated and inevitable sequelae to expression of the rage symbolized by his fantasy of defecating on the world: further loss in the transference of the paternal object. In addition, this conflict about inundating the world mirrored the themes of overstimulation and parental deprivation so prominent during his crisis of rapprochement and heightened the aggressive components of Mr. R.'s dilemma.

The theme of loss assumed prominence in the two final recurrences of the symptom in the terminal phase of the analysis. The patient had developed a serious and nonsexual relationship with a woman, re-creating the oedipal triangle once again, with the analyst experienced as father. At this point in the analysis, the emergence of frankly oedipal issues served several functions: (1) to convince me that more work was necessary; (2) to defend further against, while at the same time continuing to search for, gratification of the homosexual transference; (3) to introduce aspects of the maternal transference; and (4) to signal a new resolution of anal and phallic conflicts so that a new effort at mastering the oedipal dilemmas could be attempted, this time with a more benign superego.

In the first occurrence of the symptom during this phase, Mr. R. identified the stresses and dynamics as being quite similar to the very first onset: increased pressure of instinctual demands that he yearned for the soon-to-be-lost analyst to help modulate. In the context of termination, the final appearance of the compulsion again represented a regression from the pressures of his growing attachment to H. Fire imagery led to a recognition of the incestuous wishes for his mother, but this led to sadistic, anal, masturbatory fantasies, a report of the sensations of anal burning, and an angry exacerbation of the symptom. His fury at me for abandoning him led rapidly to intensely sadistic fantasies toward his mother and a reconstruction of the anal traumas he had so vigorously kept from awareness (but which he also announced by his compulsion to return home and check his stove). At the anal level of organization, the conflict with the maternal object was between holding onto her so as not to lose her, on the one hand, and inundating her with his body products, on the other. And at the phallic level, the conflict over possessing mother was expressed in his fantasies of violence toward and mutilation of women. The conjunction of a regression from phallic themes with material relating to separation and loss had led to an exacerbation of the symptom picture. At each level, the aggressive aspects of the material was consistent with what would be expected from early difficulties in separation and the repeated overstimulation by his mother coupled with the deprivations by both parents. The importance of the final reappearance lay in the recovery from repression of the genetic origins of both trends and the abreaction of the repressed, drive-organized complex of thoughts associated with infantile traumas. Once all components were identified, Mr. R. felt in control of the symptom and was able to terminate the analysis with a sad comfort.

Insofar as the analytic situation requires an outpouring of associations, the end result of which is giving up deeply held and highly charged material and the loss of a firmly established and intimate relationship, it replicated the patient's central dilemma. Remember here the patient's early use in the analysis of an excessive rhetorical style, verbosity, and impossibly long dreams. There, outpouring became inundation. This replication facilitated the development of the symptom by intensifying from the outside Mr. R.'s latent conflict. Although he had organized his life and chosen his objects in such a way as to insure the repetition of the conflict, the abstinence and, in a certain sense, the inevitable deprivations of the analytic situation deprived him of the usual sources of gratification. But the presence of the analyst, perhaps represented at the end of the mental image of the stove's being turned off, also replaced his absent father in assisting with understanding and control of his intensely conflicted feelings toward his mother. This combination of abstinence and presence facilitated an internal reorganization whereby the drives, derivatives, and representations were reexamined, expressed in transitory form, and finally changed. In a sense, the partial internalization referred to by Mahler et al. was completed, and Mr. R.'s indecision about terminating was resolved. This change was associated with structural changes in the form of a more benevolent superego and a more coherent, less conflicted ego which permitted a reevaluation by the more adult or mature ego, instead of the old, structuralized infantile solution. This allowed the patient to resume his progress again toward modified interpersonal and vocational goals.

In addition to confirming analytic hypotheses of symptom formation, the material points toward including conflicts around separation and loss in the etiological mechanism of transitory symptom formation. It may be that these conflicts contribute to the elaboration of what Luborsky meant by an altered or larger background upon which the classical mechanism of symptom formation can unfold. As Breuer and Freud (1893–95) postulated in *Studies on Hysteria,* this raises the further question as to whether or not the presence of such states is a prerequisite for symptom formation in general. Finally, the appearance of neurotic symptoms in a patient with character pathology suggests clues to the relation between character and symptom, as well as offering technical data about their simultaneous analysis.

BIBLIOGRAPHY

ALEXANDER, F. (1923). The castration complex in the formation of character. *Int. J. Psychoanal.,* 4:11–45.

ARLOW, J. A. (1963). Conflict, regression and symptom formation. *Int. J. Psychoanal.,* 44:12–22.

BERGLER, E. (1946). Use and misuse of analytic interpretation by the patient. *Psychoanal. Rev.,* 33:416–441.

BETTELHEIM, B. & SYLVESTER, E. (1949). Physical symptoms in emotionally disturbed children. *Psychoanal. Study Child,* 3/4:353–368.

BLUM, H. P. (1979). On the concept and consequence of the primal scene. *Psychoanal. Q.,* 48:27–47.

Breuer, J. & Freud, S. (1893–95). Studies on hysteria. *S.E.,* 2:215–221.

DUNBAR, H. F. (1938). *Emotions and Bodily Changes.* New York: Columbia Univ. Press.

FENICHEL, O. (1945). *The Psychoanalytic Theory of Neurosis.* New York: Norton.

FERENCZI, S. (1912). Transitory symptom-construction during the analysis. In *Sex in Psychoanalysis,* pp. 193–212. New York: Robert Brunner, 1950.

FREUD, S. (1908). Character and anal erotism. *S.E.,* 9:167–175.

——— (1909). Notes upon a case of obsessional neurosis. *S.E.,* 10:153–318.

——— (1912). Types of onset of neurosis. *S.E.,* 12:227–238.

——— (1913). The disposition of obsessional neurosis. *S.E.,* 12:311–326.

——— (1918). From the history of an infantile neurosis. *S.E.,* 17:3–122.

——— (1921). Group psychology and the analysis of the ego. *S.E.,* 18:67–143.

——— (1926). Inhibitions, symptoms and anxiety. *S.E.,* 20:77–178.

GLOVER, E. (1924). Active therapy and psycho-analysis. *Int. J. Psychoanal.,* 5:269–311.

——— (1935). A developmental study of the obsessional neurosis. *Int. J. Psychoanal.*, 16:131–144.

——— (1955). *The Techniques of Psychoanalysis*. New York: Int. Univ. Press.

GREENACRE, P. (1952). *Trauma, Growth and Personality*. New York: Int. Univ. Press, 1969.

HENDRICK, I. (1958). *Facts and Theories of Psychoanalysis*. New York: Alfred Knopf.

ISAKOWER, O. (1938). A contribution to the patho-psychology of phenomena associated with falling asleep. *Int. J. Psychoanal.*, 19:331–345.

KUBIE, L. S. (1950). *Practical and Theoretical Aspects of Psychoanalysis*. New York: Int. Univ. Press.

LUBORSKY, L. (1967). Momentary forgetting during psychotherapy and psychoanalysis. In *Motives and Thought*, ed. R. R. Holt, pp. 177–217. New York: Int. Univ. Press.

——— & AUERBACH, A. H. (1969). The symptom content method. *J. Amer. Psychoanal. Assn.*, 17:68–99.

MAHLER, M. S., PINE, F., & BERMAN, A. (1975). *The Psychological Birth of the Human Infant*. New York: Basic Books.

MILLER, I. (1965). On the return of symptoms in the terminal phase of psycho-analysis. *Int. J. Psychoanal.*, 46:487–501.

MUNICH, R. L. (1977). Depersonalization in a female adolescent. *Int. J. Psychoanal. Psychother.*, 6:187–199.

NAGERA, H. (1966). *Early Childhood Disturbances, the Infantile Neurosis, and the Adulthood Disturbances*. New York: Int. Univ. Press.

PANEL (1963). Symptom formation. H. Nierenberg, reporter. *J. Amer. Psychoanal. Assn.*, 11:161–172.

Pious, W. (1961). A hypothesis about the nature of schizophrenic behavior. In *Psychotherapy of the Psychoses*, ed. A. Burton, pp. 43–68. New York: Basic Books.

ROSENBLATT, B. (1963). A severe neurosis in an adolescent boy. *Psychoanal. Study Child*, 18:561–602.

SANDLER, J. & JOFFEE, W. G. (1965). Notes on obsessional manifestations in children. *Psychoanal. Study Child*, 20:425–438.

SCHILDER, P. (1938). *Psychotherapy*. New York: Norton.

SHARPE, E. F. (1930). The technique of psycho-analysis. In *Collected Papers on Psycho-Analysis*, pp. 9–106. London: Hogarth Press, 1950.

SHENGOLD, L. (1967). The effects of overstimulation. *Int. J. Psychoanal.*, 48:403–415.

WAELDER, R. (1930). The principle of multiple function. *Psychoanal. Q.*, 5:45–62, 1936.

"Lying" and "Lying"

A Case Report of a Paradoxical Reaction to the Couch

LYNN WHISNANT REISER, M.D.

THIS CASE HISTORY ILLUSTRATES HOW ASPECTS OF THE ANALYTIC setting—particularly the use of the couch—interacted with constitutional and early experiential factors in a way that seemed initially to result in a stalemated analysis. When the treatment was switched to psychoanalytic psychotherapy, the patient was able to work in an analytic mode, and it turned out that the stalemate had been due to an altered state of consciousness related to her feeling about lying on the couch. Lying on the couch had mobilized in the transference conflicts that were based in early preoedipal trauma. When she was sitting up, free of the specific anxieties associated with lying on the couch, we were able in retrospect to understand not only the patient's difficulty in communicating from the couch but also to recover memories which revealed the genetic roots of the problem.

In early spring a garden may still look like a piece of barren ground, although extensive work has been done in spading, fertilizing, and seeding. Similarly, the first work on the couch in this case ended with little signs of real growth. The garden requires cultivating, weeding, watering to bear fruit—so too in this case the harvest came later after additional work. The later work done in the psychoanalytic psychotherapy with this patient, however, built on and depended on the understanding of intense transference feelings from the previous epoch of analytic work on the couch.

Associate clinical professor, Department of Psychiatry, Yale University School of Medicine.

The use of the couch in psychoanalysis has been of interest to
analysts since Freud (1913) originally suggested that it helped to
free him from being looked at as he focused on his own associations and allowed the patient freedom from attending to visual
cues about him. Supporting and extending Freud's suggestions,
Sterba (1929), Macalpine (1950), Khan (1962), and Greenson
(1967) have discussed the role and importance of the couch in
the analytic setting.

However, the literature contains a number of cases who had
difficulty with the analytic situation—particularly with the use of
the couch (Greenson, 1965; Orens, 1965; Silber, 1977; Weissman, 1977; Greenacre, 1980). Bibring (1936) wrote about a
transference resistance linked to reality factors which is extremely difficult to overcome. She discussed this in terms of the
sex or personal characteristics of the analyst. Reality factors may
also be specifically related to the analytic setting, the position on
the couch, and inability to see the analyst's face.

Such patients had similar events in their early family history,
including early separation from mother and a depressed, withdrawn father who was unpredictably violent. Several of the patients had alcoholic and/or psychotic fathers. The transferences
were rooted both in the yearning to be reunited with mother, the
perception of father as a rival for mother's attention, and a
childhood role as special mediator with father.

Vision may assume a particular importance in such children—
in the early visual union with the mother, and in visual sur-
veillance of the untrustworthy father. Kris (1956) discusses "facial searching" in the children of depressed mothers who both
wish to coax and distract that mother from her mood and also to
watch for unpredictably angry shifts in the parent's mood.
Greenson (1965), Orens (1965), Silber (1977), and Weissman
(1977) report cases with this kind of history who need to see the
analyst's face during the part of the analytic work when they
were immersed in this kind of transference.

This case illuminates the meaning of the couch for a particular
patient, and it also suggests that a period of work on the couch
may stir up intense transference feelings which facilitate later

understanding of the patient's neurosis. Circumstances that at the time create a stalemated analysis may later provide particularly useful and illuminating insight.

CASE HISTORY

When Debbi entered treatment she was a 37-year-old white, Protestant, unmarried law student, who worked part-time as a secretary. She was an attractive, youthful, well-groomed brunette, soft-spoken, friendly, and articulate. She seemed observant and curious. She explained that she had been in treatment once before—only for 4 sessions, years ago, during a crisis with a boyfriend. She had not found that treatment helpful. Now she sought treatment again because several circumstances in her life made her feel increasingly unable to cope.

At the first meeting she stressed the effects of an automobile accident (her car had been hit from behind while she was stopped at a traffic light). Although the accident had occurred some 6 months earlier, she continued to suffer anxiety attacks with flashbacks of the accident, frequently when driving. She had trouble sleeping and difficulty concentrating, particularly on her schoolwork. She also commented that she was back in a familiar unsatisfactory relationship with a boyfriend. She hoped to understand herself better and to change.

We agreed to begin treatment, meeting for 4 months twice a week with Debbi sitting in a chair. During this time Debbi presented her past history and current concerns in a vivid and lively way. As she described herself and her past, Debbi often used precise visual descriptions of memories, dreams, and fantasies. She showed a wide and appropriate range of affect. She seemed able to move easily from the here and now to past and fantasy material. Her level of anxiety markedly decreased. I discussed analysis with her. Debbi was eager to pursue this. She could afford a moderate fee. After interrupting our meetings for my August vacation, we resumed them in September, beginning the analysis then.

In the psychotherapy sessions Debbi had been able to work in an analytic mode sitting up. After a period of time on the couch, however, it became clear that she was not able to work

consistently analytically while she was lying down. Instead
Debbi became concrete, complaining, and passively resistant. At
times, she seemed to be in a different ego state. After 264
hours, that is, 1½ years, I decided to discontinue the analysis,
and return to psychotherapy twice a week. Once again, in the
sitting position, Debbi began to work more comfortably. She
was able to remember and to work through specific memories
related to the position on the couch, clarifying in retrospect her
altered ego state in the analytic situation, as well as related aspects of transference and transference resistance. While she
was on the couch, however, these insights were not available for
her.

Although her hours on the couch had created intense affect
and resistance at the time, it seemed that without time spent
lying down she might not later have recovered and understood
the memories revived by the experience on the couch. Debbi
verbalized the memories evoked by lying down so that we were
able to understand and to consolidate gains and insights.

HISTORY ("FIRST VERSION")

Before describing the analytic process, I would like to present
the version of her life history as Debbi recounted it in the initial
sessions. Both during the analysis and particularly during the
psychotherapy that followed, she elaborated and greatly altered this presentation.

Debbi's mother, age 70, was a lawyer, nationally prominent,
and still active in her profession. She was from a respected established family. Debbi's father, age 73, was a retired chemist.
He came from an immigrant Irish family. Her paternal grandfather had been hospitalized for psychosis. Her parents met
and married after a brief courtship shortly after Debbi's mother's fiancé committed suicide.

Debbi was the youngest of three children, born just after her
father left for an assignment overseas. He rejoined the family
when she was 18 months old and lived with them for about a
year. While Debbi's father got settled in the city, Debbi's mother
took the children with her to live with her parents for a year.

After that, the family spent a summer together at a camp and then moved to the city where Debbi's father had found a position.

Debbi described her father as a big, gentle man, fond of animals. She felt she was his special favorite. At times he became silent and withdrawn and she tried very hard to cheer him up. She described her mother as a difficult women, jealous of Debbi's relationship with her father. Her mother often antagonized and nagged him. Debbi saw herself as the peacemaker between them.

Debbi was a bright student in school, excelling in art and science. In high school her first serious boyfriend was a rebellious "James Dean" type who often talked about suicide. Just after Debbi told him she was going to college rather than marry him, he did commit suicide.

Debbi graduated from high school, attended a local college, then moved to New York. She worked as a department store buyer. She had several long-term relationships with other men, each time choosing a man who, while talented and successful in his career, was distant and difficult to relate to and simultaneously had other girlfriends. When she was 27, she had traveled with one of them, Dan, to India. She became quite ill with dysentery and hepatitis—and also became pregnant. Dan was not eager to marry her and she reluctantly decided, in part because of her illness, to return to the United States and abort the child. The fetus was dead. She believed it was a male. Shortly thereafter she left New York to live with Dan in the country. A decline in her ability to function at work dates from that time.

She felt unable to cope with Dan's inaccessibility and his affairs with other women. Finally (age 29) she left him for David (age 22), who seemed more straightforward and affectionate. They lived together in a rural area for 3½ years and were talking about marriage when he, a fireman, was killed at work. A month later her father became ill. She decided then to "take charge of her life" by returning to school to learn a trade. She enrolled in law school, but continued to live in the country, surrounded by animal pets. She worked steadily as a secretary supporting herself. She made the Dean's list her first year in law school. She had several close supportive women friends. She was in frequent telephone contact, several times a week, with her parents, particularly her mother.

After a time, she resumed her old unsatisfactory relationship with Dan, and with that she began to feel increasingly fatigued and depressed. In this period, she was in a car accident—hit from behind when stopped at a traffic light. She began to have anxiety attacks and episodes of derealization. She saw a psychiatrist and several neurologists in consultation. This crisis helped bring her to a decision to seek psychotherapy, and led to the referral to me.

During the screening interviews Debbi reported three memories which seemed particularly vivid and which subsequently were referred to often and considerably revised in the retelling: (1) the death of a pet bird when she was 3; (2) an illness when she was 4; and (3) her boyfriend's suicide when she was 17. They came to be understood to represent and symbolize Debbi's central conflicts.

IMPRESSION AFTER THE SCREENING INTERVIEWS

A continuing theme in Debbi's beginning analysis was her problematic relationships with men. Two boyfriends had died violently, and she thought she had aborted a male fetus. Her relationships with women seemed more positive. She had several close girlfriends and as an adult she had a supportive relationship with her mother. She seemed to choose distant or depressed men—like her father—and to repeat the triangular competitive relationships she experienced as a child with her parents. It was unclear how significant her early disturbances in object relationships would be—her father away from home until she was 1½ years old and again from age 2½ to 4 years—and how much primitive fantasies of being cared for by the analyst and depressive features might interfere. I anticipated that her efforts to maintain contact with a silent and rejecting, perhaps depressed, father might be repeated with me and present an early or difficult transference resistance. The diagnostic impression was of a neurotic character disorder, predominantly pregenital narcissistic with hysteric features.

THE ANALYSIS

The hours on the couch, four times a week, were markedly different from the sessions that preceded them. Difficulty began the first day when, invited to use the couch, Debbi lay down on her stomach, face propped in her hands, watching me intently. I explained to her the rationale for the couch: by not seeing the analyst and being in a relaxed position, she might be more able to "see" her own thoughts, fantasies. She complied with my request to lie on her back and I did not stop to explore her responses fully. We did not really begin to understand what lying on the couch meant to her until 1½ years later when she resumed sitting on a chair.

In spite of her seeming sophistication about psychoanalysis and her previous ease at working in psychotherapy, suddenly she seemed to have become a stupid woman, unable to generalize from one day's happenings to the next. Debbi found the demands of free associating very difficult.

She expressed confusion about the "rules," began to miss sessions or came late, and did not pay her bills. She connected the "rules" with the "mustache game" she played with her father; she'd touch his mustache with her finger and he'd "play" at biting it. When he got tired of the game, he would really bite her finger, hurting her. Repeatedly shocked that he had broken "the rules," she would demand that he continue to play, she'd say to "reestablish the rules."

During this opening phase of the analysis, the first 6 or 7 months, Debbi was concerned with describing problematic relationships with her doctors, teachers, boyfriends, and father. Her father, while sensitive and giving at times, was more often depressed, withdrawn, and silent. She now added that he unpredictably became irrational, erupting in violent rages. Debbi vacillated, she either felt close to him and special, or attacked and excluded. She began to recount more stories of how she had re-created the experience of her father's outbursts by seeking out potentially violent boyfriends (for example, her boyfriend Dan left a loaded gun by her bed) and by putting herself in dangerous situations, hoping each time to be saved. Vivid stories of encounters with dangerous dogs in her sister's apartment, rapists in her own apartment, unscrupulous doctors—all repeated the same theme of being endangered while in a "safe" situation. Each episode had been perceived as unique and surprising.

By canceling sessions or showing up late Debbi found a way to engage in the "mustache game" during the analysis, repeating her teasing relationship with her father. "Do you want me to come even if I lost my job? Do you want me to be on time even if I get a speeding ticket or am in a car accident?" These plaints were ways of rebuking the "sadistic father/analyst" for hurting the child with a real bite.

Attempts to interpret her angry or negative feelings expressed in the absences, in the obsessive teasing about rules, or in her associations to "bad" doctors and teachers as related to feelings about me, were repeatedly denied, "You always take things so negatively." Debbi dealt with each incident separately, presenting each missed or canceled session as an isolated problem. Gradually it became clearer to me that there was a predictable pattern of irregular attendance which seemed to correlate with a conflict between scheduled analytic sessions and school and work commitments. Interpretation of this pattern to her, combined with rescheduling her work schedule and her analytic sessions, led to more regular attendance and a beginning understanding of a similar tendency to deal with others in her life, particularly her father and boyfriends, incident by incident.

During the second year of analysis, Debbi began to report feeling that her life was settling down. Changes in her life closely paralleled her progress in the analysis. She had failed two courses in school in the previous fall semester because of frequent absences and tardiness. During this same time in analysis she was the most absent and tardy.

Following my clarifying her vague communication about our schedule and the fee, she renegotiated her work schedule, her school courses. Her school and work evaluations improved, she got her finances in order, and for the first time paid her taxes and paid her bills to me.

In discussing her problems at work, which at first she described in terms of scheduling, she became more aware of difficulties in relationships with her bosses as she felt either the special favorite or arbitrarily ignored, and of rivalrous feelings toward female co-workers whom she blamed for reverses in her fortunes with the boss. I began to interpret the parallels between this pattern and the relationships in her family, and with me.

Interpretation of the real and symbolic issues involved in the scheduling and fee promised to alleviate some of the resistance Debbi was manifesting in her actions—and indeed she at first expressed great relief, and did begin to come to her sessions regularly. However, she often arrived 3 or 4 minutes late (symbolically late), and would then spend the rest of the session in misery, certain the tardiness was all I cared about. She declared that she felt unable to say what was on her mind and what was important to her because she was "forced" to talk about the structure. During these "tantrums" she seemed inaccessible either to interpretation or to reality-orienting interventions. Some of her behavior seemed like provocative teasing in the service of her intense interest in getting me to talk and her desperate need to know how I was reacting.

Debbi complained that my silence was provocative, particularly my "not answering questions." Her feeling reminded her of the Tar Baby story:

> Br'er Rabbit meets a Tar Baby sitting by the road—he becomes more and more fascinated, angry and provoked by the Tar Baby's silence, and finally attacks the Tar Baby to make it talk, becoming at last hopelessly stuck and at the mercy of Br'er Fox (who had put the Tar Baby there as a trap).

Debbi connected this with her impulses to tease and torment me into communicating with her, feeling stuck in the interaction herself and associating her "drowsy" state with being stuck and giving up. She also felt that she repeatedly chose "Tar Baby" boyfriends, ending up stuck, helpless, and terrified of the violent fox.

I began to interpret the similarity expressed in the transference "mustache game," and how this tactic facilitated denial that her father or boyfriend were repetitively violent.

Debbi's early maternal transference was also strong. Responding to an interpretation of her critical feelings toward me, Debbi complained, "Don't you understand—now I'm much closer and dependent on you than on my family." She was concerned with the welfare of her "babies"—ponies or pet crow; and she would like to be my "pet crow." She wished me to figure out what she needed just from her actions, as she did with her pets, and to satisfy her without being asked. (Similarly her absences from analytic sessions might mean she wished for me to understand from her actions the conflicts she encountered in scheduling.) Her sense of being cared for by my consistent presence and interest in her seemed to be part of this maternal transference, as did her wish to be part of an exclusive mother-child unit with no man present.

She had broken off her relationship with Dan during the summer break. At the end of the first year of analysis she began an affair with a famous colleague/mentor. Although he seemed in many ways similar to previous boyfriends, this relationship was separate enough from her day-to-day life that, although often distressing to her, it was not as disruptive as others had been. It became more apparent how similar the problems in her work, financial, school life, and intense initial transference were to her problems in her destructive attachments to men. Gradually, as she focused on this, she began to get some distance from her new boyfriend and began to extricate herself.

In the midst of this, she at times was able to free associate, and be curious about dreams, memories, fantasies, and feelings about me, and to wonder a bit about her own behavior during the sessions. But after a while she would again revert to her complaining, teasing behavior. For a long time it was not clear what motivated these shifts.

In a dream Debbi portrayed the analytic couch and the "structure" of the analysis—times and scheduling—as a "procrustean bed" to which she had to confine herself. In associating to this dream she declared that she was afraid to relax and say what her thoughts were—although she had initially felt this would be "easy and enjoyable" for her to do because she would "get drowsy and fall asleep." This drowsiness reminded her of a memory which recurred more and more often and which she had first told me in one of our beginning sessions.

The summer when Debbi was 4, both parents served as counselors at a camp. Debbi remembered being hospitalized for a "strep throat." She was shut into a crib, and a very sick 2-year-old was next to her. To hush Debbi's crying her parents told her to "be good and quiet like the other little girl." She felt frightened by this since she sensed the other child was silent because she was very sick and perhaps dead.

During the same hospitalization, while she was crying for her father, an unfamiliar doctor came in and took her on his knee and asked her what was wrong. She was surprised that a stranger would be so kind. He told her that her father would come to visit soon—and he did.

At that time it had seemed likely to me that this episode with the "strange doctor" who had been so kind might very well indicate potential for a positive transference. It had seemed encouraging. However, recovery of additional mnemonic revisions gave the episode the opposite cast. Rather than predicting a positive transference, it represented the difficulties that would arise, the "helpful father/doctor" actually turned out to be an abusive parent.

She subsequently repeated that she was hospitalized and confined to a crib, but added that she had been moved to and shut up in the crib, alone in an abandoned chicken house at the camp to convalesce. She remembered feeling frightened, angry at being confined, and being lied to by her mother about what would happen and how long she would be restrained. She was again repeatedly told that her father would come to take her out of the crib. When he did not come, she at first had tantrums, then she found a solution by "doing something with my mind"—going into a drowsy state in which she "didn't really think about things," but seemed to "float near the ceiling" while the hours "just passed." She felt shocked when she was abruptly taken out of the crib and expected again to be part of the world outside.

She also recalled that as an older child whenever she was being punished she would be sent to her room. There she "relaxed" in the same drowsy way. As an adult if she felt angry she would go to bed, lie down, and just drop everything in her life. (In her analysis she assumed the same drowsy state which of course sabotaged any progress she was making in her work.)

She now revealed that she had been habitually drinking after work to get to sleep, but had recently been able to stop drinking

("I think drinking was to decrease anxiety, and now I feel less anxious"). Debbi now realized that she used alcohol to put her more quickly into this drowsy state.[1] In her life outside she began consciously to resist this "giving up" retreat; she also found that she did not need to spoil her analytic work that way.

After about 1½ years of analytic work it seemed that although Debbi had benefited from the treatment and her life was going better, it was clear that her ability to work consistently in the classical analytic mode was limited. Despite some understanding and interpretation of possible motives for resistance, the difficulty persisted, expressed in hours where she continued to ruminate obsessively about "the schedule." At these times she seemed inaccessible either to reality clarification or to interpretation; paradoxically at other times she pulled back from free association expressing her fear of "the drowsy state." It seemed that perhaps she was in such marginal contact with reality that communication must be maintained through visual as well as spoken contact (Greenacre, 1954).

Debbi said that she was tempted to glance at me at the beginning and end of the sessions, but felt her curiosity was "against the rules"—that she could "learn too much" if she looked. She thought often of her silent father and of her role in the family as the one to communicate with him and to make peace between the parents. She recalled her difficulty in sorting out whether her father was silent because he was tired or angry or just lost in thought. And she was never sure whether her efforts to communicate with her silent father would result in a friendly interchange or a violent outburst. All of this surfaced in the transference in this pervasive sense of being "STUCK" with a silent father/analyst whom she tried to cajole or indirectly sleuth around to find out his/her moods.

Finally I decided to discontinue the classical analysis and to resume sessions sitting up. One week prior to this discussion Debbi had dreamed about her horses and in her associations told of how her favorite mare had been the dominant "boss" horse until Debbi put up an electric fence. In exploring the fence, the

---

1. Silber (1977) discusses the relationship of alcohol use to the "hypnoid" state.

mare had been thrown to the ground on her back in such a way that she hit the wire and was shocked every time she tried to get up, finally giving up and lying there until Debbi rescued her. After this the mare became ineffectual and timid, no longer able to lead the other horses. Debbi stressed how devastating it was to a horse to be held on its back and how this technique was used to break and control wild horses. Her close identification with this horse was pointed out as explaining the decision to try sitting up. We decided to continue meeting with Debbi sitting up rather than lying on the couch and to return to the twice a week frequency of the screening interviews.

AFTER "THE ANALYSIS"

The analytic work continued in the psychoanalytic psycho-therapy.[2] Many of the memories and transference feelings which explained Debbi's neurosis became available only after the classical analysis ended. Her ability to work in a very different way, sitting up rather than lying down, clarified much of what had taken place during the preceding years. Yet without the experience of the intense transference response while she was lying down, it is unlikely that the material could have emerged with enough power and clarity to be analyzed. Debbi's need to deny her parents' psychopathology and to present her childhood in terms of the family myth may have prevailed in a less rigorous or less depriving treatment setting.

A dramatic change followed the change in posture. Debbi initially felt very disturbed and panicked by this decision. She feared this meant that I was stopping the treatment abruptly and abandoning her—sitting up she was able to put this feeling into words.[3] I interpreted her fear of suddenly losing me as she had

2. There are some analysts who might have increased the audibility of the psychoanalytic presence and frequency of interpretations but continued with the patient on the couch (Lipton, 1977; Edelson, 1985). Some analysts would have had the patient sit up but would regard it as a temporary parameter in a perhaps lengthy analysis.

3. Greenson (1965) and Weissman (1977) both noted marked differences in freedom of associations in their patients who had difficulty working on the couch. When sitting up, both cases feared the ending of the analysis and the loss of the transference object.

experienced abrupt losses before. During all of the subsequent sessions I maintained an analytic stance.

The first hour sitting up she began by declaring that "a terrible feeling came over me when I had to lie on the couch the first time. I tried not to pay attention to it, but I started thinking about it more recently when you said I should sit up. I didn't say anything about it at the time. I was hoping I'd just get used to it."

She then began a series of associations having to do with lying on the couch and the multiple overdetermined meaning of "lying" to her. Since the decision to sit up, she had been preoccupied with thinking about the circumstances of her high school boyfriend's suicide and about her stay in the hospital at age 4. Now in both cases additional aspects of the memories were clear to her, and the events assumed a quite different cast.

In the screening, Debbi had described her boyfriend's suicide when she was a senior in high school. She remembered that on the day of his death he had asked her to drive home with him, but she had a dental appointment. He had said "Good-by" rather than "So long." She was apprehensive about this, and drove by his house. At that time, she heard a car backfire. Lying in the dentist's chair she suddenly panicked and felt that she "knew" that something terrible had happened to her boyfriend, attributing her knowledge to "E.S.P." When she got home, her mother told her that her boyfriend had committed suicide by shooting himself. Debbi felt angry at neighbors who said she was lucky to be alive herself.

This time, in recounting the happening, Debbi began to realize with horror that she had been afraid that her suicidal boyfriend would shoot her too. She now realized she had gone into his house, and the "backfire" was from her boyfriend's gun. She had left and gone to the dentist. In her earlier descriptions of the events she had changed the timing so that she was lying in the dentist's chair when her boyfriend died. She had rationalized her memory of hearing the shot at his house as a car backfiring and had explained her panic at the dentist as E.S.P. She now felt less guilty, recognizing that she had refused to go with him as self-protection and she recalled many details confirming his homicidal potential.

As a child she had been phobic about dentists because they

said, "This won't hurt," and then hurt her. Thus, the "lying" of the dentist about pain and "lying" in the dentist chair were over-determined—like the habitual lying of her parents and her experiences of lying in the crib at age 4, and her own lying about where she was when her boyfriend died. In discussing her boyfriend's suicide Debbi slowly became more aware of how disturbed she felt her father had been and of her fear of his homicidal and suicidal potential. Her need to choose psychotic boyfriends became clearer.

In thinking more about the illness when she was 4, Debbi also realized she had put together scraps of memory in a way that reversed the emotional cast. She had always remembered her mother lying when she said Debbi would not get a shot—even when Debbi was able to see the needle being prepared or ready on the bedside table. Debbi stressed now that this lie meant that she had to argue with her mother when instead she wanted mother to acknowledge the truth and comfort her. In the first version of the memory, Debbi had recalled a "friendly" doctor who took her out of her crib, comforted her. Now she stressed what she had only mentioned before: no one could locate such a doctor nor even believe that he had been at her hospital bed. She also added that she thought the doctor had undressed and hurt her before comforting her, "some kind of a sexual hurt which made it hard to urinate the next day" (or, she wondered, did he just give her a shot?). She felt most distressed by her mother's denial that anyone had been there with her or that Debbi was in pain. After that, Debbi refused to let her mother leave at night. Her mother had told her she would be asleep on a cot outside the room where Debbi couldn't see or hear her. (Debbi discussed this recently with her mother who now admitted that she had lied and that she had left.) Debbi feared that if she became drowsy and went to sleep, her mother would creep away, so she forced herself to stay awake and to engage her mother by having tantrums. Debbi connected her sense of panic in that memory with her feelings about my sitting quietly out of sight and her fear of giving up contact with me when falling asleep/free associating when she could not see that I was there. Her fear of getting drowsy/free associating on the couch became more understandable to both of us, as did her mistrust of caring people who lied to

her and abandoned her, and especially who told her that she
wouldn't be hurt by something that then hurt her. (Her earlier
preoccupation with a series of doctors who had harmed her
became clearer.)

Later she recalled that the "mustache game" had always occurred lying in bed with her father in the morning. She also
remembered sitting on his lap and "playing with his pocket,"
something she thought he enjoyed—but when she exclaimed
aloud, "What's this?!" he suddenly became angry and abruptly
threw her off. (She now thought the game must have involved
touching his penis.) She also remembered his beating her with a
hair brush and wondered about the extent of the sexual and
aggressive abuse she suffered as a child. Her mother's failure to
protect her from him and her mother's use of Debbi to placate
him added to her distress. Indeed her mother's refusing to acknowledge the nature of her father's difficulties and her mother's lying both to Debbi and to her father were essential in understanding Debbi's own use of denial.

In the next weeks she focused more on her relationship with
her father. She was surprised to see a repetitive pattern in the
way her father acted. Previously she had tried to deal with and
explain away each separate instance of irrationality and had
never admitted to herself what kind of a person he was—predictably irrational, violent, and abrupt; or silent and withdrawn.
During these moods he would be "unreachable," unable to be
reasoned with or talked with. The transference to me as father
was further clarified: when she couldn't see me, she feared a
sudden violent outburst. As an adult she related that to her own
difficulty in recognizing dangerous situations, for example, her
lack of judgment about her boyfriend's character.

Increasingly she produced evidence of having been severely
abused as a child and of feeling neglected by both parents. She
now realized that they were too involved with each other to
notice her, and saw her mother as quite different, warmer, more
direct, and more available when her father was away.

Debbi also puzzled over why, as things got better in her external world during the second year of analysis, she had become
more and more anxious and uneasy and retreated more into "a
certain state of mind" in the analysis. She had struggled with her

idea that analysis was supposed to help her "feel more secure, be more successful in reaching her goals," and recognized a foreboding that in the past, whenever her life had been free of chaos, a disaster had happened. She cited first her boyfriend's death just when she was preparing for college, and then David's death as they began to talk about marriage. She finally recalled her father's appearing, disappearing, and reappearing in her life as a small child just when things seemed settled and secure, the uprooting of the family that accompanied his coming and goings, and the sudden violent rages which might appear just when he seemed silent or calm. She had been convinced that keeping chaos in the analysis would not only keep me in closer contact with her but would forestall the peaceful time which came before disaster.

She now recognized that she saw herself as being in two states—one where she felt "rational, comfortable"; the other, the "ready alert state." Certainly both were evident in the way she interacted with me during the analytic hours. A third way of being, "the drowsy state," which she invoked when she felt endangered but helpless to escape, when she felt like she was floating near the ceiling, resembled self-hypnosis.

Debbi began to conceptualize the difference in the ways she felt and to describe them more clearly. When Debbi confronted a "paradoxical situation" where she did know how the other person would react, she entered a "ready alert state": "It begins with a physical feeling, in my stomach; it spreads to my chest; my mind becomes filled with possibilities, gets more and more confusing and upsetting; then I don't ask questions because I feel I already know the answers; that part of me handles difficult situations. The only thing then that's important is the other person, their feelings, how they'll react." This was the terrified state of mind in which she had focused on the "structure" in the analysis.

In associating to the drowsy state, Debbi reworked a series of memories centering around the "drowsy" time in the crib. She described herself as intolerant of restraint—or anesthesia— struggling to come out of confinement or anesthesia as soon as possible. An earlier memory related to this.

She had first recovered it early in our work in associating to a disturbing recurrent dream. She dreamed of "scratching pimples and having insects come out." In the spring of the year when she was 3 and living at the farm, her father came to visit. Her parents and siblings went out, leaving her alone. She decided to feed her pet bird (a baby bird they had found), but it didn't seem hungry; then she gave it a bath. When the family came home the bird was dead; her brother blamed her for its death. She felt misunderstood. Her brother buried the bird in the garden. She found it hard to believe the bird was really dead. She crept out into the garden and dug it up—and was horrified to find it covered with maggots. She then felt the dream expressed her guilt and horror about killing the bird.

She now added that at first she had thought the bird was asleep, not dead, and that it was her father's bird. Still later Debbi said that her father, not her brother, in a rage, had accused her of purposely drowning the bird. It was hard for her, at age 3, to understand how the bath was related to the "asleep"/dead bird or even what it meant to be dead. For many years thereafter, she became phobic herself about taking a bath.

In this series of dreams and memories, Debbi connected being drowsy with being "hurt in a special way"; both were related to her memory of the crib, of the "friendly doctor," abortion, and babies being killed. Her mother now told her that they had considered aborting her; both parents claimed it was the other's idea. We connected all of this with her fear of letting herself free associate, "become drowsy," lying on the couch.

Further clarification of Debbi's difficulty lying on the couch occurred about 2 months after she sat up in association to a dream that she was sitting on the couch and I was sitting in my chair. She remembered often lying on her stomach on the couch in the den at home watching TV. Her father sat in his chair where she could watch him (the position she assumed the first hour of the analysis). In this context Debbi stressed how "out of touch" her father was when angry—silent, inaccessible to reason or communication. She also remarked how anxious and preoc-cupied her mother became when her father was angry and how her mother was unable to confront him. Rather she dealt with him by being indirect, lying, or sending Debbi to deal with him. Debbi connected this—again—with her provoking me and her silent boyfriends with her indirect yet persistent questioning and with her alertness to visual cues.

Like Silber's patient (1977), Debbi was talented in art and her vision was constitutionally unusually acute (20/14). She felt that if she glanced at me at the beginning or end of the session, she would see many "clues" to how I was feeling. She asserted that this was "against the rules" while she was using the couch, although she desperately wanted the reassurance of seeing me. Debbi also was convinced that words often belied emotional states, so that it was necessary to rely on vision. Thus, Debbi was gifted with both keen vision and had life experiences which reinforced her reliance on her vision. She learned to distrust verbal information; for example, when she was told by her mother that she would not be getting a shot, yet had seen the needle being prepared and placed on the bedside table. She described this with anger at her mother for trying to deceive her and with despair that her mother, since she was pretending nothing was going to hurt Debbi, could not comfort her.

After sitting up Debbi described a recurrent nightmare she had had since childhood—a frightened feeling that someone or something which might be dangerous was standing beside her bed or just outside the door, but of being unable to wake up or open her eyes to check out whether the "thing" was friend or foe. Her "dream" then turned to focus on the terrifying struggle to wake up, open her eyes or move; she was, of course, able to hear (pavor nocturnus).[4] As Freud (1900) and Shopper (1978) have pointed out, audition is the sense organ of sleep. Debbi had powerful experiences of being able to hear but "not wake up or move," times when she felt terrified. Again a constitutional vulnerability to this sleep disorder related to her difficulty in lying on the couch, reinforcing her sense of helplessness.

---

4. Debbi described night terrors (pavor nocturnus) which occur in stage IV sleep. This state is characterized by paralysis of voluntary musculature, extreme autonomic arousal, and often a brief frightening thought, such as the idea of an intruder. Treatment is by medication, such as diazepam, to suppress stage IV sleep (Linn, 1980). It was interesting that Debbi used alcohol—a hypnotic which affects stage IV sleep—to induce sleep when she was feeling anxious.

Debbi continued to work productively twice a week sitting up for 2 years.

DISCUSSION

Three sets of circumstances converged to make work lying down on the couch particularly intense and problematic for Debbi:

1. A history of growing up with an abusive father and a mother who denied the father's pathology. Experiences of separation, physical confinement, and overstimulation as a child predisposed her to defensive use of splitting and an altered state (Fliess, 1953; Shengold, 1963, 1967, 1971; Dickes, 1965).

2. A particular history of trauma connected with being in a reclining position, and an association of lying down with the special altered state of mind.

3. A constitutionally keen vision, with a reliance on visual and nonverbal rather than auditory cues.

The real nature of Debbi's preverbal trauma—separation from her mother—had not been immediately evident in the history. She was alone with her mother until age 18 months. Debbi's considerable strengths may have dated in part from having this time away from her psychotic father. Her father returned from the service and lived with the family until she was 2½. As with so many of her memories, further understanding of the circumstances turned what had seemed an apparent positive family reunion into a time of deprivation and anxiety. Her father's rages and outbursts and her mother's anxious preoccupation with his depression brought Debbi's at first repressed early memories of being neglected, not listened to, and injured into focus.

Developmentally, 18 months was the rapprochement phase (Mahler et al., 1975) when the child began actively to explore her own motor skills and to be able to move away from the mother. Her father's reentry at this developmental stage also must have colored Debbi's sense of the importance of her locomotion and her wish to keep her mother in view.

Debbi's later experiences in the middle of the oedipal period at age 4 reinforced this early loss. Her separation from her maternal grandparents and her mother when they moved away

from the farm in the reunion with her father, immediately followed by her illness, confinement to bed, and move to another
city all repeated the earlier trauma.

Her memory of the hospital was a screen memory, perhaps
condensing several episodes of traumatization by her father.
Her need for a "good" parent to comfort her after the attack by
the "bad" one also was clear in her revision of the memory to
include the "kind stranger." Her way of dealing with me while
on the couch was characteristic of children of psychotic parents
who defensively lapse into an altered state (Shengold, 1967,
1971) in which they become unable or unwilling to connect cause
and effect, and instead concentrate their attention on responding to the dangerous parent. Dickes (1965) described similar
defensive use of altered states of consciousness to ward off sexual or aggressive affects, particularly in patients who experienced
sexual or aggressive trauma as children. Debbi came to realize
that she was seldom in a state of alertness. What she had previously considered a state of alertness was really a mild hypnoid
state (Dickes, 1965, p. 392).

She had a series of memories: the dead/asleep baby bird, the
quiet/dying little girl in the next hospital bed, her suicidal boyfriend, her abortion of a dead fetus, and finally her boyfriend's
death and the truck hitting her car from behind. All repeated
the same themes of sudden (unexpected) death and murderous
violence.

Vision assumed a particular importance for Debbi, both in the
early visual union with mother which was prematurely interrupted; and in vigilantly watching her father, using eye contact
both to cajole him out of depressed moods and to be alert to a
sudden shift of his mood into violence or rage.

Her constitutionally keen vision and vulnerability to pavor
nocturnus interacted with particular traumatic and overstimulating experiences in early life, contributing to her inability
to tolerate the deprivation of visual contact and the position of
lying on the couch. The silence of the analyst then became anxiety-provoking. On the other hand, she was better able to tolerate my silences and lack of auditory contact when in visual contact with me.

She has been able to use treatment well with the therapist as a transference object. She was not able to use auditory closeness but responded to being able to see me. Her particular history sensitized her to the couch and lying down as especially dangerous and predisposed her to retreat to an altered state.

> Thus, it may be that we should not place too much emphasis on the patient's ability to tolerate the visual deprivation of the couch. In some cases this may be indicative of a weak ego or significant ego deficiencies which would preclude an analytic approach; in other instances there may be special genetic or developmental circumstances making contact via audition conflict-laden, or where vision, for multiple reasons, is the modality of choice and audition has not been relied on as a modality of contact [Shopper, 1978, p. 299].

This case raises technical questions about the analytic setting beyond the scope of this paper. Perhaps most significant is whether this depth and kind of work could have been done at all without some time on the couch.

Finally, this case suggests that a period of analysis which seems to be leading toward a negative therapeutic reaction may be in fact not barren ground but capable of yielding a bountiful analytic harvest.

BIBLIOGRAPHY

BIBRING, G. L. (1936). A contribution to the subject of transference resistance. *Int. J. Psychoanal.*, 17:181–189.

DICKES, R. (1965). The defensive function of an altered state of consciousness. *J. Amer. Psychoanal. Assn.*, 13:356–403.

EDELSON, M. (1985). Personal communication.

FLIESS, R. (1953). The hypnotic evasion. *Psychoanal. Q.*, 22:497–511.

FREUD, S. (1900). The interpretation of dreams. *S.E.*, 4 & 5.

_____ (1913). On beginning the treatment. *S.E.*, 12:133–134.

GREENACRE, P. (1954). The role of transference. *J. Amer. Psychoanal. Assn.*, 2:671–684.

_____ (1980). Certain technical problems in the transference relationship. In *Psychoanalytic Explorations of Technique*, ed. Harold P. Blum, pp. 419–440. New York: Int. Univ. Press.

GREENSON, R. R. (1965). The working alliance and the transference neurosis. *Psychoanal. Q.*, 34:155–181.

_____ (1967). *The Technique and Practice of Psychoanalysis*. New York: Univ. Press.

KHAN, M. R. (1962). Dream psychology and the evolution of the psycho-analytic situation. *Int. J. Psychoanal.,* 43:21–31.

KRIS, E. (1956). The recovery of childhood memories. *Psychoanal. Study Child,* 11:54–88.

LINN, L. (1980). Clinical manifestations of psychiatric disorders. In *Comprehensive Textbook of Psychiatry,* ed. H. Kaplan, A. Freedman, & B. Sadock, 3rd ed., p. 1009. Baltimore: Williams & Wilkins.

LIPTON, S. D. (1977). The advantages of Freud's technique as shown in his analysis of the rat man. *Int. J. Psychoanal.,* 58:255–273.

MACALPINE, I. (1950). The development of transference. *Psychoanal. Q.,* 19:501–539.

MAHLER, M. S., PINE, F., & BERGMAN, A. (1975). *The Psychological Birth of the Human Infant.* New York: Basic Books.

ORENS, M. H. (1965). Setting a termination date. *J. Amer. Psychoanal. Assn.,* 3:651–665.

SHENGOLD, L. (1963). The parent as sphinx. *J. Amer. Psychoanal. Assn.,* 11:725–751.

———— (1967). The effect of overstimulation. *Int. J. Psychoanal.,* 48:403–415.

———— (1971). More about rats and rat people. *Int. J. Psychoanal.,* 52:277–288.

SHOPPER, M. (1978). The role of audition in the early psychic development. *J. Amer. Psychoanal. Assn.,* 26:283–310.

SILBER, A. (1977). The alcohol induced hypnoid state and its analytic corollary. *Int. J. Psychoanal. Psychother.,* 6:253–267.

SPITZ, R. A. (1956). Transference. *Int. J. Psychoanal.,* 37:380–385.

STERBA, R. (1929). The dynamics of the dissolution of the transference-resistance. *Psychoanal. Q.,* 9 (1940):363–379.

WEISSMAN, S. M. (1977). Face to Face. *Psychoanal. Study Child,* 32:421–450.

The Specter of Genetic Illness and Its Effects on Development

JUDITH A. YANOF, M.D.

IN RECENT YEARS CONSIDERABLE ATTENTION HAS BEEN GIVEN TO the issue of female sexual development. This has meant another look at prevailing theories and observational data on children. While we struggle to answer questions about the normal process of female development and its variations, we look to our psychoanalytic work with children to see if it affords us any clues that might help in this investigation.

This paper describes the analysis of a latency girl. Her family was very concerned that she might develop a hereditary deforming bone disease which her father had. As is likely, her parents gave her conflicting messages about whether this disease was a major problem. This girl had significant concerns about being damaged, and at the time her analysis began had failed to consolidate an age-appropriate female identity. She also had a learning inhibition and an inhibition of physical activity, both of which significantly interfered with her development.

Recent papers about gender identity development suggest that girls, from birth, begin a learning process from their parents and the environment that decisively determines their sense

Member, Boston Psychoanalytic Institute and Society; faculty, Psychoanalytic Institute of New England, East.

I would like to thank Drs. Anna Wolff and Herbert Goldings for numerous helpful suggestions and criticisms during the writing of this paper. Drs. Robert Gardner, Alexandra Harrison, and Morris Stambler also provided helpful comments. This paper was presented as the Annual Beata Rank Lecture in Child Analysis before the Boston Psychoanalytic Society and Institute on November 28, 1984.

of themselves as female. This has been called "primary femininity" and "core gender identity," and arises in the first year of life
(Stoller, 1968; Money and Ehrhardt, 1972; Kleeman, 1976).
Roiphe and Galenson (1981) conclude that during the second
half of the second year of life, there is a divergent sexual development for male and female children, organized around their
reactions to the anatomical sexual differences. They observed
distinctly recognizable castration reactions among girls, ranging
from mild and transient to severe and permanent. Roiphe and
Galenson observed that more severe castration reactions occurred in children who had an uncertain and fluctuating outline
of their bodies as a consequence of a birth defect, severe bodily
illness, or surgical intervention.

Harrison (1984) described her therapy with two 5-year-old
girls who had hand deformities. The physical defect became the
organizing factor for each child's sexual development. It was
confused with defective genitalia and interfered with each
child's attempt to identify with her mother and consolidate a
feminine identity.

Although the girl I am discussing did not in fact have a visible
body defect, there was a very real possibility that she might develop a bone disease that would manifest itself at some point
during her childhood before she reached puberty. It is my hypothesis that her family's understandable concern about and
attention to her body contributed to an early lack of stability in
her body image that had consequences for her later development. Anthony (1968) has stated that the body image is not
merely an "accurate mental representation of the individual's
body structure," but is a flexible, dynamic picture created by
everything affecting the individual, including "constitutional
factors, sensory impressions, environmental attitudes, together
with the person's interpretation of these influences and their
integration into his [or her] personality" (p. 1104f.).

Peter Blos (1960) in a paper on the psychological consequences of cryptorchism talks of how a "distorted, vague, and
incomplete body image exerted its pathological influence on ego
development" (p. 427). Blos feels that cryptorchism lends itself
to a situation in which the body image remains vague and indefi-
nite because of the uncertainty about when the testes might

descend spontaneously. All three children presented by Blos had learning difficulties and memory disturbances that involved forgetting as well as problems with sexual identity. The girl I am presenting experienced a similar uncertainty about her body because there was continually a question about whether a genetic disease would manifest itself. Her symptoms were remarkably similar to those described by Blos.

I will try to show through selected analytic material that Katie's body image was fraught with confusion and that she had a deep-seated fear that she was damaged. Katie used the imagery of castration and the anatomical sexual differences to express her concern about her body. Since Katie equated her sense of herself as damaged with being female, she had difficulty accepting a feminine identity and did not want to become a woman. At the same time, she was fearful of her identification with her father, who was afflicted with a genetic illness, and this fear prevented her from using normal latency sublimations because she labeled them masculine. Katie developed a defensive style in which she avoided seeing things clearly, and this contributed to a learning inhibition.

CASE REPORT

BACKGROUND

Katie was the oldest of three daughters, born to a family who had moved several years before from a city in the Southwest. Also living with the family was a maternal grandmother who had held a position of considerable prominence in that city.

Katie was originally referred to me at age 9 years by her pediatrician, who had seen her over the previous year for numerous physical complaints, including leg pains, hip pains, headaches, and eye pains. None of these symptoms could be found to have a physical basis. Both of Katie's parents were caring and involved. However, they felt overwhelmed by Katie's complaints. They were frightened that the doctors might be overlooking an important physical illness.

Katie was born by Caesarean section due to a breech presentation. The parents were told that Katie had a "hip problem" at birth for which exercises were prescribed. However, there was no mention of this on the birth record. Katie's development was otherwise normal.

Katie's father had a hereditary bone disease. This illness had resulted in several childhood bone operations and the permanent foreshortening of his left leg. To the casual observer a minor abnormality in gait was noticeable. This genetic illness had a high degree of penetrance and many members of his family had it. He was quite concerned lest his children be affected by this same condition that could, in its more severe forms, lead to disfigurement. It was the family's understanding that this illness could affect any of the long bones at any time during the period of active bone growth. From the time of Katie's infancy the father often checked her bones, running his fingers over the bone shafts to see if he could detect any abnormal growth spurs. The parents shared the same concern for Katie's two sisters.

When Katie was 5, she complained of hip pain, and it was belatedly discovered that she had streptococcal synovitis in her right hip. At that time, she was hospitalized and was placed in a body cast for 6 weeks. Although one parent had been with her at all times during the hospitalization, several painful procedures were performed and the body cast immobilized her. Yet the father remarked, with some degree of puzzlement, that Katie looked back on this time with nostalgia, and even now seemed gleeful when she reported a new symptom.

Katie's parents told me that her behavior was difficult at home, and had been so since the birth of her younger sister when she was 2½. She had temper tantrums and was stubborn and slow moving. She verbally tormented this younger sister, and was nasty to her father whom she devalued. She had a less provocative, but somewhat clingy and regressed relationship with her mother.

In school, although Katie got average marks, her work was painstakingly slow. She had great anxiety about tests and assignments, and dealt with this by "forgetting," putting things off indefinitely, and most recently by having physical symptoms. She hated to be seen as not knowing something and tried to cover up her deficiencies. She needed a parent at her side coaxing her along to produce any homework. Her learning was inhibited by a forgetting of facts and a reliance on global impressions without an attention to detail.

Katie had psychological testing before the analysis began. This showed moderate compromises in intellectual functioning. She had great difficulty with the coding and picture completion subtests. Projective tests indicated that she had a hysterical neurosis with major inhibitions in motor function.

Katie's father was a successful lawyer and a rather striking-looking man, tall and full-bearded. Her mother was a mathematics teacher whose return to full-time work after an academic leave coincided with Katie's many somatic complaints. Both parents had a long-standing interest in the handicapped whom they overtly accepted. At the same time a persistent vigilance and fear about the father's genetic illness remained part of the family dynamic.

Katie had known the medical facts about her father's bone disease for some time and was well aware that she might inherit his illness. While consciously minimizing any discomfort, she routinely checked her bones. It seemed clear that the uncertainty about whether she carried this "bad gene" and the ways it had become tied symbolically to other concerns about herself played a major part in this elusive, yet persistent, defective self image.

THINGS ARE NOT WHAT THEY SEEM

From the beginning of the analysis, Katie made clear that she saw herself as damaged, missing something, and a "have-not." In her play some body defect or injury always befell one of her characters. Her early experience of her treatment was that she was being seen because there was something wrong with her that needed fixing. However, the actual nature of the defect remained vague and elusive.

Shortly after her treatment began, there was a session in which Katie picked up the baby doll and said, "The baby is sick. I'll be the mother and you be the doctor." When I agreed, she said in a snooty, high-pitched voice that she had come to have her baby "fixed." "The baby cries all the time. Her leg is broken, I think." As I began to examine the baby's leg that I was told wasn't working in a variety of ways, the baby suddenly started dancing and jumping around, obviously having made a spontaneous recovery. Then Katie went through a similar sequence with the baby's arm and its eye. I was by now somewhat puzzled. Katie said, "It's a head problem, no, a headache problem, no, a head problem. Can't you tell?!" At this point she sounded quite exasperated and her voice was at its snootiest. "The baby has HIPSALOSIS!" I had to concede that I was not all that familiar with hipsalosis, and I asked Katie to tell me about it. "It's a strange disease," she said. "It comes from too much jumping around." "Jumping?" I asked. "No, not really, she had poisoned milk when she was little." "Oh," I said, "something happened when she was little?" Katie changed her mind again and said, "No. She inherited it. She was born with it." Then Katie turned into the snooty mother again and said in a demeaning way, "You are the one who is crazy! Not my baby! You are not even a doctor! It is obvious that there is nothing wrong with my baby. Look how fine she is!" After this attack, Katie looked a little sad, and began to put the doll away.

This doll play was an accurate representation of Katie's own symptoms, and of the sense of confusion and frustration that they caused in the family. At first, I saw the doll's spontaneous recoveries as a defensive denial of her thoughts about being damaged, and the painful affects that must have accompanied them. However, as time went on I realized that Katie was trying to tell me something more specific. Over and over again, in one form or another, she was trying to tell me: things are not what they seem.

There was a true confusion about whether something was wrong with Katie. Although her body seemed fine, it might be carrying a bad gene. This confusion and unease had occurred from the very earliest times, before Katie had an organizational context in which to put her concerns. What was wrong with her body became confused with the other things she worried might be wrong with her. For instance, her concerns about the badness of her aggressive and sexual fantasies became fused with concerns about her health.

Things not being what they seemed reflected a central confusion about her father. In Katie's child's-eye view, father's damage was greater than in the view of the world at large, where he was seen as "okay," even successful. After all, she was privy to a more exposed view of his body and subject to the influence of his unconscious feelings as well. The parents' overt response to father's handicap was that it didn't matter at all, but this was discordant with the family's unconscious response of fear and shame. This became clear to me as I watched them handle issues around Katie's psychiatric treatment. Overtly they advocated and supported it wholeheartedly, yet they were very ashamed to tell anyone about it. This attitude was communicated to Katie but in a way that she was not able to acknowledge and contributed to her confusion. In the midst of seeming openness, there was no permission to talk about certain aspects of the parents' own feeling about defect. This functioned like a family secret. There was a covert message in the family to "not know" certain things.

Curiosity begins as a physical curiosity that later gets sublimated and is enlarged to include the rest of the world (Pearson, 1952). When looking at one's own body is conflict-ridden, curiosity may be inhibited. Over the years Katie had adopted a pattern of not looking at things too closely, not remembering, and not striving to reconcile conflicting information. This pattern had been incorporated into a characteristic defensive style. In her play the ground was constantly shifting. Things changed fluidly without any attempt on Katie's part to make a coherent story or to integrate the disparate strands. A corollary was Katie's difficulty in talking about the real events of her life. She seldom did, but when she did, she had a vague, disconnected way of relating things that left out important affects or important facts, so that one missed the heart of the matter. This defensive pattern became part of her cognitive style and affected her learning. Her need to keep conflicting ideas apart and unintegrated and her need to avoid the unpleasant interfered in her work, particularly in areas where her psychological conflicts had more impact.

Over and over again, during Katie's play, I drew her attention to her shift of ground and wondered with her what thought or feeling had preceded this shift. While the analysis of this defense was at first resisted, ultimately this activity became a very important basis of our alliance. The analysis came to represent the seeking of the truth. Analysis was the place where we could talk directly, where things were what they seemed to be. Moreover, as the defense was analyzed, her vagueness disappeared and her learning slowly improved.

Although Katie at times denied any worries, she presented herself as defective and inadequate. She was constantly riddled with physical aches and pains. This exaggerated focus on her body and its functioning mimicked in an uncanny way the very concerns she and her parents were most worried about. Yet, it had both an adaptive and defensive function. Using this sick self, Katie managed to get certain regressive needs met while avoiding more conflicted positions. Being little and sick, she could avoid being angry and competitive.

Once the analysis started Katie's need to be sick at home quickly lessened and was transferred into the analytic hours. As the analysis deepened, rarely an hour went by without Katie talking about a physical complaint of one kind or another. Sometimes she twisted her leg and limped in. Sometimes she had pains that made her miserable. Sometimes there were blisters, cuts, or moles to be looked at. At times she used me as a medical consultant. At other times her complaints were a ritualistic beginning to the hours, a rite of entry, so to speak, that she mentioned with little affect.

In Katie's play, becoming sick had a prominent place as well. One frequent character is her play was a little girl whose mother was a famous and busy surgeon. In order to get this mother's attention, the little girl would resort to falling off the roof, breaking her leg, and needing an operation performed by mother. This also involved immobilization in a cast. Later in the analysis when Katie became more involved in triadic concerns, the same girl returned with the same solution, but to a whole new set of problems. Falling off the roof then brought the parents back from a second honeymoon or kept the father from having an affair with a prostitute. It was clear that getting sick covered a variety of affects. Katie's characters got sick when they were angry, when they were lonely, when they were jealous, and when they did not want to compete.

As time went on Katie and I developed our own language of affects to share her experiences. I began to point out to her that her characters were very good at getting sick, but didn't know how to get angry or sad or frightened. Katie and I then began to notice how she often felt sick instead of feeling certain feelings. Eventually a new character appeared, a ridiculous mother who always said, "Get the thermometer," whenever her child was emotionally upset. On one level this meant that Katie felt that the kind of self most acceptable to her mother was a sick self. On another level, this mother represented a part of Katie that could not tolerate her own affects and I saw this character as an acknowledgment of my interpretations. As the mother grew more ridiculous over time, it showed Katie's capacity to use her sense of humor to deal with a troubling aspect of herself.

One day, Katie walked into her analytic hour saying she had a headache and had gone to the school nurse. The nurse reprimanded her and sent her back to class. In the session, Katie attached all the magic markers end to end in a long polelike structure that bent precariously because of its length. She put it in her pants leg and said that it was a "bum" leg. She pretended that she was a woman and that there was nothing wrong with her leg, although it kept breaking. She told me, in an aside, that the leg was an artificial limb, but she had the woman deny this in the play. Evidently when the woman was 3, she and her mother had been in a car accident. Because she was 3, she assumed the leg was real, just like anyone else's. Her mother had never told her the truth about her leg. Katie coached me to confront the woman who became angrier and angrier, saying that there was nothing wrong with her. In fact she said that she was special. Her mother told her that she had extra powers; that if she touched someone with her leg, she could read their minds.

It turned out that, prior to Katie's headache, the class had been dissecting a frog that she thought was "yukky." In the session, she revealed a clear association between the frog dissection and mother's "cut" from her Caesarean births. This stirred several masochistic and sadistic fantasies involving the pregnant mother and unborn child. The anxiety accompanying these fantasies caused Katie to leave the dissection room "sick." This anxiety also gave rise to the particular defensive organization that appeared in the hour: a restitutive fantasy of being special.

The most intense affect of the hour came when Katie communicated through the lady with the "bum" leg the vital connection between being special and being handicapped, a position authorized by mother, at least according to Katie's story. There was no comfort in this position as the truth was constantly making itself apparent; the leg kept breaking off. Nevertheless, in order to stay attached to her mother, the woman had to stay in the 3-year-old position of giving up her own truth. This material reflected Katie's view that her mother valued being little, sick, and not knowing more than she valued being independent and assertive.

While this material indicated Katie's identification with her father in sharing the "bum" leg, Katie also presented the damaged aspect of her self in this sexual imagery. The woman is "missing" a leg and only has a "bum." In the story this is presumably her mother's fault. In order to keep the attachment to her mother she must avoid the knowledge of this loss and the feelings about it. She puts a phallic object into her pants to replace what is missing and erase the specter of the cut body.

WO-MAN: A DILEMMA OF SEXUAL IDENTITY

Katie's uncertainty about her body image and the association she makes between herself as damaged and herself as female had far-reaching consequences for her feminine development. One day, Katie came into the office and began to make a bird with a large beak out of clay. She had a great deal of difficulty forming one of the wings. She wanted the wings to be exactly the same, but one was always too small. The sex of the bird went through several changes before she called her Mrs. Robin consistently. Mrs. Robin started off as a traditional enough female bird. She built a nest and laid eggs. However, it soon became clear that Mrs. Robin was not interested in the task of sitting on the eggs. She instead was lured on by the wish to have great flying adventures.

It turned out that Mrs. Robin could fly in all sorts of daring ways, with fancy swoops and dives, that Katie performed with great abandon and joy. Katie confided to me that Mrs. Robin was quite like a male bird in this respect, because normally females could not do such things. I was very interested in the differences between the males and females. Mrs. Robin was a lawyer bird, and the purpose of these flights was to pick up evidence for her trials. She had been taught these special male skills by her devoted father.

At one point Katie had some second thoughts about leaving the eggs unattended, and she made a small Mr. Robin that had no beak to do this job. Suddenly in the middle of one excited swoop, Mrs. Robin dropped from the air, damaging her wing. I wondered what had happened. "She fell out of the air," said Katie. "She saw something that made her fall. The shock of it. It was a monster." "What kind of monster?" "A monster with only one eye. No. A monster with no nose. Something weird. Crazy. It was retarded." When I asked what that shocked feeling was like, Katie said, "I don't know. But she will have to stay home and be a regular woman now. She will never fly again." Katie stopped playing. I said, "You look sad. It makes you feel bad when you think about something hurt that can't be fixed. Like something lost forever." Katie said thoughtfully but without much conviction, "Well, maybe her wing will heal." Mrs. Robin did fly again, but her injured wing remained a handicap.

Katie's view of being female was synonymous with being damaged, second class, and locked into passivity: in short, something to be avoided. What Katie longed to do, the fancy swooping and diving, was, as she saw it, off limits for women and for men only. In her play, Katie maintained the fantasy that she could do whatever the men did and even more. The incredible dives had an overcompensatory quality, and it was Mrs. Robin who had the long beak. However, she could not give herself up to this fantasy completely because on some level she knew the truth about her anatomy. When she least expected it, Mrs. Robin was confronted by the "reality" of her own missing part in the form of the one-eyed, no-nosed, no-brained monster. There was, moreover, some sense that she could become further damaged from all this activity.

Under some conditions, rejecting her femininity might not have been so difficult for Katie to manage during her latency, before the full onslaught of adolescent sexual demands. Some girls become tomboys. They have little difficulty during this phase in their lives socially because they tend to be accepted by boys and girls alike. But for Katie this was impossible. She needed to put great restraint on any activity designated by her as phallic. Sports and learning were both libidinized and dealt with by severe inhibition. There were at least two reasons for this: for one, earlier unresolved aggressive conflicts were fused with these phallic aims, and, for another, Katie was as fearful of identifying with a man as with a woman. Seeing her father as damaged made a male identification as dangerous and unacceptable as a female identification. Katie seemed to see her choice as organizing herself around a damaged female configuration or a damaged male configuration.

Katie's dilemma was illustrated in the following material. She drew a picture of two sisters. She then drew the girls' mother who was strong and muscular, looking like a man, or as Katie elaborated a "Wo-Man," part man and part woman. The father came last and was a tiny, effeminate man. Katie said that the mother was happy as a Wo-Man, but she wanted her daughters to be "regular," because she thought that they would be happier. The younger girl who got good marks was a tomboy, who climbed trees and did boys' things, and wanted to be a Wo-Man like her mother. The other girl wanted to be "regular" and have dates, but she had a terrible case of acne. Being strong and active, on the one hand, and being attractive to men, on the other, seemed mutually exclusive. However, for Katie the real problem was not that she had to choose between them, but that she could not choose either of them. Each position carried too many dangers. She was truly stuck in the limbo of Wo-Man: neither man nor woman.

THE OEDIPAL TRIANGLE

In normal development a girl turns to her father in order to mitigate her disappointments with a mother who is not all that she wants her to be. Katie did not have an idealized father to turn to. She was as angry with her father as with her mother. Men were the givers of bad seeds and were the source of troubles as frequently as were mothers in Katie's fantasies. This left Katie stuck with more aggression and with less to do about it than otherwise might have been the case.

As I listened to Katie, I became increasingly aware that while there were phallic women, damaged women, damaged men, and a few boys, there was no intact masculine man. There was no idealized oedipal father anywhere in the early material. It was only through the work of analysis that Katie's father was gradually rehabilitated.

The following segment of a session was a precursor of the eventual change in Katie's view of her father. Katie began to draw a squiggle that she made into a pig. She said, "This is his tail. It covers him up. He is hiding." I wondered what he was hiding. "This! He has one big ear and one small ear. Well it's normal to have one ear shorter than the other. But his ear is very short, too short. It's an irregular ear." I asked if the pig were hiding his ear because he was embarrassed. "Oh no," said Katie, "There is a very wicked king who will kill him if he finds out about his ear. The king is prejudiced and he feels everyone should be perfect." It turned out that the pig was the king's long-lost brother and so when the king found out about the pig's ear he did not kill him. "In fact," Katie said, "in a long time from now the king will die. Then all the king's jewels will go to the pig, and the pig will take back the law that persecutes people with short ears. Then all the people with short ears will come out of hiding. And, do you know what, there are an awful lot of them."

In this story Katie and her father are the long-lost brothers. Katie had her own wicked king inside that persecuted both herself and her father for not being perfect. Yet Katie's strength clearly lay in her ability to understand the proper solution to her dilemma and to work toward that end. There will come a time, she said, when the wicked king will die and the pig can live in peace with his imperfections like everyone else. Katie saw her analysis as enabling her to achieve that end.

The improvement in Katie's view of her father went hand in hand with the improvement in her own self-esteem. As the analysis progressed, oedipal figures began to emerge. During this part of her analysis Katie wrote the diary of a Pilgrim girl she called Rebecca who lived with her mother and father. At the beginning of the story Rebecca befriends an Indian family or, more correctly, a father and daughter, Big Rein and Little Deer. Big Rein is very big and powerful. He teaches Rebecca how to grow corn, how to hunt and fish, and how to read all the wonderful secrets of nature. This enables her to take part in his world as well as her own. She in turn teaches Little Deer how to read and embroider. As time passes, Rebecca's father gets pneumonia and dies. Rebecca now must provide for herself and her mother. She is able to survive because of the vast knowledge she has acquired from Big Rein, and this is how Katie ends the story. However, in the session she said, "I was actually thinking of having Rebecca's mother die too. Then Rebecca could go off with Big Rein. But when I asked my mother about that ending, she said I shouldn't make it too tragic, so I left it the way it was."

In this story Katie, as Rebecca, chooses to remain in the masculine position with her mother, but she is now flirting with alternatives. As Katie suggested to me, it was her mother's need to keep her close that stopped her from going off with the man. Nevertheless, a large part of Katie's inability to move forward in her female development was her difficulty in leaving behind certain aspects of her dependency on her mother. Her behavior toward her mother was negativistic, but not autonomous. She was unable to enter a more separate, competitive relationship with mother.

A large portion of the analysis resided in the territory of this early relationship with her mother. During the analyst's pregnancy, through the vehicle of the transference, many of Katie's anal-sadistic fantasies and preoccupations were elaborated. Mother's Caesarean scar was evidence to Katie not only that mother was as damaged as father, but that Katie was responsible for this damage. A family "joke" had it that Katie had been "too stubborn" to turn herself around and had therefore caused this surgical assault to her mother.

In her analysis at this time Katie had a dream: "Two women were walking across an ice-skating rink. One woman was old and one was young. Suddenly a hockey player came along, knocked them down, and cut both of them with the blade of his skate. The younger one was only hurt in the leg, but the older woman was severed in two and died." Katie associated to her mother's Caesarean scar that looked like she "had been cut in two" and to the mother of a girl in her class who had had a mastectomy and then died.

There followed a period in which Katie relived the turmoil attending her younger sister's birth. There was intense anger as well as stubborn battles over appointment times followed by guilt and concern for my welfare. There emerged a plethora of sadistic fantasies to be visited on mothers and babies alike. Katie and I were able to reconstruct her emotional experience when her sister was born and she began the terrible temper tantrums.

One of Katie's stories was that a Mrs. Yanof who had been posing as a Dr. Yanof, a psychiatrist, tricked and manipulated a 3-year-old girl. This evil woman used the magic weapon of truth serum to render the girl passive and helpless. The ongoing saga was of the girl's revenge against Mrs. Yanof that involved cutting her in half and flattening her with a steamroller. This brought retaliations of various sorts, including limb amputations and operations. In these fantasies the various defects encountered were seen and experienced entirely as the result of aggressive acts.

Katie emerged from this period in her analysis more able to relinquish her little girl posture both at home with her mother and in the analysis with me. She began to view both her parents more realistically, seeing them as having their own strengths and weaknesses.

THE APPROACH OF ADOLESCENT SEXUALITY

She now turned to her conflicts over her sexuality. Katie brought in the following dream: "It was very vague. I had the sense that in the dream I did something wrong. I don't know what it was. Monica, my older cousin, was very angry at me. She gave me a dirty look and called me a pig. I think I had stolen something from her. Something valuable. Maybe an antique." Then Katie thought for a while and smiled. "Now I know what I did. I had sex. That was it. I had sex with an older boy and Monica was very mad at me. I think I must have been older too. I asked Monica a question and she could tell I had sex from what I asked. What's strange is that Monica is quite free about sex. She wouldn't be angry with me."

The oedipal nature of the dream was revealed by Katie's sense of badness for stealing someone too old who belonged to someone else. On another level, Katie was now approaching an age where she would have to make her own decisions about whether sex was good or bad. Katie began by saying the dream was "vague" and she didn't know what it was about. As she took an analytic posture, she allowed herself to remember the dream. In the dream asking questions revealed one's wishes and deeds and had the danger of making people angry with her.

As Katie's adolescence approached, I wondered how she would deal with her own body changes. Since preoccupations about height, weight, breast size, and fears about the body's functioning are the "norm" for this stage of development, I wondered how Katie's early unstable body image would affect her. Katie focused on two concerns that seemed related to her earlier preoccupations about getting her father's illness. She noticed that one breast was bigger than the other and worried that it would remain that way. She also worried that she would get scoliosis. She said that she know that this was silly, but she worried about it anyway. She knew the connection was that scoliosis was a bone disease. These worries never overwhelmed Katie's resources.

Katie was interested in being attractive to boys and took pride in her long black hair. Although she felt moderately at ease with boys as friends, she was generally reluctant to participate in heterosexual activities, like parties where kissing games might be played. She reassured herself that she was only 13 and had plenty of time to work this out.

In school she became very interested in a child development course in which she worked with preschool children and made observations about their development. She felt this was connected to her work in analysis. While school had long ago ceased to be an ordeal for Katie, this was the first year she was truly interested in her studies. Although Katie never became an athlete, she participated in physical activities with increasing satisfaction and a new sense that her body was stronger or better than she thought it had been.

At one point during the last half year of analysis, Katie had been rubbing herself between her legs in an offhanded and apparently unaware way while we were talking. When it happened on several occasions, I asked her if perhaps she had wanted to tell me something about touching herself but didn't know how to bring it up. Katie said she thought not, and then said that she had no feeling when she touched herself down there. She had wondered about it, but perhaps it was for the best anyway since she really wasn't old enough for sex.

In the following session, Katie told me that she had changed and that she now enjoyed babysitting for children. She told me that she hated, however, to have to watch Mr. Rogers on television, and she especially hated a song he sang about boys being fancy on the outside and girls being fancy on the inside. She became rather vague and sounded like the Katie of times past. She claimed that she had no idea what the song meant. Finally I told her that the song was about the sexual differences between boys and girls. "Really!" she said in amazement. She was quiet for a while and then she said, "I keep thinking of when I got sick and went to the hospital. For some reason I keep thinking of that. Now I remember. I used to have a big red tractor. It was my favorite toy. I used to straddle it and ride around very fast. I jumped around on it. When I got sick, my parents took it away. You know they took it away when I was in the hospital and they didn't say much. But when I asked about it, they told me that they thought the straddling had made my hip sick." I said to Katie, "Maybe you thought it was the good feelings between your legs when you straddled that made your hip sick. Maybe that's why you are afraid of having too many good feelings there now." Katie looked thoughtful. "I always did a special sign for my hip." She made a circle with the thumb and pointer of her left hand, and put the pointer of her right finger through it and rubbed in a circular motion. "I did a special sign for my hip to show how the bones fit together, but I never knew that meant sex until this year."

In Katie's mind, her sickness was a punishment for her sexual activity and the thoughts that accompanied it. She protected herself from further damage by inhibiting masturbatory impulses and by developing a genital hypesthesia. We can speculate that her immobilization by a body cast that prevented her from touching and jumping was also seen as a punishment made to fit the crime. There also may have been a relationship between this immobilization and Katie's later massive inhibition of body activity.

RESOLUTION

At the time Katie completed her analysis she was almost 14 years and had not yet reached menarche. Although still expressing some fears about growing up, and some fears about growing up without me, Katie generally saw herself on an equal footing with her peers. During one of her last sessions Katie spoke about how she had always felt "behind" her friends, but having an analysis made her feel that she was now ahead of them. She was ahead because she had thought about herself and her life in a way her friends had not. Put in this way, Katie saw her analysis as giving her the "something extra" she had always wanted.

Katie's ideas about her future had changed. She now wanted to have children, not only a career. She felt, however, that unlike her parents, she would stay home more while her children were growing up. She would do this even if it would be hard because she did not want her children to feel lonely like she sometimes did. She wanted to study archaeology and she had a fantasy that her work would lead her to discover a very important skeleton, a skeleton of early man. This discovery might even make her famous one day. In this creative fantasy Katie identified with the analytic work of uncovering and returning to the past in order to find and reconstruct the old bones of her defect. This then became a sublimation that she could pursue with passion.

Katie is a grown woman now. I have not heard from her since her analysis ended. Three years after her termination I ran into Katie quite by accident in a local restaurant. She was with her mother and a Mongoloid girl to whom she introduced me. She explained that she was part of a Big Sister program, evidently for retarded children, and was taking this child out for dinner. I watched her briefly as she tended to this girl in a most caring way.

DISCUSSION

Freud (1925) wrote, "The ego is first and foremost a body ego" (p. 26), by which he meant that the early ego was formed around a core of body experience. Children with congenital or early acquired body defects have distortions of their body image that affect various aspects of their ego functioning.

Although reactions to a congenital or an early acquired defect differ from person to person, some common observations have been made in the literature. Authors have observed that the body defect tends to become the organizing factor around which the body image is formed, and often distorted, and around which ego and superego development take place (Blos, 1960; Niederland, 1965; Harrison, 1984). This can be true whether the defect is big or small, visible or hidden. Often the distortion seems out of proportion to the defect (Niederland, 1965; Harrison, 1984). The defect is experienced as a narcissistic injury, is symbolically equated with badness, and becomes intermingled with other conflictual anxiety, e.g., body disintegration anxiety, castration anxiety (Blos, 1960; Niederland, 1965; Harrison, 1984). Authors mention a strong bisexual elaboration of the defect which tends to interfere with the consolidation of gender identity (Blos, 1960; Lussier, 1960; Niederland, 1965; Harrison, 1984). Another feature observed is the rich and secret fantasy life of such patients which often includes compensatory fantasies of a grandiose and unrealistic nature, such as fantasies of immortality, invincibility, or magical powers (Lussier, 1960; Niederland, 1965). In some cases, these can interfere with reality testing and object relations (Jacobson, 1959; Lussier, 1960; Niederland, 1965). The defect can also be elaborated in terms of sadomasochistic fantasies of mutilation and revenge. Marked disturbances in learning, memory, thinking, and time-space perception were reported in several boys who had cryptorchism (Blos, 1960).

In Katie's situation, not a defect itself, but the anticipation of developing a genetic illness, led to an uncertainty about the intactness of her body. The threat of this defect and the sense of her body self as defective became a central organizing focus around which Katie's development occurred. Phase-specific developmental conflicts were exaggerated or distorted as they became inextricably bound to conflicts about her body. It is in this way that Katie's experience is similar to those children who have had actual defects. The question raised by this paper is whether other children who live in the shadow of a genetic illness are subject to similar influences in their development.

Katie's early experience was one in which there was an understandable focus by her parents (although not by others) on her body. The examination of Katie's bones stirred both painful and pleasurable affects. While this was a form of special attention, the focus of the examination was anxiety-provoking and conflict-ridden. Katie denied these charged affects, but her concerns were apparent in the symbolic representation of her play. Although Katie knew the facts of her father's illness and of her own genetic vulnerability from an early age, paradoxically she remained unclear about whether and in what way she was damaged. She was unable to engage in an ongoing dialogue that would have helped her to clarify and integrate her perceptions as she became cognitively capable of such a task.

Katie developed a defensive pattern in which she kept herself in a state of confusion and avoided looking. This was generalized to many areas of potential curiosity, not just curiosity about her body. It interfered in her learning, in remembering, in attending to detail, and in integrating contradictory data.

Katie's unstable body image interfered with the stage-specific task of acknowledging and coming to terms with the anatomical sexual differences. Katie equated her female anatomy with having a missing body part, a damage, a narcissistic injury. This was associated with a deep-seated sense of inferiority and envy. Conflict about her body was expressed primarily in sexual terms. At the same time, the area of sexual conflict had a sense of concreteness and an added dimension that blocked its resolution. Her father's impaired leg and her mother's Caesarean scar were concrete evidence to Katie that neither had her parents escaped damage.

At age 5, Katie had a traumatic body experience, the streptococcal synovitis, which she interpreted as a further sign of sexual damage. She saw this illness as the consequence of her masturbatory activity and sexual fantasies. Again, she experienced the confusion of sexual conflict and body integrity.

As Katie's development proceeded, she had a serious dilemma in her attempt to consolidate her femininity. Not wanting to accept a femininity that she equated with damage, she held tenaciously to the idea that she did not have to become a woman. She wished instead to be a man or a woman with a penis. However, being a man was equally fraught with danger and damage. She therefore was conflicted about activities she considered masculine, such as learning and sports. Sadistic aggressive fantasies of bodily mutilation and revenge were also attached to competition and physical activity. This was further reason to inhibit these functions. Katie retreated into the symptomatic, but relatively safer, position of being little and sick and Wo-Man, neither man nor woman.

This paper has suggested an analogy between the development of children who have congenital or early acquired defects and those who, like Katie, live in the shadow of genetic illness. The similarity rests on the way in which conflict about the body defect tends to become an organizing factor around which development occurs and becomes confused with other phase-specific developmental conflicts. With further information about other children who anticipate genetic illness, we may learn how much of Katie's experience is in fact generalizable.

BIBLIOGRAPHY

ANTHONY, E. J. (1968). The child's discovery of his body. *Phys. Ther.* 48:1103–1114.
BLOS, P. (1960). Comments on the psychological consequences of cryptorchism. *Psychoanal. Study Child*, 15:395–429.
FREUD, S. (1923). The ego and the id. *S.E.*, 19:3–66.
HARRISON, A. (1984). Body image and self-esteem. In *The Development and Sustaining of Self-Esteem in Childhood*, ed. S. L. Ablon & J. E. Mack, pp. 90–102. New York: Int. Univ. Press.
JACOBSON, E. (1959). The "exceptions." *Psychoanal. Study Child*, 14:135–154.
KLEEMAN, J. A. (1976). Freud's views on early female sexuality in the light of direct child observation. *J. Amer. Psychoanal. Assn. Suppl.*, 24:3–27.
LUSSIER, A. (1960). The analysis of a boy with a congenital deformity. *Psychoanal. Study Child*, 15:430–453.
MONEY, J. & EHRHARDT, A. A. (1972). *Man and Woman, Boy and Girl.* Baltimore: Johns Hopkins Univ. Press.
NIEDERLAND, W. G. (1965). Narcissistic ego impairment in patients with early physical malformations. *Psychoanal. Study Child*, 20:518–534.
PEARSON, G. H. J. (1952). A survey of learning difficulties in children. *Psychoanal. Study Child*, 7:322–386.

ROIPHE, H. (1979). A theoretical overview of preoedipal development during the first four years of life. In *Basic Handbook of Child Psychiatry*, ed. J. D. Noshpitz, pp. 118–126. New York: Basic Books.

ROIPHE, H. & GALENSON, E. (1981). *Infantile Origins of Sexual Identity*. New York: Int. Univ. Press.

STOLLER, R. J. (1968). *Sex and Gender*. New York: Science House.

APPLIED PSYCHOANALYSIS

Psychoanalytic Studies and *Macbeth*

Shared Fantasy and Reciprocal Identification

HAROLD P. BLUM, M.D.

SHAKESPEARE'S MACBETH IS A LARGER THAN LIFE TRAGEDY THAT
for its brevity and rapidity of action is probably unparalleled in
its dramatic scope and study of character, motive, and conflict.
Macbeth is scrutinized not only for application of psychoanalytic
discoveries, but as an artistic depiction of the most primitive and
most advanced aspects of the human psyche which inspires as
well as illuminates psychoanalytic insights.

This paper explores *Macbeth* in terms of shared fantasies and
the reciprocal identifications intrinsic to their formation and
structure. Freud (1908) introduced shared fantasies in discussion of aesthetic communication by poets and artists and in terms
of group psychology. The poet conveyed his daydreams and
dreams to the audience, awakening similar fantasies in the audience and inviting identification with the character and content
of his own fantasy creation. Furthermore, myth, legend, and
folklore were shown to converge with the fantasies disguised in
literature and art. The primal fantasies of all cultures (Freud,
1916–17, p. 371), the universal fantasies of incest and parricide,
matricide, pregnancy, birth, death, castration, omnipotence,
etc., were all shared between writer and reader.

Shared fantasies exert a selective influence on the growth and

Clinical professor of psychiatry and training analyst, New York University.
Executive director, Sigmund Freud Archives, Inc.

development of personality functions. They facilitate, impede, or inhibit some lines of development while fostering other developmental potentials. The impact of the parents' feelings and fantasies will so selectively influence development as to make that child the child of that particular caretaker (A. Freud, 1965, p. 86) and culture. Whether shared fantasies exert unusual developmental influence will likely depend upon the identification investment and exclusive attachment of the parent, usually the mother, and the developmental phase, sensitivity, and proclivities of the child. Shared fantasies tend to shape personal, familial, and social history (Blum, 1985). The personal myth (Kris, 1956) may be overdetermined and affirmed by shared intrafamilial fantasy such as a child being chosen for great deeds to fulfill parental ambition, or for a scapegoat function, or as a replacement child, etc.

Following Freud's investigation, I shall turn to the applied analysis of *Macbeth* for elucidation of shared phallic narcissistic fantasy, though with changing developmental vicissitudes and with idealization of masculine aggression. In the course of this condensed commentary on the play, it will be clear that our understanding of *Macbeth* parallels the growth of psychoanalytic knowledge and insight. Each generation of analysts will interpret the play, like the Irma dream, in the light of new understanding which should enlarge rather than diminish its analytic and aesthetic appreciation. Freud (1916) regarded Shakespeare as the greatest of poets and used characters of Shakespeare's plays in his study of character types. Clearly intrigued by *Macbeth*, he told Ferenczi, "I have begun to study *Macbeth* which has long tormented me without my being able to find a solution" (Jones, 1955, p. 372). Freud (1916) quoted the play at great length, summarized the plot, and then referred to the "triple layer of obscurity into which the bad preservation of the text, the unknown intention of the dramatist, and the hidden purport of the legend have become condensed" (p. 323). Nevertheless, he stated that while the dramatist can overwhelm us by his art, "he cannot prevent us from attempting subsequently to grasp its effect by studying its psychological mechanism" (p. 323). Freud did not deal with methodology, although he was aware of the limits to inference with created characters (Baudry, 1984). Lady

Macbeth is given as an example of a person who is wrecked by success, "after striving for it with single-minded energy. . . . Beforehand there is no hesitation, no sign of any internal conflict in her. . . . She is ready to sacrifice even her womanliness to her murderous intention" (p. 318). Lady Macbeth is ultimately destroyed by the very "vaulting ambition which overleaps itself" (I, 7), in the crimes committed in order to become queen and make her husband king. Oedipal victory could not be tolerated since it resulted in unconscious guilt and self-punitive destruction.

Actually, Freud gave several explanations for the basic motives in the play in addition to unconscious oedipal guilt, and these complementary and competing explanations have been largely overlooked. In this connection he also pointed to the disappointment of childlessness "to break the woman down and drive the man to defiant rage" (p. 322) so that childlessness drives the couple to crime. Freud comments that only a childless person could kill children, a remark that is strangely contradictory to his awareness of parental infanticide and filicide. In another explanation, Macbeth's childlessness and Lady Macbeth's barrenness are poetic justice, talion punishment for their crimes against the sanctity of generation so that childlessness is not the cause but the consequence of the crime.

The father-son relationship is also invoked by Freud with the murder of Duncan clearly noted as parricide. In Banquo's case Macbeth kills the father while the son escapes, and Macduff's children are killed while the father escapes. Lady Macbeth would have killed Duncan herself had he not resembled her father, and suspicion for his murder falls on his sons: "who cannot want the thought how monstrous it was for Malcolm and for Donaldbain to kill their gracious father? Damn fact!; so the sons of Duncan are thought to have murdered their father, the King, and Banquo's son, Fleance, is under suspicion and fleeing from his father's death" (III, 6). In putting her husband in her father's place, Lady Macbeth is clearly implying a hidden incestuous relationship. It seems to me that there can be no doubt that the play expresses derivatives of oedipal conflict with talion punishment for oedipal crimes. The punishment is childlessness, castration, and death, as Freud indicated. Parricide is virtually a manifest theme.

Numerous other explanations of this extraordinary drama have been offered. Calef (1969) invoked the concept of one crime, parricide, defending against another crime, incest, and the need to conceal and destroy the fruits of incestuous transgression. More recently, authors have discussed the play in terms of preoedipal themes, disregarding the earlier oedipal formulations. Newer work builds on Freud's formulation that Macbeth and Lady Macbeth are split characters which are not completely understandable until brought together into a unity. Macbeth is weak-willed and acts like a feminine man, and is goaded to brutal, fearless masculinity by his wife, while she is unsexed and becomes a masculine woman. Freud (1916, p. 324) noted: "It is he who has the hallucination of the dagger before the crime; but it is she who afterwards falls ill of a mental disorder. . . . Macbeth does murder sleep . . . and so 'Macbeth shall sleep no more'; but we never hear that *he* slept no more, while the Queen . . . rises from her bed and, talking in her sleep, betrays her guilt. It is he who stands helpless with bloody hands, lamenting that 'all great Neptune's ocean' will not wash them clean, while she comforts him: 'A little water clears us of this deed'; but later it is she who washes her hands . . . and cannot get rid of the bloodstains: 'All the perfumes of Arabia will not sweeten this little hand.' . . . she becomes all remorse and he all defiance . . . like two disunited parts of a single psychical individuality, and it may be that they are both copied from a single prototype." Extending Freud's formulations, I wish to emphasize the importance of both oedipal and preoedipal determinants. I shall comment on the relationship of the different developmental phases to each other.

The understanding of this extraordinary, enigmatic drama is enlarged through consideration of the shared, phallic-narcissistic fantasy of the Macbeths, a fantasy system which undergoes regressive and progressive transformation. The Macbeths are paired as husband-wife, and unconsciously as mother-son. Lady Macbeth is the bewitching oedipal mother, but she is also the incompletely separated preoedipal mother. Lady Macbeth is not fully differentiated from Macbeth or from the witches. She is the most real and differentiated witch, the least and greatest, most benign and malignant of the witches. The witches reproject

Macbeth's forbidden fantasies and ruthless ambition. The apparent validation of the witches' prophecies is comparable to the validation of shared fantasies of reciprocal projection and identification across indistinct boundaries.

Lady Macbeth is initially more determined and unscrupulous than Macbeth, who is conflicted and hesitant to perpetrate parricide-regicide. Lady Macbeth uses Macbeth as her own deadly instrument, her dagger, her murdering minister. Macbeth is initially overwhelmed by Duncan's murder, while Lady Macbeth remains concerned only with the details of what is to be done to maintain appearances and fabricate a cover-up. Darkness and blood pervade the drama, and the murder is carried out as a primal scene, with the stabbing in the dead of night, uncertain as to who committed the crime and blood dripping down the stairs until Macbeth will stand in a sea of blood. All Scotland bleeds, and forms become blurred in a murky, sleepless, sinister atmosphere. As Lady Macbeth grows remorseful, she still believes that a little water will dissolve the guilt. Fearful of attempts at retaliation and seeing others now trying to usurp the very throne which he has just seized, Macbeth descends into violent assaults as he becomes a hardened criminal.

The many references to Macbeth's being planted and full of growth (I, 4) and to the "pendant bed and procreant cradle of her castle" (I, 6) contrast with Macbeth's sterility and his extinction of life and lineage. One murder begets another, and Macbeth destroys rather than creates, unable to stop, though he has "supped full of horrors" (V, 5). Banquo is murdered, and then Lady Macduff and her children are murdered as Macbeth attempts to annihilate Macduff's entire extended family. Lady Macbeth collapses into suicidal depression, and poetic intuition of rudiments of analytic therapy follow. Macbeth admonishes her physician, "cure her of that. Can'st thou not minister to a mind diseased, pluck from the memory a rooted sorrow, raise out the written troubles of the brain." And the doctor replies, "Therein the patient must minister to himself" (V, 3). Believing in his invulnerability, Macbeth proclaims, "I bear a charmed life" (V, 7). According to the witches' prophecies he cannot be vanquished by "any man of woman born" and is safe so long as Burnham Wood comes not to Dunsinane Castle. Macbeth goes off to his final battle with avenging forces. The armies advance using Burnham Wood as camouflage and Macbeth is beheaded by the avenging Macduff who "was from his mother's womb untimely ripped" (V, 8). The curtain falls as the rightful heir is restored to the throne.

Macbeth is a study of regicide, as Hamlet, with attempts to usurp the throne, the paternal position, power, and penis. Critics have also noted the relationship of Macbeth to the Elizabethan era. Freud commented on Elizabeth's childlessness which resulted in her making the son of Mary Stuart, whom she had executed, her successor to the throne. Freud noted that this was similar to the prophecy of the Weird Sisters that Macbeth would be King without successors but that Banquo's children should succeed to the crown. Macbeth laments, "Upon my head . . . a fruitless crown . . . a barren sceptre in my grip" (III, 1). Macbeth is incensed and violently jealous, since he wishes to found a dynasty. When's Banquo's eight descendants appear to Macbeth in the witches' cavern, he exclaims, "What, will the line stretch out to the crack of doom" (III, 1). His jealousy of parents and envy of their progeny contribute to his destructive rage against parents and children, particularly those in the dynastic line.

The promptings of the Weird Sisters, the witches, are closely related to the instigation, provocation, and goading of his wife. Lady Macbeth is an awesome figure, one of the great characters of literature. Macbeth readily succumbs to Lady Macbeth's influence, and at the same time struggles to free himself from the dangers of her domination and femininity. If Lady Macbeth is wife and mother, the pair form a mother-son latent relationship, but one of a very special type. Barron (1960) first noted that they were not only a composite character, they failed to differentiate from each other and had failed to achieve separate identities. Actually, the separation-individuation issues are intertwined with the oedipal themes and give a particular cast to the oedipal drama. Muslin (1984) explicates the play in terms of self psychology and sees Lady Macbeth as a selfobject. Following the murder of Duncan, Muslin presumes that Lady Macbeth undergoes fragmentation of the cohesive self. Macbeth then loses her as an idealized parental selfobject responsible for his own self-cohesiveness and narcissistic equilibrium.

To my mind, important transformations occur at the beginning of the play, prior to Duncan's murder, and continue in an unfolding sequence. Macbeth is involved with the witches at the inception of the drama as they reflect his own grandiose ambitions which are shared in letter and speech with Lady Macbeth. Lady Macbeth is transformed, almost at once, from devoted wife to the bewitching, beguiling, seductive, oedipal mother and then to the archwitch, the preoedipal mother. Lady Macbeth becomes a mirror of Hecate, Goddess of Witches. Hecate admonishes the witches, "all you have done hath been but for a wayward son, spiteful and wrathful, who as others do, loves for his own ends, not for you" (III, 5). The preoedipal witch-mother is both an idealized and persecutory narcissistic object. "Fair is foul and foul is fair" (I, 1), and the drama is replete with reversals, splits, bisexuality, and paired opposite identifications. Regressive transformations are punctuated by some progressive reorganization which makes it easier for the audience to identify with the villainous heroes (antiheroes) of the drama.

The rampant entitlement, seizure, and abuse of power begin as a *folie à deux*. Peering through the thick fog on the heath that envelopes the play, Macbeth's descent into barbaric cruelty and tormented tyranny parallels that of Lady Macbeth. Semen and milk turn into blood. Lady Macbeth, anticipating ambitious fulfillment with "her dearest partner of greatness" (I, 5), nevertheless fears his nature, "it is too full of the milk of human kindness" (I, 5). She is ready to pour spirits into his ear, "and chastise with the valor of my tongue all that impedes thee" (I, 5). Lady Macbeth then undergoes one of the most dramatic and terrifying transformations in literature, "Come, you spirits that tend on mortal thoughts, unsex me here, and fill me, from the crown to the toe, topped full of dirous cruelty! Make thick my blood. Stop up the access and passage to remorse, that no compunctuous visitings of nature shake my sole purpose. . . . Come to my woman's breasts and take my milk for gall, you murdering ministers" (I, 5). Unsexed, she is a masculinized woman like the bearded witches of ambiguous gender. She represents the murderous preoedipal mother, with both phallic and castrating attributes. She will then go on to ridicule her husband's vacillation, impugning his masculinity, and asserting those gripping lines which Freud also cited, "I have given suck, and know how tender 'tis to love the babe that milks me; I would, while it was smiling in my face, have plucked my nipple from his boneless gums, and dashed the brains out, had I so sworn as you have done to this" (I, 7).

These lines, so applicable to child abuse and infanticide (Blum, 1980), may also serve as a developmental metaphor crucial to a deeper understanding of the drama. The child may always have felt threatened and pressured to meet his mother's expectations, or projected such demands onto her. He fears betrayal or being dethroned by his mother or a rival at her breast. Motherliness unpredictably disappears, to be replaced by a devouring oral envy and greed. As Lady Macbeth is milked, she is depleted of nurturance and kindness; both Macbeths become mercilessly cruel. Lady Macbeth discards her conscience with her baby, although her unconscious superego will later assert itself with savage force and overpowering punishment. It is unconsciously fitting that as the instigating mother figure, the power behind the throne, she assumes the guilt. There is splitting between good and evil, male and female, creativity and destruction, generativity and sterility. Everything that is cruel, merciless, and murderous is associated with masculinity; everything compassionate, tender, motherly, and merciful is feminine (Martin, 1984).

Macbeth is initially the proxy agent and passive partner to Lady Macbeth's ruthless, phallic narcissism. He tries to cling to the passive position of the child without responsibility, directed by others and external forces. "If chance will have me king, why chance may crown me, without my stir" (I, 3). As he disengages from his initially dominant and controlling wife-mother, he emerges as the ruthless, omnipotent tyrant, unable to experience real grief or guilt, but experiencing persecutory visions and afraid of external retaliation. He wishes for and fears merger and femininity and defends to the death (or separation merger) his masculine autonomy. His regressively transformed witch-mother represents the infantile dangers institutionalized in witchcraft. (It is significant that suicides in the Elizabethan era could be ambivalently regarded as martyrs or as demonic sinners. "Sinful" suicides could be buried at night by crossroads with a stake driven through the heart [Forbes, 1970]. Lady Macbeth's suicide would then confirm her as a witch, and her death would match as well as atone for Duncan's midnight stabbing murder.)

The unintegrated bisexuality is of critical importance and related to the incomplete separation-individuation and lack of oedipal resolution. Lady Macbeth is disappointed in womanhood, hostile to her own mother and her child. Men also inevitably fail her, as Macbeth is later failed by his wife and the witches. She idealizes only her own possessed, illusory, omnipotent penis, her husband-son. Macbeth recognizes her masculine drive, identifies with it, and tells her to "bring forth men-children only! For thy undaunted mettle should compose nothing but males" (I, 7). He will ambivalently live out her grandiose omnipotent fantasies, redeem her disappointments, and be the weapon that avenges her fantasied injuries. (Banquo has a similar shared fantasy enjoining his son to revenge [III, 3].) There is a hidden shared fantasy that this son is his mother's phallus and omnipotent object.

If we look at Lady Macbeth's tormenting dialogue, the dialogue (Spitz, 1965) between mother and infant, he is massively threatened by nonconformity with her aspirations and will be thoroughly rewarded, yet threatened anew, with compliance. At the very moment when his smile should elicit maternal affection and increasing attachment, the infant is faced with malignant loss of face, breast, and nurturance. The smile and eye contact do not elicit the reciprocal smile which should be an organizer for the mother as well as the infant. The infant's smile is negatively perceived and becomes an aversive cue, evoking insufferable demand and feelings of angry accusation in the mother. Instead of providing a holding environment (Winnicott, 1965), she will cast the child down, just as later, "The sweet milk of concord" (IV, 3) will be poured into hell. Actually, the play is replete with images of mothers turning into witches and milk into gall. Security and safety are offered only to be suddenly and unpredictably withdrawn; such an unreliable frame of reference tends to impede differentiation and the achievement of self and object constancy. The witches themselves, bearded, undifferentiated, demonic, and divided from more mature nurturant images of motherhood, are unmistakably both maternal and antimaternal. As with betrayal at the breast (Erikson, 1959; Bachmann, 1978), Macbeth imbibes the witches brew, inspires their air and is inspired by their prediction, and swallows the narcissistic supplies which he demands. The cauldrons represent pregnancy, the breast, and feeding, but the milk is poison and the brew is intoxicating and toxic. The witches and Macbeth have the shared fantasy of phallic-narcissistic grandeur and ruthless entitlement, murder, and retaliation.

Macbeth disengages from Lady Macbeth only to turn to the witches and from the witches back to Lady Macbeth and then to a "bold, bloody resolute" and rageful independence. The witches continue Lady Macbeth's threatening dialogue and dichotomy between murdering and nurturing infants: "finger of birth-strangled babe, ditch delivered by a drab" and "sow's blood that have eaten her nine farrow" (IV, 1) illustrate that the theme of childlessness also refers to infanticide. The sow is the preoedipal witch who cannot feed, but feeds on and as a cannibal devours her offspring. The infanticidal Lady Macbeth vicariously lives on and through the oedipal Macbeth who is the son who killed the father and the father who kills the son.

Many representations are split into opposites. The wicked witches augur harm, but Edward the Confessor's prophecies heal. Lady Macduff is the split-off nurturant mother who tries to support and comfort her children. Duncan is the venerated father who is trusting and trustworthy. Macbeth, distrustful and destructive, is the parricidal son and filicidal father. Macduff is both the deserting father who has failed to protect and the avenging father, the superego precursor, who will make Macbeth pay for his horrible crimes. But Macduff has been untimely ripped from his mother's womb, an exception in the form of a Caesarean birth, untainted with incestuous passage through the birth canal and a child who could not have been expected to live in that era. Only a Caesar could then survive a Caesarean birth. He is the avenger of the children whose lives were early aborted, on the oral level representing rivals at the breast, who are omnipotently destroyed by a voraciously greedy and envious Macbeth. Macbeth's narcissistic rage requires that the envied rival should disappear without possible return or replication; the extended family of kinsmen must also be killed, akin to genocide, so that no avenger could arise. Macbeth is the babe that milked Lady Macbeth of human kindness, the toddler whose rage threatens to consume and destroy everyone and everything. Macbeth retains awareness of some potential for moral revulsion, but his oral-narcissistic rage predominates: "I have supped full with horrors: Direness, familiar to my slaughterous thoughts, cannot once start me" (V, 5). Like Macbeth, Duncan's horses turn wild and devour each other after Duncan's murder (II, 4). The sterility of the Macbeths is associated with the infantile depletion and consuming destruction.

It is also possible to understand that to be untimely ripped from the womb is a metaphor for premature separateness with increased separation anxiety, oral regression, and coercion of the preoedipal mother to whom omnipotence is delegated. Helplessness is magically avoided by incorporating or being incorporated by the omnipotent witch, i.e., through merger with the preoedipal mother who is and who controls life and death. The drama depicts, with consummate artistic perception, the great dilemmas of separation-individuation (Mahler et al., 1975) in concert with oedipal conflict. Macbeth, as the conquering hero toddler, becomes painfully aware of separateness, helplessness, and vulnerability. The more he recognizes how dependent and vulnerable he is, the more he turns to the witches for omnipotent reassurance and protection (Muslin, 1984). Their prophecies assure his invulnerability. If he is their sword, they are his shield. But they simultaneously threaten omnipotent retaliation, superego precursors that both reward and punish (Mahler and McDevitt, 1980). He can only be vanquished by someone like Macduff who has mastered the vulnerability of sudden premature separation. His magical dyadic orbit is omnipotently secure, and his space cannot be invaded nor lost through merger so long as Burnham Wood comes not to Dunsinane. The daggers in men's smiles (Bachmann, 1978), the treachery present in every form of intimacy, and the primal scene of mutual destruction (bodies locked in deadly combat) overweigh the unbridled narcissism of a frightened, enraged child who lacks self-definition and confidence, and the assurance of oral-narcissistic supplies. Macbeth attempts to ward off the awareness of anxiety, separateness, and helplessness, entreating and coercing the witches, holding on to them, darting away from them, having no comprehension or control of their mysterious appearance and disappearance. He is remorseless and furious when his magic fails and his mother will not function as an extension of himself and does not automatically understand or fulfill his unspoken wishes. "Be these juggling fiends no more believed" (V, 8). Reality has mercilessly intruded and the mighty tyrant has fallen from grace. Extreme disillusionment follows after infantile awe and idealization. Reality and omnipotence coexist and clash.

How are the crises to be resolved? Development will be determined by the prophecies which Macbeth drinks from the witches' cauldron. Here is a beautiful poetic metaphor for the character of the ego being determined by identification modeled on oral incorporation. Macbeth and Lady Macbeth demonstrate reciprocal identifications between marriage partners, parents, and parent and child. Macbeth drinks in her ruthlessness and infanticidal rage, as she appears to be drained and deprived. He is identified either with an object distorted by the projection of his own oral aggression or possibly with a mother who has undergone a profound oral regression concomitant with maternity. Lady Macbeth is identified with an ambivalently hated and feared mother and is unable to be consistently holding and nurturant. She is perceived as threatening rather than protective, perhaps threatened by a demanding infant with low frustration tolerance and circular, contagious anger within the dyad. Macbeth and his Lady cannot soothe or console each other. Macbeth's identification with Lady Macbeth's murderous attitudes may also be understood as an identification with the aggressor and her aggression. As in the formation of the superego, the identifications are based upon the parents' real and fantasied qualities; the image of a tyrannical, sadistic, and punitive parent may be based upon a child's primitive defenses and impulses, on problems in the child or the maternal environment, or on special problems within that particular dyadic relationship. The dyadic dimension of the drama may be read with emphasis on the demanding mother, the insatiable child, the particular mix and match, or the regressive relationship and reciprocal identification. Where there are serious preoedipal fixations and separation-individuation is incomplete, there tends to be a distortion of the oedipus complex and often a fusion of oedipal and pre-oedipal issues (Kernberg, 1980). Parental images, normally split in the family romance, undergo extremes of idealization and devaluation. Castration anxiety covers and simultaneously represents separation anxiety, and phallic aims and objects continue preoedipal strivings as represented in the breast-penis equation. Oedipal disappointment and jealousy are likely to be intolerable since they are infiltrated with unresolved narcissistic frustration and oral greed, envy, and rage. The intensified and validated oedipal and castration fantasies present in each partner of a sterile couple are associated in *Macbeth* with much earlier, unresolved, parental ambivalence and infanticidal attitudes. The "milk of human kindness" has been depleted and replaced by a consuming exploitation and annihilation of narcissistic objects and oedipal rivals. Macbeth is the sterile child whose demands, envy, and rage can destroy the whole family. Macbeth is one of the rare dramas that approaches the theme of genocide, suggesting major underlying motives. Sterility is a motive, representation, consequence, and retribution for his villainy.

Macbeth has gone to the three Weird Sisters, the past, present, and future, and Freud's three fateful visions of mother, "to know by the worst means the worst" (III, 4). He received feedback steeped in omnipotence and in the blood of consuming hostility. After Lady Macbeth's demise, Macbeth is again prematurely separated, "She should have died hereafter. There would have been time for such a word" (V, 5). With separation and separateness he is alone with his inner anxieties and demons. As he acknowledges loss while defending against its affective meaning, time and life are suspended as "tomorrow, tomorrow, and tomorrow creeps in its petty pace from day to day, to the last syllable of recorded time" (V, 5). Deadened and dehumanized, he does not mourn but proclaims in anger and apathy that life is "a tale told by an idiot, full of sound and fury, signifying nothing" (V, 5). But in the age of psychoanalysis, even nothing has significance (Lewin, 1948). Nothing may mean the absent penis or flatus, but may also represent the helplessness of separateness (Abrams and Shengold, 1974). The shared phallic-narcissistic fantasies which dominate the unresolved oedipal conflicts have their roots here in preoedipal dyadic issues. The unavailable narcissistic object is devalued and discarded. Macbeth repudiates his feminine identification, struggles against any weakness which is seen as being like a "baby girl" (III, 4), and simultaneously denies separation, castration, and death anxiety. His narcissism demanded descendants and now demands immortality through not dying. As the drama concludes, the cruel and remorseless coercion of the deflated toddler gives way, and the curtain falls on the "watchful tyranny . . . of this dead butcher and his fiend-like queen" (V, 8). The drama, ranging from the most profound and advanced levels of philosophical thought to the dyadic beginnings of the dialogue, grips the audience in shared fantasy and trial identification. Development may become deviant in the very vulnerable dyadic phase and wrecked if the postoedipal reorganization does not eventuate in reparative correction and benevolent transformation. "The instruments of darkness tell us truths" (I, 3). Macbeth illuminates analytic understanding of extreme hostility and sterility versus the harmony and fertility that are nurtured by the "milk of human kindness" and the internalization of benevolent parental attitudes and authority.

BIBLIOGRAPHY

ABRAMS, S. & SHENGOLD, L. (1974). The meaning of nothing. *Psychoanal. Q.*, 43:115–119.

BACHMANN, S. (1978). "Daggers in men's smiles." *Int. Rev. Psychoanal.*, 5:97–104.

BARRON, D. (1960). The babe that milks. *Amer. Imago*, 17:133–161.

BAUDRY, F. D. (1984). An essay on method in applied psychoanalysis. *Psychoanal Q.*, 53:551–581.

BLUM, H. P. (1980). The maternal ego ideal and the regulation of maternal qualities. In *The Course of Life*, ed. S. Greenspan and G. H. Pollock, 3:91–114. Washington, D.C.: National Institute of Mental Health.

_____. (1985). Shared fantasy and reciprocal identification. In *Unconscious Fantasy*, ed. H. P. Blum, Y. Kramer, & A. Richards. New York: Analytic Press (in press).

CALEF, V. (1969). Lady Macbeth and infanticide. *J. Amer. Psychoanal. Assn.*, 17:528–548.

ERIKSON, E. H. (1959). *Identity and the Life Cycle*. New York: Int. Univ. Press.

FORBES, T. (1970). Life and death in Shakespeare's London. *Amer. Scientist,* 58:511–520.

FREUD, A. (1965). Normality and pathology in childhood. *W.,* 6.

FREUD, S. (1908). Creative writers and day-dreaming. *S.E.,* 9:141–153.

———. (1916). Some character-types met with in psycho-analytic work. *S.E.,* 14:309–333.

———. (1916–17). Introductory lectures on psycho-analysis. *S.E.,* 15 & 16.

JONES, E. (1955). *The Life and Work of Sigmund Freud,* vol. 2. New York: Basic Books.

KERNBERG, O. F. (1980). *Internal World and External Reality.* New York: Aronson.

KRIS, E. (1956). The personal myth. *J. Amer. Psychoanal. Assn.,* 4:653–681.

LEWIN, B. D. (1948). The nature of reality, the meaning of nothing, with an addendum on concentration. *Psychoanal. Q.,* 17:524–526.

MAHLER, M. S. & McDEVITT, J. B. (1980). The separation-individuation process and identity formation. In *The Course of Life,* ed. S. Greenspan & G. H. Pollock, 1:395–406. Washington, D.C.: National Institute of Mental Health.

MAHLER, M. S., PINE, F., & BERGMAN, A. (1975). *The Psychological Birth of the Human Infant.* New York: Basic Books.

MARTIN, J. (1984). Discussion of "Macbeth," by H. Muslin. American Psychoanalytic Association.

MUSLIN, H. (1984). Macbeth. Read at the American Psychoanalytic Association.

SPITZ, R. A. (1965). *The First Year of Life.* New York: Int. Univ. Press.

WINNICOTT, D. W. (1965). *The Maturational Processes and the Facilitating Environment.* New York: Int. Univ. Press.

Nursery Rhymes

A Developmental Perspective
VINCENT P. DeSANTIS, M.D.

THE VERSES WHICH ARE RECITED AND SUNG BY CHILDREN AND PARents are so much a part of our present culture and heritage that they are usually taken for granted. When we do wonder about the characters and scenes described in these short rhymes, it is frequently because a child has asked us about them. The common questions relate to the surface of the poems such as why the old woman lives in a shoe, why London Bridge is falling down, or how a cow can jump over the moon; sometimes these questions are difficult to answer. The vivid images of the nursery songs are ambiguous and puzzling. Their compressed, epigrammatic style explains far less in the way of a story than, for example, fairy tales, and the rich symbols which bear the images of families living in shoes and livestock cavorting by moonlight seem to be all the more opaque in spite of, or perhaps because of, their long familiarity.

This paper is an attempt to unravel some of these mysteries from our childhood. Initially I comment on some general characteristics of this literature and its tradition and then consider in some detail a number of nursery rhymes from a psychoanalytic developmental point of view.

The notion of analyzing a particular genre of children's literature from a developmental perspective is not a novel one. Goldings (1974) demonstrated the important role which jump-rope

Assistant child psychiatrist, Hall-Mercer Children's Center, McLean Hospital, Belmont, MA; instructor in psychiatry, Harvard Medical School.

The author wishes to acknowledge helpful discussions of some of the ideas contained in this paper with James M. Herzog, M.D., and Bennett Simon, M.D.

rhymes can play in the development of latency-age girls. Bettelheim (1976) has argued persuasively for the influence which fairy tales exert on the imaginations of children because of their ability to address various developmental dilemmas. Both studies share with this paper an interest in a child's unconscious response to the symbols presented in rhymes and stories and the way in which these symbols encapsulate troubling ideas and affects for which the child can find no immediate resolution. According to this view, the function of a rhyme or story is to allow the child to keep the question in mind until such time as an answer can be found.

A REVIEW OF SELECTED LITERATURE

A striking characteristic of nursery rhymes and songs is their durability. In their authoritative collection, *The Oxford Dictionary of Nursery Rhymes,* Iona and Peter Opie (1951) review what little is known of the origins and history of these rhymes. The existence of simple children's verses dates back to at least Roman times, and the Opies believe that one out of four in our present collection were current in Shakespeare's youth. Although they survived primarily through oral transmission, written records demonstrate extremely heterogeneous origins. While some rhymes such as infant amusements, counting out charts, and lullabies were intended for children, by far the greater portion of rhymes derive from the songs, catches, and ballads of adults. Of course, we are also speaking of a time when childhood, as we know it, did not exist and children were exposed at a far younger age to the full range of adult experience.

The first nursery rhyme collections were published in the eighteenth century and were associated with a variety of figures who were alleged to have invented these verses for the entertainment and soothing of children. Thus, among others, *Tommy Thumb's Pretty Song Book* (c. 1744) and *Gammer Gurton's Garland* (c. 1784) competed with *Mother Goose's Melody* (c. 1765) before she established herself as the dominant persona of the genre on this side of the Atlantic; in England the primary designation remains nursery songs.

The goose imago has a venerable history and is rich in associations. The Mother Goose figure derives from an old French tradition that long predates the publication in 1697 of Perrault's collection of fairy tales which were purportedly told by La Mere Oie. German folklore also has a Fru Gosen. As Shengold (1982) has reported, the goose was traditionally regarded as a stupid, dirty animal, and "goose" was a term in the seventeenth and eighteenth century for venereal disease and also for a prostitute. The goose is vulnerable to predators, but can also be a fierce aggressor. A modern American slang term, "to goose," refers to an attack where a finger is thrust into someone's anus. The Golden Goose of Aesop and Grimm can be interpreted as containing elements of a number of issues including parent-child conflict over masturbation and anal control. The goose imago as a symbol for the inventor of the rhymes is a complex one; she is a sharp old lady of dubious background who has dirty titillating verses to both excite and sooth the young. At any rate her rhymes ought to contain all a child ever wanted to know but was afraid to ask about a multitude of subjects.

Halliwell (1849), the first to publish complete modern collections of the rhymes in the mid-nineteenth century, was also the first to call attention to numerous parallel rhymes in the Germanic and Scandinavian countries. Eckenstein (1906) pursued this comparative approach in some detail. Thus one finds many versions of Humpty Dumpty. In Saxony as follows:

> Hümpelken-Pümpelken sat on the bank,
> Hümpelken-Pümpelken fell from the bank;
> There is no doctor in England
> Who can cure Hümpelken-Pümpelken.

While in Denmark:

> Little Trille lay on the shelf,
> Little Trille fell down from the shelf.
> No one in whole land
> Can cure Little Trille.
> Opie, 1951, p. 10

The Opies believe that the numerous parallels and variations argue in favor of a common Germanic origin rather than merely being examples of translations. As we shall see, the comparative approach can frequently be helpful in clarifying the meaning of a particular rhyme.

Poems which are so durable and universal might be conceived of as fulfilling a psychological need of children and their parents. The study of children's games in the nineteenth century led Gomme (1894–98) to the conclusion that these activities helped prepare children to take on the appropriate roles which would be expected of them as adults. The study of psychological development during childhood has led to the recognition that children need to make sense of the emotional urges within themselves as well as the emotional crosscurrents in their immediate environment and that play together with gradually developing verbal skills help children articulate these issues in their early years.

The developmental line linking these two activities and allowing for continuous development through to adulthood is the capacity for symbolization. Sarnoff (1976) has studied in some detail the process by which the capacity to symbolize evolves and, in conjunction with increasing use of repression and cognitive changes, brings about the structure of latency. There is also a change from more primitive forms of memory based on images and actions (eidetic and affecto-motor memory) to a memory organized at the verbal conceptual level.

Nursery rhymes illustrate this intrapsychic process and its associated interpersonal function. In their earliest years children hear them from parents, learn to recite them, and share an experience with grownups where both meet on common ground. The rhymes are brief, contain vivid images, and frequently can be sung or played as a game. They are the first cultural experience with language used as a tool to convey a sense of the inner experience of one's body, feelings about oneself, desires for attachment, worry about separation, and the fears and hopes concerning aggressive and sexual urges.

The fact that this is a shared experience is one of the delights of this kind of verbal play. Children express feelings quite openly about the descriptions contained in the rhymes. In addition, they will frequently ask the parents questions about the dilemmas presented by the verses. Sometimes parent or child will respond spontaneously to the material at a conscious or unconscious level. Thus the father of an assertive, confident 4-year-old girl read to her:

> Little Miss Muffet,
> Sat on a tuffet,
> Eating her curds and whey;
> There came a big spider
> Who sat down beside her

Coming to the last line, which usually reads "And frightened Miss Muffet away," he changed it to: "And she slapped the hell out of him." The girl, picking up the cue, later changed the third line to "Eating her curds out of the way," and her laughter about her own change underscored her enjoyment about the sense of active mastery which she felt.

A 3-year-old boy of more cautious temperament who was just beginning to share his mother with a new sibling changed "Yankee Doodle" from:

> Yankee Doodle came to town
> Riding on a pony:
> He stuck a feather in his cap,
> And called it macaroni.

To the following version:

> Yankee Doodle stayed at home
> He didn't ride his pony.
> He cooked some spaghetti on the stove
> And called it macaroni.

Although with time the language of the rhymes and some of the imagery have become more obscure so that we may not know that a tuffet is a cushion or that macaroni refers to "something that might be worn by a fop, a macaroni" (Baring-Gould, 1962), children and grownups still respond to the overall emotional tone of the verses. It is part of the nursery rhyme literary style to describe striking images, preposterous or unrealistic situations, or downright nonsense. As we shall see, this is because, as in dreams, this form is well suited to the disguise of unconscious conflicts.

As in dreams, there is frequently no resolution of the anxiety. The manifest scenes depicted by the rhymes include all manner of aggressive acts including murder, drowning, assault, and cannabilism: the entire range of sexual experiences is treated in more disguised form. And yet the events of a nursery rhyme are rarely if ever the source of a nightmare. The capacity of the rhymes to contain the anxiety is remarkable, especially when one compares it with other forms of children's literature. Fairy tales usually have a denouement which provides some reassurance to the child that a way through life's predicaments can be found, and, although fables may end on an anxiety-provoking note, there is at least a clear resolution. The fact that there is a moral to the story is supportive to the child's superego. A few nursery rhymes, particularly those with a rather straightforward oedipal content, such as Tom the Piper's Son who was beaten for stealing a pig, and the Knave of Hearts who met a similar fate from the King for stealing the Queen's Tarts, have this quality, but most do not.

A final aspect of the rhymes which is beyond the scope of my presentation is the music and pictures which accompany them. These elements capture the attention of young children because they are geared to the eidetic and affecto-motor memory processing typical of this age. The presence of these formal elements grounds the rhymes more securely in the realm of primary process than is the case in other types of children's literature.

SOME NURSERY RHYMES

As we turn to the rhymes themselves, we move into a strange world where we may initially lose our bearings. It will be necessary to explore and chart the new territory on its own terms. This may be comparable to what the child experiences in trying to make sense of his new environment. As a child must, we will follow the method of attempting to find linkages which help to articulate latent themes from the scenes described in the rhymes.

> Rub a dub dub
> Three men in a tub
> And who do you think they be?
> The butcher, the baker,

The candlestick-maker
Turn'em out knaves all three.
Opie, p. 376

This is one of a number of rhymes dealing with the theme of separation at various stages of development. This is not immediately obvious until these verses are compared with other rhymes. Initially "Rub a dub dub" seems to be a puzzling image of 3 grown men crowded into a somewhat ridiculous and inappropriate vessel or container. A similar situation is depicted in:

Three wise men of Gotham,
They went out to sea in a bowl,
And if the bowl had been stronger
My song would have been longer.
Opie, p. 193

It seems clear then that an attempt to travel in this fashion can be quite risky. Gotham, a village near Nottingham, England, has been notorious for centuries because of the supposed stupidity and folly of its inhabitants. It is a Danish rhyme that provides the link between such a poorly planned journey and the theme of a child's separation from the parents.

Jørgen from Jutland
sailed in a pot.
The pot split,
Jørgen cried
mother, mother once again.
Hertz and Clante, p. 34; my tr.

Danes have traditionally regarded the simple inhabitants of rustic Jutland as "Gothamites." Here a boy tries to go to sea in a kitchen pot only to discover that he is not ready to sever his ties to home; he calls for his mother just as he did when he was little and really dependent upon her. The image of a pot from the family kitchen suggests the explanation for his lack of success: what served as the source of oral supplies in early years cannot be a solid foundation so long as it remains external to the child. Sometimes a fairy tale will treat an issue similar to that contained in a nursery rhyme. Thus, the story of "The Three Pigs" also describes an attempt to separate from the home and the

way in which this endeavor requires that each pig build a structure adequate to the task. In "The Three Pigs" the structure
which is needed must protect the developing psyche from the
ravages of uncontrolled instinctual impulses as symbolized by
the wolf. In the rhymes above, it is the water, one of the elements, and by poetic extension, the sea, which represents the
dangerous id forces which may capsize the vessel.

Thus, "Rub a dub dub" depicts a trio in a quandary similar to
that of the pigs; the wish of the 3 men to take on an adult role is
incompatible with the attainment of this goal in the cramped
and slightly ludicrous confines of the tub. If the child stays too
long in the tub, he will outgrow it—it will become too small to
sustain his development. The dangers inherent in such prolonged dependence are touched on by an alternate reading:

> Rub a dub dub,
> Three men in a tub,
> And how do you think they got there?
> The butcher, the baker,
> The candlestick-maker,
> They all jumped out of a rotten potato
> T'was enough to make a man stare.
> Opie, p. 376

Here the vegetable which stays in the ground beyond its time
symbolizes the unhealthy aspects of staying bound to home beyond the appropriate season. Stagnation threatens if the hatch-
ing is delayed too long.

In his study of fairy tales, Bettelheim (1976) reminded us
that the use of the number 3 carries a sexual connotation.
Thus, 3 enumerates the visible genitalia for each sex (for boys,
the testes and the penis, for girls, the breasts and vagina).

The first line of "Rub a dub dub" suggests masturbation and,
as parents frequently observe, the nightly bath is an ideal occasion for this activity. A child is naked, and ordinary water play
and washing provide some indirect stimulation to the genital
area. The opportunity for further experimentation by direct
manipulation is not usually passed up. The 3 tradesmen of
these verses also manipulate organic matter and are frequently
pictured holding the productions of their handiwork—a sau-

sage, a loaf of bread, and a candle. These results of rub-a-dub-
dub activity would lead onlookers to "stare" from outrage or
perhaps admiration. The spectacle of the 3, engaging as a
group in this manipulation and phallic exhibitionism, is reminiscent of certain sexual practices of early adolescent boys. This
normal process of reworking negative oedipal feelings must, as
Blos (1967) has emphasized, be transcended; that is, the adolescent must move beyond longings for a dependent relationship
with the same-sex parent toward heterosexual intimacy. The
nursery rhyme can be interpreted as supporting this view that
too much rub-a-dub-dub activity in the narcissistic shell of the
tub will hinder separation and loosening of incestuous object
ties.

The way in which apparently homoerotic concerns can mask
heterosexual interests is paralleled in the history of the rhyme
whose earliest version is:

> Hey rub a dub, ho! rub a dub, three maids in tub,
> And who do you think were there?
> The butcher, the baker, the candlestick-maker,
> and all of them gone to the fair?
> Opie, p. 376

Apparently then the original trio were observing a sideshow of
doubtful propriety. From a developmental perspective, however, what is being described is scoptophilia, the desire to look,
which is the normal sexual curiosity of children about anatomic
differences. An especially fascinating mystery for both sexes is
the nature of the female genitalia—that is, what is actually in the
tub. Another issue is the social rules for access to a tub, i.e., how
societal roles are integrated with an individual's sexual needs.

The rhymes, considered together here, illustrate the psychological complexity that can be compressed into a few lines of
verse which are easy for a child to remember, in part because of
the amazing and even absurd images. Until the child can grasp
for himself these issues in an integrated fashion he has the advantage of having at his disposal ready-made verbal play designed to conserve these images and affects. This verbal play has
served a similar function for a parent. Thus, the rhymes contain
the highly charged material in such a way that it remains avail-

able over time to the child's evolving ability to process symbols both consciously and unconsciously.

The ambiguity of the rhymes reflects the complexity of the themes which they contain. The trio sits in the tub which they must outgrow. They are struggling with the urgency of their sexual desires and facing the tasks of consolidating gender identity and resolving narcissistic issues so as to achieve a stable integrated self.

The rhymes do not point forward to resolutions of these conflicts but contain some hints that will be reassuring to children. The rhymes remind a child that grownups have been through this uncomfortable process and that they also felt like "Gothamites" at one time. The conglomeration of fragments which do not quite fit suggests the role of seasoning or development in aiding some ultimate integration. The tradesman's occupations involve turning 3 basic raw materials (carbohydrate, protein, and fat), 3 building blocks of even more complex organisms, into socially appropriate and useful products; the child is encouraged to hope that he has within himself the right makings and that the skill in shaping these resources can be acquired.

Confidence about the sense of oneself as a separate individual leads the way to the discovery about who the child is as a boy or girl. Children are preoccupied with their bodies and want to compare them with those of the same-sex parent whose secondary sex characteristics often are greatly admired. The exhibitionism and scoptophilia of this phallic-narcissistic phase (Edgcumbe and Burgner, 1975) are quite apparent in a number of rhymes. The eagerness to display what one has oneself and to view the opposite sex is well expressed in the following:

> Ride a cock-horse to Banbury Cross
> To see a fine lady upon a white horse;
> Rings on her fingers and bells on her toes,
> And she shall have music wherever she goes.
> Opie, p. 65

For the little girl the metaphor may often be that of something capable of sustaining growth or bearing fruit in the future.

> How does my Lady's garden grow?
> How does my Lady's garden grow?

> With silver bells and cockle shells,
> And pretty maids all in a row.
> Opie, p. 301

> I had a little nut tree
> Nothing would it bear
> But a silver nutmeg
> And a golden pear;

> The king of Spain's daughter
> Came to visit me
> And all for the sake
> Of my little nut tree.
> Opie, p. 330f.

The boy's more aggressive thrusting behavior literally merits the designation phallic; the way in which he attempts to assess the value of his instrument is illustrated in the following Danish rhyme:

> Abel, you spendthrift,
> What does your saber cost?
> 2.20 marks
> If it's good.

> If you want one of copper,
> Go to my brother-in-law.
> If you want one of glass,
> Then you're [lit. go to] a clown!
> Hertz and Clante, p. 21

His worry is, of course, that the instrument may not have the strength or value required; this anxiety can and does at times lead to overstimulation and clowning. However, he does believe that initiative is rewarded.

> Little Jack Horner
> Sat in a corner
> Eating a Christmas pie;
> He put in his thumb,
> And pulled out a plum,
> And said, What a good boy am I.
> Opie, p. 234

The anxiety that this will not work out so well is expressed in the well-known "Simple Simon":

> Simple Simon met a pieman
> Going to the fair;
> Says Simple Simon to the pieman,
> Let me taste your ware.
>
> Says the pieman to Simple Simon,
> Show me first your penny;
> Says Simple Simon to the pieman,
> Indeed I have not any.
> Opie, p. 385

When a boy asks his father about whether he can grow up to be like him, the father may welcome this admiration or instead he may doubt or even deny that his son has the currency, the where-withal, to accomplish this. The problems may, however, also stem from the boy's closeness to the mother and from her expectations of him.

> Simple Simon went a-fishing
> For to catch a whale.
> All the water he had got
> Was in his mother's pail.

The sad conclusion implied in the well-known first two verses is made explicit in the last verse.

> Simple Simon went to look
> If plums grew on a thistle;
> He pinched his finger very much
> Which made poor Simon whistle.

A more hopeful note for children's realistic acceptance of imperfections in themselves is struck in the following rhyme:

> There was a crooked man, and he walked a crooked mile,
> He found a crooked sixpence against a crooked style;
> He bought a crooked cat, which caught a crooked mouse,
> And they all lived together in a little crooked house.
> Opie, p. 289

A person's own effort produces the currency with which family life and domestic ties can be acquired. A boy who together with his brother had had minor orthopedic problems which required modified footwear demanded an explanation of this rhyme and in response to the most general statement about people not always being as well made as they would wish, exclaimed, "I really like my special shoes!"

Peller (1959) has pointed out that well-known children's stories frequently help a child achieve denial in fantasy of the two great polarities, male-female and old-young. Thus in a story like *Winnie the Pooh*, there is a group of "loyal friends" (Pooh and the other animals) and a "magician-protector" (Christopher Robin), but the distinctions between boys and girls and grownups and children are glossed over or blurred.

Of course, comforting as this denial is, it cannot for long assuage children's anxiety about the anatomic difference between the sexes. If for a boy the feelings are organized around whether he can hold on to what he has or whether it is good enough, the girl must struggle with whether it is good enough to be without one, what it is exactly she has instead, and how this all came about. The saga of Little Bo Peep touches on several of these issues.

> Little Bo Peep has lost her sheep
> And can't tell where to find them;
> Leave them alone, and they'll come home,
> And bring their tails behind them.
> Opie, p. 93

Historically the term Bo Peep refers both to the infant amusement peekaboo and the game of hide-and-seek. The girl's initial hope then is that what at first appears to be missing will turn out to have been there all along; far from being something which she lost, it will prove on closer examination to be there after all (the sheep will come home on their own). Sheep's tails are frequently cut off soon after birth and this "castration" is thought to have some hygienic value. The resulting stub may be hard to see in the folds of wool on the rump. Another confusion for the girl is the close proximity of the ano-genital openings. This ambiguity and the possible reluctance to look in a dirty, smelly place are explored and resolved in the following rhyme which is usually suppressed in modern collections:

> When I was a young Maid, and
> Wash't my mother's dishes,
> I putt my finger in my _____ and
> Pluck't out little Fishes.
> Baring-Gould, p. 31

The discovery of one's animal nature, one's id, may be symbolized in rhymes and fairy tales by creatures of the sea, the place where life first arose.

The explanation that a girl had it once but doesn't have it now because she lost it appears in the following rhyme which adds further support to the idea that this "loss" may mark the beginning of a girl's search for her sexuality.

> Lucy Locket lost her pocket,
> Kitty Fisher found it;
> Not a penny was there in it
> Only a ribbon round it.
> Opie, p. 279

This rhyme introduces, in addition, the complexity of a girl's adolescent sexual development. The little girl, Lucy, who "loses" something which boys have, struggles with secrets which seemed "locked" up inside her both literally and figuratively. Like Simple Simon, she has no penny in it, only a feminine pocket which might wrap around something of value. The teenage Lucy will struggle with the issue of how loose or locked up the ribbon should be around the pocket. Lucy's kittenish alter ego who is "on the catch" suggests a different kind of strategy which is successful. The rhyme substantiates the girl's hope that something *was* there all along, but it provides no clear definition of what she possesses.

In some rhymes, as in fairy tales (such as Sleeping Beauty and Snow White), the time which must pass before an individual reaches maturity can be symbolized by sleep.

> Little Bo Peep fell fast asleep
> And dreamt she heard them bleating;
> But when she awoke she found it a joke,
> For they were still all fleeting.
>
> Then up she took her little crook,
> Determined for to find them;
> She found them indeed, but it made her heart bleed
> For they'd left their tails behind them.

The second of these stanzas indicates a progression. Instead of merely relying on fantasy and wish fulfillment, Bo Peep takes an active role, symbolized here by the crook, in searching for a solution. Thus she has moved from the passive denial of the first verse and from the preparation through the dream (which symbolizes the internal work which has been accomplished over time) to the point where she can probe more deeply with her crook into the mystery of her sexuality.

Kestenberg (1975) has described the difficulty a girl faces organizing the information about genitalia which are internal and therefore invisible and yet which may give rise to inner physical sensations. Here Bo Peep is able to act on her curiosity: impelled by the urge for mastery she does probe internally. The bleeding which may follow symbolizes the anxiety which may be felt about a number of experiences. These include the onset of menarche as well as the fear or the experience of hymeneal tear either during the girl's own manipulations or during initial experiences with intercourse. Menarche may help to define the internal genitalia, and the physical experience of intercourse may add pieces to the complex mosaic of her sexuality, but these gains do not resolve the narcissistic tension. The sheep are back, but they are not as they were before.

Sheep appear frequently in the rhymes to disguise sexual themes. Their wool comes off to be spun into clothing, and they call attention to the human body under the clothing. The famous, relatively modern American rhyme, "Mary Had a Little Lamb," is unabashed celebration of a little girl's narcissistic investment in her body image. The exhibitionism described puts one in mind of the way girls of 3 or 4 will lift up their dresses almost as a form of greeting. The interest in body hair is great and the wish for it was touched on in "I had a little nut-tree." The acquisition of pubic hair is the subject of the following rhyme:

> Baa, Baa black sheep
> Have you any wool?
> Yes sir, yes sir,
> Three bags full;
> One for the master,
> And one for the dame,
> And one for the little boy
> Who lives in the lane.
> Opie, p. 88

An alternate reading for the next-to-last line is "but none for the little boy who lives in the lane" (*Mother Goose's Melody*, 1765, p. 59). Both are psychologically true, because whereas during the first resolution of oedipal issues a child must accept that there is a difference between adults and children, he knows then (and can later experience the fact) that he will develop into an adult like his parents.

Another child whose sheep are untended, a little boy who may cry from frustration if awakened before he is ready to accomplish all that he might like, is Little Boy Blue.

> Little Boy Blue
> Come blow your horn,
> The sheep's in the meadow,
> The cow's in the corn;
> But where is the boy
> Who looks after the sheep?
> He's under the haycock,
> Fast asleep.
> Will you wake him?
> No, not I,
> For if I do
> He's sure to cry.
> Opie, p. 98.

Here the question is also raised of whether the child's pleasurable activities "under the haycock" distracted him from the realities which need to be faced. In addition, a parent's overprotectiveness may reinforce this narcissistic dawdling or fail to provide the needed awakening.

Children are, of course, asked to look after their younger silbings and even when the request is not an inappropriate abdication of parental responsibilities, the older sibling has strongly ambivalent feelings concerning it. The tender solicitude of Bo Peep toward the missing sheep may defend against her less kindly feelings toward her charges. The arrival of a younger sibling of the opposite sex may also coincide with the heightened interest in anatomic differences; a little girl in this situation will form her own conclusions about what value parents seem to place on a baby brother and his various attributes.

Competition with a brother as well as her parent's attitudes toward femininity may complicate a girl's search for a sexual identity which she can acknowledge and which merits her confidence. This is indeed a complicated game of hide-and-seek; Bo Peep's search continues.

> It happened one day as Bo Peep did stray
> Into a meadow hard by,
> There she espied their tails side by side,
> All hung on a tree to dry.

In a landscape just past the bounds of her usual explorations she encounters fertile grazing pasture and a tree with the tails hanging from it like branches. This stanza conveys to a little girl a solution to the mystery by way of a riddle. Although the reproductive organs are close to the vagina, the little girl cannot discover for herself anything about their appearance. Their function is even more mysterious, although menarche can and does provide some definition; Bo Peep experiences this in the third verse where it also serves to reinforce the differentiation between anal and genital openings (i.e., the source of the bleeding does locate the "tails" as being "behind"). The riddle contained in this stanza is the metamorphosis of the sheep tail phallus into a wet tree branch. In the last stanza we learn that this transformation must be bidirectional.

> She heaved a sigh, and wiped her eye
> And over the hillock went rambling,
> And tried what she could, as a shepherdess could
> To tack again each to its lambkin.

The peekaboo infant amusement and the hide-and-seek games are related, then, in that one line of development in the discovery of woman's sexuality leads to pregnancy and childbirth. For Bo Peep, this allows her to consolidate one aspect of female adult narcissism. She feels first a "shepherdess" when some of the earlier confusion can be organized by her exertions on the hillocks (which includes the laborious breathing and crying) and by ministrations to her redefined charges, the lambkins. The riddle is solved when the apparent lack of something in a girl reveals itself as a veritable internal tree of life with one branch attached to an infant.

A general discussion of female psychological development and the relative theoretical weight which should be attached to organizing principles such as anxiety about the anatomical difference, possible envy, and the wish for a child is beyond the scope of this presentation. The rhyme takes no position on these highly debated issues. Rather it helps the child and the parent to bear the complexity and ambiguity inherent in the developmental process. The Bo Peep rhyme differs from most nursery songs in that it is an extended story which permits some elaboration and resolution of the conflicts. It is the emphasis on perseverance in the uncovering of inner resources which is supportive of both the grownup's parenting and the child's growth. For Bo Peep, the wish to explore provided her with the instrument of mastery, the crook, and this came finally to symbolize adult adaptation to a world where socially useful activity and caring for others are valued.

The sociology of the nursery setting would be an interesting study in and of itself. Psychoanalysts have long been interested in the relationship between the persons in charge of the nursery and their wards. The nurse could be an older unmarried woman or, as in Dickens's *Dombey and Son,* a woman separated from her husband and children; a particular stereotype, however, is that of the sexually preoccupied and possibly sexually active adolescent girl. For the nurse in her loneliness or sexual frustration the rhymes would serve a particular purpose and have particular meaning. Bergman's *Fanny and Alexander* depicts nursery life at the turn of the century with tensions around oedipal and incestuous issues, and a nursery rhyme is used in one sexually explicit context to embellish the scene.

A number of rhymes treat the vicissitudes of heterosexual relationships during adolescence and may primarily address the developmental needs of the nurses and only secondarily provide diversion for their wards. The usual subject of these rhymes is how best to approach the opposite sex. An old folk song which has entered the nursery-rhyme literature describes one way of broaching the subject.

> Where are you going to, my pretty maid?
> I'm going a-milking, sir, she said.

May I go with you, my pretty maid?
You're kindly welcome, sir, she said.
Opie, p. 281

As things progress, greater persuasion may be needed and the boy might invoke an old charm of milkmaids for refractory cows.

Cushy cow, bonny, let down thy milk,
And I will give thee a gown of silk;
A gown of silk and a silver tee [cow-tie],
If thou wilt let down thy milk to me.
Opie, p. 137

The fascination and repulsion which the girl feels about her own desires is well described in the following:

There was a lady loved a swine,
Honey, quoth she,
Pig-hog wilt thou be mine?
Hough, quoth he.

I'll build thee a silver stye,
Honey, quoth she.
And in it thou shalt lie
Hough, quoth he.

Pinned with a silver pin,
Honey, quoth she.
That thou may go out and in,
Hough, quoth he.

Wilt thou have me now,
Honey? quoth she.
Speak or my heart will break
Hough, quoth he.
Opie, p. 261

The original song from the time of James I was even more direct:

There was a Lady lov'd a hogge, hony quoth shee.
Won't thou lie with me tonight? oug, quoth he.
Opie, p. 262

The integration of sexuality into a love relationship is described in the well-known courtship rhyme sung by a considerably more articulate lover to a girl whose name suggests that she may have been capable of more self-restraint than the aforementioned lady.

> Curly locks, curly locks,
> Wilt thou be mine?
> Thou shalt not wash dishes
> Nor yet feed the swine,
> But sit on a cushion
> And sew a fine seam,
> And feed upon strawberries,
> Sugar and cream.
> Opie, p. 140

The varieties of sexual experience depicted in the rhymes include masturbation, erection, premature ejaculation, impotence, and frigidity, and male to male anal intercourse. The feelings which accompany these events range from elation to despair, from exhaustion to chagrin. Again it is clear that one reason the rhymes have endured is that they have addressed the concerns of the older and younger denizens of the nursery.

SOME FAMOUS RHYMES

A few nursery rhymes found in every collection are as ambiguous as they are well known. Rhymes such as "London bridge is falling down," "Three blind mice," "Hey diddle diddle, the cat and the fiddle," and others are so familiar that they seem to be permanent fixtures in the landscape of everyone's childhood. Learned by rote like religious incantations or the pledge of allegiance to the flag, they are too close to us to prompt much reflection. When we do consider them, we may be disturbed by their violent or unrealistic content. For this reason some parents prefer not to have children hear them. Frequently they are as incomprehensible as they are brief.

I believe that this handful of popular rhymes represents a prototype of the nursery-rhyme genre in that these rhymes rely so much on primary process, the child's archaic mode of experience. For this reason our responses to them are more unconscious and personal; their appeal rests more on their ability to evoke a powerful response from children, adults, and analytic interpreters than on their meaning being transparent. For these rhymes the kind of analysis we have been pursuing up to now must be at the same time more tentative and more adventurous because the degree of disguise is so much greater.

As an illustration of these ideas I have chosen two rhymes which contain descriptions of aggressive themes in the relationship between parents and children. The first is a single-parent family where the situation is a bit out of hand:

> There was an old woman who lived in a shoe
> She had so many children, she didn't know what to do;
> She gave them some broth without any bread;
> She whipped them all soundly and put them to bed.
> Opie, p. 434

The symbol of the shoe stems from an ancient cultural heritage. It is preserved in the custom of throwing a shoe after the bride for good luck as she embarks on her honeymoon; a slipper plays a central role in one of the best known fairy tales, *Cinderella*. In nursery rhymes this symbol has a similar significance and appears in the following lament with a male counterpart:

> Cock a doodle doo!
> My dame has lost her shoe,
> My master's lost his fiddlestick,
> And knows not what to do.
> Opie, p. 128

The old woman seems to be in the opposite predicament. Having lived in her shoe to such an extent that she has too many family responsibilities, she is a depriving and abusive parent. Of course, all mothers seem this way to children at some time: she seems to pay too much attention to the others and to be unable to provide what the child needs. Bettelheim (1976) has pointed out how the wicked stepmother imago, so frequent in fairy tales, is a distortion which may aid the child in his efforts at separation. Another version of this rhyme is as follows:

> There was an old woman, and she liv'd in a shoe,
> She had so many children, she didn't know what to do.
> She crumm'd 'em some porridge without any bread;
> And she borrow'd a beetle, and she knocked 'em all o' the head.

> Then out went th' old woman to bespeak 'em a coffin,
> And when she came back, she found 'em all a-loffeing.
> Opie, p. 435

The Shakespearean word for laughing also occurs in "Old Mother Hubbard," the story of a well-intentioned and conscientious parent who is teased for 14 verses by her dog, and all for want of a bone in the cupboard.

> Old Mother Hubbard
> Went to the cupboard
> To fetch her poor dog a bone;
> But when she came there
> The cupboard was bare
> And so the poor dog had none.
>
> She went to the baker's
> To buy him some bread;
> But when she came back
> The poor dog was dead.
>
> She went to the undertaker's
> To buy him a coffin;
> But when she came back
> The poor dog was laughing.
> Opie, p. 317

There are other rhymes and fairy tales concerning a woman who needs a bone in her cupboard, and Old Mother Hubbard's efforts to please could be interpreted on a number of levels. Her good humor persists to the end, but another parent might more easily succumb to the rage provoked by these sadistic torments from demanding children. The proverbial bad mother may then retaliate because the children really are bad; that is, there may be a good reason for the old woman in the shoe to become angry and set a firm limit with her children.

The woman of the shoe also has difficulty containing her sexual urges, and the deprivation and "abuse" may be two modes which she employs to address this problem; she may deny herself, or may refuse to give in to the sexual desires with which her shoe is teeming, or she may resort to strenuous "abuse," whether "self-abuse" or promiscuity, which also takes its toll. The theme of being on fire with these urges, which can be in conflict with parenting goals, is treated in a rhyme with numerous variants and parallels.

> Ladybird, ladybird, fly away home,
> Your house is on fire, your children will burn.
> Eckenstein, p. 92

The Swedish word for Ladybird is the Virgin Mary keybearer (Jungfru Marias Nyckelpiga—actually "key girl") and refers to the myth that of all the animals it was the ladybird who came to the Virgin's aid and found the keys to heaven which Mary had lost; thus the ladybird mother was once a child who achieved mastery and overcame the lack of a bone in the cupboard. In some versions of the Ladybird rhyme a boy survives:

> All but one, and he is Tum,
> And he lies under the grindelstone.
> Eckenstein, p. 93

The grindelstone or grindstone belongs to a mill and a chain of associations from comparative folklore sketches in the image of a powerful boy with no father who possesses a hammer like a flat stone mace. The boy's hammer, which is properly the instrument of a miller, symbolizes masculine aggressive impulses which are necessary for survival and the part of his heritage derived from his father. A variant of the Ladybird song from Saxony addresses the issue of the father's whereabouts, and the mother's position.

> Fly, beetle, fly, Father has gone to war,
> Mother has crept into the shoe,
> She has broken her left leg.
> Eckenstein, p. 100

The broken left leg has, of course, been bitten by the stork who brings babies and mention of it merely confirms mother's maternal status. The reason for mother's deprivations and her frustrations is clearer now. Father is engaged in the business of the world, while she, cramped and confined by maternal obligations, tries to nourish their children with warmth from the hearth without allowing internal and interpersonal tensions to ignite. When things are stretched to the limit and there is no father, that is, no miller to grind the flour, life for the children is quite monochromatic, all broth and no bread; in addition, the aggressive, sadistic impulses may be given full rein because of inadequate containing and modulating forces from a male parent (Herzog, 1980).

The most gruesome such scene is contained in the following rhyme:

> Three blind mice, see how they run!
> They all ran after the farmer's wife,
> Who cut off their tails with a carving knife,
> Did you ever see such a thing in your life,
> As three blind mice?
> Opie, p. 306

The number 3 has, of course, oedipal resonance, and this gory scene may be a blinding and castration from the farmer because of the scoptophilia and sexual attraction toward his wife by the young ones. An obscure version from 1609 provides a connection with the Miller and reinforces the impression that the lady is the violent one.

> Three blinde Mice, three blinde Mice
> Dame Julian, Dame Julian
> The Miller and his merry old Wife,
> Shee scrapte her tripe licke thou the knife.
> Opie, p. 306

Tripe refers to belly or intestine but also to "any poor, worthless (usually offensive) matter, thing or person." Does this simply mean that one of these women castrated herself and after this self-inflicted humiliation offered someone a triumphal but possibly dangerous taste of the experience? It brings to mind Kaplan's speculations (1976) concerning a Medusa complex; she hypothesized that self-debasing behavior by juvenile delinquent girls could be used defensively to attack or humiliate an onlooker. Since the first 3 lines of the rhyme have a bawdy lilt, the final line is even more shocking. The associations between sexuality and aggression are, of course, a constant childhood concern, and the power of this rhyme derives from the combination of excitement and fright about these impulses which it conveys.

The relationship between sexuality and aggression is a complicated one for children and some adults. Both famous rhymes discussed above deal with some aspect of this association as it relates what one might broadly denote as oedipal and counteroedipal themes. Here are the many images of the parent-child relationship: the bad, sadistic, depriving parent and the good but ineffectual and masochistic parent; the erotically stimulating parent; the frightening parent who may attack or behave in a self-destructive way; the absent parent who remains a powerful force in the child's mind; and the child who is a victim, a tormentor, or capable of self-rescue, and able to nurture.

In contrast to rhymes discussed earlier, the story of these last two rhymes is even more difficult to translate into the kind of psychoanalytic story constructed earlier. Although this high degree of ambiguity creates difficulties for explications, it can be a characteristic of the rhymes which make the deepest imprint on young and old minds alike. When the disguise is so complete and the stories so fragmentary, much more is left up to the imagination of the listener.

CONCLUSION

This survey has attempted to display the value of not only approaching each rhyme on its own terms, but also treating it as part of a larger organic whole. Thus, children and parents have available to them an amalgamation of many rhymes capable of generating a multiplicity of interpretations, and the rhymes as a whole are well constituted so as to serve all of us in our different moods and different positions in the life cycle.

Any selection of rhymes for study would be dependent upon the observer's interests, and clearly other linkages between rhymes could be explored than the ones treated here. A welcome addition to the studies in this presentation would be information about rhymes which are important to child and adult patients and the way in which responses to this body of literature is intertwined with psychopathology (Petty, 1953).

The fact that the rhymes, like children's games, have endured for centuries in forms with a slow rate of change suggests that they express some basic transcultural and transhistorical equations. As such they can be considered to be a kind of clinical material worthy of study. They represent the articulation of raw experience as it is transformed by language and culture with a simplicity which puts them within the reach of a shared developmental rendezvous point for both parents and children. At this rendezvous point these universal experiences can be articulated in the psychological context of the family with the specific colorations and nuances which apply at that moment to that parent-child pair.

BIBLIOGRAPHY

BARING-GOULD, W. & C. (1962). *The Annotated Mother Goose.* New York: Bramhall House.
BETTELHEIM, B. (1976). *The Uses of Enchantment.* New York: Knopf.
BLOS, P. (1967). The second individuation process of adolescence. *Psychoanal. Study Child,* 22:162–186.
ECKENSTEIN, L. (1906). *Comparative Studies in Nursery Rhymes.* London: Duckworth.
EDGCUMBE, R. & BURGNER, M. (1975). The phallic-narcissistic phase. *Psychoanal. Study Child,* 30:161–180.
GOLDINGS, H. J. (1974). Jump-rope rhymes and the rhythm of latency development in girls. *Psychoanal. Study Child,* 29:431–450.
GOMME, A. B. (1804–98). *The Traditional Games of England, Scotland, and Ireland.* New York: Dover, 1964.
HALLIWELL, J. O. (1849). *Popular Rhymes and Nursery Tales.* London: John Russell Smith.
HERTZ, G. J. & CLANTE, I. (1971). *Dig og mig og vi to . . . børnerim og sange.* Copenhagen: Carlsen.
HERZOG, J. M. (1980). Sleep disturbance and father hunger in 18- to 28-month-old boys. *Psychoanal. Study Child,* 35:219–233.
KAPLAN, E. B. (1976). Manifestations of aggression in latency and preadolescent girls. *Psychoanal. Study Child,* 31:63–78.
KESTENBERG, J. S. (1975). *Children and Parents.* New York: Aronson.
Mother Goose's Melody. London: Christopher, c. 1765.
OPIE, I. & P. (1951). *The Oxford Dictionary of Nursery Rhymes.* New York: Oxford Univ. Press.
PELLER, L. F. (1959). Daydreams and children's favorite books. *Psychoanal. Study Child,* 14:414–433.
PERRAULT, C. (1697). *Histoires au Contes du temps passe.* Paris.
PETTY, T. A. (1953). The tragedy of humpty dumpty. *Psychoanal. Study Child,* 8:404–412.
SARNOFF, C. (1976). *Latency.* New York: Aronson.
SHENGOLD, L. (1982). Anal erogeneity. *Int. J. Psychoanal.,* 63:331–345.

Twinship Themes and Fantasies in the Work of Thornton Wilder

JULES GLENN, M.D.

A RECENT BIOGRAPHY, *THE ENTHUSIAST,* BY GILBERT A. HARRISON (1983) fortifies the hypothesis that Wilder's life and work were influenced by his having been a survivor of a pair of twins. Goldstone (1975) and Friedman (1952) had noted that the author of *The Bridge of San Luis Rey* (1927) had a twin brother who died a few hours after his birth. Now Harrison provides us with important addenda: "Born prematurely and a twin, he had a precarious start. His identical brother, though perfectly formed, was stillborn, too frail to be cried or patted into life, and there was doubt whether Thornton himself would survive. For weeks during that first hot summer he was carried about on a pillow and fed limewater" (p. 17).

In this paper I will draw on facts of Wilder's history, activities, and fantasies, which Harrison learned from many sources, including Wilder's personal journals, to delineate how the famous author's twinship affected his personality and writings. Drawing on his work, I will describe two of his books, *The Bridge of San Luis*

Clinical professor of psychiatry, New York University Medical Center. Training and supervising analyst, The Psychoanalytic Institute, New York University Medical Center.

I want to express my appreciation for the helpful comments of those who have read and discussed drafts of this paper. They include Drs. Harold P. Blum, Isidor Bernstein, Stanley Grossman, Eugene Halpert, Milton Jucovy, and Eugene Kaplan who compose the study group in Great Neck where we discussed my paper, and Dr. Jacob A. Arlow. In addition, Drs. Francis Baudry, Theodore Jacobs, Shelley Orgel, and Leonard Shengold as well as professors Richard Goldstone and Arthur Zeiger were kind enough to offer extensive critiques of the article.

627

Rey (1927) and *Theophilus North* (1973), which are particularly relevant to our topic and which Wilder actually connected with his twinship.

The circumstances of Wilder's life and birth and the content of some of his writing suggest the following hypotheses: After Thornton learned of his twinship, he wondered why he had survived and his brother died. Could his brother have been punished for something bad Theophilus had done? Or could his twin Theophilus, "dear to the gods or God" (Webster, 1956) and lover of God (Wilder, 1973), have been rewarded by going to heaven with its peace (Theophilus's nickname was Pax!)? He attributed his sibling's death and his own survival to a super-natural force and felt grateful but guilty. But for the grace of God it could have been Thornton who died. Because he was glad that his brother and not he had died, it was as though he himself had killed his sibling. But he nevertheless envied Theophilus for being in heaven and wanted to join him there. Feeling remorse, he tried to atone and undo the tragedy by becoming a rescuer of people in difficulty. He could also keep his brother alive through reproducing him in the form of a character in a novel or play and by identifying with his dead sibling in his creations. The identifi-cation was not always useful, as he confused his possibly pun-ished brother and himself and assumed his guilt. And the identi-fication served as a self-punishment. Inner forces to separate himself from his twin made for a certain distance and aloofness in himself and some of his characters.

I am not suggesting that Thornton Wilder's guilt at his broth-er's death or fear of its implications appeared at birth. At that time no child possesses the cognitive capacity to understand the facts or the significance of a dead infant. Rather I believe the knowledge acquired later of his brother's catastrophe—and his own fortuitous survival—organized complicated and even con-tradictory fantasies. The fantasies contained references to his relationship with his parents and his other siblings as well. These included antagonistic feelings toward his overbearing, moral-istic, distant, but in some ways kind father, with whom he also identified; wishes to save his mother from the cruel and possibly sexual treatment of his father; affectionate attachment to mother and sisters. The twin fantasies served defensive screening and organizing functions.

There is a marked difference between the experience of twins who are raised in close proximity and those of a twin who learns that his identical counterpart died at birth. Each of the twins raised together sees and feels and hears another similar person going through developmental stages at the same time. Each touches and gratifies the other, offsetting frustration by parents. On the other hand the twins may suffer parental neglect as mother can feed or otherwise care for only one at a time. Excessive stimulation and frustration may interfere with the development of self and object representations, reality testing, and secondary process thinking. The presence of the gratifying twin may interfere with oedipal gratification, parental cathexis, and oedipal resolution. Superego deficiencies may occur through the twins' being considered special, exceptions, and as a result of failures of oedipal resolution. Supplementing these experiential determinants are the things the twins hear and learn about twinship—that they come from one egg which splits, for instance (Arlow, 1960; Glenn, 1966; Joseph, 1975). A twin like Wilder, who does not live with his sibling, must build his picture of their fantasied relationship out of thinner and more intellectual material.

Eissler (1968) has suggested that applied analytic studies can cast light not only on creative processes and products through the application of psychoanalytic knowledge and theory, but can also provide data and hypotheses that advance analytic science.

Previous studies have revealed that twin fantasies involve not one but a variety of genetic and dynamic constellations. These include attempts to resolve oedipal conflicts and to provide reassurance against castration anxiety, separation anxiety, and loneliness (Burlingham, 1952; Tyson, 1980), narcissistic desires for and fears of the presence of doubles (Rank, 1914), needs to overcome narcissistic imbalance and enhance the stability of the sense of self (Kohut, 1971), and regressive wishes for symbiotic attachment (Tyson, 1980). Twin fantasies can appear with marked intensity in adopted children (Glenn, 1974b; Berlin, 1985), when there is multiple mothering (Kramer, 1985), when a child has twin siblings (Bernstein, 1980), or when the child's parent is a twin, especially when a strong libidinal attachment exists (Coen and Bradlow, 1982).

THE BRIDGE OF SAN LUIS REY AND THE SURVIVOR THEME

On July 20, 1714, the fictional bridge of San Luis Rey collapsed and with it five people fell to their destruction. The first thought of many a survivor was to calculate mentally "how recently he had crossed by it and how soon he had intended crossing by it again" (Wilder, 1927, p. 3f.). A person would say "to himself with secret joy: 'within ten minutes myself!'" (p. 5). Wilder put aside these forbidden thoughts—close to those he himself might have had when he learned of his birth and his brother's death—and through Brother Juniper, who observed the bridge's destruction, asks, "Why did this happen to *those* five?" (p. 5) Juniper tries to discover any pattern that would show whether God had intended the death of the five persons on the bridge and for what reasons. Could their demise have been punishment for some evil intent or act? Or could it have been a reward for virtue? Brother Juniper "thought he saw in the same accident the wicked visited by destruction and the good called early to Heaven. He thought he saw pride and wealth confounded as an object lesson to the world, and he thought he saw humility crowned and rewarded for the edification of the city" (p. 130). The individuals, however, were not necessarily totally sinful or entirely good; indeed, one woman who had previously fought a losing battle with her hateful disposition toward her daughter found love before she died.

As the book ends we come to realize that the death of the victims touched those who lived as well. The living came to love the dead and perhaps then perform good acts. An Abbess, suffering loss, wonders about its significance and thinks, "But soon we shall die and all memory of those five will have left the earth, and we ourselves shall be loved for a while and forgotten. But the love will have been enough; all those impulses of love return to the love that made them. Even memory is not necessary for love. There is a land of the living and a land of the dead, and the bridge is love, the only survival, the only meaning" (p. 139).

Implied in these words is the idea that for the living love bridges the way to the dead, and also perhaps—though Wilder explicitly has denied it—that the living can reach, have contact, union with the dead they love.

The five people who died are Dona Maria, Marquesa of Montemayor; Pepita, her servant; Esteban, a twin whose brother had died; Uncle Pio who, Pygmalionlike, had trained a local beauty, Camila Perichole, to be a great actress; and Jaime, her son.

I shall concentrate on Esteban, the twin who probably is the central character of the novel, the one most identified with the author. Indeed, there is striking evidence that this is so. Prior to the publication of *The Bridge of San Luis Rey* Wilder noted in his journal "that one of the principal ideas behind my work is the fear of catastrophe (especially illness or pain), and a preoccupation with the claim of a religion to meet the situation" (Harrison, 1983, p. 103). That he viewed the birth of his brother and himself as a catastrophe is confirmed by a fictional date he assigned to the collapse of the bridge. Although he finally made the fateful day "Friday noon, July the twentieth, 1714," in an early version the data was April 17, his own birthday (p. 105).

Wilder was aware that his twinship had an impact. Replying to an inquiry by Friedman (1952), Wilder noted, "I was an identical twin. . . . That left me very attentive to twinship" (p. 72). And during a lecture following the publication of *The Bridge,* he described his "amused and affectionate speculation as to what it would be like to have an identical self going about the world with one, writing perhaps, collaborating perhaps. But before I knew it, those tranquil speculations turned out in the book to be more and more serious" (Harrison, p. 117).

The fact that one of the twins of the novel was named Manuel further supports the contention that the story is about Theophilus and Thornton. Manuel is Spanish for Emmanuel which means "God with us" (Webster, 1956), almost a synonym for "beloved of God."[1] (For the curious I will add that Esteban, the other twin's name, is Spanish for Stephen, which means "crown.")

Manuel and Esteban were identical twin foundlings raised in

1. Dr. Leonard Shengold brought this to my attention.

the Convent of Santa Maria Rosa de los Rosas by the Abbess, Madre Maria del Pilar, who came to love them. They worked hard at the convent, cleaning, running, and polishing, but eventually became scribes and copyists for the choirmasters. The boys, taciturn, developed a secret language, a "symbol of their profound identity" (p. 51). "*Love* is inadequate to describe the tacit . . . oneness of these brothers" (p. 52). Indeed, they experienced a mutual telepathy. They felt all persons except the twins were strange and hostile. At the same time they avoided looking at each other, even walking together in public. Eventually the love of the Perichole, the Peruvian actress, came between them. Manuel, attracted to her, became her scribe and periodically wrote private love letters for her which he promised not to reveal even to Esteban. Because Esteban was deeply hurt and Manuel feared losing him, he decided to give up the Perichole, not write for her anymore. He denied that he loved her because he had never come close to consummating a relationship with the actress.

Tragedy came upon them as Manuel injured his knee when a piece of metal pierced his flesh. The infection that ensued was painful, especially when Esteban followed the barber's advice and ministered painful compresses. Manuel, delirious, cursed and asked God to condemn his brother to hell, only to deny responsibility for his damnations. When Manuel died, Esteban, distraught, refused to view his brother's body. Once he took on his brother's name and identity. He longed to die but could not commit suicide. In a poorly disguised attempt at self-destruction, he ran into a burning house to rescue someone but escaped unharmed. He agreed to go on a long sea journey in which the captain would give him dangerous jobs on the ship. On the way to Lima to start the voyage, Esteban crossed the bridge and died.

It is apparent that the twinship of Manuel and Esteban dominated their lives, that they felt like one and could not bear separation. Esteban longed to be reunited with his beloved brother and wished to die to achieve it. With the collapse of the bridge he achieved this aim. The bridge took him to heaven and to Manuel. Mystically, but in accord with the principles of over-determination and multiple functions, the collapse of the bridge represented the birth of the twins, in which they were separated, as well as the bridge that would reunite them.

Studies of the bridge as a more or less universal psycho-analytic symbol (Ferenczi, 1921; Freud, 1933; Lewin, 1933; Friedman, 1952; Shengold, 1980) have revealed it can possess a panoply of related meanings. It can represent "the male organ, which unites the two parents in sexual intercourse; but after-wards it develops further meanings which are derived from this first one. In so far as it is thanks to the male organ that we are able to come into the world at all, out of the amniotic fluid, a bridge becomes the crossing from the other world (the unborn state, the womb) to this world (life); and, since men also picture death as a return to the womb (to the water), a bridge also ac-quires the meaning of something that leads to death" (Freud, 1933, p. 24).

I suggest that in Wilder's case the bridge symbolized the birth canal from which the twins emerged, a meaning consonant with the fact that Wilder equated the collapse of the bridge and the catastrophic birth of his twin and himself. I have seen two pa-tients to whom a bridge represented a birth canal, and passage over the bridge meant birth and danger. One patient imagined herself giving birth and identified with the baby. Her bent knees as she lay supine looked like the overhead supports that span the bridge. She also pictured herself in her car crossing the bridge as the baby was being born. The birth meant to her a calamitous separation from her beloved mother, who had died and whom she wanted to be with. Another patient with a fear of crossing bridges pictured the configuration of the Tappan Zee Bridge as similar to that of the birth canal which he was traversing; as one crossed the span, one rode upward and then downward to the exit. For him birth was separation from mother and castration. Being in the birth canal represented intercourse with mother, a seductive woman, which demanded castration as a punishment. As in Freud's (1933) description, the bridge was associated with birth and death, but the route to the symbol was different.

The symbol of the bridge cannot be separated from the sym-bol of the aqueous chasm below into which the person who crosses the bridge may fall to his death. Falling into the body of water has been shown to represent death, a punishment for

incest and castration. As the water reminds one of the baby's
amniotic surround, it symbolizes birth and entrance into the
mother's body as a preoedipal infant or an oedipal child
(Lewin, 1933). We may surmise that Wilder's learning of his
twinship evoked fantasies that the image of the falling bridge
made vivid.

Before discussing Theophilus North and rescue fantasies, I
note that questions of survival appear in Wilder's plays. *Our
Town* asserts that mankind will continue its course despite death
and difficulty. Goldstone (1975) underlines its "inherent optimism derived from its native soil" (p. 141). "The play," he
writes, "somehow provided hope and promise for the American future. . . . *Our Town* has been determined by a people with
faith in itself, in the nation's capacity to survive. . . . When the
faith, the survival, the principles go, presumably another nation will come into being" (p. 141f.). Interestingly enough, in
Act I, Wilder engages the audience's optimism by having first a
doctor and later the stage manager announce the birth of twins.
Unlike Theophilus who perished, each twin survives and adds
to the populace.

The Skin of Our Teeth depicts even more forcefully humanity's
repeated ability to endure even when confronted by devastating conditions—the ice age, the flood, war. As Goldstein (1965)
states, "The title itself announces the theme, which is that no
matter how hard pressed or frightened, the human race has
power to survive its great adventure in a world where physical
nature and its own internal conflicts pose endless threats" (p.
118). In addition to the survival motif, the plays reveal Wilder's
unremitting desire to rescue people, which manifests itself in a
savior theme that we will examine in *Theophilus North*. *The Skin
of Our Teeth* was "calculated to encourage the troubled public of
1942" (p. 118) during World War II.

THEOPHILUS NORTH AND THE RESCUE THEME

We know from our clinical work that we should apply psychoanalytic symbolism with caution. I have therefore relied on Wilder's comments on the bridge and birth as well as patients'
associations in discussing its significance. I will be less cautious

as I note that *Theophilus North,* Wilder's last novel, starts with what analysts have found to be a symbol of pregnancy and birth, the number 9 (Freud, 1923), which recurs during the story. In the first chapter the protagonist describes his nine ambitions. The second chapter compares Newport, Rhode Island, where the events of the novel occur, and Troy: each of the cities is composed of nine cities which the author describes. A later chapter in the book is about an estate called "Nine Gables" and North describes a later section as "Nine Gables Part II." The symbolism serves to alert us to the impact of Wilder's unusual birth on the tales he will spin.

Theophilus North is a young man born in Wisconsin, raised in China and Berkeley, a graduate of Yale who had been to Europe for a year after graduation and who had taught at a boys' preparatory school in New Jersey for three years, a background almost identical to Wilder's. Further similarities between author and protagonist include their fathers' being editors and then holding diplomatic posts in China. The Theophilus of the novel comes to Newport to earn money as a tutor of and reader to the wealthy. Not incidentally he goes about rescuing people in difficult circumstances. Almost every chapter describes such a salvation. I select only a few of the adventures.

When engaged to read family letters for an elderly Miss Norine Wyckoff, Theophilus discovers that because rumor has it that her mansion is haunted, she cannot keep servants or entertain properly. First he uncovers the origin of the rumor. Many years ago when Miss Wyckoff's parents spent a great deal of time away from their Newport home, the servants had cavorted wickedly. A young boy of 12, Bill Owens, had observed their banquets and orgies and even believed they practiced cannibalism. Later, Owens spread debasing stories of what he had seen. Meanwhile Mr. Wyckoff had returned, surprised his servants, and fired them. Owens's tales and their exaggerations reached employment agencies and Wyckoff became unable to hire help. The belief that the house was haunted grew from the reports of the servants' behavior.

The mystery solved, North set about replacing the malicious rumors with good ones. He maneuvered a gossip columnist, whose pen name was Flora Deland, to publish glorious tales of the Wyckoff place—stories of its wonderful ventilation due to its remarkable architecture, of its magnificent acoustics which made Paderewski weep and which enticed Thomas Edison to supervise the recording of Nellie Melba's voice there. North even succeeded in getting Miss Deland to write about a miraculous and saintly healer who had lived in the house. These corrective rumors served to rehabilitate the mansion, make it sought after as a source of employment, and restore Miss Wyckoff to a prestigious and happy life. In addition, through her inspiring and generous columns, different from those she had written in the past, Flora gains a respect she had longed for.

In "Nine Gables" Theophilus acquires a position reading to an old, physically restricted, and seemingly ill man. Dr. James Bosworth's family, especially his daughter Sarah, is for the most part leary of North's entrance into the home and his intimacy with Dr. Bosworth as they study Berkeley together. They keep a sharp eye on the two. Their purpose is to keep Dr. Bosworth in check, keep him from entering any relationship that might end in his distributing his wealth to fortune hunters, female or male, intent on marriage or eager to acquire money for philanthropies. To that end they convince him he is ill with a kidney ailment and cannot leave the house lest he be incontinent or become sicker.

Theophilus North pretends he has been a truck driver and hence knows of remedies for the kidney trouble which plagues drivers. He passes pills and some sort of contraption to control Dr. Bosworth's incontinence. With the help of the man's granddaughter Persis who gets him a new younger doctor not in cahoots with the family, North succeeds in convincing Dr. Bosworth that he is not ill, that he can leave the house, visit the buildings he admires, drink whiskey, and enjoy life. Some time later North meets Dr. Bosworth and learns he has abandoned his plan for an Academy of Philosophers but is planning to build and endow a clinic for the young physician.

The reader will note that in most of the stories, Theophilus rescues not one but several people in need. Perhaps this configuration refers to a wish that both he and his twin be rescued, and to his desire to rescue his mother as well.

After rescuing Dr. Bosworth, Theophilus also saves Persis and a German diplomat, who marry. In chapter 10, Theophilus encourages a brilliant young man who had lost his feet in an accident to go to college and to date women. In the same story, Agnes, the girl he goes out with—a twin!—becomes relieved as she realizes her deceased husband might have died honorably in the war and not immorally as she had feared. In chapter 11, Theophilus rescues both a husband and wife from the misery of childlessness by having intercourse with the woman.

Wilder's preoccupation with rescue fantasies was present in a number of his novels, including *The Cabala* and *Heaven's My Destination*. It also appears in several of his plays. *The Matchmaker* is about a woman who arranges other persons' lives and in the end her own.

Heaven's My Destination was a comic treatment of a character who had traits similar to Theophilus North. Wilder asserted that the book was autobiographical, at least in the sense that it attempts to come to terms with early influences in his life (Goldstone, 1953). It chronicles events in the life of George Brush when he was 23 to 24 years of age. Brush is a fundamentalist Baptist traveling salesman of educational books who is intent on propounding his ideas and improving people's lot. His unbelievably naïve and bumbling interventions succeed in antagonizing people and even landing him in jail. He is a firm believer in God and an opponent of smoking and the theory of evolution. He refuses to accept interest from banks. He is a follower of Gandhi who believes in *ahimsa* and even takes a vow of silence. In one episode, Brush gets into serious difficulty when he attempts to reform a thief by telling him where the victim's cash is and even giving him money. Innocently and with the most Christian of motives, he abets the petty criminal's escape and appears to be holding up the store. In another episode he advises a young lady on how to improve herself by finding true belief and giving up evils like smoking. He succeeds in throwing her into hysterics.

The tale takes a depressing turn when Brush loses his faith and becomes so dejected and ill he almost dies. In a physical recovery at the end of the book, he sadly regains his beliefs and returns to his old ways, blundering along in his picaresque journey through life.

In *The Cabala,* the protagonist's attempts at rescue fail. For instance, his attempts to rescue young Marcantonio from an

immoral and promiscuous life by encouraging a strict and pu-
ritanical conscience end in the youth's punishing himself by suicide for engaging in incest with his half sister.

The reader might well be skeptical of my suggestion that
Theophilus North is about Thornton Wilder and his twin were
it not for the fact that his twin's name was Theophilus. Knowing that, one can readily see significance in the fact that the
name Theophilus North contains the names of both brothers,
Theophilus and Thornton, the first five letters of the latter
being an anagram of North. Confirming the suggestion that
Theophilus North is an amalgam of the two, Harrison (1983)
writes:

> The twin relationship had long been pondered. The-
> ophilus . . . and Todger (Thornton) were bound together in an
> unstable coexistence. Todger carried the burden of his father's
> New England ethos, whose watchword was duty—self-im-
> provement and the improvement of others. Theophilus was
> eager to explore other roads—adventure, enjoyment. Todger
> was the excellent student, one who set an example to mis-
> guided fellows who bring grief and shame on their parents.
> "But it should be remembered at the same time," Thornton
> wrote, "that these twins were mixed-up young men." Todger
> had his curiosities, too. Nor was Theophilus a mere hedonist;
> he had his share of quixotic idealism. Identical twins, Thorn-
> ton noted, are not just amalgamations of the characteristics in-
> herited from their ancestors . . . but are one man's packet of
> characteristics in two editions: "If your name (say) is George,
> there are two Georges. Outwardly you and your brother re-
> semble one another exactly. . . . In George One and George
> Two there are only the same inherited traits distributed differ-
> ently. . . ." In his journal, Thornton remarked, "It was some
> time before the author of this book became fully aware that he
> was a mixed package" [p. 368]

In addition Goldstone (1975) observes that "Wilder told inter-
viewers . . . that Theophilus was his alter ego, his opposite—
what his twin brother might have been like had he lived" (p.
261).

The question arises as to who the rescuer in *Theophilus North*
is. Was it Thornton or his deceased twin brother? It seems quite
likely that Thornton Wilder himself, out of wishes to undo his

brother's death, to rescue him retrospectively, was the savior. Indeed, as Harrison reports, Thornton Wilder was an inveterate advice giver in real life. He intended and often succeeded in setting people on the right road, getting them proper connections, etc.

In a chapter entitled "Throwing Out Lifelines," Harrison describes quite a few rescue missions. "Thornton threw out lifelines, but he expected the one at the other end to take hold. . . . He didn't argue with the sufferer, seldom criticized. . . . And although he thought that his heart got colder with the years, the testimony to his constancy and helpfulness is so abundant that his self-deprecation has to be questioned" (p. 305).

A specific example: "Reading . . . that John Sweet, a member of the *Our Town* cast in London in 1944, had decided to give up the stage, he wrote him a four-page letter urging him to think carefully about leaving the theater . . . and when Sweet came to New York he was taken to the Century Club and given notes to five producers. Thornton did the same for scores of young artists" (p. 306).

Earlier in the biography Harrison points out that Wilder "would aid refugees fleeing Nazi Germany and Austria, providing affidavits of support enabling them to obtain American visas, welcoming them at the dock in New York, handing them five hundred dollars, arranging hotel accommodations, taking them to dinner and sending them theater tickets" (p. 210).

Several considerations lead me to believe that the savior was his twin as well as Thornton. First, the name Wilder chose for the rescuer in *Theophilus North* contained the names of both twins, and Wilder actually stated that North was what his twin might have been. Second, each twin was in desperate need of saving. Theophilus, sadly, died in early infancy and, according to the family tale, Thornton was close to death after his birth. As Thornton grew up, his father considered him socially and physically fragile. We have seen that Wilder must have wished he had saved his brother. Most likely he imagined and hoped that his brother, dear to God and lover of God[2] certainly a

2. Although Webster (1956) defines Theophilus as dear to the gods or God, Wilder (1973) has one character define it as "one who loves God" (p. 238).

favored person, could perform a similar miracle, return to earth and, Christlike, save Thornton. As noted above, entries in Wilder's journals suggest that he conceived of the two as a single united being.

The concluding chapter of *The Cabala* appears to confirm the idea that Wilder harbored the fantasy that Theophilus returned to earth, entered and fused with Thornton, making a Godlike rescuer of the earth-bound man, who acquired the rescuing qualities of the one who lived in heaven.

Elizabeth Grier, a spokeswoman for an elite Roman group, the Cabala, tells the writer nicknamed Samuele that when a god of antiquity died, "his godhead was passed on to someone else; no sooner is Saturn dead than some man somewhere feels a new personality descending upon him like a straight-jacket" (p. 219). For instance, she says, reading a document to the author, a certain Hollander became the god Mercury in 1912. Similarly, she implies, Samuele is a man transformed into a god. Indeed, the name Samuele itself, like Theophilus, connotes a godlike quality. It means "His name is *El* (God)" (Webster, 1956).[3] Samuele, who, during the novel, attempted several rescues, protests that he is not a deity, but later he appears convinced that Elizabeth Grier is correct. As he sails home to the United States, he muses that "Mercury is not only the messenger of the gods; he is the conductor of the dead as well. If in the least part his powers had fallen to me I should be able to invoke spirits" (p. 226). He then does make the dead arise. At his wish Virgil appears before him—or so he imagines—and they engage in conversation. Praising death, Virgil says, "Are you still alive? . . . How can you endure it? . . . Oh, what misery to be a man. Hurry and die!" (p. 230).[4]

We have come full turn. As in *The Bridge of San Luis Rey,* death and union are goals and glory. The god has died and entered the living man who in turn must die.

3. I thank Dr. Shelley Orgel for calling this to my attention.
4. Goldstein interprets this episode as signifying that the members of the Cabala were gods. He fails to see that Elizabeth Grier believed that Samuele too is a god.

Past History, Oedipal Issues, Separation Issues

Since Wilder did not have the actual experience of having a twin but heard of his brother from his family, we may surmise that other experiences imbued his twinship with additional cathexis. It could serve as a defensive and organizing screen to deal with conflicts arising in other areas. As Burlingham (1952) has pointed out, fantasies of having a twin, like family romance fantasies, serve to express and defend against disappointments with and frustrations of oedipal wishes. The presence in imagination of a twin from whom one is *not* separated also defends against feelings and fears of loss. Indeed, she noted in remarks about *The Bridge of San Luis Rey* that Esteban and Manuel reunite in death. Twin fantasies, she stated, also protect one from fears of castration and death. Through the imaginary companion, one can feel complete, powerful, and invulnerable. There may be a preoedipal factor here. The imaginary companion may symbolize a lost mother with whom one wishes to unite.

In attempting to tease out the factors which determined the intensity of Wilder's fantasy that his twin was often (or always?) present, we can first note that the Wilder family appears to have made much of the fact that Thornton had a twin who died. The fact that they not only gave him a name but also a nickname, Pax, suggests that the family talked about Theophilus to a remarkable degree. It would be helpful to know how old Thornton was when he heard of his twinship, but this information is not available. Nor do we know whether the twins were truly identical or whether the parents invented this.

Parental preoccupation with Thornton's twinship may have provided sufficient basis for us to understand Wilder's defensive use of a twin fantasy to overcome the disappointment with one's family that is commonplace. Nevertheless we should examine the circumstances of his life to try to ascertain whether the usual preoedipal and oedipal frustrations motivated his twin fantasy or whether there were unusually intense disappointments.

We do possess information about Wilder's parents' traits and historical data about his relations with and separation from his parents and siblings. We tread less solid ground when we try to gauge the impact of his preoedipal and oedipal experiences and fantasies on his adult personality, his homosexuality, and his writings. Be that as it may, we must attempt to place Wilder's twinship in the broader context of his life.

Thornton Wilder was born in Madison, Wisconsin, where he and his family lived for 9 years.[5] Then his father, editor of the *Wisconsin State Journal,* a newspaper, was appointed consul general in Hong Kong. Amos Wilder found his position rewarding and spent 7 years in the Orient, but to Mrs. Wilder it was tiring. In 6 months she and the children (Amos, Jr., Thornton, and two younger girls, Charlotte and Isabel) returned to the United States. They lived in Berkeley, California. The father wrote frequently—every week—but Thornton did not see him for 3 years when his father came home for two visits on a brief, strained leave. A third sister, Janet, was born when Thornton was 13. Soon thereafter his mother, Thornton, and his sisters returned to China where Wilder and Charlotte attended boarding school for a year, from almost 14 to 15. From 15 to 16 Thornton boarded at the Thatcher School in California. Then his mother returned to Berkeley, this time from Italy, and Thornton, reunited with her, attended public high school once more until he started Oberlin at 18. He transferred to Yale, from which he was graduated. When Thornton was 17, his father left China but lived in New Haven away from the family.

Wilder may have been pleased to get his critical father out of his hair, but he was unhappy at Chefoo, the school in China. There they rebuked and even hit him for ignorance in Greek, Latin, mathematics, and history, subjects he had less acquaintance with than his fellow students—although he was knowledgeable in many areas.

He saw his sister Charlotte for only a few minutes once a week, and told his mother in his letters of the poor food—a crust of bread, "dishwater," and "weeds." At one point he remarked on how "hard and callous" (Harrison, p. 27) the Wilders were with their repeated leavetakings. Later he attempted to deny his unhappiness. " 'We Wilders,' he would say in 1918, 'never know we

---

5. Again we find the significant number 9 that appeared in *Theophilus North.* Again it signifies separation, this time from father at age 9.

are happy until the period has faded almost out of memory. How blissful I must have been at Chefoo—and how wretched'" (p. 23). On another occasion he reassured his mother about *her* loneliness. "'I am there, I *am* . . . Before long you will see me— know I will see *you*'" (p. 27).

At the Thatcher School, Thornton was looked down on, was considered a "freak," and would have been elected most likely to fail in life, a contrast to his athletic older brother Amos who was chosen as most likely to succeed. He did not shine academically, athletically, or socially. He was in fact "jumpy." His literary interests appeared alien to his teachers who considered him pretentious.

I dwell on this outline of events for it demonstrates the many separations from both parents. He lived apart from his father from 9 on and away from his mother from almost 14 to 16. The importance of loss and reunion, which we have attributed to Thornton's losing his twin, most likely derived in part from his loss of his parents. The intense emotions about his twin must have involved defensive displacement of feelings from his parents to the twin he never actually knew. The preoccupation with his twinship must have served to hide or mute or compensate for feelings of deprivation and antagonism about his parents' repeated desertion of him. We can imagine he wished to be rescued from the schools in which he felt so unhappy.

In addition, the rescue theme has origins in the author's relationship with his father. Wilder, Sr., with whom his son identified, was a preacher and saver. When he was separated from his family, he wrote repeated letters of advice. As an editor he took a strong moral stand against corruption and drink. As an employer he meddled in the lives of his workmen. He would even examine the mouths of reporters and get them to a dentist if he saw a defective tooth. As a father he preached orally when he was with his children and by letter when he was not. "If he could not shape his children's lives by being with them, Papa counted on the persuasive power of the written word and on his return to Shanghai did his best to guide them by exhortation. . . . Singing in the Episcopal choir was not as wholesome as regular attendance at one's own place of worship (Congregational). The children should shun bad books, bad pictures, bad stories" (Harrison, p. 21). Father even made two of them sign a pledge to abstain from alcohol when Thornton was 15. Isabel said that George Brush, the moralistic meddling salesman of *Heaven's My Destination,* was based on their father.

It is not surprising to learn that Thornton had an uneasy ambivalent relationship with his father. "Thornton took from him a desire to shape and improve lives, a facility with language, a histrionic virtuosity, moral energy" (p. 13f.). When father visited Berkeley, "the togetherness was strained. . . . Papa was sure that his son needed his protective arms. . . . Thornton would have no way of defending or supporting himself" in "the cruel world" (p. 20f.). During adolescence Thornton wanted to "get out of that feeling that he was 'always being hurt by father and always hurting him'" (p. 36). Goldstone (1975) writes of Wilder's "lifelong resentment of his father . . . [which] erupts in the final scene of *The Skin of Our Teeth*" (p. 184).

Toward the end of the play, Mr. Antrobus and his son Henry return home after World War II. Henry had risen to the rank of general in the enemy army. He hates his father and wants to destroy the books that Mr. Antrobus loves and depends on to increase and spread knowledge. Father and son engage in a dramatic confrontation. Henry is defiant and provocative as Mr. Antrobus threatens to shoot him. He will have nothing to do with his father's type of peace in which he could be told what to do. At this point the actors lose control and start to fight with each other. Sabina, the maid, tries to halt the action. "Stop! Stop! Don't play the scene. You know what happened last night. Stop the play. . . . Last night you almost strangled him." The actor who plays Henry apologizes and explains that his outburst stemmed from his relationship with his father who had whipped him, restricted him, and even locked him up. Enraged, he felt he had to kill or be killed. After this cathartic outburst, the story itself continues.

In *The Eighth Day* oedipal murder actually occurs. George Lansing shoots his father because he believes he mistreated his mother as well as himself. The murder is followed by his suffering pangs of conscience which he cannot suppress.

Thornton's parents got along poorly. His mother declared her husband "a ruthless dictator" who announced three days before his wedding "that he had no tenderness left in him" because he had previously been jilted by another woman. Because of the long separations "there was *not enough understanding* between us to survive the strain" which continued (Harrison, p. 14). Thornton's mother worked hard caring for her children and keeping house, but, as we have seen, she was not averse to leaving them— and father. Thornton was close to, loved, his mother, who had artistic, musical, and literary interests. He said she was "like one of Shakespeare's girls—'a star danced and under it I was born'" (p. 15). She encouraged her son along literary lines, and he read his work to her. "Every one of Thornton's pages was read aloud to his mother" (p. 34) when they lived together in Berkeley.

Wilder's direct and indirect comments about his oedipus complex, although not conclusive in themselves, will cast light on the matter. Impressed with psychoanalytic findings, including the oedipus complex, Wilder once wrote to Timothy Findley, a Canadian playwright-novelist: "As to your question of sex in the novel, I'm a Freudian. I think it's intermingled with everything" (p. 314). Indeed, the author "often acknowledged his indebtedness to Freud" (p. 139). He met the psychoanalyst, then 79, for a half-hour talk in Vienna in 1935 and called himself a Freudian thereafter. At the end of the interview, as reported by Harrison, Freud said something that indicates his awareness of Wilder's difficulties with women (and also possibly of his wish that Wilder court his daughter, as Goldstone [1975] suggested). Freud regretted that Anna had not been there. "She is older than you, you do not have to be afraid. She is a sensible, reasonable girl. You are not afraid of women? . . . Are you married, may I ask?" (p. 140).

In *Theophilus North,* Wilder indirectly acknowledges his oedipus complex. In that novel, the protagonist, Wilder's alter ego as we have seen, says that Freud told him of a complex similar to Charles Marlow's in Goldsmith's *She Stoops to Conquer.* Marlow could function sexually with women of the lower class but not with women of his own station in life. "He [Freud] then went on to point out to me the relation of the problem to the Oedipus-Complex and to the incest-taboo under which 'respectable' women are associated with a man's mother and sisters— 'out of bounds'" (p. 170 of the biography; p. 4 of *Theophilus*

North). Theophilus suffered from that inhibition. Although these words of Freud would appear to arise solely from Wilder's imagination, Goldstone (1975) asserts that Freud actually said something of the sort: "Wilder had conversations with Freud which, according to Wilder, were on the identical subject of Theophilus's discussions" (p. 263.).

On another occasion Wilder wrote "We [the Wilders] all come up out of the great well which is the Oedipus-Complex." He blamed his father for the family's being "crazy as coots." "It's Father who is neurotic, not Ma" (p. 140).

Indeed, Wilder was inhibited. He practiced homosexuality, and his affairs, according to Harrison, were brief and lacked intensity. One such sexual act—with Samuel Steward, a Gertrude Stein scholar—"was so hurried and reticent, so barren of embrace, tenderness or passion that it might never have happened" (p. 166). Another of Thornton's companions said that "any physical encounter was brief, awkward, left Thornton slightly discomfited and probably remorseful. In each instance, practical counsel was offered: 'There was always something of a preacher about him'" (p. 167). Here we find Wilder to be like Theophilus North, the rescuer, and, as I have suggested, the twin who rescues—either the dead twin or the surviving one. Could he also have identified with his father, a preacher, and treated his lover as Thornton had been or wished to be treated, a not uncommon homosexual constellation?

Wilder justified his lack of passion by saying one should reserve one's energies for artistic endeavors. Friends called him "priestly," "fastidious," "neuter," "asexual," or even "antisexual." Perhaps his lack of closeness and intimacy stems from a desire to separate his self representation from that of his dead brother as well as oedipal inhibitions. This implies a fear of fusion with love objects stemming from a variety of sources.

We must be cautious in evaluating and explaining the lack of passion Harrison asserts is characteristic of Wilder. Goldstone (personal communication) believes Harrison, as an authorized biographer, errs in his characterization. Nevertheless, even a passionate man can be inhibited.

Searching through *The Bridge of San Luis Rey* for evidence of oedipal inhibition related to twinship, I find that the suggestions of a developing oedipal attachment appear when Manuel becomes the admiring scribe of an older and beautiful woman, the Perichole. This love could not be consummated. He had to break off his relationship with the actress lest he hurt his brother too much. The twins' love for each other prevailed over the forbidden oedipal wishes. Perhaps Wilder's fantasies about loyalty to Theophilus had a similar inhibiting effect.

I am assuming that the particular configuration of Thornton's oedipus complex involved images of desertion by both parents and resentment and longing as well as images derived from his fantasies about his twin. He pictured his father as cruel and overbearing to his mother and the children. Still he loved and emulated his father, and adored and sought the admiration of his mother. Living with his mother without the diluting and modulating influence of his father after the age of 9 must have intensified his oedipal wishes. Wilder reacted to these emotions of love and hate with fears of injury and feelings of disappointment. Because of their intensity and his own capacities and propensities, he evolved a number of defensive and adaptive maneuvers. He developed intense rescue fantasies. He became homosexual. He was inhibited in certain areas and at times perhaps lacked passion. Still his drives expressed themselves in his enthusiasm for his work and in his social interchanges with people, an excitement that led Harrison to entitle his biography *The Enthusiast.*

Although we have insufficient information to decide on the genesis and dynamics of Wilder's homosexuality, we may assume that one aspect involved defense against the oedipus complex which led him to feminine identification. Even as a child he would act out female roles in plays, a practice his father objected to. We may also assume his feminine identification was supported by his longing for his absent father. Again it seems likely that his attachment to his imaginary male twin, which served to damp his intense feelings of longing, love, and hate, also acted to accent his homosexuality. Here we see a narcissistic aspect; loving his alter ego was a form of self love.

Rescue fantasies, as we know from analyses, usually encompass desires to save mother from a cruel sexual father (Freud, 1910), and we may assume this is true of Wilder. Displacing his

wishes to rescue mother to his twinship, he integrated his unconscious needs to rescue mother and to rescue his twin into a larger
gestalt, which he expressed in his life and work.

Wilder's devotion to literature derived in part from his keeping contact with his parents through letter writing. It also derived from his identification with his parents. He identified with
his father as a parent he lived with for 9 years, and as a lost
parent he wanted to be with and as an aggressor he needed to
defend himself against. (His identification also manifested itself
in his preaching, his savior attitude, and possibly his lack of
sexual passion.) He identified with his mother whom he loved
and whom he tried to keep himself from being angry at when she
left him. He probably also identified with her as a means of
avoiding forbidden sexual feelings toward his mother.

His father was a writer, an editor, who kept in touch with his
family through letters throughout his long separation. Thornton wrote to his parents when away from them. When with his
mother he read his literary endeavors to her. Such writing *for* a
parent or other person is common in creative people and can
propel their artistic achievements. Greenacre (1957) has described producing for "collective alternates," imagined or real
people, and Meyer (1967, 1972) has said that the author seeks a
"secret sharer" to write for. I have suggested (1974a) that a twin
may use his living sibling or his representation as the object for
whom he writes. Quite possibly Wilder wrote not only for his
parents but also for his imagined twin brother, an unconscious
displacement from his mother and father or "collective alternates."[6]

Writing then became a sublimation of the means Thornton
used to keep contact with absent people and thus avoid antag-

6. Since this article was written *The Journals of Thornton Wilder* (1985) have
been published. Unfortunately, the editor has omitted "passages of introspec-
tion and self-analysis, including dreams" (p. xxv), even excerpts that Harrison
(1983) has provided. Isabel Wilder, in her introduction to the volume, adds
substance to the idea that Wilder wrote for his twin, at least when he composed
his journal. "He talked of it as one did of a person or of an animate crea-
ture. . . . Sometimes . . . Thornton would say, 'Gotta go and tell it to the Journal.'" Isabel imagined "Thornton's pen scratching or his voice talking to his
twin" (p. xvii).

onism to them as deserters. A prolific writer, he kept a journal in which he wrote regularly. Wilder created many characters who, like himself, were writers. The *Ides of March* consists for the most part of letters and journals composed by Caesar and by others. The twins of *The Bridge of San Luis Rey* enscribed letters for others. The Marquesa of that book wrote extensively to her daughter who lived far from her in Europe. John Ashley of *The Eighth Day* could not write to his family from whom fate separated him, but his son George became a newspaper columnist and hoped he would reach his father through that medium.

The fantasies about twinship most certainly influenced Wilder's oedipal fantasies. So too did his oedipal wishes have an impact on his concerns about twinship. I suggested earlier that Wilder felt guilty about his twin's death because of hostility toward Theophilus, but it wasn't clear why he should be antagonistic to his brother. It appears likely that Wilder's antagonism toward both parents as deserters and toward his father as an oedipal rival was displaced onto his twin brother (in his fantasy also an abandoner) when he learned of him. Most likely there was a displacement of antagonism from his older brother Amos, whom his father preferred as more robust and worldly. Similarly we would expect that affectionate feelings toward parents and siblings—his three sisters and his brother—were transferred to the representation of his twin. The twinship, significant in itself, was thus enhanced by additional cathexis.

SUMMARY

Two important motifs appear in Thornton Wilder's work: the survivor theme and the rescue theme. In this paper, evidence is mobilized to demonstrate that both derive from the circumstances of Wilder's birth. He was the survivor of a pair of twins. His brother Theophilus died a few hours after his birth and Wilder was said to have been a frail child whose life was in peril. The survivor theme indicates that the author wondered why one twin would live and the other die, that he felt guilty about his good fortune and about associated hostile feelings, probably derived from oedipal feelings, and that he wished to undo and master the calamitous birth. The rescue theme, in which the protagonist saves one or several persons from tragedy, is not only an attempt at reversing the catastrophic birth, but also derives from oedipal wishes. Issues having to do with the twinship and oedipal desires intertwine. In Wilder's case, disappointment in his parents who fought with one another and deserted him influenced the configuration of his oedipal wishes. His twin fantasies derived from and were intensified by his defenses against feelings of rage and oedipal love.

BIBLIOGRAPHY

ARLOW, J. A. (1960). Fantasy systems in twins. *Psychoanal. Q.*, 29:175–199.
BERLIN, R. (1985). A child analytic termination with an adopted child. Read at the Psychoanalytic Association of New York.
BERNSTEIN, B. A. (1980). Siblings of twins. *Psychoanal. Study Child*, 35:135–154.
BURLINGHAM, D. T. (1952). *Twins*. New York: Int. Univ. Press.
COEN, S. J. & BRADLOW, P. A. (1982). Twin transference as a compromise formation. *J. Amer. Psychoanal. Assn.*, 30:599–620.
EISSLER, K. R. (1968). The relation of explaining and understanding in psychoanalysis. *Psychoanal. Study Child*, 23:141–171.
FERENCZI, S. (1921). The symbolism of the bridge. In *Further Contributions to the Theory and Technique of Psycho-Analysis*, ed. J. Rickman, tr. J. I. Suttie, pp. 352–356. London: Hogarth Press, 1926.
FREUD, S. (1910). A special type of choice of object made by men. *S.E.*, 11:165–175.
––––––– (1923). A seventeenth-century demonological neurosis. *S.E.*, 19:73–105.
––––––– (1933). New introductory lectures on psycho-analysis. *S.E.*, 22:5–182.
FRIEDMAN, P. (1952). The bridge. *Psychoanal. Q.* 21:49–80.
GLENN, J. (1966). Opposite sex twins. *J. Amer. Psychoanal. Assn.* 14:736–759.
––––––– (1974a). Anthony and Peter Shaffer's plays. *Amer. Imago*, 51:270–292.
––––––– (1974b). The adoption theme in Edward Albee's *Tiny Alice* and *The American Dream*. *Psychoanal. Study Child*, 29:413–429.
GOLDSTEIN, M. (1965). *The Art of Thornton Wilder*. Lincoln: Univ. Nebraska Press.
GOLDSTONE, R. H. (1953). An interview with Thornton Wilder. *Paris Rev.*, 15:36–57.
––––––– (1975). *Thornton Wilder*. New York: Dutton.
GREENACRE, P. (1957). The childhood of the artist. *Psychoanal. Study Child*, 12:47–72.
HARRISON, G. A. (1983). *The Enthusiast*. New Haven & New York: Ticknor & Fields.

JOSEPH, E. D. (1975). Psychoanalysis—science and research. *J. Amer. Psychoanal. Assn.*, 23:3–31.

KOHUT, H. (1971). *The Analysis of the Self.* New York: Int. Univ. Press.

KRAMER, S. (1985). The fantasy of having a twin. Presented at 16th Annual Symposium on Child Development, Margaret S. Mahler Symposium Series.

LEWIN, B. D. (1933). The body as phallus. *Psychoanal. Q.* 2:24–47.

MEYER, B. C. (1967). *Joseph Conrad.* Princeton: Princeton Univ. Press.

––––– (1972). Some reflections on the contribution of psychoanalysis to biography. *Psychoanal. & Contemp. Sci.*, 1:373–391.

RANK, O. (1914). *The Double.* Chapel Hill: Univ. North Carolina Press, 1971.

SHENGOLD, L. (1980). Some reflections on a case of mother/adolescent son incest. *Int. J. Psychoanal.*, 61:461–476.

TYSON, P. (1980). The gender of the analyst in relation to transference and countertransference manifestations in prelatency children. *Psychoanal. Study Child*, 35:321–338.

WEBSTER, N. (1956). *New International Dictionary of the English Language*, 2nd ed. Springfield, Mass: Meriam.

WILDER, T. N. (1926). *The Cabala.* New York: Albert & Charles Boni.

––––– (1927). The bridge of San Luis Rey. In *The Stories of Thornton Wilder.* London: Longmans, Green, 1934.

––––– (1935). *Heaven's My Destination.* New York: Harper.

––––– (1938). *Our Town.* New York: Coward-McCann.

––––– (1942). *The Skin of Our Teeth.* New York: Harper.

––––– (1948). *The Ides of March.* New York: Harper.

––––– (1955). The matchmaker. In *Three Plays.* New York: Harper.

––––– (1967). *The Eighth Day.* London: Longmans, Green.

––––– (1973). *Theophilus North.* New York: Harper & Row.

––––– (1985). *The Journals of Thornton Wilder, 1939–1961*, ed. D. Gallup. New Haven: Yale Univ. Press.

Index